A CONSUMER'S GUIDE TO PRESCRIPTION MEDICINES

Dr Barrington Cooper & Dr Laurence Gerlis
Consultant Pharmacist: Dawn Hurrell

with a Foreword by
T P Astill LLB, BPharmS, FRPharmS, FBIM
Director, National Pharmaceutical Association

NEW EDITION

Fully revised to reflect the latest prescribing practices

hamlyn

Edited by Neil Curtis
Designed by Richard Garratt

This edition published in 2001 by Hamlyn,
a division of Octopus Publishing Group Limited,
2–4 Heron Quays,
Docklands,
London E14 4JP

A CIP catalogue record of this book is available from the British Library

ISBN 0 600 60305 9

Printed and bound in Finland by WS Bookwell OY

10 9 8 7 6 5 4 3 2 1

In the introductory sections of this book, it has been emphasized that *A Consumer's Guide to Prescription Medicines* must **not** be used for self-prescription. Nor is it intended to be a substitute for the advice of a prescribing physician or the instructions on the medicine's package.

Every effort has been made to ensure that the information contained in the book is as accurate and up-to-date as possible at the time of going to press but medical and pharmaceutical knowledge continue to progress, and the use of a particular medicine may be different for every patient. And **remember** that many natural or over-the-counter remedies may contain powerful constituents that could interact adversely with a prescription medicine. **Always** consult your medical practitioner or other qualified medical specialist for advice.

The authors, editors, consultants, and publishers of this book can not be held liable for any errors or omissions, nor for any consequences of using it.

Preface to the fourth edition

In updating this book again we have found significant changes in the prescription medicines available in the United Kingdom. There have been more older products deleted than new products entered, indicating a marked rationalization in the Pharmacopoeia. The new products available are very exciting: for example, we have medicines to treat neurological conditions such as multiple sclerosis and motor neurone disease for which specific drugs are available for the first time.

There is now a number of drugs given by self-injection and this enables us to include more injectable preparations in this edition.

In publishing this book we have maintained our principle of not replacing the role of the doctor in publishing this book and, thus, most anti-cancer preparations and injectable drugs are not included. This distinction is becoming more and more difficult, however, as the pace of development and public awareness accelerates.

New delivery systems, modified-release formulations, and new biotechnology products add to an exciting range of medicines that doctors can prescribe. This book remains unique in providing information to the public on so broad a spectrum of prescription medicines, and we believe this will help patients with management in an age of increasingly evidence-based medicine.

While we accept alternative medicines and indeed encourage some of our patients to consider these alternatives, it is worth remembering that every drug in this book has had to prove quality and consistency of manufacture, mode of action, and significant clinical benefit in a range of controlled clinical trials, as well as having been fully documented regarding safety. The regulatory environment for medicines has never been more stringent, and it is a great tribute to the scientists, clinical researchers, and the pharmaceutical industry to be able to offer such a variety of medicines to the clinician.

We live in a time when there is greater emphasis on lifestyle factors involved in health, greater use of complex new science, such as biogenetics, to treat illness and an increasing awareness of the importance of informed consent by the patient to medical procedures. These and other changes present a bewildering array of information; we have rewritten this book in order to maintain an up-to-date and accessible resource so that patients may continue to be as fully informed as possible in sustaining the vital relationship of partnership between doctors and patients.

We extend our gratitude to Dawn Hurrell, Neil Curtis, and Richard Garratt for their significant roles in producing this book.

Dr Barrington Cooper
10 Devonshire Place
London
W1G 6HS

Dr Laurence Gerlis
21 Devonshire Place
London
W1G 6HZ

2001

Foreword

It is no exaggeration to say that the last fifty years have seen a revolution in pharmacy and medicine. In the 'good old days', the family doctor would write a prescription which was usually in the form of a recipe and, quite deliberately, in semi-legible handwriting so that the patient could not read it – just in case the patient was able to decipher the writing, the names of the ingredients were in abbreviated Latin! The pharmacist would look at the prescription, nod sagely, and disappear out of sight behind his dispensary screen to make the pills or to mix the ingredients of the ointment or medicine. The name of the product never appeared on the label because everyone, including most patients, felt that it was undesirable for ordinary people to know what had been prescribed. It can now be revealed that what was in the bottle was probably innocuous and pharmacologically ineffective. The curative power of medicine in those days derived in large measure from the mystery and mystique which surrounded its preparation, coupled always with the doctor's bedside manner and confident reassurance.

Since then, there has been an enormous increase in scientific knowledge, especially of the way in which chemical substances affect the organs of the human body and of the way in which the body itself works. Antibiotics and other anti-infective agents have also been discovered, with the result that many hitherto fatal diseases have either disappeared altogether or can now be cured easily. Those who criticize the pharmaceutical industry forget too readily the former ravages of tuberculosis, polio, meningitis, septicaemia, typhoid fever, endocarditis, and other killing and crippling diseases. Many people suffering from asthma, epilepsy, hormone deficiency, or allergy can now lead a normal life whereas they would previously have been severely handicapped, confined to a wheelchair, or dead at an early age. Modern advances in surgery, such as organ transplants, have also been made possible by the drugs which control the body's natural tendency to reject 'invaders'.

Alongside this pharmaceutical revolution, there has also been a consumer revolution. Nowadays, you want to **know** what kind of drugs you are taking, and rightly so. While some people may regret the passing of the age of medicinal mystique, most of us prefer to be told precisely what is wrong with us and what is being provided to put us right. We want to know what effect the medicine is likely to have, what side effects might occur, and what precautions we need to take to ensure that the medicine behaves as it should. The modern medicine is certainly a powerful weapon for good, but it is also often complex in its chemistry and formulation. It is important, therefore, that patients are properly informed about their medicines, not only for their own peace of mind, but also so that the product gives them the maximum possible benefit with the minimum risk of harm.

For these reasons, I warmly welcome this new book by Dr Cooper and Dr Gerlis. In simple language it tells us what we need to know about our prescribed medicines. It reinforces and supplements what we have been told by our doctor and pharmacist; it will help us to understand why a particular medicine has been selected; and it tells us how it should be used. As the authors emphasize in their introduction, the book is **not** intended to be a substitute for professional advice. You should not hesitate to talk to your doctor or pharmacist if you are in serious doubt about any aspect of your treatment. But this book is a very usable source of reference and will fill reassuringly many gaps in our knowledge. It will help to remove those little apprehensions which many of us feel when we leave the surgery with the prescription and the pharmacy with our medicine.

T P Astill LLB, BPharmS, FRPharmS, FBIM
Director, National Pharmaceutical Association

How the book works

Apart from some injectables and a small number of other medicines and appliances, all medicines which may be commonly prescribed by general practitioners in the United Kingdom (through the National Health Service or private practice) should be found in this book. Most medicines prescribed by hospital doctors are also included although some which are highly specialized have been omitted.

The medicines are arranged in strict alphabetical order throughout with brand names, generic names, and any commonly used medical terms contained within the same sequence.

Some drugs are required to be prescribed by their generic (scientific) names only, and it is then up to the dispensing pharmacist to select a particular manufacturer's product. Other products are prescribed by brand names. In this book the main description of any preparation is generally to be found under its generic name, with brand names cross-referenced to the main generic entry (e.g. propranolol and Inderal). In the description of the generic product, brand names are also given when they are available. There is also a move to change British Approved Names (BANs) to Recommended International Non-proprietary Names (RINNS). In this book the main entry remains under the BAN but RINNS have again been cross-referenced where applicable (e.g. bendrofluazide and bendroflumethiazide). It should therefore be a simple matter to find details about a medicine, no matter what name is used on the prescription, by following the links made in the cross-referencing.

The name of the medicine is given in **bold** type at the beginning of each entry, with the name of the manufacturing company in brackets on the next line. A short paragraph then follows describing the physical nature of the medicine (e.g. tablet, capsule, suspension, etc.), what type of medicine it is (e.g. antibiotic, corticosteroid, etc.), and what it is used for (e.g. to treat bacterial infections of the nose, throat etc.). Next the strengths (e.g. 10 mg, 0.5% etc.) are given followed by the usual dosages (**NB** if these differ from those indicated by your doctor, **always** follow the doctor's recommendations). There is also a section to indicate whether the medicine is available through the NHS, by private prescription, or over the counter (purchased without a prescription). Please be aware that some of those products available 'over the counter' will be restricted to sale through pharmacies. Items available through the NHS or 'over the counter' may be available only to certain groups of patients, and this is indicated where relevant. The components of the preparations are given in terms of their scientific names for both generic and branded entries.

For extra clarity, a new departure in this edition of the book is that any possible side effects that the medicine might produce, any cautionary advice in its use, circumstances in which the medicine should not be used, or other medicines or foodstuffs with which the medicine may interact, perhaps adversely, are set out in separate boxes highlighted by appropriate symbols which are explained on each page. These sections clearly state, for example, if the medicine is not to be used for particular groups of patients, such as children or pregnant women. And for information, other products containing some of the same components are also listed as are 'compound products', that is products with the ingredient described plus one or more additional ingredients.

Note that words or phrases in SMALL CAPITAL LETTERS, such as NON-STEROIDAL ANTI-INFLAMMATORY DRUG, cross-refer to explanations of medical terms, names of groups of drugs, etc., that can be found in the alphabetical sequence elsewhere in the book.

How to use this book (including how *not* to use it)

When a doctor prescribes a medicine for a patient, then he or she will always explain carefully to the patient how it is to be used. Similarly, the pharmacist will always write instructions for the drug's dose on the container, and the name of the drug will also be clearly visible. If you look up the name in *A Consumer's Guide to Prescription Medicines*, you will be able to confirm that you have understood the doctor's instructions fully so that you can be confident you are making the best possible use of the medicine. It will also help you to anticipate and prepare for any possible side effects, and ensure that you are not taking anything else which perhaps the doctor was not made aware of and which might interact with the prescription. More importantly perhaps, the book will enable you to become better informed generally about the medicine(s) which has been prescribed to treat or prevent a particular condition.

A Consumer's Guide to Prescription Medicines is **not** a guide to self-prescription. Nor is it a 'home doctor'. The authors recognize clearly that it is the advice of the prescribing doctor, given after a careful investigation of the patient and his or her symptoms, that should always be followed by patients. If the information given in this book differs in any particular from the doctor's recommendations about a medicine, this must only be a basis for discussing such differences with the prescribing doctor or perhaps with the dispensing pharmacist.

The information contained in this book should not be followed in preference to the recommendations of the prescription even though it has been compiled by highly qualified physicians and a pharmacist using the most up-to-date sources. There are few doctors or pharmacists who do not welcome well-informed questioning by their patients, and it is the purpose of this book to add to the information already given by the prescribing physician in the surgery and on the product's labelling. On the other hand, the authors have chosen not to include the names and addresses of the manufacturers of the drugs described because it is the policy of most drug companies not to respond directly to enquiries concerning their medicines from individual patients; generally, they will refer such enquiries back to the general practitioner.

abacavir solution/tablets

A tablet or solution used as an antiviral (in conjunction with other similar drugs) to treat HIV infection.

Strengths available: a 300 mg tablet or 20 mg/ml solution.
Dose: adults 1 tablet or 15 ml solution every 12 hours.
Availability: NHS and private prescription.
Contains: abacavir.
Brand names: Ziagen.

upset stomach, fever, headache, loss of appetite, lethargy, severe allergic reactions.

in patients with liver or kidney disorders. Patients should report any breathing difficulties, cough, rash, fever, sore throat, or influenza-like symptoms to a doctor. You may be advised to have regular blood tests.

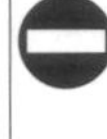
pregnant women, mothers who are breastfeeding, children, or for patients with moderate to severe liver disorder or severe kidney disease.

Abidec *see* multivitamin drops
(Warner Lambert Consumer)

Able Spacer

(Clement Clarke)
A one-piece spacer device which fits all commonly used inhalers.

Availability: NHS and private prescription, over the counter.

AC Vax *see* meningitis vaccine (A and C)
(SmithKline Beecham Pharmaceuticals)

---

acamprosate calcium tablets

A tablet used in addition to counselling, to maintain abstinence in patients with alcohol dependence.

Strengths available: 333 mg tablets.
Dose: adults over 18 years 2 tablets in the morning, 1 at noon, and 1 at night (or 2 tablets three times a day for patients over 60 kg in weight). Treatment usually started as soon as possible after alcohol withdrawal and continued for one year.
Availability: NHS and private prescription.
Contains: acamprosate calcium.
Brand names: Campral EC.

upset stomach, skin reactions, change in sexual desire.

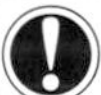
in patients continuing to abuse alcohol (treatment may fail).

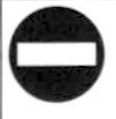
children under 18 years, elderly patients over 65 years, pregnant women, mothers who are breastfeeding, or for patients with kidney or serious liver disorders.

---

acarbose tablets
A tablet used to treat diabetes.

Strengths available: 50 mg or 100 mg tablets.
Dose: adults, 50 mg chewed with the first mouthful of food, or swallowed whole with liquid three times a day at first, increasing to 100 mg three times a day if needed after 6-8 weeks, then up to a maximum of 200 mg three times a day.
Availability: NHS and private prescription.
Contains: acarbose.
Brand names: Glucobay.

wind, bloating, abdominal pain, diarrhoea, feeling over-full after eating, rarely, liver disorders and skin reactions.

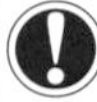
your doctor may advise regular blood tests.

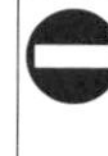
children under 12 years, pregnant women, mothers who are breastfeeding, or for patients suffering from liver or severe kidney disorders, inflammatory bowel disorders, ulcers of the colon, blocked intestines, digestive disorders, any disorders made worse by wind, or with a previous history of abdominal surgery or hernia.

pancreatin, neomycin, cholestyramine, other antidiabetic drugs, kaolin.

Accolate *see* zafirlukast tablets
(Zeneca Pharma)

Accupro *see* quinapril tablets
(Parke Davis)

Accuretic tablets *see* quinapril tablets and hydrochlorothiazide tablets
(Parke Davis)

Dose: adults 1-2 a day.

ACE-inhibitor (angiotensin-converting enzyme inhibitor)
A drug that blocks the production of water-retaining hormones, and thus functions as a DIURETIC. Example, captopril tablets.

ACE-II antagonist (angiotensin-II receptor antagonists)
A drug that acts similarly to an ACE-INHIBITOR but with a lower tendency to result in cough as a side effect. Example, losartan tablets.

---

acebutolol capsules/tablets
A capsule or tablet used as a BETA-BLOCKER to treat angina, abnormal heart rhythm, or high blood pressure.

cont.

A

Strengths available: 100 mg and 200 mg capsules, 400 mg tablets.
Dose: up to 1200 mg a day in divided doses (maximum of 800 mg a day to treat high blood pressure).
Availability: NHS and private prescription.
Contains: acebutolol.
Brand names: Sectral.
Compound preparations: Secadrex.

 cold hands and feet, sleep disturbance, slow heart rate, tiredness, wheezing, heart failure, low blood pressure, stomach upset, dry eyes, rash.

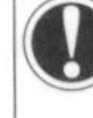 in pregnant women, and in patients suffering from diabetes, MYASTHENIA GRAVIS, kidney or liver disorders, or asthma. May need to be withdrawn before surgery. Withdraw gradually. Your doctor may advise additional treatment with DIURETICS or digoxin.

 general anaesthetics, CALCIUM-CHANNEL BLOCKERS, ALPHA-BLOCKERS, clonidine, ANTIHYPERTENSIVES, amiodarone, antidiabetics, thymoxamine, theophylline, aminophylline.

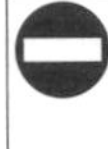 children, mothers who are breastfeeding, or for patients suffering from heart block or failure, low blood pressure, or untreated PHAEOCHROMOCYTOMA.

---

aceclofenac tablets

A tablet used as a NON-STEROIDAL ANTI-INFLAMMATORY DRUG to treat pain and inflammation in arthritis and ankylosing spondylitis.

Strengths available: 100 mg tablets.
Dose: 1 tablet twice a day.
Availability: NHS and private prescription.
Contains: aceclofenac.

 stomach upset, dizziness, itching, altered liver enzymes.

 in patients with stomach disorders, or disease of the kidney, liver, or heart.

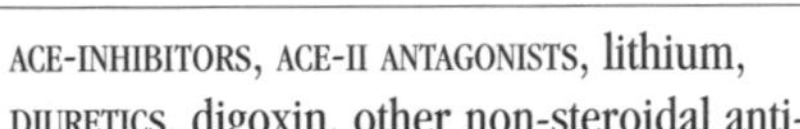 ACE-INHIBITORS, ACE-II ANTAGONISTS, lithium, DIURETICS, digoxin, other non-steroidal anti-inflammatory drugs, lithium, tacrolimus, cyclosporin, some antibiotics, phenytoin, antidiabetics, methotrexate, ANTICOAGULANTS, some antiviral drugs.

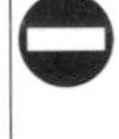 children, pregnant women, mothers who are breastfeeding, or for patients with a stomach ulcer, bleeding in the gut, moderate to severe kidney disease, or allergy to aspirin or non-steroidal anti-inflammatory drugs.

Brand names: Preservex.

---

acemetacin capsules

A capsule used as a NON-STEROIDAL ANTI-INFLAMMATORY DRUG to treat arthritis, low back pain, and pain or inflammation after operation.

Strengths available: 60 mg capsules.
Dose: 2-3 capsules a day in divided doses, with food.
Availability: NHS and private prescription.

 stomach upset, headache, dizziness, fluid retention, chest pain, itching, blood changes, noises in the ears, blurred vision.

Contains: acemetacin.
Brand names: Emflex.

in patients suffering from psychiatric disorder, epilepsy, Parkinson's disease, liver or kidney disorder, congestive heart failure, some infections, body fluid or chemical imbalance, and in elderly patients. Your doctor may advise regular blood tests and eye examinations.

ANTICOAGULANTS, other non-steroidal anti-inflammatory drugs, lithium, cyclosporin, tacrolimus, ACE-INHIBITORS, ACE-II ANTAGONISTS, antidiabetics, phenytoin, some antivirals, methotrexate, digoxin, some diuretics, some ANTIBIOTICS.

children, pregnant women, mothers who are breastfeeding, or for patients with stomach ulcer (or history of stomach ulcer), allergy to aspirin or other non-steroidal anti-inflammatory drugs, or severe allergy.

---

acenocoumarol *see* nicoumalone (alternative name)

Acepril *see* captopril tablets
(Bristol-Myers Squibb Pharmaceuticals)

---

acetazolamide tablets/modified-release capsules

A tablet or M-R CAPSULE used as a weak DIURETIC and fluid-balance drug to treat heart failure, fluid retention, premenstrual swelling, epilepsy, glaucoma, and to help prevent mountain sickness.

Strengths available: 250 mg tablets and 250 mg m-r capsules.
Dose: 250-375 mg a day or every other day in the morning at first. For premenstrual swelling, 125-375 mg a day as a single dose. For epilepsy, adults 250 mg-1000 mg a day in divided doses (children lower doses, according to body weight, maximum 750 mg a day). For glaucoma, 250-1000 mg a day in divided doses.
Availability: NHS and private prescription.
Contains: acetazolamide.
Brand names: Diamox, Diamox SR.

flushing, stomach upset, taste disturbance, thirst, headache, drowsiness, dizziness, increased urination, irritability, decreased sexual desire, chemical imbalance in body, kidney stones, abnormal skin sensations, blood changes, excitement, rash, depression, lack of appetite, confusion, liver and blood disorders, fits, sensitivity to light, temporary short sight.

in pregnant women, mothers who are breastfeeding, elderly patients, and in patients suffering from emphysema, lung blockages. Your doctor may advise that potassium supplements may be needed, and may advise regular blood and urine tests. Report any unusual rash to your doctor.

children (except for epilepsy), or for patients suffering from chronic closed-angle glaucoma, some kidney conditions, liver failure, ADRENAL insufficiency, low sodium or potassium levels, or allergy to some drugs.

cont.

aspirin, other diuretics, phenytoin, carbamazepine, ANTICOAGULANTS, alcohol, sedatives, NON-STEROIDAL ANTI-INFLAMMATORY DRUGS, lithium, pimozide, drugs affecting the blood pressure or heart rhythm, digoxin.

Acetest

(Bayer Diagnostics)

A tablet used as a reagent to test for the presence of ketones in the blood or urine. Raised ketone levels indicate an imbalance in the metabolism of fat in the body, such as occurs when a patient is suffering from diabetes.

Availability: NHS and private prescription, nurse prescription, over the counter.

acetic acid *see* Otomize

acetic acid ear spray

A spray used to treat infections of the ear canal.

Strengths available: 2% spray.
Dose: adults, 1 spray into the affected ear(s) three times a day for up to 7 days.
Availability: NHS and private prescription, over the counter.
Contains: acetic acid.
Brand names: Earcalm.

children.

acetic acid vaginal jelly

A jelly with applicator, used as an antiseptic to treat non-specific vaginal infection.

Strengths available: 0.94%.
Dose: 1 applicatorful once or twice a day for up to 2 weeks.
Availability: NHS and private prescription, over the counter.
Contains: glacial acetic acid.
Brand names: Aci-Jel.

irritation and inflammation.

in pregnant women and mothers who are breastfeeding.

children.

condoms and diaphragms (effects not known).

acetomenaphthone *see* Ketovite

acetylated wool alcohols *see* emollient preparations

acetylcysteine *see* Ilube

Acezide tablets *see* co-zidocapt tablets
(Bristol-Myers Squibb Pharmaceuticals)

Achromycin *see* tetracycline capsules and ointment
(Wyeth Laboratories)

Aci-Jel *see* acetic acid vaginal jelly
(Janssen-Cilag)

---

aciclovir cream

A cream used as an antiviral treatment for cold sores and genital herpes infections.

Strengths available: 5%.
Dose: apply every 4 hours (five times a day) for 5 days, starting at the first sign of the attack.
Availability: NHS and private prescription. (Also available over the counter to treat cold sores only.)
Contains: aciclovir.
Brand names: Zovirax. (Over the counter brands include Zovirax Cold Sore Cream, Boots Avert, Herpetad, Soothelip, Virasorb.)
Other preparations: aciclovir eye ointment, aciclovir tablets.

temporary stinging or burning, reddening and flaking of skin.

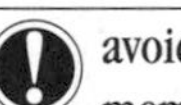
avoid contact with eyes or mucous membranes.

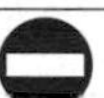
eye conditions.

---

aciclovir eye ointment

An eye ointment used as an antiviral treatment for herpes infection of the eye.

Strengths available: 3%.
Dose: insert 1 cm length of ointment inside the lower eyelid five times a day (every 4 hours), and continue for at least 3 days after healing.
Availability: NHS and private prescription.
Contains: aciclovir.
Brand names: Zovirax.
Other preparations: aciclovir cream, aciclovir suspension/dispersible tablets/tablets.

Side effects: mild smarting, superficial inflammation of the eye.

---

aciclovir suspension/tablets/dispersible tablets

A tablet or suspension used as an antiviral treatment for herpes infections such as chicken pox, shingles, cold sores, and genital herpes.

cont.

A

Strengths available: 200 mg, 400 mg, and 800 mg tablets; 200 mg, 400 mg, and 800 mg dispersible tablets; 200 mg/5 ml and 400 mg/5 ml suspensions.

Dose: for chicken pox and shingles, adults 800 mg five times a day (every 4 hours) for 7 days. To treat other herpes infections, adults 200 mg five times a day (every 4 hours) for 5 days. (Reduced doses for children and for prevention of herpes infections.)

Availability: NHS and private prescription.

Contains: aciclovir.

Brand names: Zovirax, Virovir.

Other preparations: aciclovir cream, aciclovir eye ointment.

rash, stomach upset, liver changes, blood changes, headache, dizziness, confusion and other brain reactions, tiredness.

in pregnant women, mothers who are breastfeeding, and in patients suffering from kidney damage; drink plenty of fluids.

---

acipimox capsules

A capsule used as a lipid-lowering agent to treat elevated lipid levels in the blood.

Strengths available: 250 mg capsules.

Dose: 2-3 capsules a day with meals, in divided doses.

Availability: NHS and private prescription.

Contains: acipimox.

Brand names: Olbetam.

flushes, rash, itching, stomach upset, redness, headache, general feeling of being unwell, stomach upset, dry eyes; rarely, severe allergy and breathing difficulty.

in patients with kidney disorders.

children, pregnant women, mothers who are breastfeeding, or for patients with stomach ulcer or severe kidney disorder.

Acitak *see* cimetidine tablets
(Opus Pharmaceuticals)

---

acitretin capsules

A capsule used to treat severe extensive psoriasis and other related skin disorders.

Strengths available: 10 mg and 25 mg capsules.

Dose: Initially 10-30 mg once a day for 2-4 weeks, increasing to a maximum of 75 mg a day (50 mg for Darier's disease) if needed for a further 6-8 weeks (or up to 6 months in ichthyosis and Darier's disease). Children treated only in

dryness, erosion of mucous membranes, reversible hair loss, itching, liver disorder, mood changes, blood changes, nausea, headache, drowsiness, sweating, joint or muscle pain, thickening of bones, inflamed nasal membranes, nose bleeds. sensitivity to light, changes in blood lipids, reddened skin, eye disorders (including decreased tolerance to contact lenses), scaling of feet and hands, dry eyes, inflammation of gums or vagina.

exceptional circumstances (reduced doses, with careful monitoring). Prescribed only by hospital specialists.

Availability: NHS and private prescription. (Restricted to hospital use.)

Contains: acitretin.

Brand names: Neotigason.

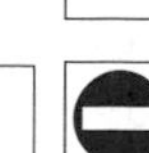

in patients suffering from diabetes. Women of child-bearing age must use effective contraception during treatment and for 2 years afterwards. Your doctor may advise regular X-rays, blood tests, and examinations. You should not donate blood for at least 1 year after the last dose. Avoid excessive exposure to sunlight and the use of sunlamps.

vitamin A, methotrexate, ANTICOAGULANTS, alcohol, skin products that soften and remove the skin surface, sedating drugs.

pregnant women, mothers who are breastfeeding, or for patients with high lipid levels, liver or kidney disorders.

Acnecide *see* benzoyl peroxide cream/gel
(Galderma)

Acnisal *see* salicylic acid lotion
(DermaPharm)

Acoflam/Acoflam Retard/Acoflam SR *see* diclofenac enteric-coated tablets/modified-release tablets
(Goldshield Healthcare)

---

acrivastine capsules

A capsule used as an ANTIHISTAMINE to treat allergic rhinitis, hayfever, and other allergies.

Strengths available: 8 mg capsules.

Dose: 1 capsule three times a day.

Availability: NHS and private prescription. (Also available over the counter to treat hayfever and allergic skin conditions only.)

Contains: acrivastine.

Brand names: Semprex. (Over-the-counter brand, Benadryl Allergy Relief.)

rarely, drowsiness.

in pregnant women and mothers who are breastfeeding.

children under 12 years, the elderly, or for patients with kidney disorders.

sedatives, alcohol.

ACT-HIB *see Haemophilus influenzae* type b vaccine
(Aventis Pasteur MSD)

ACT-HIB DTP *see* diphtheria, tetanus, pertussis, and *Haemophilus influenzae* type b vaccine
(Aventis Pasteur MSD)

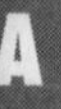

Acticin *see* tretinoin cream/gel
(Strakan)

Actinac
(Peckforton Pharmaceuticals)
A lotion used as an ANTIBIOTIC, CORTICOSTEROID, and skin softener to treat acne and associated disorders.

Dose: apply night and morning for 4 days, then at night only until 3 nights after the spots have gone.
Availability: NHS and private prescription.
Contains: chloramphenicol, hydrocortisone acetate, butoxyethyl nicotinate, allantoin, sulphur.

 severe reddening of the skin. (Side effects listed under topical corticosteroids also apply.)

 in pregnant women. (Cautions listed under topical corticosteroids also apply.) Remove jewellery before applying.

 (*see* topical corticosteroids).

---

activated dimethicone (simethicone) *see* dimethicone

Actonel *see* risedronic acid tablets
(Aventis and Proctor and Gamble Pharmaceuticals UK)

Actos *see* pioglitazone tablets
(Takeda UK)

Actrapid *see* insulin (Human Actrapid)

Acular *see* ketorolac trometamol eye drops
(Allergan)

Acupan *see* nefopam tablets
(3M Health Care)

Adalat/Adalat Retard/Adalat LA *see* nifedipine modified-release tablets/capsules/modified-release capsules
(Bayer Pharma Business Group)

---

adapalene cream/gel

A cream or gel used to treat acne.

Strengths available: 0.1%.
Dose: apply thinly once a day at bedtime, after washing and drying the skin. Condition to be reassessed after 3 months.
Availability: NHS and private prescription.
Contains: adapalene.
Brand names: Differin.

skin irritation, increased sensitivity to sunlight, temporary changes in skin pigment.

avoid application to the eyes, lips, mucous membranes, and angles of the nose. Avoid excessive exposure to sunlight and sunlamps. Women of childbearing age should use effective contraception.

skin softeners and preparations that cause peeling.

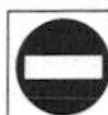
pregnant women, mothers who are breastfeeding, or for patients with severe acne, broken skin, or eczema.

Adcal-D3 *see* calcium and vitamin D tablets
(Strakan)

Adcortyl in Orabase *see* triamcinolone dental paste
(Bristol-Myers Squibb Pharmaceuticals)

Adcortyl injection *see* triamcinolone injection
(Bristol-Myers Squibb Pharmaceuticals)

Adcortyl with Graneodin *see* topical corticosteroid cream
(Bristol-Myers Squibb Pharmaceuticals)

Adgyn Combi *see* hormone replacement therapy (combined)
(Strakan)

Adgyn Estro *see* hormone replacement therapy (oestrogen-only)
(Strakan)

Adgyn Medro *see* medroxyprogesterone tablets
(Strakan)

Adipine MR *see* nifedipine modified-release tablets
(Trinity Pharmaceuticals)

Adizem SR/XL *see* diltiazem modified-release capsules
(Napp Pharmaceuticals)

---

adrenal glands

The adrenal glands are organs situated above the kidneys that produce hormones, including STEROIDS.

---

adrenaline *see* adrenaline eye drops, adrenaline injection, Ganda

---

adrenaline eye drops

Eye drops used as a SYMPATHOMIMETIC to treat glaucoma.

Strengths available: 1%, 0.5%.
Dose: 1 drop once or twice a day.
Availability: NHS and private prescription.
Contains: adrenaline.
Brand names: Eppy, Simplene.
Compound preparations: Ganda.

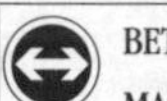 BETA-BLOCKERS, tricyclic antidepressants, MAOIS.

 pain in the eye, headache, skin reactions, temporary blurring of vision, red eye, rarely, sympathomimetic effects.

 in pregnant women, mothers who are breastfeeding, and in patients with high blood pressure, heart disease, overactive thyroid, diabetes, narrowed arteries, or who have no lens in the eye.

 children, or for patients with narrow-angle glaucoma.

---

adrenaline injection (ready to use)

A ready-to-use injection of a SYMPATHOMIMETIC drug, used for emergency treatment of severe allergy. (Also used by trained medical personnel to treat heart attack.)

Strengths available: 0.15 mg or 0.3 mg per dose.
Dose: for severe allergy, 0.15 mg-0.3 mg (according to age) injected by the intramuscular route, and repeated after 15 minutes (for adults) or 10 minutes (for children) if necessary.
Availability: NHS and private prescription.
Contains: adrenaline.
Brand names: Epipen, Min-I-Jet Adrenaline.

 anxiety, shaking, rapid or irregular heart beat, dry mouth, cold hands and feet, sweating, upset stomach, difficulty breathing.

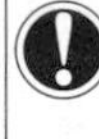 in pregnant women, the elderly, and in patients suffering from overactive thyroid, diabetes, heart disease, or high blood pressure.

 BETA-BLOCKERS, tricyclic antidepressants, entacapone, anaesthetics, ANTIHYPERTENSIVES, breathing stimulants, MAOIS, other sympathomimetics.

Aerobec/Aerobec Forte Autohaler *see* beclomethasone inhaler
(3M Health Care)

A

Aerochamber
(3M Health Care)
A one-piece spacer device used with all types of inhalers. Mask available for children and infants.

Availability: NHS and private prescription, over the counter.

Aerocrom Inhaler/Syncroner *see* sodium cromoglycate inhaler and salbutamol inhaler
(Distriphar)

Strengths available: 1 mg + 100 mcg per dose inhaler.
Dose: adults 2 puffs four times a day.

Aerolin Autohaler *see* salbutamol inhaler
(3M Health Care)

Agenerase *see* amprenavir capsules/solution
(GlaxoWellcome UK)

Agitane *see* benzhexol tablets
(DDSA Pharmaceuticals)

Ailax *see* co-danthramer suspension
(Galen)

Ailax Forte *see* co-danthramer forte suspension
(Galen)

Airomir inhaler/autohaler *see* salbutamol inhaler (CFC-free)
(3M Health Care)

Akineton *see* biperiden tablets
(Knoll)

Aknemin *see* minocycline capsules
(Crookes Healthcare)

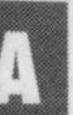

Aknemycin Plus *see* tretinoin cream and erythromycin solution
(Crookes Healthcare)

Strengths available: 0.025% + 4% solution.
Dose: adults and children, apply to affected areas once or twice a day for 9-12 weeks.

Albustix
(Bayer Diagnostics)
A plastic strip used as an indicator for the detection of protein in the urine. Protein in the urine may indicate damage to, or disease of, the kidneys.

Availability: NHS and private prescription, nurse prescription, over the counter.

---

alclometasone *see* topical corticosteroid cream/ointment

Alcoderm *see* emollient cream/lotion
(Galderma (UK))

Aldactide *see* co-flumactone tablets
(Searle)

Aldactone *see* spironolactone tablets
(Searle)

Aldara *see* imiquimod cream
(3M Health Care)

Aldomet *see* methyldopa tablets
(Merck Sharp and Dohme)

---

alendronate tablets
A tablet used to treat or prevent OSTEOPOROSIS in women after the menopause. Also used to treat osteoporosis and prevent bone loss caused by use of CORTICOSTEROIDS in men and women.

Strengths available: 5 mg and 10 mg tablets.
Dose: in women after the menopause to treat osteoporosis, 10 mg once a day; to prevent osteoporosis in women after the

rash, abdominal pain, stomach upset, muscle or bone pain, headache, stomach ulcer, sensitivity to sunlight, blood changes, eye disorders, severe allergy reactions. Report any difficulty or pain when swallowing to your doctor.

menopause, 5 mg once a day; to treat and prevent osteoporosis caused by corticosteroids, 10 mg once a day for women after the menopause who do not take HRT (or 5 mg for men, women before the menopause, or women after the menopause who take HRT). The dose is taken in the morning, 30 minutes before food or other medicines, with a full glass of water.

Availability: NHS and private prescription.

Contains: alendronate sodium (alendronic acid).

Brand names: Fosamax.

in patients suffering from stomach/ swallowing disorders, or calcium/vitamin D deficiency.

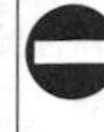
children, pregnant women, mothers who are breastfeeding, or for patients with kidney disorders, abnormal oesophagus, or delayed emptying of the stomach, or who cannot remain upright for 30 minutes.

calcium, ANTACIDS, iron supplements.

---

alendronic acid *see* alendronate tablets

---

alfacalcidol capsules/drops

Capsules or drops used as a source of vitamin D to treat bone disorders caused by kidney disease, rickets, over- or underactive parathyroid glands, low calcium levels in newborn infants, or other bone disorders.

Strengths available: 2 mcg/ml drops; 0.25 mcg, 0.5 mcg, and 1 mcg capsules.

Dose: adults and children over 20 kg body weight, 1 mcg each day at first, adjusting as needed; children under 20 kg and elderly patients, 0.05 mcg per kg each day at first.

Availability: NHS and private prescription.

Contains: alfacalcidol (vitamin D).

Brand names: AlfaD, One-Alpha.

in pregnant women, mothers who are breastfeeding, and in patients suffering from kidney failure. Your doctor may advise that calcium levels should be checked regularly. Some brands contain peanut oil.

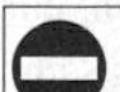
patients with high blood calcium levels.

barbiturates, digoxin, some diuretics, antacids, mineral oils, cholestyramine, colestipol, sucralfate, danazol.

AlfaD *see* alfacalcidol capsules
(Berk Pharmaceuticals)

---

alfuzosin tablets/modified-release tablets

A tablet or M-R TABLET used to treat enlarged prostate.

dizziness, vertigo, stomach upset, low blood pressure on standing, fainting, dry mouth, changes in urine flow, rapid heart rate, palpitations, fluid retention, chest pain, tiredness, drowsiness, rash, itching, flushing, headache.

cont.

Strengths available: 2.5 mg tablets; 5 and 10 mg m-r tablets.
Dose: initially 2.5 mg three times a day (elderly 2.5 mg twice a day), increasing to maximum of 10 mg each day. Using m-r tablets, either 5 mg once or twice a day (Xatral SR) or 10 mg once a day (Xatral XL).
Availability: NHS and private prescription.
Contains: alfuzosin
Brand names: Xatral, Xatral SR/XL.

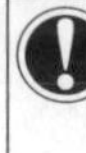 in elderly patients, and in those suffering from raised blood pressure or heart, liver, or kidney disorders. Your doctor may advise regular blood pressure checks. Treatment should be withdrawn if chest pain worsens, or 24 hours before anaesthesia. The first dose should be taken when going to bed.

 children, or for patients suffering from severe liver disorder, or with a history of low blood pressure on standing, or fainting while passing urine.

 other ALPHA-BLOCKERS, ANTIHYPERTENSIVES, some drugs used to treat heart or circulation disorders, anaesthetics, NON-STEROIDAL ANTI-INFLAMMATORY DRUGS, alcohol, sedatives.

Algesal *see* analgesic (topical)
(Solvay Healthcare)

Algicon *see* alginate liquid/tablets
(Rhône-Poulenc Rorer)

---

alginate dressing

A sterile dressing used to treat wounds, such as leg ulcers and pressure sores, which are weeping. (Various sizes available.)

Availability: NHS and private prescription, nurse prescription, over the counter.
Contains: calcium alginate or calcium sodium alginate.
Brand names: Algisite M, Algosteril, Kaltogel, Kaltostat, Melgisorb, Seasorb, Sorbalgon, Sorbsan, Sorbsan Plus, Sorbsan SA 2000, Tegagen.

---

alginate liquid/tablets/infant sachets

A liquid or tablet used as an ANTACID and reflux suppressant to treat reflux symptoms including indigestion, hiatus hernia, and oesophagitis. Infant sachets used to treat regurgitation and reflux in children.

Dose: *see* table. The doses are taken after food and at bedtime. Tablets should be chewed before swallowing.
Availability: NHS and private prescription, over the counter.

 products containing sodium may aggravate high blood pressure, kidney or heart disorders. Low-sodium products (marked * in table below) may be more suitable for these patients. Products with high sugar content († in table) may be unsuitable for diabetics.

Contains: (*see* table below).
Other preparations: Pyrogastrone.

some products not suitable for children or for patients with kidney failure. Infant sachets not suitable for premature babies, in children likely to dehydrate, or if the intestines are obstructed.

E-C TABLETS/CAPSULES, some ANTIBIOTICS, ANTIHYPERTENSIVES, some anti-epileptic treatments, iron preparations, lithium. Infant sachets not to be used with other thickening preparations.

Product	*Main ingredients*	*Dose*
Algicon Tablets * †	aluminium hydroxide, magnesium alginate, magnesium carbonate, potassium bicarbonate, sucrose	Adults 1-2 tablets four times a day.
Algicon Liquid *	aluminium hydroxide, magnesium alginate, magnesium carbonate, potassium bicarbonate, sucrose	Adults 10-20 ml four times a day.
Gastrocote Tablets †	alginic acid, aluminium hydroxide, magnesium trisilicate, sodium bicarbonate	Adults and childen over 6 years, 1-2 tablets four times a day.
Gastrocote Liquid	aluminium hydroxide, magnesium trisilicate, sodium alginate, sodium bicarbonate	Adults and older children, 5-15 ml four times a day.
Gaviscon Tablets	alginic acid, aluminium hydroxide, magnesium trisilicate, sodium bicarbonate	Adults 1-2 tablets. Children 6-12 years 1 tablet. Children 2-6 years 1 tablet.
Gaviscon Liquid	sodium alginate, sodium bicarbonate, calcium carbonate.	Adults 10-20 ml. Children 6-12 years 5-10 ml. Children 2-6 years as directed by doctor.
Gaviscon Advance Suspension	sodium alginate, potassium bicarbonate	Adults and children over 12 years 5-10 ml.
Gaviscon Infant Sachets	sodium alginate, magnesium alginate, colloidal silica, mannitol	1-2 doses (according to child's weight) after feeds.
Peptac Suspension	sodium bicarbonate, sodium alginate, calcium carbonate	Adults 10-20 ml. Children 6-12 years 5-10 ml.
Topal Tablets * †	alginic acid, aluminium hydroxide, magnesium carbonate, sucrose, sodium bicarbonate	Adults 1-3 tablets four times a day. Children half adult dose.

* *Low-sodium preparation.*   † *High sugar content – caution needed in diabetics.*

alginic acid *see* alginate liquid/tablets

Algisite M *see* alginate dressing
(Smith and Nephew Healthcare)

Algosteril *see* alginate dressing
(Beiersdorf UK)

---

alimemazine *see* trimeprazine (alternative name)

---

allantoin *see* Actinac, Alphosyl, Alphosyl HC, Anodesyn

Allegron *see* nortriptyline tablets
(King Pharmaceuticals)

---

allopurinol tablets

A tablet used as an enzyme blocker to prevent gout and kidney stones.

Strengths available: 100 mg and 300 mg tablets.
Dose: 100 mg a day at first, increasing to maintenance 100-900 mg a day (in divided doses if more than 300 mg). Colchicine or an anti-inflammatory drug should also be prescribed for the first few weeks of treatment for gout.
Availability: NHS and private prescription.
Contains: allopurinol.
Brand names: Caplenal, Xanthomax, Zyloric.

skin reaction, rash, stomach upset, acute gout. Rarely, headache, vertigo, drowsiness, hair loss, liver or kidney disorder, pins and needles, vision or taste disturbances, high blood pressure, nerve pain, general feeling of being unwell, fever, enlarged lymph glands, joint pain, blood changes, epilepsy.

in pregnant women, mothers who are breastfeeding, the elderly, and in patients suffering from kidney or liver disease. Be sure to drink plenty of fluids.

ANTICOAGULANTS, azathioprine, mercaptopurine, alcohol, sedatives.

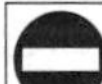
immediate treatment of gout attacks.

Almodan *see* amoxycillin capsules/syrup
(Berk Pharmaceuticals)

---

almond oil ear drops

An oil used to soften ear wax before syringing the ear.

Dose: for hard wax, use a few drops twice a day for a few days before syringing. Lie with the affected ear uppermost for a few minutes after instilling the drops.
Availability: NHS and private prescription, nurse prescription, over the counter.
Contains: almond oil.
Compound preparations: EMOLLIENT preparation (for use on skin).

Not to be used for: patients with perforated ear drum.

Alomide *see* lodoxamide eye drops
(Alcon)

---

alpha-blocker
A drug used to block some of the effects of adrenaline in the body, causing smooth muscle to relax and blood vessels to widen. Alpha-blockers are therefore useful as ANTIHYPERTENSIVES to treat high blood pressure, and to relieve symptoms of enlarged prostate gland (by relaxing muscles enough to improve urine flow). Examples prazosin, terazosin.

Alpha Keri *see* emollient bath preparations
(Bristol-Myers Squibb Pharmaceuticals)

Alphaderm *see* topical corticosteroid cream and urea cream
(Proctor and Gamble Pharmaceuticals UK)

Alphagan *see* brimonidine eye drops
(Allergan)

Alphavase *see* prazosin tablets
(Ashbourne Pharmaceuticals)

Alphosyl *see* coal tar cream/shampoo/solution
(Stafford-Miller)

Alphosyl HC *see* coal tar cream/shampoo/solution and topical corticosteroid
(Stafford-Miller)

---

alprazolam tablets
A tablet used for the short-term treatment of anxiety.

Strengths available: 0.25 mg and 0.5 mg tablets.

cont.

Dose: elderly or frail patients, 0.25 mg 2-3 times a day; adults 0.25-5 mg three times a day, up to a maximum of 3 mg each day.
Availability: private prescription only.
Contains: alprazolam.
Brand names: Xanax.

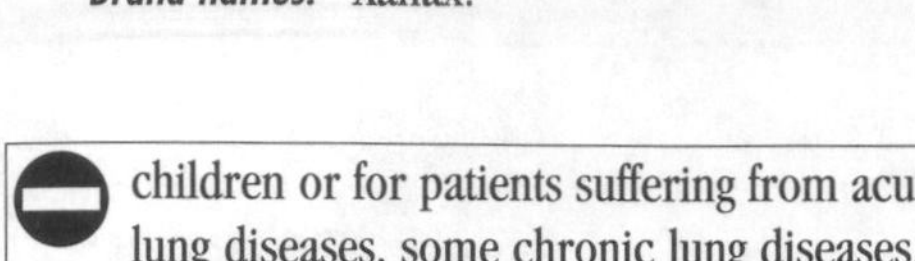

children or for patients suffering from acute lung diseases, some chronic lung diseases, severe liver disease, MYASTHENIA GRAVIS, some obsessional and psychotic disorders, or who have stopped breathing while asleep.

alcohol, other sedating drugs, some antivirals and anti-epileptic medications.

drowsiness, light-headedness, confusion, vertigo, stomach disturbances, loss of memory, aggression, headache, joint immobility, salivation changes, shaking, unsteadiness, low blood pressure, rash, changes in vision, changes in sexual desire, retention of urine, incontinence, blood changes, jaundice. Risk of addiction increases with dose and length of treatment. May impair judgement.

in the elderly, pregnant women, mothers who are breastfeeding, women during labour, and in patients suffering from lung disorders, glaucoma, kidney or liver disorders, muscle weakness, PORPHYRIA, or with a history of drug or alcohol abuse. Avoid long-term use and withdraw gradually.

alprostadil injection/urethral stick

An injection or pellet used to treat erectile impotence in men.

Strengths available: 5 mcg, 10 mcg, 20 mcg, or 40 mcg injections; 125 mcg, 250 mcg, 500 mcg, or 1000 mcg urethral sticks.
Dose: by intercavernosal injection into the penis 2.5 mcg at first, increasing in steps of 5-10 mcg to obtain a dose that produces an erection lasting not more than 1 hour, (maximum dose 40-60 mcg, maximum frequency once a day and three times in any one week); by urethral stick, 250 mcg at first, adjusted according to response (usually 125-1000 mcg per dose), maximum of two doses in 24 hours and seven in 7 days. Lower initial doses used in patients with spinal cord injury. May be self-administered after proper training.
Availability: private prescription, and on NHS prescriptions for men with certain specified causes of impotence (e.g. spinal cord

burning or pain in the penis during erection, thickening of the tissue, flushing, bruising or other reactions at injection site, pain around the anus or in the testicles, iron and protein deposits in the penis, persistent painful erection, blood pressure changes, abnormal heart rhythm, dizziness, headache, collapse, shock, urine infections, bleeding from the urethra, abnormal ejaculation, nausea, dry mouth, fainting, chest pain, weakness, influenza-like symptoms, back or pelvic pain, swollen veins in the legs.

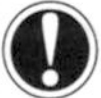

in patients suffering from tightness of the foreskin, deformed penis, thickening of the tissue of the penis, blood-clotting disorders, heart or brain blood-vessel disorders. If erection persists for more than 4 hours, medical advice should be sought. With pellet treatments, if the patient's partner is pregnant, a condom should be worn.

injury).
Contains: alprostadil.
Brand names: Caverject, Muse, Viridal Duo.

 warfarin, other treatments for impotence, ANTIHYPERTENSIVES, MAOIS.

 children or for patients suffering from sickle cell anaemia, leukaemia, some other blood disorders, some forms of cancer, or who have penile implants. The pellets should not be used by patients with some deformities, infection, or inflammation of the penis.

Altacite Plus *see* co-simalcite suspension
(Peckforton Pharmaceuticals)

Alu-Cap *see* aluminium hydroxide capsules
(3M Health Care)

aluminium acetate ear drops

Drops used as an astringent to treat inflammation of the outer ear.

Strengths available: 8% and 13%.
Dose: insert directly into the ear or saturate a gauze wick and apply into the ear.
Availability: NHS and private prescription, over the counter.
Contains: aluminium acetate.

aluminium acetate lotion

A lotion used as an astringent to treat weeping eczema and wounds.

Dose: use undiluted as a wet dressing.
Availability: NHS and private prescription, over the counter.
Contains: aluminium acetate.

aluminium chloride hexahydrate solution

A roll-on solution used to treat excessive sweating of the armpits, hands, or feet.

Strengths available: 20%.
Dose: apply if necessary at night. Wash off in the morning. Use daily at first, then reduce frequency as condition improves. Do not bathe immediately before use.
Availability: NHS and private prescription, over the counter.

 skin irritation.

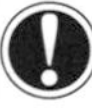 avoid the eyes and mucous membranes. Avoid contact with clothes or jewellery. Ensure that area is dry and not shaved for 12 hours before or after use.

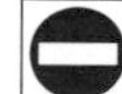 inflamed and broken skin areas.

cont.

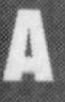

Contains: aluminium chloride hexahydrate.
Brand names: Anhydrol Forte, Driclor.

---

aluminium dihydroxyallantoinate *see* Zeasorb

---

aluminium hydroxide *see* alginate tablets/liquid, aluminium hydroxide capsules/suspension/tablets, Asilone, magnesium trisilicate compound tablets BP, Pyrogastrone

---

aluminium hydroxide capsules/suspension/tablets

A tablet/capsule or liquid used as an ANTACID to treat excess stomach acid and indigestion. The mixture and capsules are also used to lower blood phosphate levels in patients with kidney failure.

Strengths available: 500 mg tablets, 475 mg capsules.
Dose: as an antacid, adults 1-2 tablets or 1 capsule or 5-10 ml mixture four times a day and at bedtime, or as required; children aged 6-12 years, 5 ml mixture three times a day. The tablets should be chewed before swallowing. Higher doses used to lower blood phosphate levels (up to 100 ml mixture or 20 capsules per day).

 occasionally constipation.

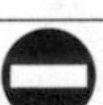 in patients with high aluminium levels in the blood.

 children or for patients with low blood phosphate levels or PORPHYRIA.

E-C TABLETS/CAPSULES, some ANTIBIOTICS.

Availability: NHS and private prescription, over the counter.
Contains: aluminium hydroxide.
Brand names: Alu-cap (capsules), Aludrox (not available on NHS).
Compound preparations: alginate liquid/tablets, Kolanticon, Maalox/Maalox TC, Maalox Plus (tablets not available on NHS), Mag-T-Co, Mucaine, Mucogel.

---

aluminium oxide *see* Brasivol

Alupent *see* orciprenaline tablets/syrup
(Boehringer Ingelheim)

Alvedon *see* paracetamol suppositories
(Novex Pharma)

Alvercol *see* Spasmonal Fibre (new name)

---

alverine capsules

A capsule used as an antispasmodic treatment for irritable bowel syndrome (and other disorders causing intestinal spasm) and period pain.

Strengths available: 60 mg and 120 mg capsules.
Dose: 60-120 mg 1-3 times a day.
Availability: NHS and private prescription, over the counter.
Contains: alverine citrate.
Brand names: Relaxyl, Spasmonal, Spasmonal Forte.
Compound preparations: Spasmonal Fibre.

 nausea, headache, itching, rash, dizziness.

 in pregnant women and mothers who are breastfeeding.

 children under 12 years or for patients without normal bowel movement.

amantadine capsules

A capsule or syrup used as an anti-parkinson/antiviral drug to treat Parkinson's disease and shingles, and to treat or prevent influenza.

Strengths available: 100 mg capsules and 50 mg/5 ml syrup.
Dose: for Parkinson's disease 100 mg each day for 7 days, then 100 mg twice a day (maximum 400 mg each day); shingles infections 100 mg twice a day for 14-28 days; influenza 100 mg each day.
Availability: NHS and private prescription.
Contains: amantadine hydrochloride.
Brand names: Lysovir, Symmetrel.

 ANTIMUSCARINICS, levodopa, stimulants, some DIURETICS, sedatives.

 skin changes, fluid retention, rash, vision, brain, and stomach disturbances, insomnia, dizziness, fits, blurred vision, reduced concentration or ability to perform skilled tasks (caution if driving). Rarely, blood disorders.

 in confused patients and in patients suffering from liver or kidney disease or congestive heart failure. Children over 10 years may be treated only for influenza.

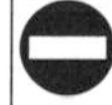 children under 10 years, pregnant women, mothers who are breastfeeding, or for patients suffering from severe kidney disease or with a history of convulsions or stomach ulcers.

Amaryl *see* glimepiride tablets
(Hoechst Marion Roussel)

Ames Lancets

(Bayer Diagnostics)
Diabetics who need to test their blood regularly can use lancets to pierce the skin, either with or without the use of a finger-pricking device.

Lancet width and length: 25G/0.5 mm (Type B).
Availability: NHS and private prescription, over the counter.

cont.

Availability: NHS and private prescription, over the counter.
Compatible finger-pricking devices: Autolet Lite, Autolet Lite Clinisafe, Glucolet.

---

amethocaine *see* amethocaine gel, Eludril

---

amethocaine gel

A gel applied to anaesthetize the skin before inserting needles into veins (e.g. for blood tests)

Strengths available: 4% gel.
Dose: apply to skin and cover with dressing for 30-45 minutes before procedure.
Availability: NHS and private prescription, over the counter.
Contains: amethocaine (tetracaine).
Brand names: Ametop.

 rash, swelling, or itching.

 avoid the eyes, ears, and mucous membranes.

 premature babies, babies under 1 month old, or for application to inflamed or injured areas of skin.

Ametop *see* amethocaine gel
(Smith and Nephew Healthcare)

Amias *see* candesartan tablets
(AstraZeneca UK)

Amiclav *see* co-amoxiclav tablets
(Ashbourne Pharmaceuticals)

Amidose Saline *see* saline solution (sterile)
(Abatron)

Amil-Co *see* co-amilozide tablets
(Baker Norton Pharmaceuticals)

Amilamont *see* amiloride solution
(Rosemont Pharmaceuticals)

Amilmaxco *see* co-amilozide tablets
(Ashbourne Pharmaceuticals)

---

amiloride tablets/solution

A tablet or solution used as a potassium-sparing DIURETIC to treat fluid retention and maintain potassium levels when used with other diuretics.

Strengths available: 5 mg tablets, 5 mg/5 ml solution.
Dose: 5-10 mg each day at first, then up to 20 mg each day.
Availability: NHS and private prescription.
Contains: amiloride.
Brand names: Amilamont.
Compound preparations: Co-amilofruse, Co-amilozide, Kalten, Moducren, Navispare.

stomach upset, rash, dry mouth, confusion, low blood pressure on standing, high potassium or low sodium levels in the blood.

in pregnant women, mothers who are breastfeeding, elderly patients, diabetics, and in patients with gout, liver or kidney disease. Your doctor may advise blood tests for potassium levels.

children or for patients suffering from high potassium levels or kidney failure.

potassium supplements, other potassium-sparing diuretics, ACE-INHIBITORS, NON-STEROIDAL ANTI-INFLAMMATORY DRUGS, carbamazepine, ANTIHYPERTENSIVES, cyclosporin, lithium.

aminophylline tablets/modified-release tablets

A tablet/M-R TABLET used as a BRONCHODILATOR to treat bronchial spasm associated with severe acute asthma, chronic bronchitis, emphysema. (The m-r tablets are also used to treat heart failure.)

Strengths available: 100 mg tablets; 100 mg, 225 mg, or 350 mg m-r tablets.
Dose: 100-300 mg 3-4 times a day after food using standard tablets, or 225 mg-450 mg twice a day using m-r tablets. Children use lower doses of m-r tablets.
Availability: NHS and private prescription, over the counter.
Contains: aminophylline.
Brand names: Amnivent, Norphyllin SR, Phyllocontin Continus.

upset stomach, headache, sleeplessness, fits, abnormal heart rhythm, skin reactions.

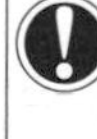
in pregnant women, mothers who are breastfeeding, the elderly, and in patients suffering from heart disease, high blood pressure, overactive thyroid, liver disease, stomach ulcer, epilepsy, fever. Patients taking m-r forms of aminophylline should remain on the same brand once stabilized. Smokers who alter their smoking habits may need dose adjusting.

patients suffering from PORPHYRIA.

cimetidine, some ANTIBIOTICS and anti-fungal treatments, CORTICOSTEROIDS, ritonavir, ANTIHYPERTENSIVES, disulfiram, zafirlukast, DIURETICS, some other bronchodilators, fluvoxamine, diltiazem, methotrexate, nizatidine, verapamil, lithium, some anti-epileptics, oral contraceptives (combined), SYMPATHOMIMETICS, sulphinpyrazone, INFLUENZA VACCINE, ticlopidine, alcohol, smoking.

A

amiodarone tablets

A tablet used as an anti-arrhythmic drug to treat heart rhythm disturbances.

Strengths available: 100 mg and 200 mg tablets.
Dose: adults 200 mg three times a day for 7 days, then 200 mg twice a day for 7 days, then usually 200 mg once a day thereafter; children as advised by doctor.
Availability: NHS and private prescription.
Contains: amiodarone hydrochloride.
Brand names: Cordarone X.

deposits on the eye surface, sensitivity to light, lung disorders, shaking, rash, nervous system, liver, heart, eye, and thyroid effects. Rarely, skin discoloration, upset stomach, vertigo, headache, nightmares, hair loss, impotence, sleeplessness, tiredness, inflamed testes, loss of co-ordination, blood changes.

in the elderly and in patients suffering from heart or kidney failure, or porphyria. Your doctor may advise thyroid, eye, and liver tests, and a chest X-ray. Treatment to be started only under specialist supervision or in hospital.

pregnant women, mothers who are breastfeeding, or for patients suffering from heart shock, some types of heart block or failure, thyroid disease, very low blood pressure, or who are allergic to iodine.

ANTICOAGULANTS, BETA-BLOCKERS, digoxin, TRICYCLIC ANTIDEPRESSANTS, phenytoin, erythromycin, tranquillizers, antimalarials, CORTICOSTEROIDS, amphoteracin, anaesthetics, co-trimoxazole, some drugs used to treat angina and high blood pressure.

amisulpride tablets

A tablet used to treat schizophrenia.

Strengths available: 50 mg or 200 mg tablets.
Dose: usually 50-800 mg each day (maximum 1200 mg). Doses over 300 mg are divided into two doses each day.
Availability: NHS and private prescription.
Contains: amisulpride.
Brand names: Solian.

weight gain, dizziness, sleeplessness, anxiety, drowsiness, lowered blood pressure on standing, agitation, upset stomach, raised levels of some hormones, parkinsonian-type symptoms, change in heart rhythm. Rarely, fits, NEUROLEPTIC MALIGNANT SYNDROME.

in the elderly and in patients with heart or circulation disorder, Parkinson's disease, kidney disorders, or epilepsy. Women of child-bearing age must use adequate contraception.

alcohol, anaesthetics, sedatives, drugs that affect heart rhythm, antidepressants, anti-epileptic treatments, ritonavir.

children under 15 years, pregnant women, mothers who are breastfeeding, or for patients with PHAEOCHROMOCYTOMA or some hormone-dependent tumours.

amitriptyline tablets/modified-release capsules/syrup

A tablet, syrup, or M-R CAPSULE used as a TRICYCLIC ANTIDEPRESSANT to treat depression with anxiety especially where sedation is valuable, and bedwetting in children.

Strengths available: 10 mg, 25 mg, and 75 mg tablets; 25 mg or 50 mg m-r capsules.
Dose: adults 75 mg a day at first, increasing to 150 mg a day if needed; elderly and adolescents 30-75 mg a day at first. To treat bedwetting in children: 7-10 years, 10-20 mg at night; 11-16 years 25-50 mg (maximum treatment period 3 months, withdrawing gradually).
Availability: NHS and private prescription.
Contains: amitriptyline hydrochloride.
Brand names: Lentizol (m-r capsules).
Compound preparations: Triptafen/Triptafen-M.

dry mouth, noises in the ears, tiredness, constipation, difficulty passing urine, blurred vision, stomach upset, palpitations, drowsiness, sleeplessness, dizziness, shaking hands, low blood pressure, weight change, sweating, fever, behavioural changes in children, confusion in the elderly, skin reactions, jaundice or blood changes, interference with sexual function, changes in heart rhythm, rash, hormone disturbances, fits, movement disorders, blood changes, breast changes in women, menstrual disorders.

in the elderly, pregnant women, mothers who are breastfeeding, and in patients suffering from heart disease, liver and kidney disorders, thyroid disease, PHAEOCHROMOCYTOMA, epilepsy, diabetes, PORPHYRIA, glaucoma, urine retention, constipation, some other psychiatric conditions. Your doctor may advise regular blood tests.

children under 7 years, children under 16 years to treat depression, or for patients suffering from recent heart attacks, heart rhythm abnormalities, severe liver disease or elevated mood.

alcohol, sedatives, MAOIS, BARBITURATES, other antidepressants, ANTIHYPERTENSIVES, tranquillizers, anti-epileptic drugs, ritonavir, entacapone, selegiline, sotalol, halofantrine, drugs affecting heart rhythm, methylphenidate.

Amix *see* amoxycillin capsules/syrup (Ashbourne Pharmaceuticals)

---

amlodipine tablets

A tablet used as a CALCIUM CHANNEL BLOCKER to treat high blood pressure and to prevent angina.

Strengths available: 5 mg and 10 mg tablets.
Dose: 5-10 mg once a day.
Availability: NHS and private prescription.
Contains: amlodipine besylate.
Brand names: Istin.

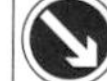
headache, fluid retention, tiredness, nausea, flushing, rash, dizziness. Rarely, itching, joint pain, muscle pain, difficulty breathing, palpitations, sleepiness, weakness, stomach upset, mood changes, increased urination, impotence, visual disturbance, gum disorders, liver changes, jaundice, breast changes in men.

cont.

in patients suffering from liver disorders, very high blood pressure, or recent heart attack.

pregnant women, mothers who are breast-feeding, or for patients with narrowed major arteries, unstable angina, or recent heart attack.

some anaesthetics, antifungals, ALPHA-BLOCKERS, ritonavir, some anti-epileptic medications, BETA-BLOCKERS, theophylline, aminophylline.

Ammonaps *see* sodium phenylbutyrate tablets/granules
(Orphan Europe (UK))

---

ammonia and ipecacuanha mixture BP

A mixture used as an expectorant to treat chesty coughs.

Dose: adults 10-20 ml 3-4 times a day.
Availability: NHS and private prescription, over the counter.
Contains: ammonium bicarbonate, ipecacuanha tincture.

---

ammonium bicarbonate *see* ammonia and ipecacuanha mixture BP

Amnivent 225-SR *see* aminophylline modified-release tablets
(Ashbourne Pharmaceuticals)

---

amobarbital *see* amylobarbitone (alternative name)

Amoram *see* amoxycillin capsules/suspension
(Eastern Pharmaceuticals)

---

amorolfine cream/lacquer

A cream or nail lacquer used as an antifungal treatment for fungal skin or nail infections.

Strengths available: 0.25% cream; 5% nail lacquer.
Dose: apply cream to skin every evening after washing for 2-3 weeks (or up to 6 weeks on the feet), continuing for 3-5 days after condition clears. The lacquer is applied to infected nails once or twice a week, after filing and washing, for 6 months (fingers) or 9-12 months (toes).

temporary burning, redness, or itching.

in pregnant women and mothers who are breastfeeding; avoid the eyes, ears, and mucous membranes. Treatment for nails should be reviewed every 3 months.

children.

9-12 months (toes).
Availability: NHS and private prescription.
Contains: amorolfine hydrochloride.
Brand names: Loceryl.

---

amoxapine tablets

A tablet used as a tricyclic ANTIDEPRESSANT to treat depression.

Strengths available: 50 mg or 100 mg tablets.
Dose: 100-150 mg a day, increasing to a maximum of 300 mg a day. Elderly patients initially 25 mg a day, increasing gradually to a maximum of 50 mg three times a day if necessary.
Availability: NHS and private prescription.
Contains: amoxapine.
Brand names: Asendis.

 children under 16 years or for patients suffering from recent heart attacks, heart rhythm abnormalities, severe liver disease.

 alcohol, sedatives, tranquillizers, adrenaline, MAOIS, BARBITURATES, ritonavir, other antidepressants, ANTIHYPERTENSIVES, cimetidine, baclofen, anti-epileptic drugs, entacapone, selegiline, methylphenidate, drugs affecting heart rhythm.

 dry mouth, noises in the ears, tiredness, constipation, difficulty passing urine, blurred vision, stomach upset, palpitations, drowsiness, sleeplessness, dizziness, shaking hands, low blood pressure, weight change, sweating, fever, behavioural changes in children, confusion in the elderly, skin reactions, jaundice or blood changes, interference with sexual function, changes in heart rhythm, rash, hormone disturbances, fits, movement disorders, blood changes.

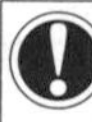 in pregnant women, mothers who are breastfeeding, and in patients suffering from heart disease, liver and kidney disorders, thyroid disease, PHAEOCHROMOCYTOMA, epilepsy, diabetes, PORPHYRIA, glaucoma, urine retention, constipation, some other psychiatric conditions. Your doctor may advise regular blood tests.

Amoxil *see* amoxycillin capsules/suspension
(Bencard)

---

amoxicillin *see* amoxycillin (alternative name)

---

amoxycillin *see* amoxycillin capsules/suspension, co-amoxiclav tablets/dispersible tablets/suspension, Heliclear, *H. pylori* eradication.

---

amoxycillin capsules/sachet/suspension

A capsule, sachet, or suspension used as a broad-spectrum penicillin antibiotic to treat respiratory, ear, nose, throat, urine, venereal, and soft tissue infections. Also for dental abscess, to prevent infection of the heart during dental procedures, and for *H. pylori* eradication. *cont.*

Strengths available: 250 mg and 500 mg capsules; 125 mg/5 ml and 250 mg/5 ml suspension; 125 mg/1.25 ml paediatric suspension; 3 g sachets.

Dose: adults 250 mg-500 mg three times a day; children up to 10 years half adult dose (infants use paediatric suspension). Short courses of higher doses used for some infections. To prevent heart infection during dental treatment: adults 3 g (children 750 mg-1500 mg) 1 hour before procedure.

Availability: NHS and private prescription.

Contains: amoxycillin trihydrate.

Brand names: Almodan, Amix, Amoram, Amoxil, Galenamox, Respillin.

Compound preparations: co-amoxiclav.

 stomach upset, rash, severe allergic reaction. Rarely, inflamed bowel, blood changes, nervous system disorders.

 in patients suffering from glandular fever, kidney disorder, leukaemia, HIV infection, and anyone with a history of allergies.

 patients who are allergic to penicillin.

 ORAL CONTRACEPTIVES (COMBINED), ANTICOAGULANTS, methotrexate.

---

amphoteracin lozenges/suspension

A tablet, suspension, or lozenge used as an antifungal treatment for infections such as thrush.

Strengths available: 100 mg tablets; 100 mg/ml suspension; 10 mg lozenges.

Dose: to treat intestinal thrush, adults 100-200 mg (children 100 mg) every 6 hours; to prevent intestinal thrush in babies, 1 ml suspension once a day; to treat thrush in the mouth, 1 lozenge dissolved slowly in the mouth (or 1 ml suspension held in the mouth) 4-8 times a day for 10-15 days (continued for 48 hours after symptoms resolve). Children should not use lozenges or tablets.

Availability: NHS and private prescription.

Contains: amphoteracin.

Brand names: Fungilin.

 occasionally stomach upset with high doses.

 children (lozenges or tablets *see above*).

---

ampicillin capsules/suspension

A capsule or suspension used as a broad-spectrum penicillin ANTIBIOTIC to treat respiratory, ear, nose, throat, urine, venereal, and soft tissue infections.

Strengths available: 250 mg and 500 mg capsules; 125 mg/5 ml and 250 mg/5 ml suspension.

Dose: adults 250 mg-1000 mg three times a day; children up to 10 years half adult dose.

 stomach upset, rash, severe allergic reaction. Rarely, inflamed bowel, blood changes, nervous system disorders.

 in patients suffering from glandular fever, kidney disorder, leukaemia, HIV infection, and anyone with a history of allergies.

Availability: NHS and private prescription.
Contains: amoxycillin trihydrate.
Brand names: Ampitrin, Penbritin.
Compound preparations: co-fluampicil.

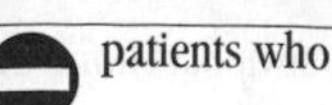
patients who are allergic to penicillin.

ORAL CONTRACEPTIVES (COMBINED), ANTICOAGULANTS, methotrexate.

Ampitrin *see* ampicillin capsules/suspension
(OPD Pharmaceuticals)

---

amprenavir capsules/solution

A capsule or solution used, in combination with other antiviral drugs, to treat HIV infection.

Strengths available: 50 mg and 150 mg capsules; 15 mg/ml oral solution.
Dose: adults and children over 12 years (and over 50 kg in weight) 1200 mg twice a day (600 mg twice a day if combined with ritonavir). Children aged 4-12 years and adults weighing less than 50 kg use lower doses, according to weight.
Availability: NHS and private prescription.
Contains: amprenavir.
Brand names: Agenerase.

stomach upset, skin disorders, tingling around the mouth, headache, shaking, sleep disorders, depressive disorders, tiredness, loss of appetite, mood disorders.

in pregnant women and in patients with liver disorders, diabetes, or haemophilia (a blood-clotting disorder). The oral solution should also be used with caution in patients with kidney disorders. Women should use barrier methods of contraception.

children under 4 years or for women who are breastfeeding. The oral solution should not be used by pregnant women or for patients with liver or kidney failure.

other antiviral drugs, rifampicin, rifabutin, calcium-channel blockers, sildenafil, statins, pimozide, ergotamine, opioid drugs, methadone, oral contraceptives, clozapine, dapsone, itraconazole, carbamazepine, cimetidine, loratadine, some tranquillizers and sedatives, dihydroergotamine, ANTACIDS, St John's wort *(Hypericum)*. Also disulfiram, metronidazole, alcohol (oral solution only).

---

amylase *see* pancreatin capsules

---

amylobarbitone/amylobarbitone sodium tablets/capsules

A tablet or capsule used as a BARBITURATE for the short-term treatment of severe sleeplessness in patients already taking these drugs.

Strengths available: 50 mg amylobarbitone tablets; 60 mg or 200 mg amylobarbitone sodium capsules.

drowsiness, hangover, dizziness, allergies, headache, shaky movements, breathing difficulties, confusion, excitement, withdrawal reactions.

cont.

Dose: 100-200 mg amylobarbitone or 60-200 mg amylobarbitone sodium at bedtime.
Availability: controlled drug; NHS and private prescription.
Contains: amylobarbitone (tablets) or amylobarbitone sodium (capsules). Also known as amobarbital or amobarbital sodium.
Brand names: Amytal, Sodium Amytal.
Compound preparations: Tuinal.

in patients suffering from liver, kidney, or lung disease. Dependence (addiction) may develop. Must be withdrawn slowly.

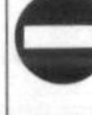
children, young adults, pregnant women, mothers who are breastfeeding, elderly or weak patients, or for those with a history of drug or alcohol abuse, or who are suffering from PORPHYRIA, or in the management of pain.

ANTICOAGULANTS, alcohol, antiviral drugs, CALCIUM CHANNEL BLOCKERS, cyclosporin, thyroxine, tibolone, theophylline, aminophylline, gestrinone, antidepressants, other sedatives, CORTICOSTEROIDS, oral contraceptives, rifampicin, phenytoin.

Amytal *see* amylobarbitone tablets
(Flynn Pharma)

Anabact *see* metronidazole gel
(Cambridge Healthcare Supplies)

---

anabolic steroid *see* page 606

Anacal ointment/suppositories
(Sankyo Pharma UK)
An ointment or suppository used as a soothing, anti-inflammatory treatment for the symptoms of haemorrhoids (piles), anal fissure, anal itch, or inflammation of the rectum.

children.

Dose: ointment applied up to four times a day; 1 suppository inserted into the rectum once or twice a day.
Availability: NHS and private prescription, over the counter.
Contains: heparinoid, lauromacrogol.

Anafranil/Anafranil SR *see* clomipramine capsules/syrup/modified-release tablets
(Novartis Pharmaceuticals UK)

A

analgesic

A preparation used to relieve pain. Example, paracetamol. Opioid analgesics are the stronger preparations which may be addictive with long-term use. Example, morphine.

analgesic (topical)

A cream, gel, or ointment applied to the skin and used as an ANALGESIC to relieve symptoms of rheumatic and muscular pain, sprains, and strains.

Dose: *see* table below.
Availability: NHS and private prescription, over the counter.
Contains: (*see* table below).

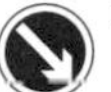 reddening of skin or rash.

 in pregnant women and mothers who are breastfeeding Avoid broken skin, lips, mucous membranes, and eyes.

 some products not suitable for younger children.

Brand	*Ingredients*	*Frequency of application*
Algesal	diethylamine salicylate	3 times a day
Balmosa	camphor, capsicum, menthol, methyl salicylate	as required
Intralgin	benzocaine, salicylamide	apply liberally
Transvasin	ethyl nicotinate, hexyl nicotinate, tetrahydrofurfuryl salicylate	2-3 times a day

Androcur *see* cyproterone tablets
(Schering Health Care)

Andropatch *see* testosterone patches
(SmithKline Beecham Pharmaceuticals)

anethol *see* Rowatinex

Angettes *see* aspirin 75 mg tablets
(Bristol-Myers Squibb Pharmaceuticals)

Angeze/Angeze SR *see* isosorbide mononitrate tablets/modified-release capsules
(Opus Pharmaceuticals)

Angiopine/Angiopine LA/Angiopine MR *see* nifedipine capsules/modified-release tablets
(Ashbourne Pharmaceuticals)

Angiozem/Angiozem CR *see* diltiazem tablets/modified-release tablets
(Ashbourne Pharmaceuticals)

Angitak *see* isosorbide dinitrate spray
(Eastern Pharmaceuticals)

Angitil SR/XL *see* diltiazem modified-release capsules
(Trinity Pharmaceuticals)

Anhydrol Forte *see* aluminium chloride hexahydrate lotion
(Dermal Laboratories)

Anodesyn ointment/suppositories
(SSL International)
An ointment or suppository used as an anaesthetic, soothing, and astringent treatment for the symptoms of haemorrhoids (piles).

Dose: the ointment applied (or 1 suppository inserted into the rectum) twice a day and after each bowel movement.
Availability: NHS and private prescription, over the counter.
Contains: lignocaine hydrochloride, allantoin.

Not to be used for: children under 12 years.

Anquil *see* benperidol tablets
(Concord Pharmaceuticals)

Antabuse 200 *see* disulfiram tablets
(Cox Pharmaceuticals)

---

antacid
A preparation that reduces the acid content of the stomach, used to relieve indigestion. Example, magnesium trisilicate mixture BP.

---

antazoline *see* Otrivine Antistin

Antepsin *see* sucralfate tablets/suspension
(Wyeth Laboratories)

---

anthraquinone glycosides *see* Pyralvex

antibiotic
A preparation that inhibits the growth of bacteria (and hence used to treat or prevent bacterial infections). Example, amoxycillin.

antimuscarinic
A drug that blocks the action of acetyl choline, a nerve transmitter. Antimuscarinics are used to reduce muscle spasm. The effects include dry mouth, difficulty passing urine, and possibly confusion. Example, hyoscine.

anticholinesterase
A drug that enhances the action of acetyl choline, a nerve transmitter. Example, pyridostigmine.

anticoagulant
A substance used to prevent the blood from clotting. Example, warfarin.

antihistamine
A preparation that blocks the histamine response in the body which occurs during an allergic reaction. Antihistamines are used to treat all types of allergy (skin rashes, hayfever, etc. Example, chlorpheniramine.

antihypertensive
A preparation used to lower blood pressure. Examples, BETA-BLOCKERS *see* atenolol; ACE-INHIBITORS *see* captopril; and CALCIUM CHANNEL BLOCKERS *see* nifedipine.

Antipressan *see* atenolol tablets
(Berk Pharmaceuticals)

Anturan *see* sulphinpyrazone tablets
(Sovereign Medical)

Anugesic HC *see* rectal corticosteroid
(Parke Davis)

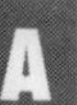

Anusol cream/ointment/suppositories

(Warner Lambert Consumer Healthcare)

A suppository, cream, or ointment used as a soothing, antiseptic, astringent treatment for the symptoms of haemorrhoids (piles), anal itch, and other rectal and anal disorders.

Dose: apply the ointment/cream (or insert 1 suppository into the rectum) twice a day and after each bowel movement.

Availability: NHS and private prescription, over the counter.

Contains: zinc oxide, bismuth oxide, peru balsam. Ointment and suppositories also contain bismuth subgallate.

Compound preparations: Anusol HC (*see* rectal corticosteroid).

Not to be used for: children.

Anusol-HC *see* rectal corticosteroid ointment/suppositories
(Kestrel Healthcare)

Apo-Go *see* apomorphine injection
(Britannia Pharmaceuticals)

---

apomorphine injection

An injection used to treat severe 'off' episodes in Parkinson's disease when the patient becomes immobile.

Strengths available: 20 mg or 50 mg ampoules, or 30 mg injector pen.

Dose: usually 3-30 mg injected subcutaneously each day in divided doses. Maximum of 10 mg per dose. May also be given by continuous injection.

Availability: NHS and private prescription.

Contains: apomorphine hydrochloride.

Brand names: Apo-Go, Britaject.

upset stomach, movement disorders, loss of balance, personality change, confusion, drowsiness, low blood pressure on standing, blood changes.

used only under specialist supervision. Treatment is started in hospital, with domperidone given for 3 days before first dose.

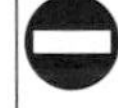

children under 18 years, pregnant women, mothers who are breastfeeding, or for patients with breathing disorders, psychiatric problems, allergy to OPIOID ANALGESICS, or severe reaction to levodopa preparations.

Caution needed with: entacapone, tranquillizers, alcohol, sedating drugs.

---

apraclonidine eye drops

An eye drop used for the short-term treatment of glaucoma that is not adequately controlled by other drugs.

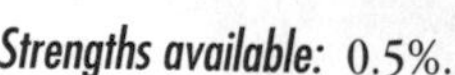

Strengths available: 0.5%.
Dose: 1 drop three times a day.
Availability: NHS and private prescription.
Contains: apraclonidine hydrochloride.
Brand names: Iopidine.
Other preparations: a preservative-free version (1%) is used to control eye pressure during laser eye surgery.

 redness, itching, discomfort, or other disorders of the eye, dry mouth or nose, disturbances of taste, headache. Rarely, drowsiness, depression, fluid retention, dizziness, slow heart rate, rash, upset stomach, euphoria, night-time disturbances.

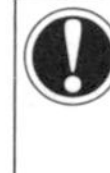 in pregnant women, mothers who are breastfeeding, and in patients with kidney disease, a history of heart disease or angina, or depression. Your doctor will advise regular checks.

 children or for patients with a history of severe heart or circulation disorder.

 TRICYCLIC ANTIDEPRESSANTS, SYMPATHOMIMETICS, MAOIS, clonidine, DIURETICS, anti-arrhythmics, digoxin, sedatives, alcohol, ANTIHYPERTENSIVES.

Apresoline *see* hydralazine tablets
(Sovereign Medical)

Aprinox *see* bendrofluazide tablets
(Sovereign Medical)

Aprovel *see* irbesartan tablets
(Sanofi Winthrop)

Aquadrate *see* urea cream
(Proctor and Gamble Pharmaceuticals UK)

Aquasept *see* triclosan liquid
(SSL International)

---

aqueous cream *see* emollient cream

---

arachis oil (peanut oil) *see* arachis oil enema, Cerumol, coal tar shampoo/solution, emollient preparations, hormone replacement – topical, Siopel, zinc cream BP

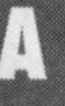

arachis oil enema

A 130 ml single-dose enema used as a faecal softener to treat faecal impaction (very severe constipation).

Dose: adults use 1 enema as required. Children over 3 years use reduced quantity, according to body weight.
Availability: NHS and private prescription, nurse prescription, over the counter.
Contains: arachis oil.
Brand names: Fletchers' Arachis Oil Retention Enema.

Caution: warm before use.

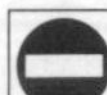
Not to be used for: children under 3 years or for patients allergic to peanuts.

Arava *see* leflunomide tablets
(Hoechst Marion Roussel)

Aricept *see* donepezil tablets
(Pfizer)

Arilvax *see* yellow fever vaccine
(Medeva Pharma)

Arpicolin *see* procyclidine syrup/tablets
(Rosemont Pharmaceuticals)

Artelac SDU *see* hypromellose single-dose units
(Nucare)

Arthrofen *see* ibuprofen tablets
(Ashbourne Pharmaceuticals)

Arthrosin *see* naproxen tablets
(Ashbourne Pharmaceuticals)

Arthrotec *see* diclofenac tablets and misoprostol tablets
(Searle)

Dose: one 50 mg tablet 2-3 times a day, or one 75 mg tablet twice a day after food.

Artificial Tears Minims

Single-dose eye drops used to treat tear deficiency (dry eyes).

Dose: as needed.
Availability: NHS and private prescription, over the counter.
Contains: hydroxyethylcellulose, sodium chloride.

Arythmol *see* propafenone tablets
(Knoll)

Asacol *see* mesalazine enteric-coated tablets
(SmithKline Beecham Pharmaceuticals)

Asasantin Retard *see* modified-release dipyridamole tablets and aspirin 75 mg tablets
(Boehringer Ingelheim)

Dose: 1 twice a day.

Ascabiol *see* benzyl benzoate application
(Rhône-Poulenc Rorer)

---

ascorbic acid tablets

A tablet used to prevent and treat scurvy, and to acidify urine.

Strengths available: 50 mg, 100 mg, 200 mg, and 500 mg tablets.
Dose: adults: prevention of scurvy, 25-75 mg a day; treatment of scurvy, at least 250 mg a day; to acidify urine, 4000 mg a day (in divided doses).
Availability: NHS and private prescription.
Contains: vitamin C.
Brand names: Redoxon (not available on NHS).
Compound preparations: Ketovite, multivitamin drops, vitamins capsules BPC.

Asendis *see* amoxapine tablets
(Wyeth Laboratories)

Aserbine cream/solution

(Forley)

A cream or solution used as a wound cleanser to treat varicose ulcers, burns, bed sores, and for cleansing wounds.

cont.

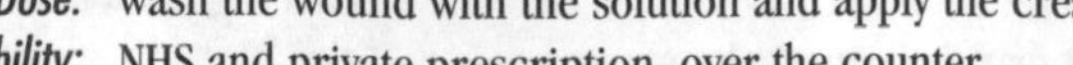

Dose: wash the wound with the solution and apply the cream twice a day.
Availability: NHS and private prescription, over the counter.
Caution: avoid the eyes.
Contains: malic acid, benzoic acid, propylene glycol, salicylic acid.

Ashbourne *see* emollient bath oil
(Ashbourne Pharmaceuticals)

Asilone suspension
(SSL International)
A suspension used as an ANTACID, anti-wind preparation to treat gastritis, stomach ulcers, indigestion, heartburn, and wind.

Dose: adults 5-10 ml after meals and at bedtime (up to four times a day).
Availability: NHS and private prescription, over the counter.
Contains: dimethicone, aluminium hydroxide, magnesium oxide.
Other preparations: Asilone Antacid liquid and tablets (not available on NHS).

Side effects: occasionally constipation.

Not to be used for: children under 12 years.

Caution needed with: ENTERIC-COATED TABLETS, some ANTIBIOTICS, iron, gabapentin, phenytoin.

Askina *see* saline solution
(B. Braun Medical)

Asmabec Clickhaler *see* beclomethasone inhaler
(Medeva Pharma)

Asmabec Spacehaler *see* beclomethasone inhaler
(Medeva Pharma)

Asmaplan *see* peak flow meter (standard range)
(Vitalograph)

Asmasal Clickhaler *see* salbutamol inhaler
(Medeva Pharma)

Asmasal Spacehaler *see* salbutamol inhaler
(Medeva Pharma)

Aspav

(Cox Pharmaceuticals)

A dispersible tablet used as an OPIOID ANALGESIC to relieve pain after operations, and other chronic pain.

Dose: 1-2 tablets dispersed in water every 4-6 hours if needed (maximum of 8 tablets in 24 hours).
Availability: NHS and private prescription.
Contains: aspirin, papaveretum.

children under 12 years, mothers who are breastfeeding, unconscious patients, or for patients suffering from bleeding disorders, severe breathing disorders, or stomach ulcers, or with a history of allergy to aspirin or anti-inflammatories

stomach upset or bleeding, allergy, asthma, confusion, addiction.

in pregnant women, women in labour, the elderly, or in patients suffering from head injury, underactive thyroid gland, asthma, impaired kidney or liver function, stomach disorders.

MAOIS, sedatives, alcohol, ANTICOAGULANTS, some antidiabetic drugs, NON-STEROIDAL ANTI-INFLAMMATORY DRUGS, methotrexate.

aspirin *see* Asasantin Retard, Aspav, aspirin 75 mg tablets, aspirin 300 mg tablets, co-codaprin tablets/dispersible tablets, Equagesic

aspirin 75 mg tablets/dispersible tablets/enteric-coated tablets

A tablet, dispersible tablet, or E-C TABLET used to prevent heart attack or stroke in patients known to be at risk.

Dose: 1-4 tablets a day.
Availability: NHS and private prescription, over the counter.
Contains: aspirin.
Brand names: Angettes, Caprin, Disprin CV (100 mg tablets), Enprin, Nu-Seals Aspirin, Postmi 75.
Compound preparations: Asasantin retard, Imazin XL, Imazin XL Forte.

stomach upset, allergy, asthma, abnormal bleeding.

in pregnant women and in patients suffering from uncontrolled high blood pressure or asthma.

children under 12 years, mothers who are breastfeeding, or for patients suffering from bleeding disorders or stomach ulcer.

NON-STEROIDAL ANTI-INFLAMMATORY DRUGS, some antidiabetic drugs, ANTICOAGULANTS, methotrexate. ANTACIDS should not be taken at the same time as e-c tablets.

aspirin 300 mg tablets/dispersible tablets/enteric-coated tablets

A tablet, E-C TABLET, or dispersible tablet used as an ANALGESIC to relieve pain, reduce fever, and treat rheumatic disease and other similar disorders.

Dose: adults: for pain, 300-900 mg every 4-6 hours as needed (maximum of 3600 mg a day); for rheumatic disease, 300-1200 mg every 4 hours (maximum 8000 mg a day); children treated only for juvenile arthritis (reduced doses according to body weight).

Availability: NHS and private prescription, over the counter. Limited quantities of dispersible tablets also available on nurse prescription.

Contains: aspirin.

Brand names: Caprin (e-c tablets), Nu-Seals Aspirin (e-c tablets).

Compound preparations: Aspav, Co-codaprin, Equagesic, Migramax.

stomach upset, allergy, asthma, abnormal bleeding, severe allergic reaction, Reye's syndrome in children. With high doses, noises in the ears, vertigo, confusion, difficulty breathing, fluid retention, blood and heart disorders, blood changes.

in pregnant women and in patients suffering from uncontrolled high blood pressure or asthma.

children under 12 years (except as above), mothers who are breastfeeding, or for patients suffering from bleeding disorders or stomach ulcer or who are allergic to any NON-STEROIDAL ANTI-INFLAMMATORY DRUG. Not to be used to treat gout.

non-steroidal anti-inflammatory drugs, some antidiabetic drugs, ANTICOAGULANTS, methotrexate. ANTACIDS should not be taken at the same time as e-c tablets.

A.T.10 *see* dihydrotachysterol solution
(Intrapharm Labs)

Atarax *see* hydroxyzine tablets
(Pfizer)

Atenix *see* atenolol tablets
(Ashbourne Pharmaceuticals)

Atenixco *see* co-tenidone tablets
(Ashbourne Pharmaceuticals)

---

atenolol tablets/syrup

A tablet or syrup used as a BETA-BLOCKER to treat angina, abnormal heart rhythm, or high blood pressure.

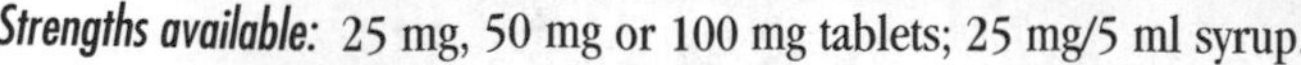

Strengths available: 25 mg, 50 mg or 100 mg tablets; 25 mg/5 ml syrup.
Dose: high blood pressure 50 mg a day; angina 100 mg a day; abnormal heart rhythm 50-100 mg a day.
Availability: NHS and private prescription.
Contains: atenolol.
Brand names: Antipressan, Atenix, Tenormin.
Compound preparations: Beta-Adalat, Co-tenidone, Kalten, Tenben, Tenif.

 cold hands and feet, sleep disturbance, slow heart rate, tiredness, wheezing, heart failure, low blood pressure, stomach upset. Rarely, dry eyes, rash, worsening of psoriasis.

 in pregnant women, mothers who are breastfeeding, the elderly, and in patients suffering from diabetes, kidney or liver disorders, MYASTHENIA GRAVIS, or with a history of allergies. May need to be withdrawn before surgery. Withdraw gradually.

 children or for patients suffering from heart block or failure, asthma, PHAEOCHROMOCYTOMA, or a history of breathing disorders.

 general anaesthetics, CALCIUM-CHANNEL BLOCKERS, ALPHA-BLOCKERS, clonidine, ANTIHYPERTENSIVES, amiodarone, antidiabetics, thymoxamine, theophylline, aminophylline.

Ativan *see* lorazepam tablets
(Wyeth Laboratories)

---

atorvastatin tablets

A tablet used in addition to diet as a STATIN to treat high cholesterol and other lipids in patients who have not responded to diet adjustment alone.

Strengths available: 10 mg, 20 mg, 40 mg, and 80 mg tablets.
Dose: 10-80 mg once a day.
Availability: NHS and private prescription.
Contains: atorvastatin calcium trihydrate.
Brand names: Lipitor.

 severe allergic reaction, headache, stomach upset, tiredness, weakness, itching, rash, cramps, dizziness, hair loss, inflamed or painful muscles, liver disorder, anaemia, pins and needles, loss of appetite, chest pain, impotence, high or low blood glucose levels, blood changes.

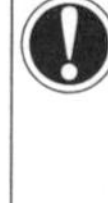 in patients with past liver disease or who have a high alcohol intake. Women of child-bearing age must use adequate contraception during treatment and for 1 month afterwards. Your doctor will advise regular blood tests. Report any unexplained muscle pain to your doctor.

 children, pregnant women, mothers who are breastfeeding, or for patients with current liver disease.

 warfarin, antifungal treatments, digoxin, cyclosporin, other lipid-lowering drugs.

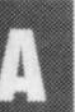

atovaquone suspension

A suspension used to treat some forms of pneumonia in patients unable to take co-trimoxazole.

Strengths available: 750 mg/5 ml.
Dose: 750 mg (5 ml) twice a day with food for 21 days.
Availability: NHS and private prescription.
Contains: atovaquone.
Brand names: Wellvone.
Compound preparations: Malarone.

rash, upset stomach, headache, fever, liver changes, blood changes (including anaemia).

in the elderly, pregnant women, and in patients suffering from diarrhoea, kidney or liver disorders, other chest diseases, or who have difficulty taking the drug with food.

rifampicin, tetracycline.

children or mothers who are breastfeeding.

---

atropine *see* atropine eye drops, co-phenotrope tablets

---

atropine eye drops/ointment

Eye drops or an eye ointment used as an ANTIMUSCARINIC preparation to dilate the pupils and treat uveitis (inflammation inside the eye).

Strengths available: 0.5% and 1% drops, 1% ointment.
Dose: used according to doctor's instructions.
Availability: NHS and private prescription.
Contains: atropine sulphate.
Brand names: Minims Atropine Sulphate (preservative-free, single dose drops).
Compound preparations: Isopto-Atropine.

disturbance of vision, temporary stinging, raised pressure inside the eye. With prolonged treatment, irritation, redness, inflammation or fluid retention in the eye. Very young or very old patients may suffer antimuscarinic effects *see* atropine tablets.

in the very young and the elderly (*see* above) and in long-sighted patients. Patients should not drive for 1-2 hours after treatment.

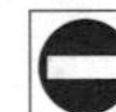
patients with narrow-angle glaucoma.

Atropine Minims *see* atropine eye drops
(Chauvin Pharmaceuticals)

---

atropine tablets

A tablet used as an ANTIMUSCARINIC treatment to relieve symptoms of stomach or intestinal spasm.

Strengths available: 600 mcg tablets.
Dose: 600-1200 mcg at night.

Availability: NHS and private prescription.
Contains: atropine sulphate.
Compound preparations: co-phenotrope.

 antimuscarinic effects, skin reactions, stomach upset, altered heart rhythm, difficulty passing urine, disturbed vision, dry mouth, intolerance of light, flushing, dry skin, confusion, dizziness.

 patients with glaucoma, MYASTHENIA GRAVIS, enlarged prostate or non-functioning intestines.

 in children, pregnant women, mothers who are breastfeeding, elderly patients, and in those with diarrhoea or inflamed bowel, high blood pressure, abnormal heart rhythm, fever, reflux oesophagitis, or heart attack.

 other antimuscarinic drugs.

Atrovent *see* ipratropium inhaler/nebulizer solution
(Boehringer Ingelheim)

Audax

(SSL International)
Drops used as an ANALGESIC and wax softener to relieve pain associated with acute inflammation of the outer or middle ear.

Dose: every four hours fill the ear with the liquid and plug it.
Availability: private prescription and over the counter.
Contains: choline salicylate, glycerol.

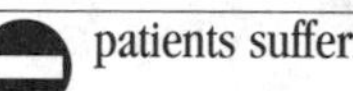 patients suffering from perforated ear drum.

Audicort

(Wyeth Laboratories)
Drops used as an ANTIBIOTIC and CORTICOSTEROID treatment for inflammation and infection of the outer ear.

Dose: 2-5 drops into the ear 3-4 times a day.
Availability: NHS and private prescription.
Contains: triamcinolone acetonide, neomycin.

 additional infection, irritation.

 in pregnant women, mothers who are breastfeeding.

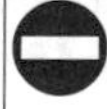 children or for patients suffering from perforated ear drum.

Augmentin *see* co-amoxiclav tablets/suspension
(Beecham Research Laboratories)

---

auranofin tablets

A tablet used as an oral gold salt to treat progressive rheumatoid arthritis which cannot be controlled effectively by NON-STEROIDAL ANTI-INFLAMMATORY DRUGS.

Strengths available: 3 mg tablets.
Dose: 1 tablet in the morning and 1 tablet in the evening for the first 3-6 months, then increase to 3 tablets a day if needed.
Availability: NHS and private prescription.
Contains: auranofin.
Brand names: Ridaura.

 upset stomach, rash, itching, inflamed bowel, inflammation of the eye or bowel, hair loss, kidney or liver disorders, blood changes, lung disorder, disturbance of taste, mouth ulcers.

 in patients suffering from kidney or liver disease, inflammatory bowel disease, rash, history of bone marrow depression. Your doctor may advise regular blood tests. Women should use adequate contraception until 6 months after end of treatment.

 children, pregnant women, mothers who are breastfeeding, or for patients suffering from severe kidney or liver disease, LUPUS, history of intestinal disorder, lung fibrosis, some forms of dermatitis, bone marrow disorders, or a history of blood disorders.

Aureocort *see* topical corticosteroid ointment
(Wyeth Laboratories)

Aureomycin *see* chlortetracycline ointment/eye ointment
(Wyeth Laboratories)

Autoclix Finger Pricking Device *see* Baylet Lancets, Cleanlet Fine Lancets, FinePoint Lancets, Milward Steri-Let/Steri-Let Ultra-Fine Lancets, Monolet Lancets, Unilet G SuperLite Lancets, Vitrex Soft Lancets
(Roche Diagnostics)

Availability: private prescription, over the counter.

Autolet Finger Pricking Devices *see* Ames Lancets, Baylet Lancets, Cleanlet Fine Lancets, FinePoint Lancets, B-D MicroFine+ Lancets, Milward Steri-Let/Steri-Let Ultra-Fine Lancets, Monolet Lancets, Unilet SuperLite Lancets, Unilet G SuperLite Lancets, Unilet GP Lancets, Unilet Universal ComforTouch Lancets, Vitrex Soft Lancets
(Owen Mumford)

Availability: private prescription, over the counter.

Autopen *see* insulin injection devices
(Owen Mumford)

Avandia *see* rosiglitazone tablets
(SmithKline Beecham Pharmaceuticals)

Avaxim *see* hepatitis A vaccine
(Aventis Pasteur MSD)

Aveeno *see* emollient bar/bath oil/cream/sachets
(Bioglan Laboratories)

Avloclor *see* chloroquine tablets
(Zeneca Pharma)

Avoca *see* silver nitrate stick
(Bray Health and Leisure (Solport)).

Avomine *see* promethazine teoclate tablets
(Manx Pharma)

Axid *see* nizatidine capsules
(Eli Lilly and Co)

Axsain *see* capsaicin cream
(Elan Pharma)

---

azapropazone capsules/tablets

A capsule or tablet used as a NON-STEROIDAL ANTI-INFLAMMATORY DRUG to treat rheumatoid arthritis, ankylosing spondylitis, and acute gout where other treatments have failed.

Strengths available: 300 mg capsules, 600 mg tablets.

Dose: 1200 mg a day in 2 or 4 divided doses (elderly 300 mg twice a day). In acute gout, initially up to 1800 mg a day reducing to 1200 mg when symptoms subside.

sensitivity to sunlight, fluid retention, stomach upset or bleeding, inflammation of the lungs or breathing difficulty, blood disorders, kidney or liver disorders, dizziness, headache, tiredness, severe allergy, hearing disturbances.

cont.

Doses are reduced in patients with kidney disorders.

Availability: NHS and private prescription.
Contains: azapropazone.
Brand names: Rheumox.

 in elderly or ill patients,and in those suffering from high blood pressure, heart failure, kidney disorders, asthma, allergy to non-steroidal anti-inflammatory drugs. Patients on long-term treatment should receive regular check-ups. Use sunblock or avoid exposure to strong sunlight.

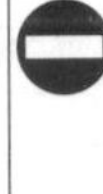 children, pregnant women, mothers who are breastfeeding, or for patients with a history of stomach ulcer, inflamed bowel, blood changes or severe kidney disorders, liver disease, porphyria. Not used to treat gout in the elderly or patients with kidney disorders.

 phenytoin, ANTICOAGULANTS, antidiabetics, digoxin, some ANTIBIOTICS, lithium, digoxin, methotrexate, cyclosporin, ACE-INHIBITORS, ACE-II ANTAGONISTS, other non-steroidal anti-inflammatory drugs, zidovudine, DIURETICS, tacrolimus.

azatadine syrup

A syrup used as an ANTIHISTAMINE and hormone blocker to treat allergic reactions such as bites and stings, itch, hayfever.

Strengths available: 0.5 mg/5 ml syrup.
Dose: adults 1-2 mg (children over 1 year 0.25-1 mg according to age) twice a day.
Availability: NHS and private prescription.
Contains: azatadine maleate.
Brand names: Optimine.

 drowsiness, reduced reactions, increased or reduced appetite, nausea, headache, ANTIMUSCARINIC effects, weakness, nervousness.

 in patients suffering from enlarged prostate, difficulty passing urine, glaucoma, stomach ulcer causing blockage, or stomach obstruction.

 sedatives, alcohol, antidepressants.

 infants under 1 year, pregnant women, or mothers who are breastfeeding.

azathioprine tablets

A tablet used to suppress the rejection of newly transplanted organs by the body's immune system. Also used to treat MYASTHENIA GRAVIS, inflamed bowel, and rheumatoid arthritis.

Strengths available: 25 mg and 50 mg tablets.
Dose: up to 5 mg per kilogram of body weight at first but generally 1-4 mg/ kg a day in divided doses according to condition.
Availability: NHS and private prescription.
Contains: azathioprine.
Brand names: Immunoprin, Imuran, Oprisine.

 general weakness, rash, dizziness, stomach upset, fever, joint and muscle pain, liver or kidney damage, heart rhythm disturbance, low blood pressure, bone marrow effects such as bruising or bleeding (must be reported to the doctor immediately), hair loss, infections. Rarely, inflammation of pancreas or lungs.

 in the elderly, pregnant women, and in patients suffering from liver or kidney disorder, infection, or where there is excessive exposure to the sun. You must have regular check-ups and blood tests.

 patients with allergy to this drug or mercaptopurine.

 allopurinol, rifampicin, warfarin, co-trimoxazole, trimethoprim, CORTICOSTEROIDS.

azelaic acid cream

A cream used to treat acne.

Strengths available: 20% cream.
Dose: apply once or twice a day and rub in. Use only once a day for the first week on sensitive skin. Continue for up to 6 months. Maximum of 10 g a day.
Availability: NHS and private prescription.
Contains: azelaic acid.
Brand names: Skinoren.

 irritation. Rarely, sensitivity to light.

 in pregnant women and mothers who are breastfeeding. Avoid the eyes.

azelastine eye drops

Eye drops used as an ANTIHISTAMINE to treat and prevent symptoms of seasonal allergic conjunctivitis.

Strengths available: 0.05% drops.
Dose: adults and children over 4 years, 1 drop in each eye 2-4 times a day.
Availability: NHS and private prescription.
Contains: azelastine hydrochloride.
Brand names: Optilast.

 irritation of the eye, disturbance of taste.

 children under 4 years or for patients wearing contact lenses.

azelastine nasal spray

A nasal spray used as an ANTIHISTAMINE to treat hayfever and rhinitis.

Strengths available: 0.1% spray.
Dose: adults and children over 5 years 1 spray in each nostril twice a day.
Availability: NHS and private prescription. Also available over the counter to treat hayfever in adults and children over 12 years.
Contains: azelastine hydrochloride.
Brand names: Rhinolast, Rhinolast Hayfever (available over the counter).

 nasal irritation, disturbance of taste.

 in pregnant women and mothers who are breastfeeding.

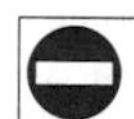 children under 5 years.

B

azithromycin capsules/tablets/suspension

A tablet, capsule, or suspension used as an ANTIBIOTIC to treat respiratory, soft tissue, skin, ear, and genital infections.

Strengths available: 250 mg capsules, 500 mg tablets, 200 mg/5 ml suspension.
Dose: adults 500 mg once a day for 3 days. For genital infections, 1000 mg as a single dose. Children up to 10 ml suspension once a day, according to age and weight. The dose should be taken with food.
Availability: NHS and private prescription.
Contains: azithromycin dihydrate.
Brand names: Zithromax.

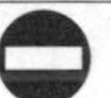 patients with any liver disorder.

 stomach upset, liver changes, rash, fluid retention, shock, loss of appetite, severe allergic reaction, dizziness, vertigo, fits, headache, drowsiness, kidney disorders, altered heart rhythm, weakness, pins and needles. Rarely, blood changes, taste disturbance, hearing disorders, severe skin disorder.

 in pregnant women, mothers who are breastfeeding, and in patients with kidney or liver damage, PORPHYRIA, or who have heart rhythm abnormalities.

 drugs altering heart rhythm, rifabutin, ANTICOAGULANTS, reboxetine, digoxin, cyclosporin, ergotamine, ANTACIDS, alcohol, sedatives.

Azopt *see* brinzolamide eye drops
(Alcon)

Babyhaler

(GlaxoWellcome UK)
A spacer device with mask used with Becotide-50 and Ventolin inhalers for children and infants.

Availability: private prescription, over the counter.

---

bacitracin *see* Cicatrin, Polyfax

---

baclofen tablets/liquid

A tablet or liquid used as a muscle relaxant to treat voluntary muscle spasticity caused by stroke, cerebral palsy, meningitis, multiple sclerosis, spinal cord damage.

Strengths available: 10 mg tablets; 5 mg/5 ml liquid.
Dose: adults 5 mg three times a day after food at first, increasing gradually to a maximum of 100 mg a day if needed. Children, up

 upset stomach, sedation, drowsiness, confusion, dizziness, muscle tiredness, reduced alertness, low blood pressure, disorders of heart, lungs, or circulation, sleeplessness, headache, fits, pins and needles, shaking, muscle pain or weakness, problems with urination. Rarely, visual disturbance, rash, taste disturbance, sweating or liver disorder, change in blood sugar level.

to 60 mg a day, according to weight, as advised by doctor.
Availability: NHS and private prescription.
Contains: baclofen.
Brand names: Baclospas, Balgifen, Lioresal.

 alcohol, procainamide, quinidine, sedatives, NON-STEROIDAL ANTI-INFLAMMATORY DRUGS, treatments for Parkinson's disease, fentanyl.

 in the elderly, pregnant women, mothers who are breastfeeding, and in patients suffering from epilepsy, stroke, liver or kidney disorder, diabetes, mental disorders, breathing problems, difficulty passing water, or with a history of stomach ulcer. Withdraw treatment gradually.

 patients with a current stomach ulcer.

Baclospas *see* baclofen tablets
(Ashbourne Pharmaceuticals)

Bactigras *see* chlorhexidine dressings
(Smith and Nephew Healthcare)

Bactroban *see* mupirocin cream/ointment/nasal ointment
(SmithKline Beecham Pharmaceuticals)

Balgifen *see* baclofen tablets
(Berk Pharmaceuticals)

Balmosa *see* analgesic (topical)
(Pharmax)

Balneum *see* emollient bath oil
(Crookes Healthcare)

Balneum Plus *see* emollient bath oil
(Crookes Healthcare)

---

balsalazide capsules

A capsule used to treat (and maintain remission of) ulcerative colitis (an inflammatory bowel disorder).

Strengths available: 750 mg capsules.
Dose: 3 capsules three times a day with food to treat symptoms (for maximum of 12 weeks); 2 capsules twice a day (maximum 8 a day) to maintain remission.
Availability: NHS and private prescription.

cont.

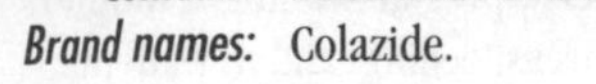

Contains: balsalazide sodium.
Brand names: Colazide.

stomach upset, headache, abdominal pain, gallstones, allergic reactions, worsening of colitis, rash, lupus-like symptoms, kidney disorders. Rarely, blood disorders, inflamed pancreas, blood disorders, liver disorders.

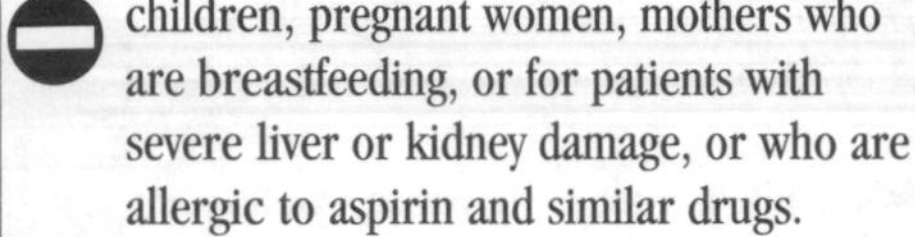
children, pregnant women, mothers who are breastfeeding, or for patients with severe liver or kidney damage, or who are allergic to aspirin and similar drugs.

in patients suffering from bleeding disorders, stomach ulcer, kidney or liver disorders, or asthma. Your doctor may advise regular blood and urine tests. Report any unexplained bruising, bleeding, fever, tiredness, or sore throat to your doctor.

digoxin, methotrexate.

Bambec *see* bambuterol tablets
(AstraZeneca UK)

---

bambuterol tablets

A tablet used as a BRONCHODILATOR to treat reversible airways disease and asthma.

Strengths available: 10 mg and 20 mg tablets.
Dose: 10-20 mg once a day at bedtime.
Availability: NHS and private prescription.
Contains: bambuterol hydrochloride.
Brand names: Bambec.

low potassium levels, shaking hands, headache, widening of blood vessels, cramps, altered heart rhythm, nervousness, severe allergic reaction.

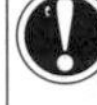
in mothers who are breastfeeding and in patients suffering from kidney damage, weak heart, irregular heart rhythm, high blood pressure, overactive thyroid, diabetes. In severe asthmatics blood potassium levels should be checked regularly.

children, pregnant women, or for patients suffering from severe liver failure.

BETA-BLOCKERS, theophylline, aminophylline, SYMPATHOMIMETICS.

Baratol *see* indoramin tablets
(Shire Pharmaceuticals)

---

barbiturate

A sedative drug used to treat the most severe cases of sleeplessness and epilepsy. Examples, amylobarbitone and phenobarbital.

Baxan *see* cefadroxil capsules/suspension
(Bristol-Myers Squibb Pharmaceuticals)

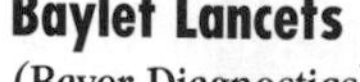

Baylet Lancets

(Bayer Diagnostics)

Diabetics who need to test their blood regularly can use lancets to pierce the skin, either with or without the use of a finger-pricking device.

Lancet width and length: 25G/0.5 mm (Type A).
Availability: NHS and private prescription, over the counter.
Compatible finger-pricking devices: Autoclix, Autolet Mini, B-D Lancer 5, Glucolet, Hypolance, Microlet, Penlet II Plus, Soft Touch. (Autolet Lite and Autolet Lite Clinisafe also compatible, but not recommended by manufacturers.)

BCG *see* tuberculosis vaccine

B-D Lancer 5 Finger Pricking Device *see* Cleanlet Fine lancets, Baylet lancets, B-D Microfine+ lancets, Vitrex Soft lancets

(BD U.K.)

Availability: private prescription, over the counter.

B-D Micro-Fine+ Needles *see* insulin injection devices

(BD U.K.)

B-D Micro-Fine+ Lancets

(BD U.K.)

Diabetics who need to test their blood regularly can use lancets to pierce the skin, either with or without the use of a finger-pricking device.

Lancet width and length: 30G/0.3 mm (Type A).
Availability: NHS and private prescription, over the counter.
Compatible finger-pricking devices: Autolet Mini, B-D Lancer 5, Glucolet, Hypolance, Microlet, Penlet II Plus, Soft Touch.

B-D Safe Clip *see* insulin injection devices

(BD U.K.)

B-D Ultra *see* insulin injection devices

(BD U.K.)

B

becaplermin gel
A gel used to treat skin ulcers in diabetic patients.

Strengths available: 0.01% gel.
Dose: clean the ulcer and apply the gel once a day, and then cover it with a gauze dressing moistened with saline. Continue treatment until ulcer heals (or maximum of 20 weeks, with check-up at 10 weeks).
Availability: NHS and private prescription.
Contains: becaplermin.
Brand names: Regranex.

 infection, ulceration, red rash, fluid retention, pain.

 in patients with infected ulcers, inflammation of the bone or bone marrow, nearby blood vessel disease, or a history of skin cancer.

 pregnant women, mothers who are breast-feeding, or patients with skin cancer near the ulcer.

 other preparations applied to the skin.

Beclazone inhaler/Easi-breathe *see* beclomethasone inhaler
(Baker Norton Pharmaceuticals/Norton Healthcare)

Beclo-Aqua *see* corticosteroid nasal spray
(Galen)

Becloforte *see* beclomethasone inhaler
(Allen and Hanburys)

---

beclometasone *see* beclomethasone (alternative name)

---

beclomethasone nasal spray *see* corticosteroid nasal spray

---

beclomethasone *see* beclomethasone inhaler, corticosteroid nasal spray, topical corticosteroid cream/ointment

---

beclomethasone inhaler
An aerosol (or other inhalation device) used as a CORTICOSTEROID to prevent asthma.

Strengths available: 50 mcg, 100 mcg, 200 mcg, and 250 mcg per dose. Other strengths available in alternative devices, *see* below.
Dose: adults 400-800 mcg daily; children 100-400 mcg daily. (Adult dose may be increased to 2000 mcg daily in severe cases.) Total daily intake usually divided into 2-4 equal

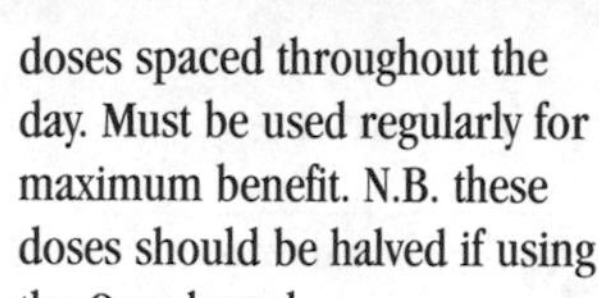

doses spaced throughout the day. Must be used regularly for maximum benefit. N.B. these doses should be halved if using the Qvar brand.

Availability: NHS and private prescription.

Contains: beclomethasone dipropionate.

Brand names: Beclazone, Becloforte, Becotide, Filair, Qvar.

Compound preparations: Ventide.

Other devices: Aerobec and Beclazone Easi-breathe (breath-activated inhaler device), Asmabec Clickhaler (dry powder inhaler), Asmabec Spacehaler (lower velocity device), Becodisks (disks of powder for inhalation), Becotide Rotacaps (capsules of powder for inhalation); Becloforte Integra (with spacer device).

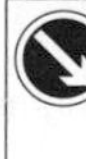 hoarseness, thrush in the mouth and throat, difficulty breathing. High doses may give rise to general corticosteroid side effects (*see* prednisolone tablets) or glaucoma. Rarely, rash or severe allergic reaction.

 in pregnant women, patients transferring from corticosteroids taken by mouth, and those suffering from tuberculosis of the lung or undergoing stressful events (such as infection or surgery).

 250 mcg strength products not recommended for children.

 with high doses, ANTICOAGULANTS.

Beclomist *see* corticosteroid nasal spray
(Co-Pharma)

Becodisk *see* beclomethasone inhaler
(Allen and Hanburys)

Beconase *see* corticosteroid nasal spray
(Allen and Hanburys)

Becotide *see* beclomethasone inhaler
(Allen and Hanburys)

Bedranol SR *see* propranolol modified-release capsules
(Lagap Pharmaceuticals)

Begrivac *see* influenza vaccine
(Wyeth Laboratories)

---

bendrofluazide tablets

A tablet used as a DIURETIC to treat fluid retention and high blood pressure.

B

Strengths available: 5 mg and 10 mg tablets.
Dose: fluid retention, 5-10 mg a day or every other day; high blood pressure, usually 2.5 mg each morning.
Availability: NHS and private prescription.
Contains: bendrofluazide (bendroflumethiazide).
Brand names: Aprinox, Neo-Bendramax, Neo-Naclex.
Compound preparations: Corgaretic, Inderetic, Inderex, Neo-Naclex K, Prestim, Tenben.

low blood pressure on standing, mild stomach upset, reversible impotence, inflamed pancreas, gout, liver disorders, low potassium levels and other blood changes, allergy, rash, sensitivity to light, or tiredness.

in pregnant women, mothers who are breastfeeding, the elderly, and in patients suffering from liver or kidney disorders, diabetes, gout, lupus.

patients suffering from severe kidney or liver disorders, Addison's disease, raised blood calcium/uric acid levels, low blood potassium/sodium levels, or PORPHYRIA.

NON-STEROIDAL ANTI-INFLAMMATORY DRUGS, antidiabetics, drugs which alter heart rhythm, carbamazepine, halofantrine, pimozide, digoxin, lithium, ANTIHYPERTENSIVES.

---

bendroflumethiazide *see* bendrofluazide (alternative name)

Benerva *see* thiamine tablets
(Roche Consumer Health)

Benoral *see* benorylate tablets/suspension
(Sanofi Winthrop)

---

benorilate *see* benorylate (alternative name)

---

benorylate tablets/suspension/sachets

A tablet or suspension used as an ANALGESIC for relief of pain and inflammation, fever, and arthritis.

Strengths available: 750 mg tablets; 4 g/10 ml suspension; 2 g sachets.
Dose: for mild to moderate pain 2 g twice a day; for rheumatic disease up to 8 g a day in divided doses (reduced doses for the

stomach upset, asthma, allergy. Rarely, blood disorders, inflamed pancreas, abnormal bleeding, hearing disorders, vertigo, confusion, severe allergy, fluid retention, and heart inflammation.

elderly).

Availability: NHS and private prescription, over the counter.
Contains: benorylate.
Brand names: Benoral.

aspirin, paracetamol, NON-STEROIDAL ANTI-INFLAMMATORY DRUGS, ANTICOAGULANTS, methotrexate.

in the elderly, pregnant women, and in patients suffering from impaired kidney or liver function, alcohol dependence, indigestion, dehydration, or uncontrolled high blood pressure.

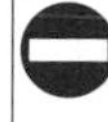
children under 12 years, mothers who are breastfeeding, or for patients suffering from blood clotting disorders or stomach ulcers, or those with a history of allergy to aspirin or suffering from asthma.

---

benperidol tablets

A tablet used as a sedative to control unacceptable sexual behaviour.

Strengths available: 0.25 mg tablets.
Dose: 1-6 tablets a day in divided doses. (Elderly use half dose initially.)
Availability: NHS and private prescription.
Contains: benperidol.
Brand names: Anquil.

in pregnant women, mothers who are breastfeeding, and in patients with heart or blood vessel disorders, infections, breathing disorders, Parkinson's disease, epilepsy, infection, kidney or liver disorders, underactive thyroid, MYASTHENIA GRAVIS, glaucoma, prostate disorders, some blood disorders, and in elderly patients.

alcohol, sedating drugs, anaesthetics, drugs that affect the heart rhythm, halofantrine, TRICYCLIC ANTIDEPRESSANTS, ritonavir.

muscle spasms, restlessness, shaking hands, changes in sexual function, dry mouth, urine retention, blurred vision, heart rhythm disturbance, low blood pressure, weight change, low body temperature, breast swelling, menstrual changes, nasal congestion, nightmares, insomnia, depression, agitation, liver disorders, blood and skin changes, eye disorders, stomach upset, drowsiness, constipation, sensitivity to light. Rarely, fits or NEUROLEPTIC MALIGNANT SYNDROME (a condition of high body temperature, varying level of consciousness, unstable blood pressure, incontinence, and rigid muscles).

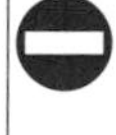
children, unconscious patients, or for patients with Parkinson's disease (or similar movement disorders), PHAEOCHROMOCYTOMA, depression, or allergy to similar drugs.

---

benserazide *see* co-beneldopa capsules

---

benzalkonium chloride *see* Conotrane, Drapolene, emollient preparations, Ionil T, Timodine

---

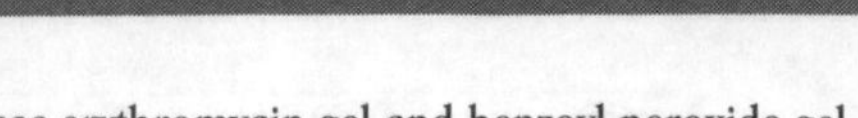

Benzamycin *see* erythromycin gel and benzoyl peroxide gel
(Bioglan Laboratories)

benzatropine *see* benztropine (alternative name)

benzhexol tablets/syrup

A tablet or syrup used as an ANTIMUSCARINIC treatment for Parkinson's disease, and similar symptoms caused by medication.

Strengths available: 2 mg and 5 mg tablets; 5 mg/5 ml syrup.
Dose: 1 mg each day, increasing gradually to 5-15 mg a day, in 3-4 divided doses.
Availability: NHS and private prescription.
Contains: benzhexol (trihexyphenidyl hydrochloride).
Brand names: Agitane, Broflex.

 other antimuscarinic or sedating drugs.

 antimuscarinic effects, confusion, agitation, rash with high doses, rapid heart rate.

 in the elderly, pregnant women, mothers who are breastfeeding, and in patients suffering from heart or blood vessel disease, liver or kidney disorders, or prostate disorder.

 children or for patients suffering from untreated urine retention, glaucoma, or intestinal blockage.

benzocaine *see* analgesic (topical)

benzoic acid *see* Aserbine, benzoic acid compound ointment BP

benzoic acid compound ointment BP

An ointment used as an antifungal preparation to treat infections such as ringworm.

Dose: apply twice a day.
Availability: NHS and private prescription, over the counter.
Contains: benzoic acid, salicylic acid, emulsifying ointment.

benzoin tincture *see* Metanium

benzoyl peroxide cream/gel

A cream or gel used as an antibacterial and skin softener to treat acne.

Strengths available: 2.5%, 5%, and 10% preparations.
Dose: usually apply once or twice a day starting with the weakest strength preparation and

gradually increasing strength if necessary.
Availability: NHS and private prescription, over the counter.
Contains: benzoyl peroxide.
Brand names: Acnecide, Brevoxyl, Panoxyl.
Compound preparations: Benzamycin, Quinoped, Quinoderm (with potassium hydroxyquinoline sulphate).

irritation, redness, peeling.

keep out of the eyes, nose, and mouth; may bleach fabrics and hair on contact; avoid excessive exposure to sunlight after treatment.

---

benzthiazide *see* Dytide

---

benztropine tablets

A tablet used as an ANTIMUSCARINIC treatment for Parkinson's disease, and similar symptoms caused by medication.

Strengths available: 2 mg tablets.
Dose: adults, initially 0.5 mg (¼ tablet) a day, increasing gradually to maximum of 6 mg a day (usually 1-4 mg a day); children 3-12 years, as advised by doctor.
Availability: NHS and private prescription.
Contains: benztropine maleate.
Brand names: Cogentin.

other antimuscarinic or sedating drugs.

antimuscarinic effects, confusion, sedation, agitation, rash with high doses.

in children, the elderly, pregnant women, mothers who are breastfeeding, and in patients suffering from heart or blood vessel disease, liver or kidney disorders.

children under 3 years or for patients suffering from untreated urine retention, glaucoma, or intestinal blockage.

---

benzydamine cream *see* non-steroidal anti-inflammatory drug (topical)

---

benzydamine mouthwash/spray

A solution used as a NON-STEROIDAL ANTI-INFLAMMATORY DRUG to treat pain and inflammation in the mouth and throat.

occasionally, numbness or stinging.

Strengths available: 0.15% solution.
Dose: rinse or gargle with 15 ml mouthwash (or use 4-8 puffs of spray) every 90 minutes-3 hours for up to one week. (Children aged 6-12 years use 4 puffs of spray; children aged under 6 years use 1 puff of spray.)
Availability: NHS and private prescription, over the counter.
Contains: benzydamine hydrochloride.
Brand names: Difflam.

---

benzyl alcohol *see* Sudocrem

benzyl benzoate *see* benzyl benzoate application BP, rectal corticosteroid preparations, Sudocrem

benzyl benzoate application BP

An emulsion used as an insect-destroying drug to treat scabies.

Strengths available: 25% emulsion.

Dose: apply the emulsion to the whole body, repeat treatment next day without bathing, then wash off 24 hours later. (A third application may occasionally be required.) The head and neck are sometimes excluded from treatment – follow your doctor's instructions carefully.

Availability: NHS and private prescription, over the counter.

Contains: benzyl benzoate.

Brand names: Ascabiol.

irritation, burning. Rarely, rash.

in pregnant women and mothers who are breastfeeding. Keep out of the eyes and avoid mucous membranes.

children or for application to broken or infected areas of skin.

benzyl cinnamate *see* Sudocrem

Beta-Adalat *see* atenolol tablets and nifedipine modified-release tablets
(Bayer Pharma Business Group)

Dose: 1 capsule once or twice a day.

beta-blocker (ß-blocker)

A drug that blocks some of the effects of ADRENALINE in the body. Beta-blockers are used to treat angina, high blood pressure, and other conditions. Example, atenolol tablets.

Beta-Cardone *see* sotalol tablets
(Medeva Pharma)

Beta-Prograne *see* propranolol modified-release capsules
(Tillomed Laboratories)

Betacap *see* topical corticosteroid scalp application
(Dermal Laboratories)

Betadine *see* povidone-iodine solution/paint/cream/gargle/mouthwash/ointment/spray/shampoo/skin cleanser/vaginal gel/pessaries/vaginal cleansing kit
(SSL International)

Betagan *see* levobunolol eye drops
(Allergan)

---

betahistine tablets

A tablet used as a histamine-type drug to treat vertigo, tinnitus (noise in the ears), and hearing loss caused by Ménière's disease.

Strengths available: 8 mg and 16 mg tablets.
Dose: 16 mg three times a day at first, then 24-48 mg a day in divided doses.
Availability: NHS and private prescription.
Contains: betahistine dihydrochloride.
Brand names: Serc.

stomach upset, rash, headache, itching.

in pregnant women, mothers who are breast-feeding, and in patients suffering from asthma or with a history of stomach ulcers.

children or for patients suffering from PHAEOCHROMOCYTOMA.

---

betaine hydrochloride *see* Kloref

Betaloc/Betaloc SA *see* metoprolol tablets/modified-release tablets
(AstraZeneca UK)

---

betamethasone *see* betamethasone eye drops/eye ointment/tablets, corticosteroid nasal drops, rectal corticosteroid, topical corticosteroid cream/ointment/lotion/mousse/scalp application

---

betamethasone drops/ointment *see also* corticosteroid nasal drops

Drops used as a CORTICOSTEROID to treat inflammation of the ear, nasal passages, or eyes where infection is not present. The ointment is used as an alternative (or in addition) to drops in the eye.

Strengths available: 0.1% drops; 0.1% ointment.
Dose: 2-3 drops into each nostril or ear every 2-3 hours, or 1-2 drops into the affected eye(s) every 1-2 hours. The ointment should be applied below the lower eyelid 2-4 times a day or just at night if used in addition to drops.

cont.

B

Availability: NHS and private prescription.
Contains: betamethasone sodium phosphate.
Brand names: Betnesol, Vista-Methasone.
Compound preparations: Betnesol-N, Vista-Methasone-N (both with neomycin, for infected conditions. Addition of neomycin carries risk of deafness. Drops are used up to six times a day in the eye, four times a day in the ear, or three times a day in the nose. Do not use in the ear if the eardrum is perforated).

irritation, burning. General corticosteroid effects with prolonged use, *see* prednisolone tablets. In the eye: thinning of the cornea, cataract, rise in eye pressure. In the nose: *see* corticosteroid nasal drops.

in pregnant women, mothers who are breastfeeding, and in patients recovering from nasal surgery (if used in the nose); do not use for longer than necessary, especially in pregnancy.

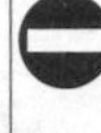
patients suffering from infected conditions. Do not use in the eye to treat patients with glaucoma or where soft contact lenses are worn.

---

betamethasone scalp application *see* topical corticosteroid

---

betamethasone tablets/dispersible tablets

A tablet used as a CORTICOSTEROID to suppress inflammation and allergies. It is useful in conditions such as asthma, rheumatoid arthritis, and fluid retention in the brain.

Strengths available: 0.5 mg tablets; 0.5 mg dispersible tablets.
Dose: adults, usually 0.5-5.0 mg each day. Children use reduced doses.
Availability: NHS and private prescription.
Contains: betamethasone or betamethasone sodium phosphate.
Brand names: Betnelan, Betnesol.

in pregnant women, mothers who are breastfeeding, and in patients who have had recent bowel surgery or who are suffering from inflamed veins, psychiatric disorders, thinning of the bones, stomach ulcers, tuberculosis or other infections, high blood pressure, glaucoma, epilepsy, diabetes, underactive thyroid, liver disease, stress. Withdraw gradually. Avoid contact with chicken pox for 3 months after treatment ends and seek medical attention if exposed.

high blood sugar, thin bones, mood changes, stomach ulcers, fluid retention, potassium loss, high blood pressure, menstrual irregularity, hairiness, increased likelihood of infection, euphoria, depression, sleeplessness, aggravation of schizophrenia and epilepsy, eye disorders, thinning of skin, acne, bruising, blood changes, stomach upset, inflamed pancreas, muscle abnormality, suppression of the ADRENAL GLANDS, ulcerated or infected oesophagus, general feeling of being unwell, hiccups, reduced growth in children.

infants under 1 year or for patients who have untreated infections.

live vaccines, some ANTIBIOTICS and anti-epileptics, ANTICOAGULANTS, antidiabetics, some antifungals, digoxin, cyclosporin.

betaxolol eye drops

Eye drops used as a BETA-BLOCKER to treat glaucoma and some other causes of high pressure in the eye. Some of the preparation may be absorbed into the body (*see* side-effects, cautions, etc. as for betaxolol tablets).

Strengths available: 0.25% (suspension – with or without preservative); 0.5% (solution).
Dose: 1 drop into the affected eye(s) twice a day.
Availability: NHS and private prescription.
Contains: betaxolol hydrochloride.
Brand names: Betoptic.

temporary discomfort or redness in the eye, dry eyes. Rarely, disorders of the cornea.

in pregnant women, mothers who are breastfeeding, and in patients with a history of breathing disorders, diabetes, overactive thyroid, or those being given a general anaesthetic.

verapamil, diltiazem, nifedipine, amiodarone.

children or for patients using soft contact lenses or suffering from some heart diseases.

---

betaxolol tablets

A tablet used as a BETA-BLOCKER to treat high blood pressure.

Strengths available: 20 mg tablets.
Dose: 20-40 mg a day. (Elderly patients 10 mg at first.)
Availability: NHS and private prescription.
Contains: betaxolol hydrochloride.
Brand names: Kerlone.

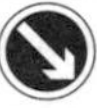
cold hands and feet, sleep disturbance, slow heart rate, tiredness, wheezing, heart failure, low blood pressure, stomach upset. Rarely, dry eyes, rash, worsening of psoriasis.

in pregnant women, mothers who are breastfeeding, the elderly, and in patients suffering from diabetes, kidney or liver disorders, MYASTHENIA GRAVIS, or with a history of allergies. May need to be withdrawn before surgery. Withdraw gradually.

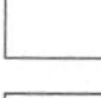
children or for patients suffering from heart block or failure, asthma, PHAEOCHROMOCYTOMA, or a history of breathing disorders.

general anaesthetics, CALCIUM-CHANNEL BLOCKERS, ALPHA-BLOCKERS, clonidine, ANTIHYPERTENSIVES, amiodarone, antidiabetics, thymoxamine, theophylline, aminophylline.

---

bethanechol tablets

A tablet used to treat urinary retention or reflux oesophagitis.

Strengths available: 10 mg and 25 mg tablets.
Dose: adults 10-25 mg 3-4 times a day, before food. Children use reduced doses as directed by the doctor.
Availability: NHS and private prescription.
Contains: bethanechol chloride.

nausea, vomiting, sweating, stomach cramps, blurred vision, slow heart rate.

cont.

B

Brand names: Myotonine.

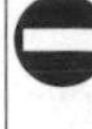
pregnant women, mothers who are breast-feeding, or for patients suffering from asthma, overactive thyroid, urinary or intestinal blockage, stomach ulcer, vagus nerve disorders, slow heart rate, recent heart attack, epilepsy, Parkinson's disease, low blood pressure.

Betim *see* timolol tablets
(Leo Pharmaceuticals)

Betnelan *see* betamethasone tablets
(Medeva Pharma)

Betnesol/Betnesol-N *see* betamethasone drops/ointment, betamethasone dispersible tablets, corticosteroid nasal drops
(Medeva Pharma)

Betnovate *see* rectal corticosteroid ointment, topical corticosteroid cream/lotion/ointment/scalp application
(GlaxoWellcome UK)

Betoptic *see* betaxolol eye drops
(Alcon)

Bettamousse *see* topical corticosteroid scalp application
(Medeva Pharma)

---

bezafibrate tablets/modified-release tablets

A tablet or M-R TABLET used as a lipid-lowering drug to treat high blood lipids (triglycerides and cholesterol).

Strengths available: 200 mg tablets; 400 mg m-r tablets.
Dose: 1 standard 200 mg tablet three times a day, or 1 m-r tablet once a day. Doses taken after food.
Availability: NHS and private prescription.
Contains: bezafibrate.
Brand names: Bezalip (standard tablets), Bezalip Mono; Liparol 400XL and Zimbacol XL (m-r tablets).

stomach upset, muscle aches, rash, itching, headache, tiredness, vertigo, dizziness, hair loss. Rarely, blood changes or impotence.

in patients with kidney disease. Your doctor may advise change of diet or lifestyle.

 children, pregnant women, mothers who are breastfeeding, or for patients suffering from severe kidney or liver disease, or gall bladder disorders.

 ANTICOAGULANTS, antidiabetic drugs, MAOIS, other drugs used to reduce cholesterol.

Bezalip/Bezalip Mono *see* bezafibrate tablets/modified-release tablets
(Roche Products)

Bi-Carzem SR *see* diltiazem modified-release capsules
(Tillomed Laboratories)

Biocare Glucose VT
(Biocare)
A reagent strip used to detect visually blood glucose levels. Blood-glucose monitoring enables individual patients suffering from diabetes accurately to control blood glucose and manage their condition.

Availability: NHS, private prescription, over the counter.

Binovum *see* oral contraceptive (combined)
(Janssen-Cilag)

Bioplex *see* carbenoxolone granules
(Provalis Healthcare)

Bioral *see* carbenoxolone gel
(Merck Consumer Health Products)

Biorphen *see* orphenadrine liquid
(Alliance Pharmaceuticals)

biotin *see* vitamin H

biperiden tablets
A tablet used as an ANTIMUSCARINIC treatment for Parkinson's disease and similar symptoms caused by medication.

Strengths available: 2 mg tablets.
Dose: initially 1 mg twice a day, increasing gradually to 3-12 mg a day (divided into three *cont.*

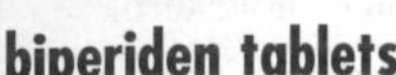

biperiden tablets

A tablet used as an ANTIMUSCARINIC treatment for Parkinson's disease and similar symptoms caused by medication.

antimuscarinic effects, confusion, drowsiness, agitation, rash with high doses.

in the elderly, pregnant women, and in patients suffering from heart or blood vessel disease, liver or kidney disorders.

children, mothers who are breastfeeding, or for patients suffering from untreated urine retention, glaucoma, or intestinal blockage.

other antimuscarinic or sedating drugs, alcohol.

Strengths available: 2 mg tablets.
Dose: initially 1 mg twice a day, increasing gradually to 3-12 mg a day (divided into three doses). Elderly patients use lower doses.
Availability: NHS and private prescription.
Contains: biperiden hydrochloride.
Brand names: Akineton.

bisacodyl tablets/suppositories

An E-C TABLET or a suppository used as a stimulant laxative to treat constipation.

abdominal cramps. Anal irritation with suppositories.

avoid prolonged use.

patients suffering from intestinal blockage.

no ANTACIDS should be taken within 1 hour of the tablets.

Strengths available: 5 mg e-c tablets; 5 mg and 10 mg suppositories.
Dose: adults, 1-2 tablets (rarely up to 4 tablets) at night, or 1 x 10 mg suppository in the morning. Children under 10 years, 1 tablet at night or 1 x 5 mg suppository in the morning.
Availability: NHS and private prescription, nurse prescription, over the counter.
Contains: bisacodyl.
Brand names: various brands available over the counter (e.g. Dulcolax) but not on NHS.

bismuth oxide *see* Anusol, rectal corticosteroid

bismuth subgallate *see* Anusol, rectal corticosteroid

bisoprolol tablets

A tablet used as a BETA-BLOCKER to treat angina, high blood pressure, and (in addition to ACE-INHIBITORS, DIURETICS, and digoxin) for heart failure.

cold hands and feet, sleep disturbance, slow heart rate, tiredness, wheezing, heart failure, low blood pressure, stomach upset. Rarely, dry eyes, rash, worsening of psoriasis.

Strengths available: 1.25 mg, 2.5 mg, 3.75 mg, 5 mg, 7.5 mg, and 10 mg tablets.

Availability: NHS and private prescription.
Contains: bisoprolol fumarate.
Brand names: Cardicor, Emcor, Monocor.
Compound preparations: Monozide.

 general anaesthetics, CALCIUM-CHANNEL BLOCKERS, ALPHA-BLOCKERS, clonidine, ANTIHYPERTENSIVES, amiodarone, antidiabetics, thymoxamine, theophylline, aminophylline.

 in pregnant women, mothers who are breastfeeding, the elderly, and in patients suffering from diabetes, kidney or liver disorders, MYASTHENIA GRAVIS, or with a history of allergies. May need to be withdrawn before surgery. Withdraw gradually.

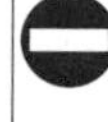 children, or for patients suffering from heart block or failure, asthma, PHAEOCHROMOCYTOMA, or a history of breathing disorders.

Blemix *see* minocycline tablets
(Ashbourne Pharmaceuticals)

BM Accutest

(Roche Diagnostics)

A plastic reagent strip used, in conjunction with Accutrend, Accutrend Alpha, and Accutrend GC meters, to detect blood glucose levels. Blood-glucose monitoring enables individual patients suffering from diabetes accurately to control blood glucose and manage their condition.

Availability: NHS and private prescription, nurse prescription, over the counter.

BM Test 1-44

(Roche Diagnostics)

A plastic reagent strip used, either visually or – more accurately – in conjunction with the Reflolux S meter, to detect blood glucose levels. Blood-glucose monitoring enables individual patients suffering from diabetes accurately to control blood glucose and manage their condition.

Availability: NHS and private prescription, nurse prescription, over the counter.

Bocasan

(Oral B Laboratories)

A sachet of granules used as a disinfectant to treat gingivitis and inflamed mouth.

Dose: dissolve 1 sachet of granules in 30 ml warm water and rinse out the mouth three times a day after meals. (Maximum of 7 days use.)
Availability: NHS and private prescription.
Contains: sodium perborate.

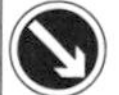 possible absorption of borate with prolonged use.

 children under 5 years or for patients suffering from kidney disease.

Bonjela *see* choline salicylate dental gel
(Reckitt Benckiser (Healthcare Division))

---

borneol *see* Rowachol, Rowatinex

---

bran *see* Trifyba

Brasivol

(Stiefel Laboratories (UK))
A paste used as an abrasive to treat acne.

Strengths available: 38.09% (no. 1 strength), and 52.2% (no. 2 strength).
Dose: wet the area then rub in vigorously for 15-20 seconds, rinse and repeat 1-3 times a day. (Start with no. 1 strength and progress, if necessary, to no. 2.)
Availability: NHS and private prescription, over the counter.
Contains: aluminium oxide.

 irritation of skin.

 avoid contact with the eyes.

 children or for patients suffering from visible superficial arteries or veins on the skin.

Brevinor *see* oral contraceptive (combined)
(Searle)

Brevoxyl *see* benzoyl peroxide cream
(Stiefel Laboratories)

Brexidol *see* piroxicam capsules
(Trinity Pharmaceuticals)

Bricanyl/Bricanyl SA *see* terbutaline inhaler/tablets/modified-release tablets/syrup
(AstraZeneca UK)

---

brimonidine eye drops

Eye drops used to treat glaucoma or other causes of high pressure in the eye.

Strengths available: 0.2% drops.
Dose: 1 drop in the affected eye(s) every 12 hours.

Availability: NHS and private prescription.
Contains: brimonidine tartrate.
Brand names: Alphagan.

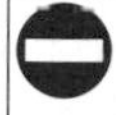 patients wearing contact lenses (leave lenses out for 15 minutes after use).

 alcohol, antidepressants, MAOIS, other sedating drugs.

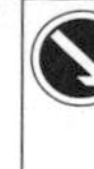 redness, stinging, inflammation, or itching in the eye, blurred vision. Rarely, swelling of the eye or lid, allergic reactions, dry mouth, headache, taste disturbance, tiredness, dizziness, drowsiness, depression, dry nose, irregular heart beat.

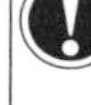 in pregnant women, mothers who are breast-feeding, and in patients with severe heart or circulation disease, Raynaud's syndrome, low blood pressure on standing, liver or kidney disease, depression.

brinzolamide eye drops

Eye drops used to treat glaucoma and high pressure inside the eye.

Strengths available: 10 mg/ml.
Dose: 1 drop 2-3 times a day. If used in conjunction with another eye preparation, administer at least 5 minutes apart.
Availability: NHS and private prescription.
Contains: brinzolamide.
Brand names: Azopt.

 children under 18 years, patients with liver disorder, patients wearing contact lenses (wait 15 minutes before inserting lenses).

 acetazolamide.

 temporary blurring of vision, discomfort in the eye, increased blood supply to the eye, alteration of taste, headache. More rarely, dry eyes, pain, inflammation, discharge, or itching of the eye, infection of the eye or lid, tired eyes, abnormal vision, chest pain, hair loss, dry mouth, upset stomach, skin inflammation or abnormal sensation, depression, dizziness, runny nose, difficulty breathing, inflammation of the chest or throat, nose bleeds, coughing up blood.

 in pregnant women, patients whose eye surfaces may be damaged (e.g. contact lens wearers), and diabetics.

Britaject *see* apomorphine injection
(Britannia Pharmaceuticals)

Britlofex *see* lofexidine tablets
(Britannia Pharmaceuticals)

Broflex *see* benzhexol syrup
(Alliance Pharmaceuticals)

bromazepam tablets

A tablet used for the short-term treatment of anxiety.

Strengths available: 1.5 mg and 3 mg tablets.
Dose: elderly 1.5-9.0 mg a day in divided doses; adults 3-18 mg a day in divided doses.
Availability: private prescription only.
Contains: bromazepam.
Brand names: Lexotan.

 drowsiness, light-headedness, confusion, vertigo, stomach disturbances, loss of memory, aggression, headache, joint immobility, salivation changes, shaking, unsteadiness, low blood pressure, rash, changes in vision, changes in sexual desire, retention of urine, incontinence, blood changes, jaundice. Risk of addiction increases with dose and length of treatment. May impair judgement.

 children or for patients suffering from acute lung diseases, some chronic lung diseases, severe liver disease, MYASTHENIA GRAVIS, some obsessional and psychotic disorders, or who have stopped breathing while asleep.

 in the elderly, pregnant women, mothers who are breastfeeding, women during labour, and in patients suffering from lung disorders, glaucoma, kidney or liver disorders, muscle weakness, PORPHYRIA, or with a history of drug or alcohol abuse. Avoid long-term use and withdraw gradually.

 alcohol, other sedating drugs, some antivirals and anti-epileptic medications.

bromocriptine capsules/tablets

A tablet or capsule used as a hormone blocker to treat Parkinson's disease, infertility, cyclical benign breast disease, and other disorders caused by raised hormone levels. Also used to dry up breast milk.

Strengths available: 1 mg and 2.5 mg tablets; 5 mg or 10 mg capsules.
Dose: 1-40 mg a day depending on condition. (Low doses used initially, gradually increasing if necessary.)
Availability: NHS and private prescription.
Contains: bromocriptine mesylate.
Brand names: Parlodel.

 low blood pressure on standing, dizziness, upset stomach, headache, drowsiness, poor circulation. With high doses, confusion, hallucinations, movement disorders, dry mouth, leg cramps, lung changes.

 in patients with a history of mental disorder, or suffering from severe heart or circulation disorder, kidney or liver damage, Raynaud's syndrome, or PORPHYRIA. Your doctor may advise regular check-ups. Women should be given regular gynaecological examinations and use adequate contraception.

 children, women with complications of pregnancy, or for patients who are allergic to ergotamine. Mothers who are breastfeeding should not breastfeed if they continue to produce milk. Should not be given to women who have recently given birth if they also have high blood pressure.

 alcohol, other sedating drugs, phenylpropanolamine (an ingredient in some cough, cold, and hayfever remedies available over the counter).

brompheniramine tablets/modified-release tablets/elixir

A tablet used as an ANTIHISTAMINE treatment for allergy symptoms such as hayfever or itchy rashes.

Strengths available: 4 mg tablets; 2 mg/5 ml elixir; 12 mg M-R TABLETS.
Dose: adults 4-8 mg (children up to 4 mg according to age) 3-4 times a day using standard tablets or elixir; using m-r tablets, adults 12-24 mg twice a day (children aged 6-12 years 12 mg at bedtime or twice a day if needed).
Availability: NHS and private prescription, over the counter.
Contains: brompheniramine maleate.
Brand names: Dimotane.
Compound preparations: various cough and cold remedies available over the counter contain brompheniramine (e.g. Dimotapp, Dimotane Co, Robitussin Night-time), Dimotane Plus.

 drowsiness, reduced reactions, dizziness, excitation, movement disorders, headache, ANTIMUSCARINIC effects. Rarely, heart rhythm disturbances, severe allergic reaction, sensitivity to sunlight, confusion, depression, fits, shaking, sweating, muscle pain, pins and needles, liver disorders, hair loss, sleep disturbances.

 in the elderly, pregnant women, mothers who are breastfeeding, and in patients with enlarged prostate, difficulty passing urine, glaucoma, epilepsy, or liver disease.

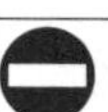 patients with severe liver disease. M-r tablets not suitable for children under 6 years.

 other sedating drugs, alcohol, antidepressants.

Bronchodil *see* reproterol inhaler
(ASTA Medica)

---

bronchodilator

A substance that enlarges the airways bringing relief in conditions such as asthma and bronchitis. Example, salbutamol tablets or inhaler.

Brufen/Brufen Retard *see* ibuprofen syrup/tablets/granules/modified-release tablets
(Knoll)

Buccastem *see* prochlorperazine buccal tablets
(Reckitt and Colman Products)

---

buclizine *see* Migraleve Pink tablets

Budenofalk *see* budesonide enteric-coated capsules
(Provalis Healthcare)

---

budesonide *see* budesonide modified-release capsules/enteric-coated capsules, budesonide inhaler, corticosteroid enema and corticosteroid nasal spray

budesonide modified-release capsules/enteric-coated capsules

A M-R or E-C CAPSULE used as a CORTICOSTEROID to treat inflammatory bowel disorders, such as Crohn's disease or ulcerative colitis.

Strengths available: 3 mg e-c or m-r capsules.
Dose: 1 e-c capsule three times a day, or 3 m-r capsules once a day (before breakfast) for up to 8 weeks. (Dose reduced for last 2 weeks of treatment.)
Availability: NHS and private prescription.
Contains: budesonide.
Brand names: Budenofalk, Entocort CR.
Other preparations: Entocort Enema *see* corticosteroid enema.

 general corticosteroid effects *see* prednisolone tablets.

 *see* prednisolone tablets.

 children or for patients with untreated infections.

 ANTACIDS, live vaccines, some ANTIBIOTICS and anti-epileptics, ANTICOAGULANTS, antidiabetics, some antifungals, digoxin.

budesonide inhaler

An aerosol (or other inhalation device) used as a CORTICOSTEROID to prevent asthma. (Nebulizer solution also used to treat croup.)

Strengths available: 50 mcg or 200 mcg per dose. Other strengths available in alternative devices, *see* below.
Dose: adults usually 200 mcg twice a day (maximum 1600 mcg daily). Children under 12 years, usually 50-400 mcg twice a day. Nebulizer solution dose is usually 1-2 mg twice a day for adults, or 0.5-1 mg for children) twice a day, with half doses for maintenance. Must be used regularly for maximum benefit in asthma. Croup is treated with a single 2 mg dose of nebulizer solution (or 2 doses of 1 mg, 30 minutes apart).
Availability: NHS and private prescription.
Contains: budesonide.
Brand names: Pulmicort (200 mcg aerosol), Pulmicort LS (50 mcg aerosol).
Other devices: Pulmicort Respules (nebulizer solution), Pulmicort Turbohaler (a dry-powder inhalation device).

 hoarseness, thrush in the mouth and throat, difficulty breathing. High doses may give rise to general corticosteroid side effects (*see* prednisolone tablets) or glaucoma. Rarely, rash or severe allergic reaction.

 in pregnant women, patients transferring from corticosteroids taken by mouth, and in patients undergoing stressful events (such as infection or surgery).

patients suffering from tuberculosis of the lung. (Nebulizer solution not recommended for asthma in children under 3 months.)

(high doses) ANTICOAGULANTS.

budesonide nasal spray *see* corticosteroid nasal spray

bumetanide tablets/liquid

A tablet used as a DIURETIC to treat fluid retention associated with congestive heart failure, liver and kidney disease, including nephrotic syndrome.

Strengths available: 1 mg and 5 mg tablets; 1 mg/5 ml liquid.
Dose: usually 1 mg in the morning, increased or repeated during the day if necessary in more severe cases.
Availability: NHS and private prescription.
Contains: bumetanide.
Brand names: Burinex.
Compound preparations: Burinex A, Burinex K.

low blood potassium, magnesium, or sodium, stomach upset, rash, cramps, blood changes, breast enlargement, gout, high blood sugar, muscle pain. Rarely, sensitivity to light.

in pregnant women, mothers who are breastfeeding, and in patients suffering from kidney or liver damage, diabetes, gout, enlarged prostate, or impaired urination.

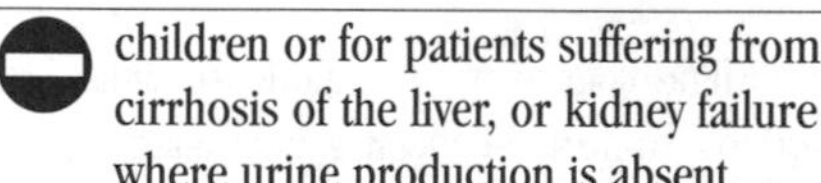
children or for patients suffering from cirrhosis of the liver, or kidney failure where urine production is absent.

ANTIHYPERTENSIVES, NON-STEROIDAL ANTI-INFLAMMATORY DRUGS, drugs affecting heart rhythm, some ANTIBIOTICS, antidiabetics, halofantrine, pimozide, digoxin, lithium.

buprenorphine sublingual tablets

A sublingual tablet used as an OPIOID to control pain and to treat addiction to other opioid drugs.

Strengths available: 0.2 mg, 0.4 mg, 2 mg, and 8 mg sublingual tablets.
Dose: to relieve pain, 0.2 mg-0.4 mg every 6-8 hours as needed (children use reduced doses). To treat opioid addiction, initially 0.8-4 mg once a day increasing to 32 mg if necessary and reducing gradually until withdrawn. The tablets are dissolved under the tongue.
Availability: controlled drug; NHS and private prescription.
Contains: buprenorphine hydrochloride.
Brand names: Subutex (treating addiction), Temgesic (pain control).

drowsiness, upset stomach, sweating, dizziness, breathing difficulty, low blood pressure, difficulty passing urine, dry mouth, headache, vertigo, flushing, change in heart rhythm, mood changes, rash, itching, addiction, reduced sexual desire.

in pregnant women, women in labour, mothers who are breastfeeding, elderly or weakened patients, and in those suffering from breathing, kidney, or liver problems, low blood pressure, underactive thyroid, enlarged prostate, or epilepsy. (Higher doses not suitable for some of these categories.)

MAOIS, alcohol, sedating drugs, ritonavir.

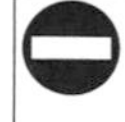
children under 6 months (for pain) or 16 years (for treating addiction), alcoholics, or for patients with head injury, reduced breathing ability, or at risk of non-functioning intestines.

B

bupropion tablets

A tablet used (in conjunction with motivational support) as an aid to stopping smoking in patients addicted to nicotine.

Strengths available: 150 mg tablets.
Dose: 150 mg once a day for 6 days, then 150 mg twice a day (with at least 8 hours between doses). Treatment continued for 7-9 weeks.
Availability: NHS and private prescription.
Contains: bupropion hydrochloride.
Brand names: Zyban.

stomach upset, shaking, sweating, agitation, taste disorders, headache, dizziness, depression, anxiety, disturbed concentration, fits, severe allergic reaction, muscle or joint pain, fever, rash, sleeplessness, dry mouth, change in heart rate, increased blood pressure, flushing, chest pain, weakness, confusion, loss of appetite, noises in the ears, visual disturbance, fainting, low blood pressure on standing.

children under 18 years, pregnant women, mothers who are breastfeeding, or for patients with a history of epilepsy, eating disorders, severe liver disease, or some psychiatric disorders, or tumours.

in the elderly and in patients with a history of head injury, alcohol abuse, nervous system tumours, diabetes, liver or kidney disorders, or in patients who have recently stopped taking drugs such as diazepam.

MAOIS, nicotine-replacement therapy, theophylline, aminophylline, CORTICOSTEROIDS, antidepressants, antidiabetic drugs (including insulin), tranquillizers, levodopa, some anti-epileptics, antimalarials, stimulants, appetite suppressants, BETA BLOCKERS, captopril, cimetidine, orphenadrine, OPIOID ANALGESICS, some ANTIBIOTICS and ANTIHISTAMINES.

Burinex *see* bumetanide tablets
(Leo Pharmaceuticals)

Burinex A *see* bumetanide tablets and amiloride tablets.
(Leo Pharmaceuticals)

Strengths available: 1 mg + 5 mg tablets
Dose: 1-2 tablets a day.

Burinex K *see* bumetanide tablets and potassium chloride tablets
(Leo Pharmaceuticals)

Strengths available: 500 mcg + 573 mg tablets.
Dose: 1-4 tablets a day.

Buscopan *see* hyoscine butylbromide tablets
(Boehringer Ingelheim)

---

buserelin injection/nasal spray

A nasal spray or injection used to treat endometriosis and infertility.

Strengths available: 150 mcg or 100 mcg per dose nasal spray; 1 mg/ml injection.
Dose: for endometriosis, 1 application of nasal spray in each nostril three times a day for up to 6 months, starting on first or second day of cycle. (For other conditions as advised by doctor.)
Availability: NHS and private prescription.
Contains: buserelin acetate.
Brand names: Suprecur, Suprefact.

hot flushes, vaginal dryness, stomach upset, vaginal bleeding, anxiety, sleeplessness, lack of concentration, loss of sexual desire, emotional upset, headache, breast tenderness, alteration of breast size, ovarian cyst, abdominal pain, thirst, appetite changes, blood and liver changes, hearing disorders, palpitations, worsening of high blood pressure, dry skin and eyes, acne, back and limb pain, muscle or joint discomfort and pain, nasal irritation. Long-term use may increase risk of brain tumour.

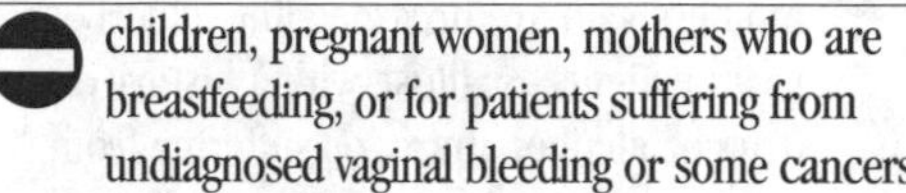
children, pregnant women, mothers who are breastfeeding, or for patients suffering from undiagnosed vaginal bleeding or some cancers.

in patients who may later develop thinning of the bones, and in depressed patients. A non-hormonal method of contraception must be used throughout treatment.

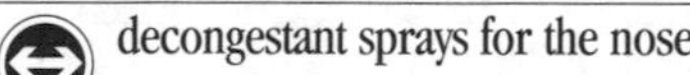
decongestant sprays for the nose.

Buspar *see* buspirone tablets
(Bristol-Myers Squibb Pharmaceuticals)

buspirone tablets

A tablet used for the short-term treatment of anxiety.

Strengths available: 5 mg and 10 mg tablets.
Dose: 5 mg 2-3 times a day at first, increasing every 2-3 days to a maximum of 45 mg a day; usual maintenance 15-30 mg a day in divided doses.
Availability: NHS and private prescription.
Contains: buspirone hydrochloride.
Brand names: Buspar.

dizziness, headache, nervousness, excitement, nausea. Rarely, rapid heart rate, chest pain, confusion, dry mouth, sweating, tiredness. May affect ability to drive or perform skilled tasks.

in patients with a history of kidney or liver disease.

children, pregnant women, mothers who are breastfeeding, or for patients suffering from severe kidney or liver disease, epilepsy.

alcohol, MAOIS.

Butacote *see* phenylbutazone enteric-coated tablets
(Novartis Pharmaceuticals UK)

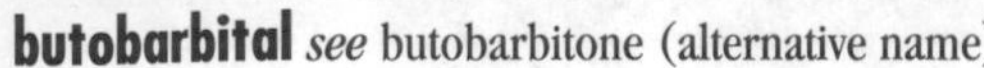

butobarbital *see* butobarbitone (alternative name)

butobarbitone tablets

A tablet used as a BARBITURATE to treat severe sleeplessness in patients already taking these drugs.

Strengths available: 100 mg tablets.
Dose: 1-2 tablets at bedtime.
Availability: controlled drug; NHS and private prescription.
Contains: butobabitone (butobarbital).
Brand names: Soneryl.

 drowsiness, hangover, dizziness, allergies, headache, shaky movements, breathing difficulties, confusion, excitement, withdrawal reactions.

 in patients suffering from liver, kidney, or lung disease. Addiction may develop. Must be withdrawn slowly.

 children, young adults, pregnant women, mothers who are breastfeeding, elderly or weak patients, or those with a history of drug or alcohol abuse, or suffering from PORPHYRIA, or in the management of pain.

 ANTICOAGULANTS, alcohol, antiviral drugs, CALCIUM-CHANNEL BLOCKERS, cyclosporin, thyroxine, tibolone, theophylline, aminophylline, gestrinone, antidepressants, other sedatives, CORTICOSTEROIDS, oral contraceptives, rifampicin, phenytoin.

butoxyethylnicotinate *see* Actinac

Cabaser *see* cabergoline tablets
(Pharmacia and Upjohn)

cabergoline tablets

A tablet used as a hormone blocker to suppress breast milk production in women as a treatment for some types of infertility, and (in conjunction with other drugs) to treat Parkinson's disease.

Strengths available: 0.5 mg, 1 mg, 2 mg, and 4 mg tablets.
Dose: in Parkinson's disease, 1 mg a day, increased gradually to 2-6 mg a day; to suppress breast milk, 1 mg on the first day after childbirth, or 0.25 mg every 12 hours for 2 days if milk has already been produced; to treat infertility, 0.5 mg a week in 1-2 doses, increasing if necessary to a maximum of 4.5 mg a week (usual maintenance 1 mg a week).
Availability: NHS and private prescription.
Contains: cabergoline.

dizziness, vertigo, headache, tiredness, breast pain, stomach upset, hot flushes, depression, weakness, pins and needles, rarely palpitations, nosebleeds, vision disturbances, swollen hands and feet, abdominal pain, angina, pain and redness of the skin, movement disorders, confusion, fluid surrounding the lungs, low blood pressure at first.

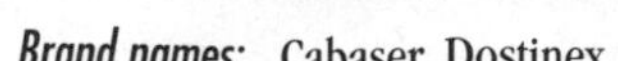

Brand names: Cabaser, Dostinex.

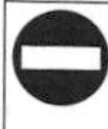 children under 16 years, pregnant women, mothers who are breastfeeding, or for patients suffering from weak liver function, toxaemia of pregnancy, raised blood pressure during pregnancy, some mental disorders, or who are allergic to ergotamine.

 alcohol, levodopa.

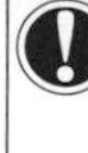 in patients suffering from kidney, liver, or heart disease, Raynaud's syndrome, stomach ulcer or bleeding, raised blood pressure, mental disorders. Before treatment pituitary function should be tested. Your doctor will advise regular blood tests. Stop treatment at least a month before trying to conceive. Use only non-hormonal methods of contraception.

Cacit *see* calcium carbonate tablets
(Proctor and Gamble Pharmaceuticals UK)

Cacit D3 *see* calcium and vitamin D tablets
(Proctor and Gamble Pharmaceuticals UK)

---

cadexomer iodine ointment/sachets

A paste or powder used as an absorbent, antibacterial treatment for leg ulcers and wounds.

Dose: apply three times a week, or change when saturated. Maximum of 150g paste in any 1 week. Not to be used for more than 3 months at a time.
Availability: NHS and private prescription, nurse prescription, over the counter.
Contains: cadexomer iodine.
Brand names: Iodoflex, Iodosorb.

 absorption of iodine into the body if large areas treated.

 in patients suffering from thyroid disorders. Not suitable for children.

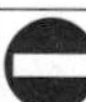 children under 2 years, pregnant women, mothers who are breastfeeding, or for patients suffering from some thyroid disorders.

 lithium, some antidiabetics.

Cafergot *see* ergotamine tablets
(Alliance Pharmaceuticals)

---

caffeine *see* Cafergot

Calaband *see* zinc paste and calamine bandage
(SSL International)

Caladryl *see* calamine lotion/cream
(Warner Lambert Consumer Healthcare)

calamine and coal tar ointment BP

An ointment used to treat chronic eczema and psoriasis.

Dose: apply 1-3 times a day.
Availability: NHS and private prescription, over the counter.
Contains: calamine, strong coal tar solution, zinc oxide, hydrous wool fat, white soft paraffin.

 irritation, acne-like skin eruptions, sensitivity to light.

 avoid broken or inflamed skin. Stains hair, skin, and fabrics.

calamine lotion/aqueous cream/oily lotion

A lotion, oily lotion, or aqueous cream used to treat itchy skin conditions.

Dose: apply when required.
Availability: NHS and private prescription, nurse prescription, over the counter.
Contains: calamine.
Compound preparations: Caladryl (with diphenhydramine, an ANTIHISTAMINE), calamine and coal tar ointment, Vasogen, zinc paste clioquinol, and calamine bandage BP 1993, zinc paste and calamine bandage.

Calanif *see* nifedipine capsules
(Berk Pharmaceuticals)

Calceos *see* calcium and vitamin D tablets
(Provalis Healthcare)

Calcette *see* calcium carbonate tablets
(Ashbourne Pharmaceuticals)

Calcicard CR *see* diltiazem modified-release tablets
(Norton Healthcare)

Calcichew/Calcichew Forte *see* calcium carbonate tablets
(Shire Pharmaceuticals)

C

Calcichew D3/Calcichew D3 Forte *see* calcium and vitamin D_3 tablets
(Shire Pharmaceuticals)

Calcidrink *see* calcium carbonate sachets
(Shire Pharmaceuticals)

---

calciferol tablets

Tablets used as a vitamin D_2 supplement to prevent or treat vitamin D deficiency.

Strengths available: 0.25 mg or 1.25 mg tablets.
Dose: 0.01 mg daily to prevent deficiency; up to 2.5 mg daily to treat deficiency (depending on condition).
Availability: NHS and private prescription, over the counter.
Contains: ergocalciferol (vitamin D).
Compound preparations: calcium and vitamin D tablets.

 loss of appetite, upset stomach, weight loss, excessive urine output, sweating, headache, thirst, vertigo, raised calcium and phosphate levels, lack of energy.

 in infants, pregnant women, and mothers who are breastfeeding. Patients receiving high doses may need regular blood tests.

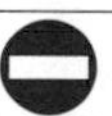 patients suffering from high calcium levels in the blood or some malignant diseases.

 other vitamin D preparations.

---

calcipotriol cream/ointment/scalp lotion

An ointment, cream, or scalp lotion used as a vitamin D treatment for psoriasis.

Strengths available: ointment and cream 50 mcg/g; scalp lotion 50 mcg/ml.
Dose: adults, apply once or twice a day (children, twice a day). Maximum of 100 g per week for adults, 50 g per week (children aged 6-12 years), 75 g per week (children 12-16 years).
Availability: NHS and private prescription.
Contains: calcipotriol.
Brand names: Dovonex.

 irritation, redness, dermatitis, sensitivity to light, worsening of psoriasis, itching, (high blood calcium levels with high doses).

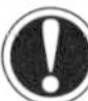 in pregnant women and mothers who are breastfeeding. Avoid use on the face. Wash hands after use.

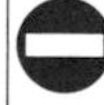 children under 6 years or for patients with disorders of calcium metabolism.

Calcisorb *see* sodium cellulose phosphate sachets
(3M Health Care)

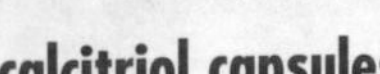

calcitriol capsules

A capsule used as a vitamin D treatment for correcting calcium and phosphate metabolism in patients suffering from bone disease caused by kidney disorder, and to treat established OSTEOPOROSIS.

Strengths available: 0.25 mcg and 0.5 mcg capsules.
Dose: kidney disorder, initially 0.25 mcg a day or on alternate days, increasing to 0.5-1.0 mcg a day; osteoporosis, 0.25 mcg twice a day.
Availability: NHS and private prescription.
Contains: calcitriol.
Brand names: Rocaltrol.

 loss of appetite, upset stomach, weight loss, excessive urine output, sweating, headache, thirst, vertigo, raised calcium and phosphate levels, lack of energy.

 in pregnant women and mothers who are breastfeeding. Patients receiving high doses may need regular blood tests.

 children or for patients suffering from high calcium levels in the blood, or some malignant diseases.

 other vitamin D preparations.

---

calcium 500 *see* calcium carbonate tablets (Martindale Pharmaceuticals)

---

calcium acetate tablets

A tablet used as a phosphate binder to treat high levels of phosphate in the blood.

Strengths available: 1 g tablets.
Dose: adjusted as needed for the individual.
Availability: NHS and private prescription.
Contains: calcium acetate.
Brand names: Phosex.

 upset stomach, high blood calcium levels.

 in pregnant women and nursing mothers. Your doctor will advise regular blood tests.

 patients with high levels of calcium in the blood or urine.

---

calcium alginate *see* alginate dressings

---

calcium carbonate tablets/sachets

A tablet, chewable tablet, effervescent tablet, or effervescent granules used as a calcium supplement to treat calcium deficiency, OSTEOPOROSIS, and to regulate blood phosphate levels in patients with kidney failure.

Strengths available: 1.25 g tablets; 1.25 g or 2.5 g chewable tablets; 1.25 g effervescent tablets; 2.5 g effervescent granules.
Dose: usually 1.25 g-3.75 g a day.
Availability: NHS and private prescription,

 mild stomach upset.

over the counter.
Contains: calcium carbonate.
Brand names: Cacit, Calceos, Calcette, Calcichew, Calcichew Forte, Calcidrink, Calcium-500.
Compound preparations: alginate liquid, calcium and vitamin D tablets, Sandocal, Titralac (with glycine – also used as a phosphate binder in renal failure).
Other preparations: Didronel PMO (combined pack).

in patients with kidney disorders or sarcoidosis.

patients with high levels of calcium in the blood or urine, some tumours, overactive parathyroid glands.

C

calcium and vitamin D tablets/chewable tablets/effervescent granules

A tablet, chewable tablet, or effervescent granules used as a calcium and vitamin D supplement to treat OSTEOPOROSIS.

Strengths available: variable.
Dose: varies according to condition but usually 1-2 tablets or sachets a day.
Availability: NHS and private prescription, over the counter.
Contains: calcium (as carbonate, lactate, phosphate) and vitamin D (as ergocalciferol or cholecalciferol – also known as colecalciferol).
Brand names: Adcal-D3, Cacit D3, Calcichew D3, Calcichew D3 Forte, Calceos, calcium and ergocalciferol tablets.

mild stomach upset. In high doses, loss of appetite, weight loss, excessive urine output, sweating, headache, thirst, vertigo, raised calcium and phosphate levels, lack of energy.

in pregnant women, mothers who are breast-feeding, and in patients suffering from kidney disorders or sarcoidosis. Patients receiving high doses may need regular blood tests.

children or for patients suffering from high calcium levels in the blood, or some malignant diseases.

other vitamin D preparations.

calcium channel blocker

A preparation used to block the flow of calcium into cells. This relaxes blood vessels and slows the rate of nerve conduction in the heart. These drugs are therefore useful in preventing angina, and in treating high blood pressure (ANTIHYPERTENSIVES). They are also used to correct abnormal heart rhythm. Examples, diltiazem, nifedipine, verapamil.

calcium folinate tablets

A tablet used as a folinic acid treatment for megaloblastic anaemia. Also used in emergency treatment of methotrexate poisoning.

Strengths available: 15 mg tablets.
Dose: for anaemia, 15 mg once a day.
Availability: NHS and private prescription.

in pregnant women and mothers who are breastfeeding.

cont.

Contains: calcium folinate.
Brand names: Leucovorin, Refolinon.

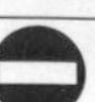 patients where vitamin B_{12} is deficient.

 methotrexate, phenobarbital, phenytoin, primidone.

calcium glubionate *see* Calcium Sandoz

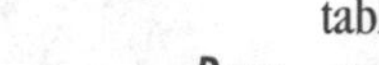

calcium gluconate tablets

A tablet or effervescent tablet used as a calcium supplement to treat calcium deficiency or OSTEOPOROSIS.

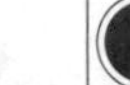

Strengths available: 600 mg tablets; 1 g effervescent tablets.
Dose: as advised by doctor.
Availability: NHS and private prescription, over the counter.
Contains: calcium gluconate.

mild stomach upset.

in patients with kidney disorders or sarcoidosis.

patients with high levels of calcium in the blood or urine, some tumours, overactive parathyroid glands.

---

calcium hydrogen phosphate *see* Vitamin Tablets for Nursing Mothers

---

calcium lactate tablets

A tablet used as a calcium supplement to treat calcium deficiency or OSTEOPOROSIS.

Strengths available: 300 mg tablets.
Dose: as advised by doctor.
Availability: NHS and private prescription, over the counter.
Contains: calcium lactate.

 mild stomach upset.

 in patients with kidney disorders or sarcoidosis.

 patients with high levels of calcium in the blood or urine, some tumours, overactive parathyroid glands.

---

calcium lactate gluconate *see* Sandocal

---

calcium lactobionate *see* Calcium Sandoz

---

calcium phosphate sachets

A powder in sachets used as a calcium supplement to treat calcium deficiency or OSTEOPOROSIS.

Strengths available: 3.3 g sachets
Dose: as advised by doctor.
Availability: NHS and private prescription, over the counter.
Contains: calcium lactate.
Brand names: Ostram.

 mild stomach upset.

 in patients with sarcoidosis.

 children or for patients with high levels of calcium in the blood or urine, some tumours, overactive parathyroid glands, kidney malfunction.

---

calcium polystyrene sulphonate *see* polystyrene sulphonate resin

---

Calcium Resonium *see* polystyrene sulphonate resin
(Sanofi Winthrop)

Calcium Sandoz *see* Sandocal
(Alliance Pharmaceuticals)

Calcort *see* deflazacort tablets
(Shire Pharmaceuticals)

Calmurid *see* urea cream
(Galderma (UK))

Calmurid HC *see* urea cream and topical corticosteroid cream
(Galderma (UK))

Calpol Paediatric/Six Plus *see* paracetamol suspension
(Warner Lambert Consumer Healthcare)

CAM *see* ephedrine syrup/tablets
(Cambridge Healthcare Supplies)

C

Camcolit *see* lithium tablets/modified-release tablets
(Norgine)

camomile *see* emollient preparations

camphene *see* Rowachol, Rowatinex

camphor *see* analgesic (topical)

Campral EC *see* acamprosate calcium
(Lipha Pharmaceuticals)

candesartan tablets

A tablet used as an ACE-II ANTAGONIST to treat high blood pressure.

Strengths available: 2 mg, 4 mg, 8 mg, and 16 mg tablets.
Dose: initially 4 mg once a day (2 mg in patients with liver or kidney disorders), adjusted according to response. (Maximum of 16 mg a day.)
Availability: NHS and private prescription.
Contains: candesartan cilexetil.
Brand names: Amias.

 anaesthetics, NON-STEROIDAL ANTI-INFLAMMATORY DRUGS, cyclosporin, DIURETICS, lithium, potassium.

 low blood pressure, high potassium levels, sore throat, runny nose, upset stomach, dizziness, rash, liver changes, pain in back, muscles, or joints, severe allergy.

 in patients with liver, heart, or kidney disorders. Your doctor may advise regular blood tests.

 children, pregnant women, mothers who are breastfeeding, or for patients suffering from severe liver disorders or bile duct obstruction.

Candiden *see* clotrimazole cream and clotrimazole pessaries
(Akita Pharmaceuticals)

Canesten *see* clotrimazole cream/pessaries/powder/solution/spray/vaginal cream/thrush cream
(Bayer Consumer Care)

Canesten HC *see* clotrimazole cream and topical corticosteroid cream
(Bayer Consumer Care)

C

Capasal *see* coal tar shampoo and salicylic acid ointment
(Dermal Laboratories)

Dose: apply daily as necessary.

Caplenal *see* allopurinol tablets
(Berk Pharmaceuticals)

Capoten *see* captopril tablets
(Bristol-Myers Squibb Pharmaceuticals)

Capozide/Capozide LS *see* co-zidocapt tablets
(Bristol-Myers Squibb Pharmaceuticals)

Caprin *see* aspirin enteric-coated tablets
(Sinclair Pharmaceuticals)

---

capsaicin cream

A cream used as a topical ANALGESIC to treat the pain of osteoarthritis, nerve pain due to shingles, or nerve disorders due to diabetes.

Strengths available: 0.025% (for osteoarthritis) and 0.075% (for nerve pain/disorder).
Dose: apply sparingly 3-4 times a day. Review after 8 weeks in diabetics.
Availability: NHS and private prescription.
Contains: capsaicin.
Brand names: Axsain (0.075%), Zacin (0.025%).

 irritation of skin.

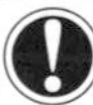 in shingles, apply only after the skin sores have healed. Do not bathe just before or after applying the cream.

 children, or on broken or irritated skin.

---

capsicum *see* analgesic (topical)

Capsuvac *see* co-danthrusate capsules
(Galen)

Capto-Co *see* co-zidocapt tablets
(Baker Norton Pharmaceuticals)

C

captopril tablets

A tablet used as an ACE-INHIBITOR to treat high blood pressure, heart failure, diabetic kidney disease in patients dependent on insulin, and as a treatment following heart attack.

Strengths available: 12.5 mg, 25 mg, and 50 mg tablets.
Dose: for high blood pressure, 6.25-12.5 mg twice a day at first (with the first dose taken at bedtime), increasing as necessary to a maximum of 50 mg three times a day; for heart failure and after heart attack, 6.25-12.5 mg at first, then 25 mg 2-3 times a day increasing to a maximum of 50 mg three times a day if needed; in diabetic kidney disease, 75-100 mg a day in divided doses.
Availability: NHS and private prescription.
Contains: captopril.
Brand names: Acepril, Capoten, Ecopace, Kaplon, Tensopril.
Compound preparations: co-zidocapt.

rash, itching, sore throat, runny nose, stomach upset, cough, blood and liver changes, kidney disorders, low blood pressure, severe allergic reaction, inflamed pancreas. Occasionally, headache, dizziness, tiredness, taste disturbance, difficulty breathing, fever, pins and needles, muscle or joint pain, sensitivity to sunlight, inflamed membranes or blood vessels, altered heart rhythm, weight loss, flushing, high blood acidity.

in the elderly, mothers who are breast-feeding, and in patients suffering from kidney disease, auto-immune diseases (such as LUPUS), severe heart failure, or with a history of severe allergies, or in patients undergoing anaesthesia or dialysis. Your doctor may advise regular blood tests.

pregnant women or for patients with some heart abnormalities, PORPHYRIA, or disorders of the blood supply to the kidney.

DIURETICS, anaesthetics, NON-STEROIDAL ANTI-INFLAMMATORY DRUGS, potassium supplements, digoxin, cyclosporin, lithium, antidiabetics.

Carace *see* lisinopril tablets
(DuPont Pharmaceuticals)

Carace Plus *see* lisinopril tablets and hydrochlorothiazide tablets
(DuPont Pharmaceuticals)

Strengths available: 10 mg + 12.5 mg and 20 mg + 12.5 mg tablets.
Dose: adults 1-2 tablets of either strength each day.

carbachol *see* Isopto Carbachol

Carbalax

(Pharmax)

A suppository used to treat constipation and to clear the bowel before surgery or diagnostic procedures.

Dose: 1 suppository 30 minutes before evacuation required.
Availability: NHS and private prescription, over the counter.
Contains: sodium bicarbonate, sodium acid phosphate (anhydrous).

 irritation.

 in elderly or weak patients.

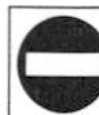 children under 12 years or for patients with acute intestinal problems.

carbamazepine tablets/chewable tablets/modified-release tablets/syrup/suppositories

A tablet used as an anticonvulsant treatment for epilepsy, as an ANALGESIC to treat trigeminal neuralgia, and to prevent manic depression in patients who do not respond to lithium.

Strengths available: 100 mg, 200 mg, and 400 mg tablets; 100 mg and 200 mg chewable tablets; 100 mg/5 ml liquid; 125 mg and 250 mg suppositories; 200 mg and 400 mg m-r tablets.
Dose: to prevent manic depression 400 mg a day at first, increasing gradually until controlled (maximum 1600 mg a day); to treat epilepsy and neuralgia, adults 100-200 mg once or twice a day at first, increasing usually to 800-1200 mg a day (maximum 2000 mg for epilepsy, 1600 mg for neuralgia), children 100-1000 mg a day depending on age.
Availability: NHS and private prescription.
Contains: carbamazepine.
Brand names: Epimaz, Tegretol, Teril Cr, Timonil Retard.

 stomach upset, loss of appetite, double vision, dry mouth, drowsiness, dizziness, confusion and agitation (in the elderly), fluid retention, low blood sodium, blood changes, rash and other skin disorders, acute kidney failure, jaundice, hair loss, hepatitis, fever, sensitivity to light, heart disturbances, depression, hypersensitivity, inflamed joints, enlarged lymph glands, impotence, reduced fertility, enlargement of male breasts, psychological changes, breathing disorders. Suppositories may be irritant.

 in the elderly, pregnant women, mothers who are breastfeeding, and in patients suffering from severe heart or circulatory disorders, liver or kidney disease, glaucoma, or with a history of blood disorders caused by other drugs. Your doctor may advise regular blood tests. Report any fever, sore throat, rash, mouth ulcers, bruising, or bleeding to your doctor immediately.

 patients suffering from heart conduction defects. PORPHYRIA, or a history of bone marrow depression.

 ANTICOAGULANTS, alcohol, CALCIUM-CHANNEL BLOCKERS, sedatives and tranquillizers, antidepressants (including MAOIS), cyclosporin, ORAL CONTRACEPTIVES, erythromycin, isoniazid, cimetidine, CORTICOSTEROIDS, danazol, doxycycline, tibolone, methadone, tramadol, clarithromycin, theophylline, aminophylline, antivirals, chloroquine, mefloquine, dextropopoxyphene, celecoxib, other anticonvulsant drugs.

C

carbaryl lotion/liquid

A liquid or lotion used as an insecticide to treat head lice.

Strengths available: 1% liquid; 0.5% lotion.
Dose: rub into dry hair and scalp, and leave to dry naturally. Shampoo off after 12 hours and comb through.
Availability: NHS and private prescription.
Contains: carbaryl (alcohol based for lotion, water based for liquid).
Brand names: Carylderm.

 irritation.

 in infants under 6 months, and in patients suffering from eczema or asthma (use liquid not lotion). Avoid contact with the eyes.

 areas of broken skin. Not for prolonged use – do not use more than once a week for 3 weeks at a time.

carbenoxolone gel

A gel used as a cell-surface protector to treat mouth ulcers.

Strengths available: 2% gel.
Dose: apply after meals and at bedtime.
Availability: NHS and private prescription, over the counter.
Contains: carbenoxolone sodium.
Brand names: Bioral.
Compound preparations: Pyrogastrone.

carbenoxolone granules

Granules supplied in sachets and used as a cell-surface protector to treat mouth ulcers.

Strengths available: 1% solution when prepared.
Dose: dissolve contents of 1 sachet in 30-50 ml warm water and use as mouth rinse three times a day and at bedtime.
Availability: NHS and private prescription.
Contains: carbenoxolone sodium.
Brand names: Bioplex.
Compound preparations: Pyrogastrone.

carbidopa *see* co-careldopa tablets

carbimazole tablets

A tablet used as an antithyroid treatment for overactive thyroid.

Strengths available: 5 mg and 20 mg tablets.

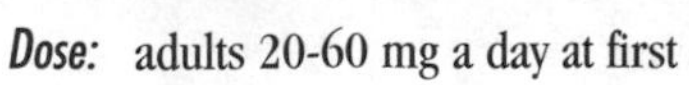

Dose: adults 20-60 mg a day at first (in divided doses), then 5-15 mg a day (or continued at 20-60 mg with supplements of thyroxine), usually for 18 months. Children use reduced doses according to doctor's instructions.
Availability: NHS and private prescription.
Contains: carbimazole.
Brand names: Neo-Mercazole.

 rash, headache, nausea, mild stomach upset, joint pain, bone marrow depression, rash, itching, jaundice. Advise the doctor immediately if you develop sore throat, mouth ulcers, tiredness, unexplained bruising, or fever.

 in pregnant women, mothers who are breastfeeding, and patients with liver disorders.

 combined carbimazole-thyroxine therapy not suitable for pregnant women.

Carbo-Dome *see* coal tar cream
(Lagap Pharmaceuticals)

---

carbocisteine capsules/syrup

A syrup or capsule used as a mucus softener to clear excessive or viscous phlegm, and to treat glue ear in children.

Strengths available: 375 mg capsules, 250 mg/5 ml or 125 mg/5 ml syrup.
Dose:
Availability: private prescription. (The syrup is available on the NHS if prescribed by generic name for children under 18 years who have a tracheostomy.)
Contains: carbocisteine.
Brand names: Mucodyne.

 stomach upset, rash.

 in pregnant women and in patients with a history of stomach ulcer.

 children under 2 years or for patients currently suffering from stomach ulcer.

---

carbomer eye drops

A liquid gel applied to the eye to treat tear deficiencies and dry eye conditions.

Strengths available: 0.2% gel.
Dose: 1 drop applied 3-4 times a day.
Availability: NHS and private prescription, over the counter.
Contains: carbomer 940 (polyacrylic acid).
Brand names: GelTears, Viscotears.

 temporary irritation and blurred vision.

 in pregnant women and mothers who are breastfeeding.

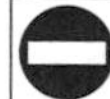 patients who wear soft contact lenses. Some brands not recommended for children.

---

cardamom *see* magnesium carbonate aromatic mixture BP

Cardene/Cardene SR *see* nicardipine capsules/modified-release capsules
(Yamanouchi Pharma)

Cardicor *see* bisoprolol tablets
(E. Merck Pharmaceuticals)

Cardilate MR *see* nifedipine modified-release tablets
(Norton Healthcare)

Cardura *see* doxazosin tablets
(Invicta Pharmaceuticals)

Carisoma *see* carisoprodol tablets
(Pharmax)

---

carisoprodol tablets

A tablet used as a sedative for the short-term treatment of muscle spasms.

Strengths available: 125 mg and 350 mg tablets.
Dose: adults 350 mg three times a day (elderly patients 175 mg three times a day or less).
Availability: NHS and private prescription.
Contains: carisoprodol.
Brand names: Carisoma.

Side effects: drowsiness, dizziness, stomach upset, headache, flushing, rash, tiredness, low blood pressure, weakness, excitement or confusion, lack of co-ordination, disturbances of vision, blood disorders, addiction, changes in sexual desire, shaking, jaundice, changes in saliva production, urine retention, or incontinence.

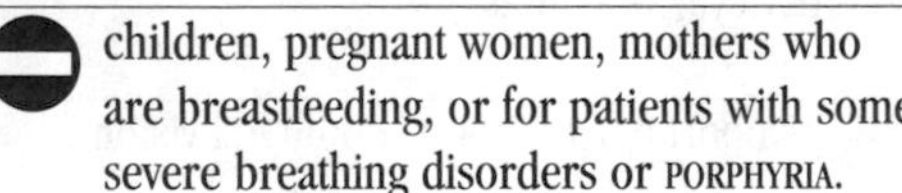

Not to be used for: children, pregnant women, mothers who are breastfeeding, or for patients with some severe breathing disorders or PORPHYRIA.

Caution: in elderly or weak patients, and in those with kidney or liver disease, breathing disorders, epilepsy, muscle weakness, or with a history of alcoholism, personality disorder, or drug addiction.

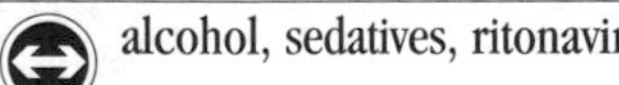

Caution needed with: alcohol, sedatives, ritonavir.

---

carmellose *see* Orabase, Orahesive, saliva (artificial)

C

carnitine solution

A solution used to treat patients with carnitine deficiency (e.g. through kidney dialysis).

Strengths available: 1 g/10 ml adult solution; 300 mg/ml paediatric solution.
Dose: as advised by doctor.
Availability: NHS and private prescription.
Contains: L-carnitine.
Brand names: Carnitor.

 upset stomach, body odour, tolerance.

 in pregnant women, mothers who are breastfeeding, and in patients with poor kidney function. Your doctor will advise regular blood and urine tests.

Carnitor *see* carnitine solution
(Shire Pharmaceuticals)

---

carteolol eye drops

Eye drops used as a BETA-BLOCKER to treat glaucoma and some other causes of high pressure in the eye. Some of the preparations may be absorbed into the body (*see* side effects, cautions, etc. as for propranolol tablets).

Strengths available: 1% or 2% drops.
Dose: 1 drop into the affected eye(s) twice a day. (Start with 1% drops and increase to 2% if necessary.)
Availability: NHS and private prescription.
Contains: carteolol hydrochloride.
Brand names: Teoptic.

 temporary discomfort or redness in the eye, dry eyes. Rarely, disorders of the cornea.

 in mothers who are breastfeeding, and in patients with diabetes, overactive thyroid, or those being given a general anaesthetic.

 children, pregnant women, or for patients using soft contact lenses, or suffering from some heart diseases, asthma, or breathing disorders.

 verapamil, diltiazem, nifedipine, amiodarone.

---

carvedilol tablets

A tablet used as a BETA-BLOCKER to treat high blood pressure, angina, and (in addition to other treatments) to treat symptoms of heart failure.

Strengths available: 3.125 mg, 6.25 mg, 12.5 mg, and 25 mg tablets.
Dose: for high blood pressure, 12.5 mg once a day at first increasing after 2 days to 25 mg once a day (maximum 50 mg once a day); for angina, 12.5 mg twice a day at first increasing to 25 mg twice a day after 2 days; for heart failure

 low blood pressure on standing, slow heart rate, dizziness, tiredness, headache, stomach upset, reduced circulation in the hands and feet, dry or irritated eyes, visual disturbance, chest pain, skin reactions, intermittent limping, influenza-like symptoms, fluid retention, changes in passing urine, skin disorders, wheezing, depressed mood, pins and needles, heart failure, blood and liver changes, stuffy nose.

cont.

3.125 mg twice a day with food at first increasing gradually to a maximum of 25 mg twice a day (50 mg twice a day in patients over 85 kg).

Availability: NHS and private prescription.
Contains: carvedilol.
Brand names: Eucardic.

 general anaesthetics, CALCIUM-CHANNEL BLOCKERS, ALPHA-BLOCKERS, clonidine, ANTIHYPERTENSIVES, amiodarone, antidiabetics, thymoxamine, theophylline, aminophylline.

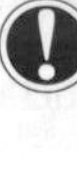 in patients with weak heart, some forms of angina, kidney disorders, MYASTHENIA GRAVIS, or who are suffering from overactive thyroid or diabetes. Patients with some forms of heart disease should have treatment withdrawn gradually. Your doctor may advise regular check-ups.

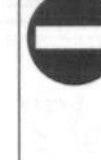 children under 18 years, pregnant women, mothers who are breastfeeding, or for patients suffering from some heart or circulation problems, PHAEOCHROMOCYTOMA, asthma, liver damage, very low blood pressure, blocked airways, or asthma.

Carylderm *see* carbaryl liquid/lotion
(SSL International)

---

castor oil *see* zinc and castor oil ointment

Catapres *see* clonidine tablets/modified-release tablets
(Boehringer Ingelheim)

Caverject/Caverject Dual Chamber *see* alprostadil injection
(Pharmacia and Upjohn)

Ceanel concentrate

(Quinoderm)

A liquid used as an antibacterial and antifungal treatment for psoriasis and scaly inflammation of the scalp.

Dose: use as a shampoo three times a week at first, then twice a week. May be used on the scalp or other skin areas if required.

 keep out of the eyes.

Availability: NHS and private prescription, over the counter.
Contains: cetrimide, undecenoic acid, phenylethyl alcohol.

Cedocard Retard *see* isosorbide dinitrate modified-release tablets
(Pharmacia and Upjohn)

---

cefaclor capsules/modified-release tablets/suspension

A capsule, M-R TABLET, or suspension used as a cephalosporin ANTIBIOTIC to treat infections (particularly urine, chest, ear, sinus, skin, or soft tissue infections).

Strengths available: 250 mg or 500 mg capsules; 375 mg m-r tablets; 125 mg/5 ml and 250 mg/5 ml suspension.
Dose: adults and children over 5 years, 250 mg-500 mg every 8 hours (adults maximum 4000 mg a day); children aged 1-12 months 62.5-125 mg (aged 1-5 years 125-250 mg) every 8 hours.
Availability: NHS and private prescription.
Contains: cefaclor monohydrate.
Brand names: Cefaclor M-R, Distaclor, Keftid, Ranbaxy.

allergy, headache, stomach upset, skin disorders, blood and liver changes, inflamed kidneys, sleep disturbance, confusion, nervousness, dizziness, tense muscles, inflamed bowel.

in pregnant women, mothers who are breast-feeding, and in patients suffering from kidney disorders or who are allergic to penicillin.

infants under 1 month or for patients suffering from PORPHYRIA or who are allergic to cephalosporin antibiotics.

ANTICOAGULANTS.

cefadroxil capsules/suspension

A capsule or suspension used as a cephalosporin ANTIBIOTIC to treat infections, (particularly urine, chest, ear, sinus, skin, or soft tissue infections).

Strengths available: 500 mg capsules; 125 mg/5 ml, 250 mg/5 ml, and 500 mg/5 ml suspension.
Dose: adults, 500-1000 mg twice a day; children, up to 500 mg twice a day (according to age and weight).
Availability: NHS and private prescription.
Contains: cefadroxil monohydrate.
Brand names: Baxan.

allergy, headache, stomach upset, skin disorders, blood and liver changes, inflamed kidneys, sleep disturbance, confusion, nervousness, dizziness, tense muscles, inflamed bowel.

in pregnant women, mothers who are breast-feeding, and in patients suffering from kidney disorders or who are allergic to penicillin.

patients suffering from PORPHYRIA or who are allergic to cephalosporin antibiotics.

ANTICOAGULANTS.

cefalexin *see* cephalexin (alternative name)

cefixime tablets/suspension

A tablet or suspension used as a cephalosporin ANTIBIOTIC to treat urine and chest infections.

Strengths available: 200 mg tablets; 100 mg/5 ml suspension.

cont.

Dose: adults and children over 10 years, 200-400 mg a day; children 6 months-10 years, up to 200 mg a day according to age and weight. Doses may be taken once a day or divided into two doses.
Availability: NHS and private prescription.
Contains: cefixime.
Brand names: Suprax.

 allergy, headache, stomach upset, skin disorders, blood and liver changes, inflamed kidneys, sleep disturbance, confusion, nervousness, dizziness, tense muscles, inflamed bowel.

 in pregnant women, mothers who are breast-feeding, and in patients suffering from kidney disorders or who are allergic to penicillin.

 infants under 6 months or for patients suffering from PORPHYRIA or who are allergic to cephalosporin antibiotics.

 ANTICOAGULANTS.

cefpodoxime suspension/tablets

A tablet or suspension used as a cephalosporin ANTIBIOTIC to treat infections (particularly urine, chest, sinus, skin, or soft tissue infections).

Strengths available: 100 mg tablets; 40 mg/5 ml suspension.
Dose: adults, usually 100-200 mg twice a day depending on infection and severity; children, up to 100 mg twice a day depending on age and weight,
Availability: NHS and private prescription.
Contains: cefpodoxime proxetil.
Brand names: Orelox.

 ANTICOAGULANTS.

 allergy, headache, stomach upset, skin disorders, blood and liver changes, inflamed kidneys, sleep disturbance, confusion, nervousness, dizziness, tense muscles, inflamed bowel.

 in pregnant women, mothers who are breast-feeding, and in patients suffering from kidney disorders or who are allergic to penicillin.

 infants under 15 days old or for patients suffering from PORPHYRIA or who are allergic to cephalosporin antibiotics. The suspension should not be used by patients suffering from PHENYLKETONURIA.

cefprozil suspension/tablets

A tablet or suspension used as a cephalosporin ANTIBIOTIC to treat chest, ear, skin, and soft tissue infections.

Strengths available: 250 mg or 500 mg tablets; 250 mg/5 ml suspension.
Dose: adults 500 mg once or twice a day (depending on infection) for 10 days; children 6 months-12 years, up to 500 mg once or twice a day depending on age, weight, and infection.
Availability: NHS and private prescription.

allergy, headache, stomach upset, skin disorders, blood and liver changes, inflamed kidneys, sleep disturbance, confusion, nervousness, dizziness, tense muscles, inflamed bowel.

Contains: cefprozil.
Brand names: Cefzil.

 children under 6 months or for patients suffering from PORPHYRIA or who are allergic to cephalosporin antibiotics.

 in pregnant women, mothers who are breastfeeding, and in patients suffering from kidney disorders, PHENYLKETONURIA, or who are allergic to penicillin.

 ANTICOAGULANTS.

---

cefradine *see* cephradine (alternative name)

---

cefuroxime suspension/tablets/sachets

A tablet, sachet, or suspension used as a cephalosporin ANTIBIOTIC to treat infections (particularly urine, chest, ear, sinus, skin, or soft tissue infections).

Strengths available: 250 mg or 500 mg tablets; 125 mg/5 ml suspension; 125 mg per sachet.
Dose: adults, usually 250-500 mg twice a day depending on condition; children over 3 months, 125 mg (over 2 years up to 250 mg) twice a day.
Availability: NHS and private prescription.
Contains: cefuroxime.
Brand names: Zinnat.

 allergy, headache, stomach upset, skin disorders, blood and liver changes, inflamed kidneys, sleep disturbance, confusion, nervousness, dizziness, tense muscles, inflamed bowel.

 in pregnant women, mothers who are breastfeeding, and in patients suffering from kidney disorders or who are allergic to penicillin.

 patients suffering from PORPHYRIA or who are allergic to cephalosporin antibiotics.

 ANTICOAGULANTS.

Cefzil *see* cefprozil suspension/tablets
(Bristol-Myers Squibb Pharmaceuticals)

Celance *see* pergolide tablets
(Eli Lilly and Co.)

Celebrex *see* celecoxib capsules
(Searle)

---

celecoxib capsules

A capsule used to treat symptoms of arthritis.

Strengths available: 100 mg and 200 mg capsules.

cont.

C

Dose: osteoarthritis 200 mg once or twice a day, rheumatoid arthritis 100-200 mg twice a day. (Elderly or other vulnerable patients maximum of 200 mg each day at first.)
Availability: NHS and private prescription.
Contains: celecoxib.
Brand names: Celebrex.

children, pregnant women (and women of childbearing age unless using effective contraception – N.B. ORAL CONTRACEPTIVES may not be appropriate, *see below*), or for patients with allergy to certain antibiotics, aspirin, or NON-STEROIDAL ANTI-INFLAMMATORY DRUGS, or history of asthma, nose disorders, or severe allergies, or those with stomach ulcers, bowel disorders, severe heart failure, or severe liver disease.

fluid retention, abdominal pain, upset stomach, dizziness, sleeplessness, sore throat, runny nose, sinusitis, infections of the respiratory system, rash. Rarely, mouth inflammation, palpitations, pins and needles, muscle cramp, tiredness, disturbance of taste, hair loss, tiredness, anxiety, depression.

in patients with liver or kidney disorders, a history of stomach or bowel disorders, heart failure, high blood pressure, fluid retention, heart or circulation disorders, and those taking DIURETICS.

warfarin, ACE-INHIBITORS, NON-STEROIDAL ANTI-INFLAMMATORY DRUGS, cyclosporin, lithium, rifampicin, carbamazepine, BARBITURATES, oral contraceptives.

Celectol *see* celiprolol tablets
(Pantheon Healthcare)

Celevac *see* methylcellulose tablets
(Shire Pharmaceuticals)

---

celiprolol tablets

A tablet used as a BETA-BLOCKER to treat high blood pressure.

Strengths available: 200 mg and 400 mg tablets.
Dose: 200-400 mg each morning.
Availability: NHS and private prescription.
Contains: celiprolol hydrochloride.
Brand names: Celectol.

children or for patients suffering from heart block or failure, severe kidney failure, PHAEOCHROMOCYTOMA, asthma, or a history of breathing disorders.

headache, dizziness, slow heart rate, tiredness, drowsiness, breathing disorders, depression.

in pregnant women, mothers who are breast-feeding, and in patients suffering from diabetes, kidney or liver disorders, MYASTHENIA GRAVIS, or with a history of allergies. May need to be withdrawn before surgery. Withdraw gradually.

general anaesthetics, CALCIUM-CHANNEL BLOCKERS, ALPHA-BLOCKERS, clonidine, ANTIHYPERTENSIVES, amiodarone, antidiabetics, thymoxamine, theophylline, aminophylline, alcohol, sedatives.

Cellcept *see* mycophenolate capsules/tablets
(Roche Products)

cephalexin capsules/tablets/syrup/suspension

A capsule, tablet, syrup, or suspension used as a cephalosporin ANTIBIOTIC to treat infections (particularly urine, chest, ear, sinus, skin, or soft tissue infections).

Strengths available: 250 mg or 500 mg capsules or tablets; 125 mg/5 ml, 250 mg/5 ml, or 500 mg/5 ml syrup; 125 mg/5 ml and 250 mg/5 ml suspension.
Dose: adults and children over 12 years, usually 1000-2000 mg a day in 2-4 divided doses (up to 4500 mg a day in severe infections); children, up to 250 mg every 8 hours according to age and weight. Adult dose to prevent urine infections, 125 mg at night.
Availability: NHS and private prescription.
Contains: cephalexin (cefalexin).
Brand names: Ceporex, Keflex.

allergy, headache, stomach upset, skin disorders, blood and liver changes, inflamed kidneys, sleep disturbance, confusion, nervousness, dizziness, tense muscles, inflamed bowel.

in pregnant women, mothers who are breast-feeding, and in patients suffering from kidney disorders or who are allergic to penicillin.

patients suffering from PORPHYRIA or who are allergic to cephalosporin antibiotics.

ANTICOAGULANTS.

cephradine capsules/syrup

A capsule or syrup used as a cephalosporin ANTIBIOTIC to treat infections (particularly urine, chest, ear, sinus, skin, or soft tissue infections).

Strengths available: 250 mg and 500 mg capsules; 250 mg/5 ml syrup.
Dose: adults, 1000-2000 mg a day in 2-4 divided doses; children, use reduced doses according to body weight.
Availability: NHS and private prescription.
Contains: cephradine (cefradine).
Brand names: Nicef, Velosef.

allergy, headache, stomach upset, skin disorders, blood and liver changes, inflamed kidneys, sleep disturbance, confusion, nervousness, dizziness, tense muscles, inflamed bowel.

in pregnant women, mothers who are breast-feeding, and in patients suffering from kidney disorders or who are allergic to penicillin.

patients suffering from PORPHYRIA or who are allergic to cephalosporin antibiotics.

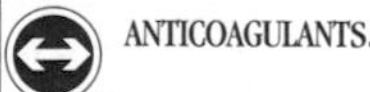
ANTICOAGULANTS.

Ceporex *see* cephalexin capsules/syrup/tablets
(Galen)

Cepton *see* chlorhexidine solution
(Eastern Pharmaceuticals)

---

cerivastatin tablets

A tablet used as a STATIN treatment to reduce cholesterol levels in patients with high cholesterol which has not reduced by dietary adjustment.

Strengths available: 100 mcg, 200 mcg, 300 mcg, and 400 mcg tablets.
Dose: 100-400 mcg once a day in the evening.
Availability: NHS and private prescription.
Contains: cerivastatin sodium.
Brand names: Lipobay.

 sleeplessness, joint pain, weakness, pins and needles, vertigo, rash, eye disorders, allergic reactions, muscle pain and inflammation, headache, stomach upset, liver changes. Report any unexplained muscle pain to your doctor.

 in patients with liver or kidney disorders. Your doctor may advise regular blood tests. Women of childbearing age should use adequate contraception during treatment and for 1 month afterwards.

 children under 18 years, pregnant women, mothers who are breastfeeding, or for patients with current liver disease.

 itraconazole, cyclosporin, other lipid-lowering drugs.

Cerumol

(LAB)

Drops used as a wax softener to remove wax from the ears.

Dose: 5 drops 10-30 minutes before syringing, or 5 drops twice a day for 3 days may enable syringing to be avoided.
Availability: NHS and private prescription, over the counter.
Contains: paradichlorobenzene, chlorbutol, arachis oil.

patients suffering from inflammation of the outer ear, dermatitis, eczema, or with perforated ear drum or allergy to peanuts.

Cetavlex *see* cetrimide cream
(Bioglan Laboratories)

---

cetirizine solution/tablets

A tablet or solution used as an ANTIHISTAMINE treatment for rhinitis and allergies.

Strengths available: 10 mg tablets; 5 mg/5 ml solution.
Dose: adults and children over 6 years, 10 mg once a day or 5 mg twice a day; children aged 2-6 years (for hayfever only)

 rarely, drowsiness, dizziness, headache, agitation, stomach upset, dry mouth.

half the adult dose.
Availability: NHS and private prescription, over the counter.
Contains: cetirizine hydrochloride.
Brand names: Zirtek.

 in patients suffering from kidney disease.

 children under 2 years, pregnant women, or mothers who are breastfeeding.

 some antidepressants, ritonavir, alcohol, sedatives.

---

cetrimide cream BP

A cream used as an antiseptic to treat minor wounds and nappy rash.

Strengths available: 0.5% cream.
Dose: apply as necessary.
Availability: NHS and private prescription, over the counter.
Contains: cetrimide.
Brand names: Cetavlex, Medicaid.
Compound preparations: Ceanel, Drapolene (with benzalkonium chloride, another antiseptic); Steripod wound and burn cleanser *see* chlorhexidine solution.

---

cetyl dimethicone *see* emollient preparations

---

cetylpyridinium chloride lozenges/mouthwash

A lozenge or mouthwash used as an antiseptic to treat infections of the mouth and throat.

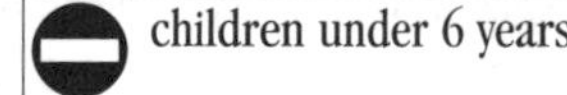 children under 6 years.

Dose: adults and children over 6 years, 1 lozenge sucked every 3 hours, or the mouthwash used (diluted or undiluted) every 3 hours (or when required) to rinse the mouth or gargle.
Availability: NHS and private prescription, over the counter.
Contains: cetylpyridinium chloride.
Brand names: Merocets.
Compound preparations: Merocaine (with benzocaine, a local anaesthetic).

Chemotrim *see* co-trimoxazole paediatric suspension

(Rosemont Pharmaceuticals)

Chemydur 60XL *see* isosorbide mononitrate modified-release tablets

(Sovereign Medical)

C

chloral mixture/elixir/tablets

A mixture, elixir, or tablet used as a sedative for the short-term treatment of sleeplessness.

Strengths available: 500 mg/5 ml mixture; 143 mg/5 ml or 200 mg/5 ml elixir; 414 mg tablets.
Dose: adults, usually 500-1000 mg at bedtime (maximum 2000 mg); children use lower doses (maximum 1000 mg). Doses should be taken with plenty of water.
Availability: NHS and private prescription.
Contains: chloral hydrate. (Welldorm tablets contain chloral betaine.)
Brand names: Welldorm.

stomach upset, wind, rash, urine changes, headache, excitement, addiction, confusion in the elderly, vertigo, lack of co-ordination, general feeling of being unwell, blood changes.

in elderly patients or in those with general debility or a history of drug/alcohol addiction or suffering from respiratory disease or some psychiatric disorders. Withdraw slowly and avoid contact with the skin.

pregnant women, mothers who are breastfeeding, or for patients suffering from heart disease, stomach inflammation, liver or kidney disorders, or PORPHYRIA. Chloral mixture should not be used for infants under 1 year (use elixir instead).

alcohol, other sedatives, warfarin.

chloramphenicol *see* Actinac, chloramphenicol capsules, chloramphenicol ear drops, chloramphenicol eye drops/ointment

chloramphenicol capsules

A capsule used as an ANTIBIOTIC to treat typhoid and other life-threatening infections.

Strengths available: 250 mg capsules.
Dose: usually 50 mg per kg body weight a day (in four divided doses). Children under 2 weeks, usually 25 mg per kg body weight.
Availability: NHS and private prescription.
Contains: chloramphenicol.

blood changes, stomach upset, nerve inflammation.

in patients with kidney or liver disorders. Not for repeated or prolonged use. Your doctor may advise regular blood tests.

pregnant women, mothers who are breastfeeding, or for patients suffering from PORPHYRIA.

ANTICOAGULANTS, some antidiabetic drugs, phenobarbital, phenytoin.

chloramphenicol ear drops

Ear drops used as an ANTIBIOTIC to treat bacterial infection of the outer ear.

Strengths available: 5% and 10% drops.

Dose: 2-3 drops into the affected ear(s) 2-3 times a day.
Availability: NHS and private prescription.
Contains: chloramphenicol.

 frequently allergic reactions.

 avoid prolonged use.

C

chloramphenicol eye drops/ointment

Drops used as an ANTIBIOTIC to treat bacterial infections of the eye.

Strengths available: 0.5% drops; 0.5% single-use drops (Minims); 1% ointment.
Dose: 2 drops or 1 application of ointment into the affected eye(s) every 3 hours or as required. Continue for 48 hours after infection subsides.
Availability: NHS and private prescription.
Contains: chloramphenicol.
Brand names: Chloromycetin, Minims Chloramphenicol, Sno-Phenicol.

temporary stinging. Rarely, anaemia.

remove contact lenses before using.

chlorbutol *see* Cerumol, Eludril, Monphytol

chlordiazepoxide capsules/tablets

A capsule or tablet used for the short-term treatment of anxiety, and as an additional treatment for the symptoms of alcohol withdrawal.

Strengths available: 5 mg and 10 mg capsules; 5 mg, 10 mg, and 25 mg tablets.
Dose: for anxiety, adults up to 30 mg a day (in divided doses) at first increasing if needed to a maximum of 100 mg a day. Elderly or frail patients use half adult dose. For other conditions, as advised by doctor.
Availability: NHS (if prescribed by generic name) and private prescription.
Contains: chlordiazepoxide.
Brand names: Librium, Tropium (neither available on NHS).

drowsiness, light-headedness, confusion, vertigo, stomach disturbances, loss of memory, aggression, headache, joint immobility, salivation changes, shaking, unsteadiness, low blood pressure, rash, changes in vision, changes in sexual desire, retention of urine, incontinence, blood changes, jaundice. Risk of addiction increases with dose and length of treatment. May impair judgement.

 in the elderly, pregnant women, mothers who are breastfeeding, women during labour, and in patients suffering from lung disorders, glaucoma, kidney or liver disorders, PORPHYRIA, muscle weakness, or with a history of drug or alcohol abuse. Avoid long-term use and withdraw gradually.

 children or for patients suffering from acute lung diseases, some chronic lung diseases, severe liver disease, MYASTHENIA GRAVIS, some obsessional and psychotic disorders, or who have stopped breathing while asleep.

 alcohol, other sedating drugs, some antivirals and anti-epileptic medications.

chlorhexidine *see* chlorhexidine dressings, chlorhexidine mouthwash/spray/dental gel, chlorhexidine solution, Eludril, emollient preparations, Naseptin, Nystaform

chlorhexidine dressings

A gauze dressing impregnated with antiseptic and used as a dressing for wounds where there may be bacterial infection.

Availability: NHS and private prescription, over the counter.
Contains: chlorhexidine acetate.
Brand names: Bactigras, Serotulle.

chlorhexidine mouthwash/dental gel/spray

A solution, spray, or dental gel used as an antibacterial treatment for gingivitis, mouth ulcers, thrush, and for mouth hygiene.

Side effects: irritation, reversible staining of teeth, swollen glands, taste changes.

Strengths available: 0.12% and 0.2% solution; 0.2% spray; 1% dental gel.
Dose: the mouthwash used to rinse the mouth for 1 minute twice a day; dental gel brushed on to the teeth twice a day; spray applied using up to 12 sprays twice a day.
Availability: NHS and private prescription, over the counter.
Contains: chlorhexidine gluconate.
Brand names: Chlorohex, Corsodyl.
Compound preparations: Eludril (with chlorbutol – an antiseptic – in mouthwash and with amethocaine – a local anaesthetic – in spray).

chlorhexidine solution/dusting powder

A solution or dusting powder used as a disinfectant for cleansing and disinfecting skin. Some preparations used as a soap substitute in acne.

Side effects: occasionally, allergic reactions.

Caution: avoid contact with the eyes.

Not to be used for: body cavities.

Strengths available: 0.05%, 0.02%, 0.25%, 0.5%, 1%, and 4% solution; 1% dusting powder.
Dose: usually applied as required (but check product labels for precise details).
Availability: NHS and private prescription, over the counter.
Contains: chlorhexidine gluconate or acetate.
Brand names: Cepton, CX Antiseptic Dusting Powder, Hibiscrub, Hibisol, Hydrex, Phiso-Med, Sterexidine, Steripod Antimicrobial Cleanser, Unisept.
Compound preparations: Hibisol (with isopropyl alcohol), Steripod Wounds and Burns Cleanser (with cetrimide), Tisept (with cetrimide), Travasept (with cetrimide).

chlormethiazole capsules/syrup

A capsule or syrup used as a sedative for the treatment of sleeplessness and agitation in the elderly, and alcohol withdrawal symptoms.

Strengths available: 192 mg capsules; 250 mg/5 ml syrup.
Dose: for sleeplessness, 1-2 capsules or 5-10 ml syrup at bedtime; for agitation, 1 capsule (or 5 ml syrup) three times a day. More complex dose schedules used for alcohol withdrawal. Used only for short periods to treat sleeplessness.
Availability: NHS and private prescription.
Contains: chlormethiazole base (capsules), chlormethiazole edisylate (syrup). Chlormethiazole also known as clomethiazole.
Brand names: Heminevrin.

 blocked or irritated nose, irritated eyes, stomach upset, severe allergy, excitement, confusion, drowsiness, headache, skin reactions, liver changes, addiction.

 in pregnant women, mothers who are breast-feeding, the elderly, and in patients suffering from long-term lung weakness, heart disease, kidney or liver disease, or with a history of drug or alcohol abuse, or personality disorders. Patients should be warned of impaired ability, and not to continue drinking alcohol while on this treatment.

 children, nor long term to treat sleeplessness.

 alcohol, other sedating drugs.

---

chlorobutanol *see* chlorbutol (alternative name)

Chlorohex *see* chlorhexidine mouthwash
(Colgate-Palmolive)

Chloromycetin *see* chloramphenicol eye drops/ointment
(Forley)

---

chloroquine tablets/syrup

A tablet or syrup used as an antimalarial drug for the prevention and treatment of malaria, and to treat rheumatoid arthritis and LUPUS.

Strengths available: 150 mg or 155 mg tablets; 50 mg/5 ml syrup.
Dose: to prevent malaria, adults 300 mg once a week (on the same day each week) starting 1 week before entering endemic area and continuing for at least 4 weeks after leaving. To treat malaria, dose determined by doctor. To treat rheumatoid arthritis or lupus, usually 150 mg a day (but determined by specialist). Children use reduced doses according to age. Doses for rheumatic disorders and *cont.*

headache, fits, stomach upset, skin disorders, hair loss, eye disorders, blood disorders, loss of hair or hair pigment, allergy.

C

C

lupus as advised by doctor.

Availability: NHS and private prescription, over the counter (if for prevention of malaria). Not generally prescribed on NHS for prevention of malaria.

Contains: chloroquine sulphate or chloroquine phosphate.

Brand names: Avloclor, Nivaquine.

Compound preparations: Paludrine/Avloclor travel pack (combined with proguanil tablets in one pack).

in pregnant women, mothers who are breastfeeding, and in patients suffering from PORPHYRIA, kidney or liver disease, severe stomach or intestinal disorder, nervous or blood disorders, MYASTHENIA GRAVIS, psoriasis, or with a history of epilepsy. The eyes should be tested before and during prolonged treatment.

amiodarone, anti-epileptic drugs, digoxin, cyclosporin.

chloroxylenol *see* Zeasorb

chlorphenamine *see* chlorpheniramine (alternative name)

chlorpheniramine tablets/syrup

A tablet or syrup used as an ANTIHISTAMINE treatment for allergies such as hayfever and nettle rash.

Strengths available: 4 mg tablets; 2 mg/5 ml syrup.

Dose: adults, usually 4 mg every 4-6 hours (maximum 24 mg a day); children aged 1-2 years, 1 mg twice a day, aged 2-5 years 1 mg every 4-6 hours (maximum 6 mg a day), aged 6-12 years 2 mg every 4-6 hours (maximum 12 mg a day).

Availability: NHS and private prescription, over the counter.

Contains: chlorpheniramine (chlorphenamine) maleate.

Brand names: Piriton.

Compound preparations: Galpseud Plus (with pseudoephedrine), Haymine (with ephedrine).

drowsiness, reduced reactions, dizziness, excitation, movement disorders, headache, ANTIMUSCARINIC effects. Rarely, heart rhythm disturbances, severe allergic reaction, skin disorders, noises in the ears, sensitivity to sunlight, confusion, depression, fits, shaking, sweating, muscle pain, pins and needles, liver disorders, hair loss, sleep disturbances.

in the elderly, pregnant women, mothers who are breastfeeding, and in patients with enlarged prostate, difficulty passing urine, glaucoma, epilepsy, or liver disease.

infants under 1 year or for patients with severe liver disease.

other sedating drugs, alcohol, antidepressants.

chlorpromazine tablets/liquid

A coated tablet or liquid used as a sedative to treat psychiatric disorders that require sedation, nausea, vomiting, persistent hiccups, and severe anxiety.

Strengths available: 10 mg, 25 mg, 50 mg, and 100 mg tablets; 25 mg/5 ml or 100 mg/5 ml liquid.
Dose: adults 25 mg three times a day at first increasing if necessary to a maximum of 1000 mg a day for psychiatric disorders or 200 mg a day for hiccups.
Availability: NHS and private prescription.
Contains: chlorpromazine hydrochloride.
Brand names: Largactil.

alcohol, sedatives, antidepressants, some antidiabetic drugs, anaesthetics, anti-epileptic medications, drugs affecting heart rhythm, ritonavir, halofantrine, sotalol, propranolol, lithium.

movement disorders, muscle spasms, restlessness, shaking, dry mouth, heart rhythm disturbance, low blood pressure, weight gain, blurred vision, impotence, low body temperature, breast swelling, menstrual changes, blood, liver, eye, and skin changes, drowsiness, apathy, nightmares, sleeplessness, depression, blocked nose, difficulty passing water. Rarely, fits.

in pregnant women, mothers who are breast-feeding, the elderly, and in patients suffering from heart, lung, or circulation disorders, epilepsy, Parkinson's disease, thyroid disorders, infections, MYASTHENIA GRAVIS, kidney or liver disease, glaucoma, enlarged prostate, or some blood disorders. Should be withdrawn gradually.

unconscious patients, or for those suffering from severe kidney or liver impairment, bone marrow depression, or PHAEOCHROMOCYTOMA.

chlorpropamide tablets

A tablet used as an antidiabetic to treat diabetes.

Strengths available: 100 mg and 250 mg tablets.
Dose: adults 250 mg (elderly 100-125 mg) a day with breakfast, adjusted to a maximum of 500 mg a day if needed.
Availability: NHS and private prescription.
Contains: chlorpropamide.

ACE-INHIBITORS, alcohol, anabolic STEROIDS, NON-STEROIDAL ANTI-INFLAMMATORY DRUGS, some ANTIBIOTICS, ANTICOAGULANTS, MAOIS, fluconazole, miconazole, some tranquillizers, BETA-BLOCKERS, nifedipine, CORTICOSTEROIDS, DIURETICS, some drugs used to lower blood cholesterol or lipids, lithium, oral contraceptives, testosterone, cimetidine, sulphinpyrazone.

allergy (including skin rash, fever, and jaundice), stomach upset, headache, flushed face after drinking alcohol, low sodium levels. Rarely, blood disorders.

in the elderly (best avoided) and in patients suffering from kidney or liver disorders.

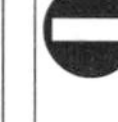
children, pregnant women, mothers who are breastfeeding, during surgery, or for patients suffering from juvenile diabetes, hormone disorders, stress, infections, PORPHYRIA, severe illness, or severe liver or kidney disorders.

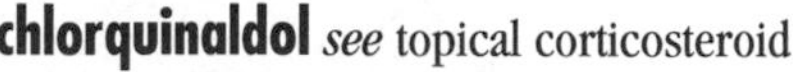
chlorquinaldol *see* topical corticosteroid

chlortalidone *see* chlorthalidone (alternative name)

---

chlortetracycline *see* chlortetracycline ointment/eye ointment, Deteclo

---

chlortetracycline ointment/eye ointment

An ointment and eye ointment used as an ANTIBIOTIC to treat eye and skin infections.

Strengths available: 3% ointment, 1% eye ointment.
Dose: apply the eye ointment into the affected eye(s) when required (3-4 times a day), and the skin ointment to the skin 1-3 times a day.
Availability: NHS and private prescription.
Contains: chlortetracycline hydrochloride.
Brand names: Aureomycin.
Compound preparations: Aureocort (*see* topical corticosteroid).

additional infection.

children, women in the last half of pregnancy, or for mothers who are breastfeeding.

---

chlorthalidone tablets

A tablet used as a DIURETIC to treat high blood pressure, heart failure, diabetes insipidus, and fluid retention.

Strengths available: 50 mg tablets.
Dose: for fluid retention, up to 50 mg a day (for short periods); for high blood pressure, 25-50 mg in the morning; for heart failure 25-200 mg in the morning; diabetes insipidus, 100 mg twice a day at first, reduced to 50 mg once a day for maintenance.
Contains: chlorthalidone (chlortalidone).
Brand names: Hygroton.
Compound preparations: co-tenidone, Kalspare.

low blood pressure on standing, mild stomach upset, reversible impotence, gout, inflamed pancreas, liver disorders, low potassium levels and other blood changes, allergy, rash, sensitivity to light, or tiredness.

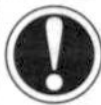

in pregnant women, mothers who are breastfeeding, the elderly, and in patients suffering from liver or kidney disorders, diabetes, gout, LUPUS.

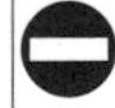

patients suffering from severe kidney or liver disorders, Addison's disease, raised blood calcium/uric acid levels, low blood potassium/sodium levels, or PORPHYRIA.

NON-STEROIDAL ANTI-INFLAMMATORY DRUGS, drugs that alter heart rhythm, antidiabetics, carbamazepine, halofantrine, pimozide, digoxin, lithium, ANTIHYPERTENSIVES.

---

cholecalciferol *see* calcium and vitamin D tablets

C

cholestyramine sachets

A powder in a sachet used as a lipid-lowering agent to treat raised cholesterol and to relieve some cases of diarrhoea and itching.

Strengths available: 4 g sachets.
Dose: adults, usually 1-6 sachets a day in divided doses according to condition (maximum 9 sachets a day). Children over 6 years, reduced doses according to age and weight.
Availability: NHS and private prescription.
Contains: anhydrous cholestyramine (colestyramine).
Brand names: Questran, Questran Light (low-sugar product).

 stomach upset, increased risk of bleeding and vitamin K deficiency with long-term use.

 in pregnant women and mothers who are breastfeeding. Patients on long-term therapy may need additional VITAMIN A, D, and K supplements.

 children under 6 years or for patients suffering from complete bile duct blockage.

 ANTICOAGULANTS. All other medications should be taken either 1 hour before or 4-6 hours after cholestyramine.

---

choline *see* Ketovite

---

choline salicylate *see* Audax, choline salicylate dental gel

---

choline salicylate dental gel

A gel applied to the mouth to relieve mouth ulcers, cold sores, mouth discomfort caused by dentures, and teething in infants.

Strengths available: 8.7% gel.
Dose: applied every 3 hours if necessary (maximum of 6 times a day). Adults use 1 cm of gel (children 0.5 cm).
Availability: NHS and private prescription.
Contains: choline salicylate.
Brand names: Bonjela.

 frequent application not advised because salicylate may be absorbed.

children under 4 months.

Choragon *see* chorionic gonadotrophin injection (Ferring Pharmaceuticals)

---

chorionic gonadotrophin injection

An injection used as a sex hormone to encourage testicles to descend in males, and to treat infertility through failure of ovulation in women, and underdeveloped sexual organs in men. Also used to stimulate the ovaries for *in vitro* fertilization.

Strengths available: 1500 unit, 2000 unit, 5000 unit, or 10,000 unit injections.
Dose: as advised by doctor.
Availability: NHS and private prescription.
Contains: human chorionic gonadotrophin (HCG).
Brand names: Choragon, Pregnyl, Profasi.

 children or for patients with some hormone-dependent tumours.

 fluid retention, headache, tiredness, over-stimulation of ovaries, multiple pregnancies, mood changes, breast swelling, skin reactions around injection site.

 in patients with heart or kidney disorders, epilepsy, migraine, asthma. Patients with hormone disorders should be treated before using this drug.

Cicatrin *see* also neomycin cream BPC
(GlaxoWellcome UK)

Dose: used up to three times a day for up to 3 weeks (cream) or 4 weeks (powder). Treatment must not be repeated within 3 months.
Contains: neomycin, bacitracin zinc, cysteine, glycine, threonine.

---

ciclosporin *see* cyclosporin (alternative name)

---

cilazapril tablets

A tablet used as an ACE-INHIBITOR to treat high blood pressure and (in addition to other treatments) heart failure.

Strengths available: 0.5 mg, 1 mg, 2.5 mg, and 5 mg tablets.
Dose: for high blood pressure, 1 mg once a day at first (0.5 mg for the elderly or patients with kidney/liver disorders) increasing to a maximum of 5 mg a day if necessary; for heart failure, 0.5 mg once a day at first (maximum 5 mg once a day).
Availability: NHS and private prescription.
Contains: cilazapril.
Brand names: Vascace.

rash, itching, sore throat, runny nose, stomach upset, cough, blood and liver changes, kidney disorders, low blood pressure, severe allergic reaction, inflamed pancreas. Occasionally, headache, dizziness, tiredness, taste disturbance, difficulty breathing, fever, pins and needles, muscle or joint pain, sensitivity to sunlight, inflamed membranes or blood vessels.

 in the elderly, mothers who are breastfeeding, and in patients suffering from kidney disease, auto-immune diseases (such as LUPUS), severe heart failure, or with a history of severe allergies, or in patients undergoing anaesthesia or dialysis. Your doctor may advise regular blood tests.

DIURETICS, anaesthetics, NON-STEROIDAL ANTI-INFLAMMATORY DRUGS, potassium supplements, cyclosporin, lithium, antidiabetics.

children, pregnant women, or for patients with some heart abnormalities, fluid in the abdomen, or disorders of the blood supply to the kidney. Not to be taken on the same day as dialysis.

Cilest tablets *see* oral contraceptive (combined)
(Janssen-Cilag)

Ciloxan *see* ciprofloxacin eye drops
(Alcon)

---

cimetidine syrup/tablets/effervescent tablets

A syrup, tablet, or effervescent tablet used as a HISTAMINE H_2-ANTAGONIST to treat stomach ulcers, hiatus hernia, indigestion, reflux of acid from the stomach into the oesophagus, and other conditions of excess acid in the stomach.

Strengths available: 200 mg/5 ml syrup; 200 mg, 400, mg and 800 mg tablets; 400 mg effervescent tablets.
Dose: adults 400-2400 mg a day depending on condition. (Children use lower doses according to age and weight.) Maintenance doses may be taken as a single daily dose (at night) but otherwise doses are usually divided (2-4 times a day).
Availability: NHS and private prescription. Low-dose tablet preparations available over the counter to treat adults for heartburn, dyspepsia, and excess stomach acid (short-term treatment only).
Contains: cimetidine.
Brand names: Acitak, Dyspamet, Galenamet, Peptimax, Tagamet, Ultec, Zita.

rash, tiredness, stomach upset, liver changes, dizziness, confusion, hair loss; rarely kidney, pancreas, bone marrow, joint, and muscle problems, headache, depression, altered bowel habit, heart rhythm disturbance, blood changes, impotence, breast swelling.

in pregnant women, mothers who are breast-feeding, middle-aged patients (or older), and in patients suffering from impaired liver or kidney function. Treatment may mask symptoms of stomach cancer.

drugs affecting heart rhythm, ANTICOAGULANTS, carbamazepine, phenytoin, sodium valproate, valproic acid, cyclosporin, theophylline, aminophylline, antidiabetics.

Cinazière 15 *see* cinnarizine tablets
(Ashbourne Pharmaceuticals)

C

cinchocaine ointment

An ointment used as a local anaesthetic and a treatment for haemorrhoids.

Dose: apply sparingly up to three times a day.
Availability: NHS and private prescription, over the counter.
Contains: cinchocaine.
Brand names: Nupercainal.
Compound preparations: various RECTAL CORTICOSTEROID products include cinchocaine.

---

cineole *see* Rowachol, Rowatinex

---

cinnarizine capsules/tablets

A tablet or capsule used as an ANTIHISTAMINE treatment for ear disorders such as vertigo, tinnitus, Ménière's disease, travel sickness, and for blood vessel disorders such as Raynaud's syndrome.

Strengths available: 15 mg tablets; 75 mg capsules.
Dose: adults, for ear disorders 30 mg three times a day; for travel sickness, 30 mg 2 hours before journey then 15 mg every 8 hours during the journey; for blood vessel disorders, 75 mg 2-3 times a day. Children aged 5-12 years may use half adult dose for travel sickness.
Availability: NHS and private prescription, over the counter.
Contains: cinnarizine.
Brand names: Cinazière, Stugeron, Stugeron Forte.

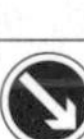 drowsiness, reduced reactions. Rarely, dizziness, excitation, movement disorders, headache, ANTIMUSCARINIC effects. Rarely heart rhythm disturbances, severe allergic reactions, skin disorders, noises in the ears, sensitivity to sunlight, Parkinson-like symptoms, confusion, depression, fits, shaking, sweating, muscle pain, pins and needles, liver disorders, hair loss, sleep disturbances.

 in the elderly, pregnant women, mothers who are breastfeeding, and in patients with enlarged prostate, low blood pressure, difficulty passing urine, Parkinson's disease, glaucoma, PORPHYRIA, epilepsy, or liver disease.

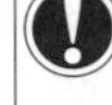 MAOIS, TRICYCLIC ANTIDEPRESSANTS, ritonavir, alcohol, other sedating drugs.

 children under 5 years.

Cinobac *see* cinoxacin capsules
(Eli Lilly and Co.)

---

cinoxacin capsules

A capsule used as a quinolone ANTIBIOTIC to treat infections of the urinary tract,

Strengths available: 500 mg capsules.
Dose: adults, 500 mg twice a day for 7-14 days. (For prevention of infection 500 mg at night.)

Availability: NHS and private prescription.
Contains: cinoxacin.
Brand names: Cinobac.

 children or for patients suffering from severe kidney disease.

 ANTICOAGULANTS, theophylline, aminophylline, cyclosporin, NON-STEROIDAL ANTI-INFLAMMATORY DRUGS, alcohol, sedating drugs.

 allergy, stomach upset, headache, dizziness, sleep disorders, skin disorders. Rarely, loss of appetite, blood changes, drowsiness, fits, confusion, depression, hallucinations, pins and needles, sensitivity to light, muscle and joint pain, disturbance of the senses, liver and kidney disorders.

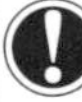 in pregnant women, mothers who are breast-feeding, and in patients suffering from kidney disease or with a history of epilepsy or liver disorders. Avoid excessive exposure to sunlight.

C

Cipramil *see* citalopram drops/tablets
(Lundbeck)

ciprofibrate tablets

A tablet used to treat high blood lipid levels which cannot be controlled by diet alone.

Strengths available: 100 mg tablets.
Dose: 100 mg each day.
Availability: NHS and private prescription.
Contains: ciprofibrate.
Brand names: Modalim.

 children, pregnant women, mothers who are breastfeeding, or for patients suffering from severe kidney or liver disease or gall-bladder disorders.

 stomach upset, muscle aches, rash, itching, headache, tiredness, vertigo, dizziness, hair loss. Rarely, blood changes or impotence.

 in patients with underactive thyroid, or kidney/liver disease. Your doctor may advise change of diet or lifestyle.

 ANTICOAGULANTS, antidiabetic drugs, other drugs used to reduce cholesterol.

ciprofloxacin eye drops

Eye drops used as an ANTIBIOTIC to treat superficial infections of the eye and surrounding areas, and ulcers on the cornea.

Strengths available: 0.3% drops.
Dose: for ulcerated cornea, 2 drops into the affected eye(s) every 15 minutes for 6 hours then every 30 minutes for the rest of the day, then 2 drops every hour on day 2, and 2 drops every 4 hours thereafter (total treatment

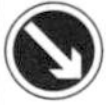 irritation, crusting of eyelids, staining or red-dening of eye, swollen eyelids, skin rash (stop treatment), bitter taste in mouth, nausea, disturbance of vision, sensitivity of eyes to light.

 in pregnant women and mothers who are breastfeeding.

cont.

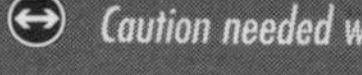

time 14-21 days); for eye infections, 1-2 drops four times a day (may be increased to 1-2 drops every 2 waking hours for the first 2 days if severe). Children over 1 year use same dose as adults.

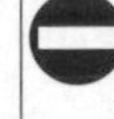
children under 1 year or for patients who wear soft contact lenses. Not to be used for more than 21 days.

Availability: NHS and private prescription.
Contains: ciprofloxacin hydrochloride.
Brand names: Ciloxan.

---

ciprofloxacin suspension/tablets

A tablet or suspension used as a quinolone ANTIBIOTIC to treat infections of the ear, nose, throat, urinary system, eyes, chest, skin, soft tissues, bone joints, stomach, and some venereal diseases.

Strengths available: 100 mg, 250 mg, and 500 mg tablets; 250 mg/5 ml suspension.
Dose: adults usually 250-750 mg twice a day. (For simple urine infections in women, 100 mg twice a day.)
Availability: NHS and private prescription.
Contains: ciprofloxacin hydrochloride.
Brand names: Ciproxin.

allergy, stomach upset, headache, dizziness, sleep disorders, skin disorders. Rarely, loss of appetite, difficulty swallowing, shaking, blood changes, drowsiness, fits, confusion, depression, hallucinations, pins and needles, sensitivity to light, muscle and joint pain, inflamed blood vessels, distortion of the senses, liver and kidney disorders, altered heart rhythm.

in patients suffering from kidney disease or with a history of epilepsy or nervous system disorders. Avoid excessive exposure to sunlight. Patients should drink plenty of fluids. Report any pain or inflammation in the limbs to your doctor.

pregnant women, mothers who are breastfeeding, or for children (except in exceptional circumstances).

ANTICOAGULANTS, theophylline, aminophylline, cyclosporin, NON-STEROIDAL ANTI-INFLAMMATORY DRUGS, glibenclamide, phenytoin, alcohol, sedating drugs.

Ciproxin *see* ciprofloxacin suspension/tablets
(Bayer Pharma Business Group)

---

citalopram drops/tablets

Drops or a tablet used as an antidepressant to treat depression and panic disorders.

Strengths available: 40 mg/ml drops, 10 mg, 20 mg, or 40 mg tablets.
Dose: adults 10-20 mg a day at first, increasing to maximum of 60 mg if necessary (elderly maximum 40 mg).
Availability: NHS and private prescription.
Contains: citalopram hydrobromide.
Brand names: Cipramil.

stomach upset, change in appetite and weight, dry mouth, nervousness, drowsiness, sweating, shaking, headache, sleeplessness, dizziness, weakness, fits, change in sexual function, movement disorders, low blood sodium levels, psychiatric disorders, heart rhythm disturbances, low blood pressure on standing, coughing, yawning, concentration and memory loss, migraine, pins and needles, vision or taste disturbances, noises in the ears, runny nose, disorders of passing urine.

in pregnant women, mothers who are breast-feeding, and in patients with epilepsy, liver or kidney disorders, or a history of heart disease, blood clotting disorders, or some psychiatric conditions. Treatment should be withdrawn slowly.

children or for patients with elevated mood.

ANTICOAGULANTS, other antidepressants, anti-epileptic treatments, ritonavir, sumatriptan, lithium, alcohol, sedatives.

C

Citramag *see* magnesium citrate powder
(Bioglan Laboratories)

---

citric acid *see* magnesium citrate powder, Mictral, oral rehydration solution, potassium citrate mixture BP, simple linctus/paediatric linctus, sodium citrate enema

---

clarithromycin *see* clarithromycin tablets/modified-release tablets/sachets/suspension, Heliclear

---

clarithromycin tablets/modified-release tablets/sachets/suspension

A tablet, M-R TABLET, sachet, or suspension used as an antibiotic to treat infections of the chest, skin, soft tissues, middle ear, and as an additional treatment for infection in patients with stomach ulcer (*see H. pylori* eradication).

Strengths available: 250 mg tablets; 500 mg m-r tablets; 125 mg/5 ml and 250 mg/5 ml suspension; 250 mg sachets.
Dose: adults 250 mg twice a day for 7 days using standard tablets or suspension, or 500 mg once a day using m-r tablets (doubled in severe infections); children up to 250 mg twice a day depending on age and weight.
Availability: NHS and private prescription.
Contains: clarithromycin.
Brand names: Klaricid.
Compound preparations: Heliclear (*see H. pylori* eradication).

stomach upset, liver changes, rash, dizziness, vertigo, headache. Rarely, low blood sugar, smell and taste disturbance, mouth disorders, hearing disorders, muscle and joint pain, severe skin disorder, liver and heart disturbances, anxiety, sleeplessness, psychiatric disorders.

in pregnant women, mothers who are breast-feeding, and in patients with kidney or liver damage, PORPHYRIA, or who have heart rhythm abnormalities.

drugs altering heart rhythm, rifabutin, ANTICOAGULANTS, reboxetine, digoxin, carbamazepine, mizolastine, antiviral treatments, tacrolimus, theophylline, aminophylline, phenytoin, cyclosporin, pimozide, ergotamine, ANTACIDS.

Clarityn *see* loratadine syrup/tablets
(Schering-Plough)

clavulanic acid *see* co-amoxiclav tablets/suspension

C

Cleanlet Fine Lancets

(Gainor Medical Europe)

Diabetics who need to test their blood regularly can use lancets to pierce the skin, either with or without the use of a finger-pricking device.

Lancet width and length: 28G/0.36 mm (Type A).
Availability: NHS and private prescription, over the counter.
Compatible finger-pricking devices: Autoclix, Autolet Mini, B-D Lancer 5, Glucolet, Hypolance, Microlet, Penlet II Plus, Soft Touch. (Autolet II, Autolet Lite, and Autolet Lite Clinisafe also compatible but not recommended by manufacturers.)

clemastine tablets/elixir

A tablet or elixir used as an ANTIHISTAMINE treatment for symptoms of allergies such as hayfever and nettle rash.

Strengths available: 1 mg tablets; 0.5 mg/5 ml elixir.
Dose: adults, 1 mg night and morning; children, 0.25-1 mg night and morning according to age and weight.
Availability: NHS and private prescription, over the counter.
Contains: clemastine hydrogen fumarate.
Brand names: Tavegil. (Other brands available over the counter but not on NHS prescription.)

drowsiness, reduced reactions, dizziness, excitation, movement disorders, headache, ANTIMUSCARINIC effects. Rarely, heart rhythm disturbances, severe allergic reaction, skin disorders, noises in the ears, sensitivity to sunlight, confusion, depression, fits, shaking, sweating, muscle pain, pins and needles, liver disorders, hair loss, sleep disturbances.

in the elderly, pregnant women, mothers who are breastfeeding, and in patients with enlarged prostate, difficulty passing urine, glaucoma, epilepsy, liver disease, or stomach/intestinal blockage.

infants under 1 year or for patients with severe liver disease.

other sedating drugs, alcohol, antidepressants.

Climagest *see* hormone replacement therapy (combined)
(Novartis Pharmaceuticals UK)

Climaval *see* hormone replacement therapy (oestrogen-only)
(Novartis Pharmaceuticals UK)

Climesse *see* hormone replacement therapy (combined)
(Novartis Pharmaceuticals UK)

clindamycin capsules

A capsule used as an ANTIBIOTIC to treat serious infections.

Strengths available: 75 mg and 150 mg capsules.
Dose: adults, 150-450 mg every 6 hours (children use reduced doses according to age and weight).
Availability: NHS and private prescription.
Contains: clindamycin hydrochloride.
Brand names: Dalacin-C.
Other preparations: clindamycin cream/lotion/solution.

 stomach upset, inflamed bowel, jaundice, blood disorders, skin reactions.

 in pregnant women, mothers who are breast-feeding, and in patients suffering from kidney or liver disease. Treatment should be stopped if diarrhoea develops.

 patients with diarrhoea or who are allergic to lincomycin.

clindamycin cream/lotion/solution

A cream (with applicators), water-based lotion, or alcoholic solution used as an ANTIBIOTIC to treat vaginal infection (with cream) or acne (with lotion/solution).

Strengths available: 2% vaginal cream; 1% lotion or solution.
Dose: for vaginal infection, 1 applicatorful of cream inserted into the vagina at night for 3-7 nights; for acne, the lotion or solution applied twice a day.
Availability: NHS and private prescription.
Contains: clindamycin phosphate.
Brand names: Dalacin, Dalacin T.
Other preparations: clindamycin capsules

 irritation, rash, dry skin. Rarely, stomach upset, inflamed bowel and diarrhoea (discontinue treatment if this occurs).

 in pregnant women and mothers who are breastfeeding. Keep out of eyes, mouth, and nose. Barrier contraceptives may not be effective with vaginal cream.

 patients allergic to lincomycin. Vaginal cream not to be used for children.

 barrier contraceptives (with vaginal cream), benzoyl peroxide (with lotion/solution).

Clinistix

(Bayer Diagnostics)

A plastic strip used for the detection of glucose in the urine. This gives an approximate estimate of blood glucose levels which may be adequate for the management of Type II diabetes.

Availability: NHS and private prescription, nurse prescription, over the counter.

Clinitar *see* coal tar cream/shampoo
(Cambridge Healthcare Supplies)

Clinitest

(Bayer Diagnostics)

A reagent tablet used for the detection of glucose and other substances in the urine. This gives an approximate estimate of blood glucose levels which may be adequate for the management of Type II diabetes.

Availability: NHS and private prescription, nurse prescription, over the counter.

Clinoril *see* sulindac tablets
(Merck Sharp and Dohme)

---

clioquinol *see* Locorten-Vioform, topical corticosteroids, Zinc paste clioquinol and calamine bandage BP 1993

---

clobazam tablets

A tablet used as a sedative to treat anxiety, tension, and agitation, and as an additional treatment for epilepsy.

Strengths available: 10 mg tablets.

Dose: adults, for anxiety 20-30 mg a day divided into three doses or as one dose at bedtime (higher doses used in hospital), and elderly patients use only up to 20 mg a day; for epilepsy 20-30 mg a day (maximum 60 mg a day). Children over 3 years may use up to half adult dose to treat epilepsy only.

drowsiness, light-headedness, confusion, vertigo, stomach disturbances, loss of memory, aggression, headache, joint immobility, salivation changes, shaking, unsteadiness, low blood pressure, rash, changes in vision, changes in sexual desire, retention of urine, incontinence, blood changes, jaundice. Risk of addiction increases with dose and length of treatment. May impair judgement.

Availability: private prescription (available on NHS prescription only if prescribed by generic name and to treat epilepsy).

Contains: clobazam.

Brand names: Frisium.

patients suffering from acute lung diseases, some chronic lung diseases, severe liver disease, MYASTHENIA GRAVIS, some obsessional and psychotic disorders, or who have stopped breathing while asleep.

in the elderly, pregnant women, mothers who are breastfeeding, women during labour, and in patients suffering from lung disorders, glaucoma, kidney or liver disorders, muscle weakness, PORPHYRIA, or with a history of drug or alcohol abuse. Avoid long-term use and withdraw gradually.

alcohol, other sedating drugs, some antivirals and anti-epileptic medications.

---

clobetasol *see* topical corticosteroid cream/ointment/scalp application

---

clobetasone *see* clobetasone eye drops, topical corticosteroid cream/ointment

---

clobetasone eye drops

Eye drops used as a CORTICOSTEROID to treat eye inflammation when no infection is present.

Strengths available: 0.1% drops.
Dose: 1-2 drops in the affected eye(s) four times a day (or every 1-2 hours in severe conditions).
Availability: NHS and private prescription.
Contains: clobetasone butyrate.
Brand names: Cloburate.

rise in eye pressure, thinning of cornea, cataract, eye infection.

avoid prolonged use in pregnant women or infants.

patients suffering from eye infections, glaucoma, corneal ulcer, or who wear soft contact lenses.

Cloburate *see* clobetasone eye drops
(Dominion Pharma)

---

clofazimine capsules

A capsule used as an anti-leprotic drug to treat leprosy.

Strengths available: 100 mg capsules.
Dose: as advised by doctor.
Availability: NHS and private prescription.
Contains: clofazimine.
Brand names: Lamprene.

skin, hair, faeces, and urine discoloration, dry skin or eyes, itching, upset stomach, headache, tiredness, sensitivity to light, skin reactions, loss of appetite and weight, eye disorders, high blood sugar, spleen and lymph gland disorders. May discolour soft contact lenses.

in pregnant women, mothers who are breastfeeding, and in patients with kidney or liver disease, diarrhoea, or abdominal pain.

C

clomethiazole *see* chlormethiazole (alternative name)

Clomid *see* clomiphene tablets
(Hoechst Marion Roussel)

clomifene *see* clomiphene (alternative name)

clomiphene tablets

A tablet used as an anti-oestrogen treatment for sterility caused by failure of ovulation.

Strengths available: 50 mg tablets.
Dose: 50 mg once a day for 5 days starting on the fifth day of the period. May be increased to 100 mg for second course of treatment. Not to be used for more than six cycles (three is usually sufficient).
Availability: NHS and private prescription.
Contains: clomiphene (clomifene) citrate.
Brand names: Clomid, Serophene.

overactive ovaries, hot flushes, uncomfortable abdomen, stomach upset, breast tenderness, headache, sleeplessness, abnormal menstrual bleeding, endometriosis, weight gain, fits, dizziness, rash, thinning hair, blurred vision.

in patients with ovarian cysts, ovary or uterus abnormalities. Pregnancy must be excluded before treatment begins.

children, pregnant women, or for patients suffering from liver disease, large ovarian cysts, womb cancer, or undiagnosed bleeding.

clomipramine capsules/modified-release tablets/syrup

A capsule, M-R TABLET, or syrup used as a TRICYCLIC ANTIDEPRESSANT to treat depression, obsessions, and phobias.

Strengths available: 10 mg, 25 mg, and 50 mg capsules; 75 mg m-r tablets; 25 mg/5 ml syrup.
Dose: adults, 10 mg a day at first for depression (25 mg for phobias and obsessions) increasing usually to 30-150 mg a day if needed. Up to 250 mg may be needed for depression. (Elderly patients maximum of 75 mg.) May be taken as a single dose at

dry mouth, noises in the ears, tiredness, constipation, difficulty passing urine, blurred vision, stomach upset, palpitations, drowsiness, sleeplessness, dizziness, shaking hands, low blood pressure, weight change, sweating, fever, confusion in the elderly, skin reactions, jaundice or blood changes, interference with sexual function, changes in heart rhythm, rash, hormone disturbances, fits, movement disorders, blood changes, breast changes in women, menstrual disorders.

in pregnant women, mothers who are breastfeeding, the elderly, or in patients suffering from heart disease, liver and kidney disorders, thyroid disease, PHAEOCHROMOCYTOMA, epilepsy, diabetes, PORPHYRIA, glaucoma, urine retention, constipation, some other psychiatric conditions. Your doctor may advise regular blood tests.

night or divided into several doses during the day.
Availability: NHS and private prescription.
Contains: clomipramine hydrochloride.
Brand names: Anafranil.

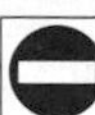
children or for patients suffering from recent heart attacks, heart rhythm abnormalities, severe liver disease, or elevated mood.

alcohol, sedatives, MAOIS, BARBITURATES, other antidepressants, ANTIHYPERTENSIVES, tranquillizers, anti-epileptic drugs, ritonavir, entacapone, selegiline, sotalol, methylphenidate, halofantrine, drugs affecting heart rhythm.

clonazepam tablets

A tablet used as an anticonvulsant to treat epilepsy.

Strengths available: 0.5 mg and 2 mg tablets.
Dose: adults, 1 mg (elderly 0.5 mg) at night for 4 nights then gradually increased to 4-8 mg a day in divided doses; children, 0.25 mg (under 5 years) or 0.5 mg (5-12 years) at first increasing to 0.5-1 mg (under 1 year), 1-3 mg (1-5 years), or 3-6 mg (5-12 years).
Availability: NHS and private prescription.
Contains: clonazepam.
Brand names: Rivotril.

drowsiness, dizziness, light-headedness, unsteadiness, aggression, irritability, psychological changes, muscle disorders, excess saliva in infants. Rarely, blood or liver disorders, May impair judgement.

in children, elderly or frail patients, pregnant women, mothers who are breastfeeding, and in patients suffering from breathing disorders, PORPHYRIA, kidney or liver disease. Treatment should be withdrawn slowly.

patients with reduced lung function.

alcohol, other sedating drugs, other anti-epileptic treatments.

clonidine tablets/modified-release capsules

A tablet or M-R CAPSULE used to treat high blood pressure and to prevent migraine, headache, or hot flushes in the menopause.

Strengths available: 25 mcg, 100 mcg, and 300 mcg tablets; 250 mcg m-r capsules.
Dose: for high blood pressure, using standard tablets 50-100 mcg three times a day increasing as needed to a maximum of 1200 mcg a day (or use 1-3 m-r capsules each day); for other conditions, 50 mcg twice a day increasing to 75 mcg twice a day if needed.

drowsiness, dry mouth, dizziness, upset stomach, rash, sleeplessness. With higher doses, fluid retention, depression, slow heart rate, Raynaud's disease, headache, and rarely impotence.

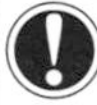
in mothers who are breastfeeding and in patients suffering from depression, Raynaud's disease, or poor circulation. Treatment with higher doses should be withdrawn slowly.

cont.

Availability: NHS and private prescription.
Contains: clonidine.
Brand names: Catapres, Dixarit.

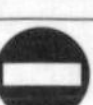 children, or for patients with PORPHYRIA.

 BETA-BLOCKERS, TRICYCLIC ANTIDEPRESSANTS, other medications used to treat high blood pressure, alcohol, sedatives.

clopamide *see* Viskaldix

clopidogrel tablets

A tablet used as an anti-platelet drug to prevent blood clots in patients with a history of blood clotting symptoms (such as stroke, heart attack, or narrowed blood vessels).

Strengths available: 75 mg tablets.
Dose: 75 mg once a day. Do not begin treatment until 7 days after stroke or a few days after heart attack.
Availability: NHS and private prescription.
Contains: clopidogrel hydrogen sulphate.
Brand names: Plavix.

 bleeding, stomach upset, stomach ulcers, liver disorders, headache, dizziness, rash and itching, blood changes, vertigo, pins and needles.

 in pregnant women and in patients with liver or kidney disease or at risk of bleeding. Report any unusual bleeding to your doctor.

 mothers who are breastfeeding, or for patients with abnormal bleeding, unstable angina, or who have undergone some types of heart surgery.

 warfarin, aspirin, NON-STEROIDAL ANTI-INFLAMMATORY DRUGS.

Clopixol *see* zuclopenthixol tablets
(Lundbeck)

Closteril *see* diclofenac modified-release tablets
(Pharmalife Healthcare Services)

Clostet *see* tetanus vaccine
(Medeva Pharma)

Clotam Rapid *see* tolfenamic acid tablets
(Provalis Healthcare)

clotrimazole cream/powder/solution/spray

A cream, powder, solution, and spray used as an antifungal treatment for fungal infections of the skin and outer ear.

Strengths available: 1% cream, powder, solution, and spray.

Dose: apply 2-3 times a day until 14 days after the infection has cleared. (The solution is used to treat outer ear infections.)

Availability: NHS and private prescription, over the counter. Cream also available on nurse prescription.

Contains: clotrimazole.

Brand names: Candiden, Canesten, Masnoderm. (Other brands marketed specifically for sale over the counter.)

Compound preparations: Canesten-HC and Lotriderm (*see* topical corticosteroids).

Other preparations: clotrimazole pessaries/vaginal cream/thrush cream.

Side effects: rarely, skin irritation or allergy.

---

clotrimazole pessaries/vaginal cream/thrush cream

A pessary or vaginal cream used as an antifungal treatment for fungal infections of the vagina, such as thrush.

Strengths available: 100 mg, 200 mg, and 500 mg pessaries; 2% thrush cream for application to external areas; 10% vaginal cream for internal use.

Dose: 1 pessary or 1 applicatorful of vaginal cream inserted into the vagina at night. (100 mg and 200 mg pessaries require repeat doses for a further five and two nights respectively.) The 2% cream may be applied to external areas twice a day (and to partner's penis).

Availability: NHS and private prescription, over the counter.

Contains: clotrimazole.

Brand names: Candiden, Canesten.

Compound preparations: Canesten HC (for skin conditions *see* topical corticosteroids).

Other preparations: clotrimazole cream/powder/spray/solution.

Side effects: rarely, irritation or allergy.

Caution: may cause damage to barrier contraceptives (condoms and diaphragms).

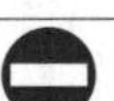

Not to be used for: children.

Caution needed with: barrier contraceptives (*see* above).

---

clozapine tablets

A tablet used as a sedative to treat schizophrenia.

Strengths available: 25 mg and 100 mg tablets.

Dose: 12.5-25 mg on first day increasing to a maximum of 900 mg a day. (Usual maintenance dose 150-300 mg a day in divided doses.)

cont.

Availability: NHS and private prescription.
Contains: clozapine.
Brand names: Clozaril.

 children, pregnant women, mothers who are breastfeeding, or for patients suffering from severe kidney or liver disease, bone marrow disorders, alcoholism, drug intoxication, uncontrolled epilepsy, drowsiness or reduced reactions, reduced activity of the nervous system, severe circulation problems, inactive bowel, heart failure, or for those in a coma or with a history of drug-induced blood disorder.

 in the elderly and in patients with a history of epilepsy, or suffering from enlarged prostate, heart or circulation disorders, Parkinson's disease, glaucoma, liver disease or intestinal abnormality. Report any symptoms of infection to your doctor. You will need regular blood tests.

 blood and skin changes, drowsiness, watering of the mouth or dry mouth, blurred vision, disturbed heart beat, tiredness, dizziness, headache, difficulty passing urine, incontinence, stomach upset, difficulty swallowing, liver disorders, temporary upset of automatic body functions, low blood pressure on standing, persistent painful erection, weight gain, increased blood sugar levels, fits, changes in temperature regulation, Parkinson-like shaking, inactive bowel, confusion, anxiety, agitation. Rarely, severe heart or breathing disorders, high blood pressure, inflamed pancreas, blood clots, enlarged glands, NEUROLEPTIC MALIGNANT SYNDROME.

 carbamazepine, some ANALGESICS and ANTIBIOTICS, other sedating drugs, alcohol, antidepressants, anti-epileptic treatments, halofantrine, ritonavir, lithium, other drugs which can cause blood disorders, drugs that affect heart rhythm.

Clozaril *see* clozapine tablets
(Novartis Pharmaceuticals UK)

---

co-amilofruse tablets *see* amiloride tablets and frusemide tablets

Strengths available: 2.5 mg + 20 mg, 5 mg + 40 mg, and 10 mg + 80 mg tablets.
Dose: 1 tablet each morning.
Brands: Froop-Co, Fru-Co, Frumil, Frumil Forte, Frumil LS, Lasoride.

---

co-amilozide tablets *see* amiloride tablets and hydrochlorothiazide tablets

Strengths available: 2.5 mg + 25 mg and 5 mg + 50 mg tablets.
Dose: for high blood pressure, up to 5 mg + 50 mg a day; for heart failure and fluid retention up to 2 x 5 mg + 50 mg a day.
Brands: Amil-Co, Amilmaxco, Moduret-25, Moduretic, Synuretic, Zida-Co.

---

co-amoxiclav tablets/dispersible tablets/suspension
A tablet, dispersible tablet, or suspension used as a penicillin antibiotic to treat infections.

Strengths available: 375 mg and 625 mg tablets; 375 mg dispersible tablets; 125/31 mg and 250/62 mg suspension for three times daily use; 400/57 mg suspension for twice daily use.
Dose: adults, 375 mg in tablet (or dispersible tablet) form three times a day, or one 625 mg

tablet three times a day for severe infections; children aged 1-6 years 5 ml of 125/31 suspension (aged 6-12 years 5 ml of 250/62 suspension) three times a day, or up to 10 ml of 400/57 suspension twice a day (according to age, weight, and severity of infection). Course of treatment should not exceed 14 days (or 5 days for dental infections).

Availability: NHS and private prescription.

Contains: amoxycillin trihydrate and clavulanic acid.

Brand names: Amiclav, Augmentin, Augmentin Duo.

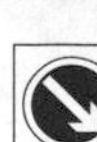 stomach upset, severe allergic reaction, liver disorders, skin reactions, inflamed blood vessels. Rarely, inflamed bowel, blood changes, dizziness, fits, headache. Teeth may be stained by suspension.

 in pregnant women and in patients suffering from glandular fever, kidney or liver disorder, leukaemia, HIV infection, and anyone with a history of allergies.

 patients who are allergic to penicillin or who have a history of jaundice or liver disorders after taking penicillin antibiotics.

 ORAL CONTRACEPTIVES (COMBINED), ANTICOAGULANTS, methotrexate.

---

co-beneldopa capsules/dispersible tablets/modified-release capsules *see also* levodopa tablets

A capsule, dispersible tablet, or M-R CAPSULE of levodopa combined with benserazide which enhances the action of the levodopa.

Strengths available: 62.5 mg, 125 mg, and 250 mg capsules; 62.5 mg and 125 mg dispersible tablets; 125 mg m-r capsules. (62.5 mg is equivalent to 50 mg levodopa, 125 mg to 100 mg levodopa, and 250 mg to 200 mg levodopa).

Dose: the equivalent of 50 mg levodopa 3-4 times a day at first increasing to a maximum of 800 mg levodopa equivalent a day in divided doses. M-r capsules used in same doses to give smoother response to symptoms (maximum total of 1200 mg levodopa equivalent).

Brands: Madopar, Madopar CR.

Co-Betaloc *see* metoprolol tablets and hydrochlorothiazide tablets

(Searle)

Dose: 1-3 tablets a day.

Long-acting preparations: Co-Betaloc SA (dose 1 tablet each day).

---

co-careldopa tablets *see also* levodopa tablets

A tablet or M-R TABLET of levodopa combined with carbidopa, which enhances the action of the levodopa.

Strengths available: 62.5 mg, 110 mg, 125 mg, and 275 mg tablets; 125 mg and 250 mg m-r tablets. (62.5 mg is equivalent to 50 mg levodopa, 110 mg and 125 mg to 100 mg levodopa, 250 mg and 275 mg to 250 mg levodopa).

Dose: the equivalent of 50-100 mg levodopa 3-4 times a day at first increasing to a maximum of 800 mg levodopa equivalent a day in divided doses. M-r tablets used to give smoother response to symptoms. (Dose adjusted according to response.)

Brands: Sinemet, Sinemet CR, Half Sinemet CR.

co-codamol capsules/sachets/tablets/effervescent tablets *see* codeine tablets and paracetamol tablets

Strengths available: 8 mg + 500 mg or 30 mg + 500 mg tablets, capsules, and effervescent tablets; 30 mg + 500 mg sachets.

Dose: as for paracetamol tablets. (30 mg strength not suitable for children.)

Availability: NHS and private prescription. Lower strength also available over the counter.

Brands: Kapake, Medocodene, Migraleve Yellow, Solpadol, Tylex, Zapain. Some additional brands of lower strength available over the counter but not on NHS.

Compound preparations: Migraleve Pink tablets.

co-codaprin tablets/dispersible tablets *see* aspirin 300 mg tablets and codeine tablets

Strengths available: 400 mg + 8 mg tablets or dispersible tablets.

Dose: adults 1-2 tablets every 4-6 hours (maximum of 8 a day). Not suitable for children.

co-cyprindiol tablets

A tablet used as an anti-androgen and oestrogen to treat severe acne and hairiness in women.

Strengths available: 2 mg + 35 mcg tablets.

Dose: 1 tablet a day (taken in sequence from the pack) for 21 days followed by 7 days without treatment. Treatment is withdrawn when condition clears, and repeated if it recurs.

Availability: NHS and private prescription.

Contains: cyproterone acetate and ethinyloestradiol.

Brand names: Dianette.

in women over 35 years, overweight or immobile patients, smokers, or those suffering from high blood pressure, diabetes, varicose veins or other blood vessel disorder, inflammatory bowel disorders, some blood disorders, sickle-cell anaemia, asthma, migraine, depression, kidney disease, multiple sclerosis, womb diseases. Your doctor may advise you not to smoke and to have regular examinations. You should stop treatment at the first sign of serious symptoms such as severe headache or jaundice. Treatment should be stopped 4 weeks before surgery. Depending on when you start the course, you may need additional (barrier) contraceptives for the first 7 days.

enlarged breasts, bloating and fluid retention, cramps, leg pains, mood change, reduction in sexual desire, headache, upset stomach, vaginal erosion, discharge and bleeding, jaundice, weight gain, skin changes, muscle twitches, raised blood pressure, liver disorder, altered menstrual pattern. Rarely, sensitivity to sunlight. Contact lenses may irritate. There is a slightly increased risk of blood clots (particularly with products containing gestodene or desogestrel) but this is still lower than the risk of blood clots during pregnancy. Also a slightly increased risk of breast cancer but this may be due to earlier diagnosis through regular examinations. Risk of womb and ovary cancer is decreased.

pregnant women, mothers who are breastfeeding, women over 50 years, patients with a history of heart disease or blood clots, or for those suffering from liver disorders, some cancers, severe migraine or migraine associated with visual disturbance, temporary blocking of blood vessels in the brain, PORPHYRIA, undiagnosed vaginal bleeding, or some ear, skin, and kidney disorders.

ACE-INHIBITORS, rifampicin, some other ANTIBIOTICS, anticoagulants, antidepressants, antidiabetics, some antifungal treatments, ANTIHYPERTENSIVES, modafinil, griseofulvin, BARBITURATES, phenytoin, primidone, carbamazepine, ethosuximide, chloral hydrate, celecoxib, cyclosporin, tretinoin, CORTICOSTEROIDS, tacrolimus, theophylline, aminophylline, lansoprazole, topiramate.

co-danthramer capsules/suspension

A suspension or capsule used as a laxative to treat constipation in terminally ill patients.

Strengths available: standard (25 + 200 mg) or strong (37.5 + 500 mg) capsules; standard (25 + 200 mg in 5 ml) or strong (75 + 1000 mg in 5 ml) suspension.

Dose: adults 1-2 capsules of either strength, or 5-10 ml of standard suspension, or 5 ml of strong suspension, taken at night. Children may use up to 5 ml of standard suspension.

Availability: NHS and private prescription, nurse prescription.

Contains: poloxamer 188 and danthron (dantron).

Brand names: Ailax, Ailax Forte, Danlax.

colouring of urine and skin around the anus. Skin irritation in incontinent patients.

in incontinent patients.

any patients other than those who are terminally ill.

co-danthrusate capsules/suspension

A suspension or capsule used as a laxative to treat constipation in terminally ill patients.

Strengths available: 50 + 60 mg capsules; 50 + 60 mg in 5 ml suspension.

Dose: adults 1-3 capsules or 5-15 ml suspension at night. Children over 6 years may use 1 capsule or 5 ml suspension.

Availability: NHS and private prescription, nurse prescription.

Contains: docusate sodium and danthron (dantron).

Brand names: Capsuvac, Normax (capsules not available on NHS prescription).

colouring of urine and skin around the anus. Skin irritation in incontinent patients.

in incontinent patients.

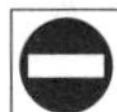

children under 6 years or for patients other than those who are terminally ill.

co-dergocrine tablets

A tablet used as an additional treatment for elderly patients suffering from dementia.

Strengths available: 1.5 mg and 4.5 mg tablets.
Dose: 1.5 mg three times a day or 4.5 mg once a day before meals.
Availability: NHS and private prescription.
Contains: co-dergocrine mesylate.
Brand names: Hydergine.

 headache, stomach upset, flushing, rash, blocked nose, dizziness, low blood pressure on standing.

 in patients suffering from slow heart rate.

 children.

co-dydramol tablets *see* dihydrocodeine tablets and paracetamol tablets

Strengths available: 20 mg + 500 mg or 30 mg + 500 mg tablets.
Availability: NHS and private prescription. (Lower strengths available over the counter.)
Dose: as for paracetamol tablets. Not suitable for children.
Brands: Remedeine, Remedeine Forte.

co-fluampicil capsules/syrup *see* ampicillin capsules and flucloxacillin capsules

A combination ANTIBIOTIC used particularly for skin infections.

Strengths available: 250 mg + 250 mg capsules; 125 mg + 125 mg in 5 ml syrup.
Dose: adults 1-2 capsules (children 5-10 ml syrup) every 6 hours, according to severity of infection.
Brands: Magnapen.

co-flumactone tablets *see* spironolactone tablets. (*See also* bendrofluazide tablets for side effects etc. of hydroflumethiazide.)

A combination DIURETIC used to treat heart failure.

Strengths available: 25 mg + 25 mg or 50 mg + 50 mg tablets (spironolactone with hydroflumethiazide).
Dose: 1-8 of the weaker tablets or 1-4 of the stronger tablets each day.
Brands: Aldactide.

co-methiamol tablets

A tablet used as an ANALGESIC, with antidote to protect against liver damage, used to treat pain or fever.

Strengths available: 100 mg + 500 mg tablets.
Dose: adults 2 tablets every 4 hours (up to 8 a day).
Availability: NHS and private prescription.
Contains: methionine and paracetamol.
Brand names: Paradote.

 rarely, rash, blood changes, inflamed pancreas, liver or kidney damage with overdose.

 in pregnant women, mothers who are breast-feeding, alcoholics, and in patients with liver or kidney disorders.

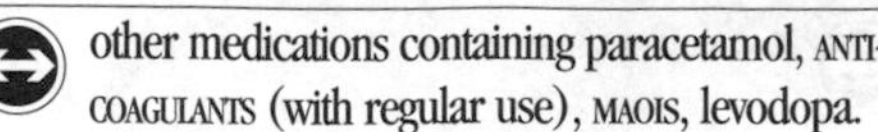
other medications containing paracetamol, ANTI-COAGULANTS (with regular use), MAOIS, levodopa.

children under 12 years.

co-phenotrope tablets

A tablet used to slow down intestinal contents and as an OPIOID and ANTIMUSCARINIC to treat diarrhoea.

Strengths available: 2.5 mg + 25 mcg tablets.
Dose: adults, 4 tablets a day at first then 2 every 6 hours; children 4-8 years, 1 tablet three times a day; children 9-12 years 1 tablet four times a day; children 13-16 years 2 tablets three times a day.
Availability: NHS and private prescription.
Contains: diphenoxylate hydrochloride, atropine sulphate.
Brand names: Lomotil, Tropergen.

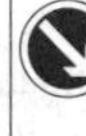
drowsiness, upset stomach (particularly constipation), antimuscarinic effects, sweating, dizziness, breathing difficulty, low blood pressure, difficulty passing urine, dry mouth, headache, vertigo, flushing, change in heart rhythm, mood changes, rash, itching, addiction, reduced sexual desire.

in pregnant women, women in labour, mothers who are breastfeeding, elderly or weakened patients, and in those suffering from breathing, kidney, or liver problems, dehydration, body fluid imbalance, low blood pressure, underactive thyroid, enlarged prostate or epilepsy. (Higher doses not suitable for some of these categories.)

children under 4 years, alcoholics, or patients with head injury, jaundice, inflamed bowel, or those at risk of non-functioning intestines.

MAOIS, alcohol, sedating drugs, ritonavir.

co-prenozide modified-release tablets *see* oxprenolol tablets and cyclopenthiazide tablets

Strengths available: 160 mg + 250 mcg tablets.
Dose: 1-2 tablets once a day.
Brands: Trasidrex.

co-proxamol tablets *see* dextropropoxyphene capsules and paracetamol tablets

Strengths available: 32.5 mg + 325 mg tablets.
Dose: adults 2 tablets 3-4 times a day. Not suitable for children.
Brands: Distalgesic (not available on NHS prescription).

co-simalcite suspension

A liquid used as an ANTACID and anti-wind preparation to treat wind, excess stomach acid, gastritis, indigestion, and stomach ulcers.

Strengths available: 125 mg + 500 mg in 5 ml suspension.
Dose: adults 10 ml (children aged 8-12 years 5 ml) between meals and at bedtime.

children under 8 years.

cont.

Availability: NHS and private prescription.
Contains: activated dimethicone, hydrotalcite.
Brand names: Altacite Plus.

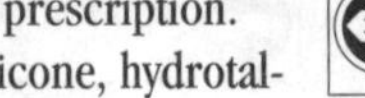
E-C TABLETS/CAPSULES.

co-tenidone tablets *see* atenolol tablets and chlorthalidone tablets

Strengths available: 100 + 25 mg or 50 + 12.5 mg tablets.
Dose: adults 1 tablet (of either strength) each day. (Not suitable for children.)
Brands: Atenixco, Tenchlor, Tenoretic, Tenoret-50.

co-triamterzide tablets *see* triamterene capsules and hydrochlorothiazide tablets

Strengths available: 50 mg + 25 mg tablets
Dose: 1-4 tablets a day.
Brands: Dyazide, TriamaxCo, Triam-Co.

co-trimoxazole suspension/tablets

A tablet or suspension used as an ANTIBIOTIC to treat some forms of pneumonia, rare bacterial infections, and parasitic infections. Also occasionally used to treat urine, chest, or ear infections if other antibiotics are not suitable.

Strengths available: 480 mg or 960 mg tablets; 480 mg or 240 mg in 5 ml suspension.
Dose: usually adults, 960 mg every 12 hours; children aged 6 weeks-5 months 120 mg every 12 hours, aged 6 months-5 years 240 mg every 12 hours, aged 6-12 years 480 mg every 12 hours.
Availability: NHS and private prescription.
Contains: trimethoprim, sulphamethoxazole (sulfamethoxazole).
Brand names: Chemotrim, Septrin.

upset stomach, mouth or tongue inflammation, rash, blood changes, folate (vitamin) deficiency. Rarely, skin changes, liver or pancreas disorders, inflamed bowel, headache, depression, kidney disorders, fits, lack of co-ordination, nerve inflammation or meningitis, vertigo, noises in the ears, muscle or joint pain, breathing disorders.

in the elderly, pregnant women, mothers who are breastfeeding, and in patients suffering from kidney disease, asthma, or sensitivity to light, Drink plenty of non-alcoholic fluids. Your doctor may advise regular blood tests during prolonged treatment.

infants under 6 weeks (except for pneumonia treatment) or for patients suffering from severe kidney or liver disease, PORPHYRIA, or blood disorders.

amiodarone, ANTICOAGULANTS, some antidiabetic drugs, phenytoin, pyrimethamine, cyclosporin, azathioprine, methotrexate.

C

co-zidocapt tablets *see* hydrochlorothiazide tablets and captopril tablets
A combination product used to simplify treatment when patients are stabilized on the two ingredients in the same proportions.

Strengths available: 12.5 mg + 25 mg or 25 mg + 50 mg tablets.
Brands: Acezide, Capozide, Capto-Co.

---

coal tar cream/gel/lotion/paste/shampoo/solution
A cream, gel, lotion, paste, shampoo, or solution used to treat chronic eczema, psoriasis, and scaly scalp disorders.

Dose: usually applied 1-3 times a day starting with lower-strength preparations. (See individual product labels for precise details.)
Availability: NHS and private prescription, over the counter.
Contains: coal tar solution or extract.
Brand names: Alphosyl shampoo, Carbo-Dome, Clinitar, Exorex, Gelcotar, Pentrax, Polytar, Psoriderm bath emulsion, T-Gel.
Compound preparations: with salicylic acid, Capasal (also contains coconut oil), coal tar and salicylic acid ointment BP, Cocois (also contains sulphur), Gelcosal, Ionil T (also contains benzal-konium chloride), Pragmatar (also contains sulphur), Psorin; with allantoin, Alphosyl cream and lotion; with emollients, Polytar emollient (also contains arachis or peanut oil); with hydrolysed animal protein, Polytar Plus (also contains arachis or peanut oil); with zinc pyrithione, Polytar AF (also contains arachis or peanut oil); with lecithin, Psoriderm cream/lotion; with TOPICAL CORTICOSTEROIDS, Alphosyl HC; with menthol, Denorex; with zinc oxide, zinc and coal tar paste BP, zinc paste and coal tar bandage.

irritation, acne-like skin eruptions, sensitivity to light. Stains skin, hair, and clothing.

avoid the eyes, mucous membranes, genital and rectal areas. Some Polytar products contain arachis (peanut) oil – not suitable for patients with peanut allergy.

areas of broken, infected, or inflamed skin.

---

coal tar and salicylic acid ointment BP *see* coal tar ointment and salicylic acid ointment

---

Cobalin-H *see* hydroxocobalamin injection
(Link Pharmaceuticals)

Cocois *see* coal tar ointment
(Medeva Pharma)

---

coconut oil *see* Capasal, emollient preparations

C

Codafen *see* ibuprofen modified-release tablets and codeine tablets
(Napp Pharmaceuticals)

Strengths available: 300 mg + 20 mg M-R TABLETS.
Dose: adults usually 1-2 (maximum 3) tablets every 12 hours.

codeine tablets/syrup

A tablet or syrup used as an OPIOID ANALGESIC to treat pain and diarrhoea.

Strengths available: 15 mg and 30 mg tablets; 25 mg/5 ml syrup.
Dose: 30-60 mg every 4 hours when needed (maximum of 2400 mg a day). Children use reduced doses according to age and weight.
Availability: NHS and private prescription.
Contains: codeine phosphate.
Compound preparations: co-codamol, co-codaprin, Codafen, Diarrest, Kaodene, Migraleve.

 drowsiness, upset stomach (particularly constipation), sweating, dizziness, breathing difficulty, low blood pressure, difficulty passing urine, dry mouth, headache, vertigo, flushing, change in heart rhythm, mood changes, rash, itching, addiction, reduced sexual desire.

 in pregnant women, women in labour, mothers who are breastfeeding, elderly or weakened patients, and in those suffering from breathing, kidney, or liver problems, low blood pressure, underactive thyroid, enlarged prostate or epilepsy. (Higher doses not suitable for some of these categories.)

 MAOIS, alcohol, sedating drugs, ritonavir.

 children under 1 year (for pain) or 4 years (for diarrhoea), alcoholics, or for patients with head injury, reduced breathing ability, or at risk of non-functioning intestines.

codeine linctus/paediatric linctus

A linctus used as an OPIOID cough suppressant to treat dry coughs. (Sugar-free versions available for diabetics.)

Strengths available: 15 mg/5 ml linctus; 3 mg/5 ml paediatric linctus.
Dose: adults, 5-10 ml standard linctus; children aged 5-12 years 2.5-5 ml standard linctus; children aged 1-5 years 5 ml paediatric linctus – all doses taken 3-4 times a day.
Availability: NHS and private prescription. Also available over the counter if the dose does not exceed 15 mg.
Contains: codeine phosphate.
Brand names: Galcodine.

 constipation. Rarely, difficulty breathing with large doses.

 in patients with asthma, kidney disorders, or a history of drug addiction.

 infants under 1 year or for patients suffering from liver disease or breathing difficulties.

 MAOIS, alcohol, sedating drugs, ritonavir.

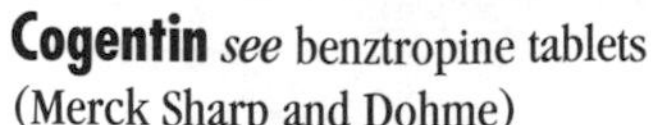

Cogentin *see* benztropine tablets
(Merck Sharp and Dohme)

Colazide *see* balsalazide capsules
(Shire Pharmaceuticals)

---

colchicine tablets

A tablet used to treat gout or to prevent attacks while other therapy is initiated.

Strengths available: 0.5 mg tablets.
Dose: 1 mg at first then 0.5 mg every 2-3 hours until relief is obtained or until vomiting/diarrhoea occurs or until a total of 6 mg (12 tablets) has been taken. The course should not be repeated within 3 days. To prevent attacks, 0.5 mg 2-3 times a day.
Availability: NHS and private prescription.
Contains: colchicine.

 upset stomach, abdominal pain, bleeding in the stomach or intestine, rash, kidney and liver damage, hair loss, blood disorders, nerve inflammation, muscle disorders.

 in elderly patients and in patients suffering from stomach, intestinal, liver, heart, or kidney disorders.

 children, pregnant women, mothers who are breastfeeding.

 cyclosporin.

---

colecalciferol *see* cholecalciferol (alternative name)

Colestid *see* colestipol sachets
(Pharmacia and Upjohn)

---

colestipol sachets

Granules in a sachet used as a lipid-lowering agent to treat raised lipid levels.

 stomach upset, increased risk of bleeding and vitamin K deficiency with long-term use.

Strengths available: 5 g sachets.
Dose: adults, 5-30 g in liquid each day (in one single dose or divided into two doses). Children as advised by doctor.
Availability: NHS and private prescription.
Contains: colestipol hydrochloride.
Brand names: Colestid.

 in pregnant women and mothers who are breastfeeding. Patients on long-term therapy may need additional VITAMIN A, D, E, and K supplements.

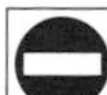 ANTICOAGULANTS. All other medications should be taken either 1 hour before or 4-6 hours after colestipol.

---

colestyramine *see* cholestyramine (alternative name)

Colifoam *see* corticosteroid enema/internal foam
(Stafford-Miller)

---

colistimethate sodium *see* colistin (alternative name)

---

colistin tablets/syrup/injection (for inhalation)

A tablet, syrup, or injection (for inhalation) used as an ANTIBIOTIC to treat some stomach infections and to prepare the bowel before surgery.

Strengths available: 1.5 million unit tablets; 250,000 units/5 ml syrup; 1 million or 500,000 unit injection.
Dose: by mouth, adults 1-2 tablets (children 5-30 ml syrup according to age) every 8 hours. By inhalation, dose determined by doctor and administered via a nebulizer.
Availability: NHS and private prescription.
Contains: colistin sulphate (tablets and syrup), colistin sulphomethate (or colistimethate) sodium (injection for inhalation).
Brand names: Colomycin.

 pins and needles, vertigo, breathing difficulty, kidney damage, muscle weakness. Rarely, changes in blood vessels, slurred speech, visual or mental disturbances.

 in patients suffering from kidney disorder or PORPHYRIA.

 pregnant women, mothers who are breast-feeding, or for patients suffering from MYASTHENIA GRAVIS.

---

colloidal oatmeal *see* emollient preparations

---

colloidal silica *see* alginate sachets

Colofac/Colofac MR *see* mebeverine tablets/modified-release tablets
(Solvay Healthcare)

Colomycin *see* colistin syrup/tablets
(Pharmax)

Colpermin *see* peppermint oil enteric-coated capsules
(Pharmacia and Upjohn)

Combivent *see* ipratropium inhaler and salbutamol inhaler
(Boehringer Ingelheim)

Strengths available: 20 mcg + 100 mcg per dose.
Dose: adults 2 puffs four times a day. Not suitable for children.
Other products: Combivent nebulizer solution (additional possible side effect of glaucoma with nebulized product).

Combivir *see* lamivudine tablets and zidovudine tablets
(GlaxoWellcome UK)
Used as combination treatment for HIV infection.

Strengths available: 150 mg + 300 mg tablets.
Dose: adults 1 tablet twice a day. Not suitable for children.

Comtess *see* entacapone tablets
(Orion Pharma (UK))

Condyline *see* podophyllotoxin solution
(Ardern Healthcare)

---

conjugated oestrogen *see* hormone replacement therapy (oestrogen-only), hormone replacement therapy – topical

---

Conotrane
(Yamanouchi Pharma)
A cream used as an antiseptic and barrier preparation to protect the skin from water, nappy rash, and bed sores.

Dose: apply several times a day or after every nappy change.
Availability: NHS and private prescription, nurse prescription, over the counter.
Contains: benzalkonium chloride, dimethicone.

Contimin *see* oxybutynin tablets
(Berk Pharmaceuticals)

---

contraceptive pill *see* oral contraceptives

C

Convulex *see* sodium valproate/valproic acid tablets/modified-release tablets/syrup/liquid
(Pharmacia and Upjohn)

---

copper acetate *see* Cuplex

Coracten SR/XL *see* nifedipine modified-release capsules
(Medeva Pharma)

Cordarone X *see* amiodarone tablets
(Sanofi Winthrop)

Cordilox *see* verapamil tablets/modified-release tablets
(Norton Healthcare)

Corgard *see* nadolol tablets
(Sanofi Winthrop)

Corgaretic *see* nadolol tablets and bendrofluazide tablets
(Sanofi Winthrop)

Strengths available: 40 mg + 5 mg or 80 mg + 5 mg tablets.
Dose: 1-2 tablets (of either strength) a day.

Corlan *see* hydrocortisone pellets
(Medeva Pharma)

Coro-Nitro *see* glyceryl trinitrate spray
(Roche Products)

Corsodyl *see* chlorhexidine dental gel/mouthwash/spray
(SmithKline Beecham Consumer Healthcare UK)

---

corticosteroid *see* corticosteroid enema/internal foam, corticosteroid nasal drops/spray, steroid, topical corticosteroid, rectal corticosteroid. *See also* page 606

---

corticosteroid enema/internal foam

An enema or foam used as a CORTICOSTEROID applied internally into the rectum to treat ulcerative colitis and other internal inflammatory conditions of the intestines.

Dose: (*see* table below).
Availability: NHS and private prescription.
Contains: (*see* table below).

 corticosteroid effects, *see* prednisolone tablets.

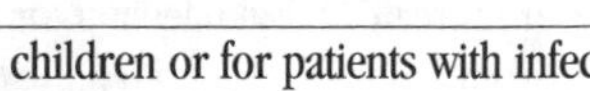 children or for patients with infected conditions, perforated or obstructed bowel.

 in pregnant women. Not for prolonged use.

Product	*Ingredient*	*Dose*
Colifoam aerosol	hydrocortisone	one application made into the rectum once or twice a day for 2-3 weeks, then once a day on alternate days.
Entocort enema	budesonide	1 enema inserted into the rectum at bedtime for 4 weeks.
Predenema	prednisolone	1 enema inserted into the rectum at bedtime for 2-4 weeks. (May be continued if good response.)
Predfoam	prednisolone	one dose applied into the rectum once or twice a day for 2 weeks. (May be continued for another 2 weeks if good response.)
Predsol Retention Enema	prednisolone	1 enema inserted into the rectum at bedtime for 2-4 weeks. (May be continued if good response.)
Predsol Suppositories*	prednisolone	1 suppository inserted into the rectum twice a day after bowel movement.

**used to treat complications of Crohn's disease.*

corticosteroid nasal drops/spray

Nasal drops or spray used as a CORTICOSTEROID to prevent and treat inflamed nasal passages and hayfever. (Some products also used to treat nasal polyps.)

Dose: (*see* table below). Must be used continuously for maximum effect.
Availability: NHS and private prescription. Some brands also available over the counter (marked * in table) only for the treatment of hayfever in adults over 18 years

 dryness and irritation of the nose and throat, nose bleeds, disturbance of taste and smell. Rarely, ulceration, glaucoma, and allergic reaction (severe allergy occasionally from budesonide). High doses may give rise to general corticosteroid side effects (*see* prednisolone tablets)

cont.

and for a maximum of 3 months.

Contains: (*see table below*).

Compound preparations: Betnesol-N and Vista-Methasone-N (both with neomycin for infected conditions – not to be used for more than 7 days without improvement); Dexa-Rhinaspray Duo (with tramazoline, a SYMPATHOMIMETIC for congestion) – for additional side-effects of this product *see* ephedrine nasal drops.

 in pregnant women, mothers who are breast-feeding, and in patients with nasal infection or who are transferring from corticosteroids taken by mouth. Particular care needed after nasal surgery.

 patients with unhealed wounds after nasal surgery, or untreated nasal infection, or those suffering from tuberculosis of the lung. Most products not suitable for young children.

ANTICOAGULANTS (with high doses).

Product	*Brand names*	*Dose*
beclomethasone (beclometasone) nasal spray	Beclo-Aqua, Beclomist*, Beconase, Beconase Allergy*, Nasobec, Nasobec Hayfever*, Zonivent Aquanasal	Adults and children over 6 years, 2 sprays in each nostril twice a day reducing to 1 spray twice a day for maintenance.
betamethasone nasal drops	Betnesol, Vista-Methasone	2-3 drops into each nostril 2-3 times a day. Not for prolonged use in infants.
budesonide nasal spray	Rhinocort Aqua	Adults and children over 12 years, 2 sprays in each nostril once a day or one spray in each nostril twice a day reducing to 1 spray in each nostril once a day for maintenance. (Also used to treat nasal polyps – a spray in each nostril twice a day for up to 3 months.)
dexamethasone nasal spray	Available only as combination product Dexa-Rhinaspray Duo *see* above	Adults and children over 12 years, 1 spray into each nostril 2-3 times a day (maximum of 6 times a day); children 5-12 years 1 spray in each nostril up to twice a day. Maximum of 14 days treatment.
flunisolide nasal spray	Syntaris	Adults and children over 14 years, 2 sprays in each nostril twice a day (maximum 3 times a day), reducing for maintenance; children 5-14 years initially 1 spray in each nostril up to 3 times a day.

Product	*Brand names*	*Dose*
fluticasone nasal spray (or drops to treat polyps)	Flixonase	Adults and children over 12 years, 2 sprays (children 4-11 years 1 spray) in each nostril each morning increasing to twice daily if needed; for polyps in adults, 6 drops into each nostril once or twice a day and assess after 4-6 weeks.
mometasone nasal spray	Nasonex	Adults and children over 12 years, 2 sprays in each nostril once a day increasing to 4 sprays if necessary and reducing to 1 spray for maintenance; children 6-11 years, 1 spray in each nostril once a day.
triamcinolone nasal spray	Nasacort	Adults and children over 12 years, 2 sprays in each nostril once a day reducing to 1 spray for maintenance; children 6-12 years, 1 spray in each nostril once a day.

* *available over the counter.*

cortisone tablets

A tablet used as a CORTICOSTEROID to treat Addison's disease, and as a replacement therapy after removal of the adrenal glands.

Strengths available: 25 mg tablets.
Dose: usually 25-37.5 mg a day (maximum of 300 mg a day).
Availability: NHS and private prescription.
Contains: cortisone acetate.
Brand names: Cortisyl.

high blood sugar, thin bones, mood changes, stomach ulcers, fluid retention, potassium loss, high blood pressure, menstrual irregularity, hairiness, increased likelihood of infection, euphoria, depression, sleeplessness, aggravation of schizophrenia and epilepsy, eye disorders, thinning of skin, acne, bruising, blood changes, stomach upset, inflamed pancreas, muscle abnormality, suppression of the ADRENAL GLANDS, ulcerated or infected oesophagus, general feeling of being unwell, hiccups, reduced growth in children.

in pregnant women, mothers who are breast-feeding, and in patients who have had recent bowel surgery or who are suffering from inflamed veins, psychiatric disorders, thinning of the bones, stomach ulcers, tuberculosis or other infections, high blood pressure, glaucoma, epilepsy, diabetes, underactive thyroid, liver disease, stress. Withdraw gradually. Avoid contact with chicken pox for 3 months after treatment ends and seek medical attention if exposed.

children or for patients who have untreated infections.

live vaccines, some ANTIBIOTICS and anti-epileptics, ANTICOAGULANTS, antidiabetics, some antifungals, digoxin, cyclosporin.

Cortisyl *see* cortisone tablets
(Hoechst Marion Roussel)

Cosopt *see* dorzolamide drops and timolol drops
(Merck Sharp and Dohme)

Strengths available: 2% + 0.5% drops.
Dose: 1 drop in the affected eye(s) twice a day.

Coversyl *see* perindopril tablets
(Servier Laboratories)

Cozaar *see* losartan tablets
(Merck Sharp and Dohme)

Cozaar Comp *see* losartan tablets and hydrochlorothiazide tablets
(Merck Sharp and Dohme)
A combination treatment used to simplify treatment of patients already stabilized on the two ingredients in the same proportions.

Strengths available: 50 mg + 12.5 mg tablets.

Creon *see* pancreatin capsules/sachets
(Solvay Healthcare)

Crinone *see* progesterone vaginal gel
(Serono Laboratories (UK))

Crixivan *see* indinavir capsules
(Merck Sharp and Dohme)

Cromogen *see* sodium cromoglycate inhaler/nebulizer solution
(Baker Norton Pharmaceuticals)

---

crotamiton cream/lotion

A cream or lotion used to treat scabies and itchy skin conditions.

Strengths available: 10% cream and lotion.

Dose: for scabies, apply to the body, apart from the head and face, after a hot bath and repeat every day for 3-5 days (bathe before each application and after end of treatment). For itching, apply 2-3 times a day (or once a day in children under 3 years).

 keep out of the eyes, and avoid areas of broken skin.

 children under 3 years (except on advice of doctor) or for patients with weeping skin conditions.

Availability: NHS and private prescription, nurse prescription, over the counter.
Contains: crotamiton.
Brand names: Eurax.
Compound preparations: Eurax-Hydrocortisone (*see* topical corticosteroid).

Crystacide *see* hydrogen peroxide cream
(Medeva Pharma)

---

crystal violet paint BP 1980

A purple solution used as a disinfectant to treat burns, boils, ulcers, and some skin infections where the skin is not broken.

Strengths available: 0.5% solution.
Dose: use undiluted as directed.
Availability: NHS and private prescription, over the counter.
Contains: crystal violet (gentian violet).

 ulceration of mucous membranes.

 stains skin and clothing.

 application to mucous membranes or broken skin.

Cuplex *see* salicylic acid collodion
(Smith and Nephew Healthcare)

Curatoderm *see* tacalcitol ointment
(Crookes Healthcare)

Cutivate *see* fluticasone cream/ointment
(GlaxoWellcome UK)

CX Antiseptic Dusting Powder *see* chlorhexidine dusting powder
(Adams Healthcare)

---

cyanocobalamin injection

An injection used as a VITAMIN B_{12} supplement to treat various anaemias.

Strengths available: 1000 mcg per injection.
Dose: as advised by doctor.
Availability: NHS (when prescribed as generic) and private prescription.
Contains: cyanocobalamin (vitamin B_{12}).
Brand names: Cytamen (not available on NHS).
Other preparations: cyanocobalamin tablets and liquid (not available on NHS).

 itching, skin disorders, fever, hot flushes, nausea, dizziness. Rarely, severe allergy.

 chloramphenicol.

---

cyclizine tablets

A tablet used as an ANTIHISTAMINE to treat vomiting, nausea, vertigo, and inner ear disorders.

Strengths available: 50 mg tablets.
Dose: adults and children over 12 years, 50 mg up to three times a day; children 6-12 years 25 mg up to three times a day.
Availability: NHS and private prescription, over the counter.
Contains: cyclizine hydrochloride.
Brand names: Valoid.
Compound preparations: Diconal, Migril.

 drowsiness, reduced reactions. Rarely, dizziness, excitation, movement disorders, headache, ANTIMUSCARINIC effects. Rarely, heart rhythm disturbances, severe allergic reaction, skin disorders, noises in the ears, sensitivity to sunlight, Parkinson-like symptoms, confusion, depression, fits, shaking, sweating, muscle pain, pins and needles, liver disorders, hair loss, sleep disturbances.

 in the elderly, mothers who are breastfeeding, and in patients with enlarged prostate, severe heart failure, low blood pressure, difficulty passing urine, Parkinson's disease, glaucoma, epilepsy, or liver disease.

 MAOIS, TRICYCLIC ANTIDEPRESSANTS, some ANALGESICS, ritonavir, alcohol, other sedating drugs.

 children under 6 years, pregnant women.

Cyclo-progynova *see* hormone replacement therapy (combined)
(ASTA Medica)

Cyclodox *see* doxycycline capsules
(Berk Pharmaceuticals)

Cyclogest *see* progesterone suppositories
(Shire Pharmaceuticals)

C

cyclopenthiazide tablets

A tablet used as a DIURETIC to treat fluid retention and high blood pressure.

Strengths available: 500 mcg tablets.
Dose: fluid retention, 250-500 mcg each morning (up to 1000 mcg in heart failure); high blood pressure, 250 mcg at first increasing to 500 mcg if necessary.
Availability: NHS and private prescription.
Contains: cyclopenthiazide.
Brand names: Navidrex.
Compound preparations: Co-prenozide, Navispare.

 NON-STEROIDAL ANTI-INFLAMMATORY DRUGS, drugs that alter heart rhythm, carbamazepine, halofantrine, antidiabetics, pimozide, digoxin, lithium, ANTIHYPERTENSIVES.

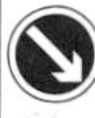 low blood pressure on standing, mild stomach upset, reversible impotence, inflamed pancreas, gout, liver disorders, low potassium levels and other blood changes, allergy, rash, sensitivity to light or tiredness.

 in pregnant women, mothers who are breast-feeding, the elderly, and in patients suffering from liver or kidney disorders, diabetes, gout, LUPUS.

 patients suffering from severe kidney or liver disorders, Addison's disease, raised blood calcium/uric acid levels, low blood potassium/sodium levels, PORPHYRIA, or who are allergic to similar drugs.

cyclopentolate eye drops

Eye drops used as an ANTIMUSCARINIC pupil dilator for eye examinations and to treat eye inflammation.

Strengths available: 0.5% and 1% drops. Also available as single-use drops.
Dose: according to doctor's instructions.
Availability: NHS and private prescription.
Contains: cyclopentolate hydrochloride.
Brand names: Minims Cyclopentolate (preservative-free, single-dose drops), Mydrilate.

 patients with narrow-angle glaucoma.

 disturbance of vision, temporary stinging, raised pressure inside the eye. With prolonged treatment, irritation, redness, inflammation or fluid retention in the eye. Very young or very old patients may suffer antimuscarinic effects, *see* atropine tablets.

 in the very young and the elderly (*see* above) and in long-sighted patients. Patients should not drive for 1-2 hours after treatment.

cycloserine capsules

A capsule used with other drugs to treat tuberculosis when other treatments have failed.

Strengths available: 250 mg capsules.
Dose: adults, 250 mg every 12 hours for 2 weeks increasing, if necessary, to a maximum of 500 mg every 12 hours; children use reduced doses according to body weight.
Availability: NHS and private prescription.

 headache, vertigo, drowsiness, dizziness, shaking hands, fits, mental disorder, rash, anaemia, liver changes, heart failure.

cont.

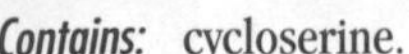
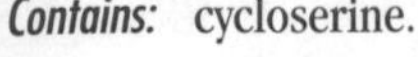

Contains: cycloserine.

alcoholics or for patients suffering from severe kidney failure, epilepsy, depression or other mental disorders, PORPHYRIA.

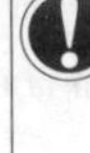
in pregnant women, mothers who are breast-feeding, and in patients suffering from kidney damage. Your doctor may advise regular blood tests.

alcohol, sedatives, phenytoin.

---

cyclosporin capsules/liquid

A capsule or liquid used to suppress the immune system and to treat severe skin disorders and rheumatoid arthritis. Also used to prevent rejection following transplants or grafts.

Strengths available: 10 mg, 25 mg, 50 mg, and 100 mg capsules; 100 mg/ml liquid.
Dose: as advised by specialist.
Availability: NHS and private prescription.
Contains: cyclosporin (ciclosporin).
Brand names: Neoral, SangCya.

kidney or liver disorders, high blood pressure, shaking, stomach upset, swollen gums, hair growth, tiredness, muscle weakness or cramp, muscle disease, burning sensation. Rarely, blood changes, gout, fluid retention, fits, headache, rash, anaemia, weight gain, inflamed bowel or pancreas, menstrual changes, pins and needles, nerve disorders, confusion, malignant disease.

ACE-INHIBITORS, NON-STEROIDAL ANTI-INFLAMMATORY DRUGS, ANTIBIOTICS, carbamazepine, phenobarbital, phenytoin, primidone, antifungals, chloroquine, ticlopidine, ritonavir, ursodeoxycholic acid, diltiazem, nicardipine, verapamil, nifedipine, colchicine, prednisolone, methylprednisolone, some DIURETICS, danazol, some lipid-lowering drugs (STATINS), progestogen treatments (such as ORAL CONTRACEPTIVES), potassium, cimetidine, neomycin, orlistat, celecoxib, St John's Wort (*Hypericum*).

in pregnant women, mothers who are breast-feeding, and in patients suffering from chicken pox or shingles, PORPHYRIA, or with high potassium/uric acid levels. Your doctor may advise regular tests during treatment. Patients should not switch from one brand to another once stabilized. Avoid excessive exposure to sunlight.

patients suffering from malignant diseases, infection, uncontrolled high blood pressure, or kidney damage.

Cyklokapron *see* tranexamic acid tablets
(Pharmacia and Upjohn)

Cymevene *see* ganciclovir capsules
(Roche Products)

---

cyproheptadine tablets

A tablet used as an ANTIHISTAMINE and ANTIMUSCARINIC treatment for symptoms of allergies (such as hayfever and itchy skin) and migraine.

Strengths available: 4 mg tablets.
Dose: for allergies, adults 4 mg 3-4 times a day up to a maximum of 32 mg a day (children aged 2-14 years, 2-4 mg 2-3 times a day according to age, maximum 12 mg a day up to 6 years and 16 mg a day up to 14 years). For migraine (adults only), 4 mg initially followed by another 4 mg after 30 minutes if necessary and repeated every 4-6 hours.
Availability: NHS and private prescription, over the counter.
Contains: cyproheptadine hydrochloride.
Brand names: Periactin.

drowsiness, reduced reactions, dizziness, excitation, movement disorders, headache, antimuscarinic effects, weight gain. Rarely, heart rhythm disturbances, severe allergic reaction, skin disorders, noises in the ears, sensitivity to sunlight, confusion, depression, fits, shaking, sweating, muscle pain, pins and needles, liver disorders, hair loss, sleep disturbances.

in the elderly, pregnant women, and in patients with enlarged prostate, difficulty passing urine, asthma, overactive thyroid, heart or circulation disorders, high blood pressure, glaucoma, epilepsy, or liver disease.

children under 2 years, mothers who are breastfeeding, or for patients with severe liver disease, intestinal blockage, or suffering from an asthma attack.

other sedating drugs, alcohol, antidepressants.

cyproterone tablets

A tablet used as an anti-androgen to treat severe hypersexuality and sexual deviation in men.

Strengths available: 50 mg tablets.
Dose: 150 mg twice a day after food.
Availability: NHS and private prescription.
Contains: cyproterone acetate.
Brand names: Androcur.
Compound preparations: co-cyprindiol tablets.

tiredness, depression, weight gain, breast enlargement, changes in hair pattern, difficulty breathing, thinning of bones, liver disorders, reduced sperm production, and reversible infertility. Acne may clear.

in patients suffering from diabetes. This product is NOT a male contraceptive. Patients must give consent to treatment. Your doctor may advise regular blood and sperm tests.

men under 18 years, where bones and testes have not reached full development, or for patients suffering from liver disease, sickle-cell anaemia, severe diabetes, malignant or wasting disease, severe chronic depression, or with a history of blood clots.

Cystagon *see* cysteamine capsules
(Orphan Europe (UK))

D

cysteamine capsules

A capsule used to treat nephropathic cystinosis (a kidney disorder).

Strengths available: 50 mg, 100 mg, and 150 mg capsules.
Dose: as advised by doctor. Capsules may be opened and sprinkled on to food but do not add to acidic drinks.
Availability: NHS and private prescription (specialist supervision).
Contains: cysteamine (mercaptamine).
Brand names: Cystagon.

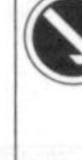
bad breath, body odour, stomach upset, bleeding or ulcers in the stomach or intestines, liver changes, fits, hallucinations, itchy rash, other kidney disorders, loss of appetite, tiredness, fever, rash, dehydration, drowsiness, high blood pressure, headache, depression, nervousness, brain or blood disorders.

in children under 6 years. Your doctor may advise regular blood tests, and adjust doses of other medications.

pregnant women, mothers who are breast-feeding, or for patients who are allergic to penicillamine.

alcohol, sedating drugs.

Daktacort *see* miconazole cream and topical corticosteroid
(Janssen-Cilag)

Daktarin *see* miconazole cream/powder/spray and miconazole oral gel
(Janssen-Cilag)

Dalacin *see* clindamycin cream
(Pharmacia and Upjohn)

Dalacin C *see* clindamycin capsules
(Pharmacia and Upjohn)

Dalacin T *see* clindamycin lotion
(Pharmacia and Upjohn)

Dalivit *see* multivitamin drops
(Eastern Pharmaceuticals)

Dalmane *see* flurazepam capsules
(ICN Pharmaceuticals)

danazol capsules

A capsule used as a hormone inhibitor to treat endometriosis (a womb and menstrual disorder), heavy periods, and non-malignant breast disorders.

Strengths available: 100 mg and 200 mg capsules.
Dose: 100-800 mg a day (in divided doses) according to condition.
Availability: NHS and private prescription.
Contains: danazol.
Brand names: Danol.

nausea, dizziness, vertigo, rash, backache, flushing, muscle spasm, reduction in size of breasts, weight gain, male hormone effects, fluid retention, hair loss, headache, emotional disturbance, blood and thyroid changes, visual disturbances, liver disorders, inflamed pancreas, menstrual changes, skin disorders including sensitivity to sunlight, changes in sexual desire, stomach or lung pain, vaginal dryness, inflamed and painful joints.

children, pregnant women, mothers who are breastfeeding, or for patients suffering from PORPHYRIA, severe kidney, liver, or heart disease, blocked blood vessels, some tumours, undiagnosed vaginal bleeding.

in the elderly and in patients suffering from heart, liver, or kidney disorder, epilepsy, blood disorders, migraine, diabetes, a tendency to gain weight, high blood pressure, or other circulatory disorders, or who have a history of blood clots. Non-hormonal methods of contraception should be used.

ORAL CONTRACEPTIVES, ANTICOAGULANTS, carbamazepine, cyclosporin.

Danlax *see* co-danthramer suspension
(Sovereign Medical)

Danol *see* danazol capsules
(Sanofi Winthrop)

---

danthron *see* co-danthramer capsules/suspension, co-danthrusate capsules/suspension

---

Dantrium *see* dantrolene capsules
(Proctor and Gamble Pharmaceuticals UK)

---

dantrolene capsules

A capsule used as a muscle relaxant to treat chronic or severe muscle spasms.

Strengths available: 25 mg or 100 mg capsules.
Dose: 25 mg a day at first increasing to a maximum of 100 mg four times a day if needed.
Availability: NHS and private prescription.

cont.

Contains: dantrolene sodium.
Brand names: Dantrium.

 weakness, tiredness, drowsiness, diarrhoea, dizziness, loss of appetite, nausea, headache, rash. Rarely, fits, heart rhythm disturbances, constipation, difficulty swallowing, disturbance of vision or speech, sleeplessness, depression, fever, difficulty breathing, blood pressure disturbance, changes in urine (and ability to pass urine), liver disorder, lung disorders, heart inflammation.

 children or for patients suffering from liver disease, short-term muscle spasm, or where spasticity is useful for movement.

 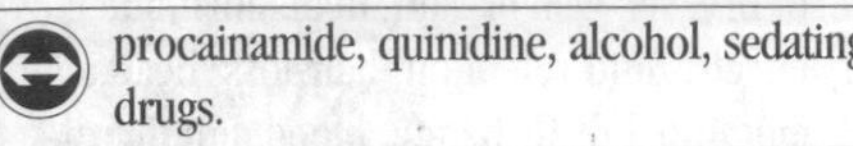 procainamide, quinidine, alcohol, sedating drugs.

 in pregnant women and in patients suffering from lung or heart disease. Your doctor may advise checks on your liver before and 6 weeks after treatment.

---

dantron *see* danthron (alternative name)

Daonil *see* glibenclamide tablets
(Hoechst Marion Roussel)

---

dapsone tablets

A tablet used as an anti-leprotic treatment for leprosy and herpes-like dermatitis.

Strengths available: 50 mg and 100 mg tablets.
Dose: as advised by doctor.
Availability: NHS and private prescription.
Contains: dapsone.
Compound preparations: Maloprim.

 liver disease, stomach upset, headache, dizziness, rapid heart rate, sleeplessness, rash or other skin disorder, nerve pain, blood changes, loss of appetite, mental disorders.

 in pregnant women and in patients suffering from heart or lung disease, anaemia, glucose 6PD deficiency (an inherited disorder). This treatment should be given only under specialist advice and should be discontinued if rash, fever, and blood disorders develop.

 patients suffering from PORPHYRIA.

Daraprim *see* pyrimethamine tablets
(GlaxoWellcome UK)

DDAVP *see* desmopressin tablets/nasal solution
(Ferring Pharmaceuticals)

D

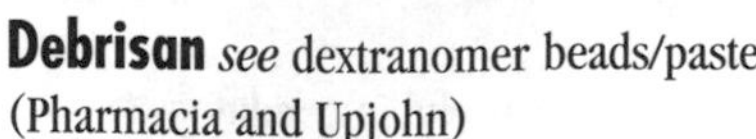

Debrisan *see* dextranomer beads/paste
(Pharmacia and Upjohn)

Debrisoquine tablets

(Cambridge Laboratories)
A tablet used to treat high blood pressure.

Strengths available: 10 mg tablets.
Dose: adults 10 mg once or twice a day increasing gradually to a maximum of 60 mg a day (or 120 mg in severe cases).
Availability: NHS and private prescription.
Contains: debrisoquine sulphate.

 anaesthetics, sedatives, alcohol, SYMPATHOMIMETICS (including those contained in cough and cold remedies).

 low blood pressure, fluid retention, stuffy nose, headache, interference with sexual function, drowsiness.

 in pregnant women and in patients with narrowed blood vessels in the heart or brain, asthma, or a history of stomach ulcers.

 children.

Decadron *see* dexamethasone tablets
(Merck Sharp and Dohme)

Decubal Clinic *see* emollient cream
(Dumex)

---

deferiprone tablets

A tablet used to treat iron overload in patients with certain types of anaemia.

Strengths available: 500 mg tablets.
Dose: as advised by doctor.
Availability: NHS and private prescription.
Contains: deferiprone.
Brand names: Ferriprox.

 reddish colour in urine, blood disorders, upset stomach, increased appetite, joint pain.

 in patients with poorly functioning immune system, or hepatitis C. Your doctor will advise regular blood tests. Report any signs of infection (such as sore throat, fever, influenza-like symptoms) to your doctor.

 some ANTACIDS, VITAMIN C.

 children under 6 years, pregnant women, or mothers who are breastfeeding.

deflazacort tablets

A tablet used as a CORTICOSTEROID to suppress inflammation and allergies. It is useful in conditions such as asthma, rheumatoid arthritis, and LUPUS.

Strengths available: 1 mg and 6 mg tablets.
Dose: adults, usually 3-18 mg a day (maximum 120 mg a day). Children use reduced doses.
Availability: NHS and private prescription.
Contains: deflazacort.
Brand names: Calcort.

in pregnant women, mothers who are breast-feeding, and in patients who have had recent bowel surgery or who are suffering from inflamed veins, psychiatric disorders, thinning of the bones, stomach ulcers, tuberculosis or other infections, high blood pressure, glaucoma, epilepsy, diabetes, underactive thyroid, liver disease, stress. Withdraw gradually. Avoid contact with chicken pox for 3 months after treatment ends and seek medical attention if exposed.

high blood sugar, thin bones, mood changes, stomach ulcers, fluid retention, potassium loss, high blood pressure, menstrual irregularity, hairiness, increased likelihood of infection, euphoria, depression, sleeplessness, aggravation of schizophrenia and epilepsy, eye disorders, thinning of skin, acne, bruising, blood changes, stomach upset, inflamed pancreas, muscle abnormality, suppression of the ADRENAL GLANDS, ulcerated or infected oesophagus, general feeling of being unwell, hiccups, reduced growth in children.

patients who have untreated infections.

live vaccines, some ANTIBIOTICS and anti-epileptics, ANTICOAGULANTS, antidiabetics, some antifungals, digoxin, cyclosporin.

Delfen *see* nonoxynol foam
(Janssen-Cilag)

Deltacortril *see* prednisolone enteric-coated tablets
(Pfizer)

---

demeclocycline capsules

A capsule used as a TETRACYCLINE ANTIBIOTIC to treat chest and soft tissue infections, and to treat low blood sodium levels caused by high levels of anti-DIURETIC hormone.

Strengths available: 150 mg capsules.
Dose: for infections, 150 mg four times a day, or 300 mg twice a day. (Up to 1200 mg a day used for low sodium levels.) The dose to be swallowed with plenty of fluid while sitting or standing.
Availability: NHS and private prescription.
Contains: demeclocycline hydrochloride.

stomach upset, irritation of the oesophagus, reddening of skin, headache, disturbed vision, sensitivity to light, additional infections, pressure on the brain, reversible diabetes insipidus, liver disorders, inflamed pancreas or bowel.

in patients suffering from liver or kidney disorders. Discontinue if reddening of skin occurs.

Brand names: Ledermycin.
Compound preparations: Deteclo.

 children under 12 years, pregnant women, mothers who are breastfeeding, or for patients suffering from LUPUS.

 milk, ANTACIDS, iron supplements, ANTI-COAGULANTS, ORAL CONTRACEPTIVES.

Demix *see* doxycycline capsules
(Ashbourne Pharmaceuticals)

De-Noltab *see* tripotassium dicitratobismuthate tablets
(Yamanouchi Pharma)

Denorex *see* coal tar shampoo
(Whitehall Laboratories)

Depixol *see* flupenthixol tablets
(Lundbeck)

Depo-Medrone/ Depo-Medrone with Lidocaine *see* methylprednisolone injection
(Pharmacia and Upjohn)

Deponit *see* glyceryl trinitrate patches
(Schwarz Pharma)

Depo-Provera *see* medroxyprogesterone injection
(Pharmacia and Upjohn)

Derbac-M *see* malathion liquid
(SSL International)

Dermalo *see* emollient bath additive
(Dermal Laboratories)

Dermamist *see* emollient spray
(Yamanouchi Pharma)

Dermestril *see* hormone replacement therapy (oestrogen-only)
(Strakan)

Dermol *see* emollient lotion
(Dermal Laboratories)

D

Dermovate/Dermovate-NN *see* topical corticosteroid cream/ointment/scalp application
(GlaxoWellcome UK)

Deseril *see* methysergide tablets
(Alliance Pharmaceuticals)

desmopressin tablets/nasal spray/nasal solution

A tablet, nasal spray, or nasal solution used as a hormone to treat diabetes insipidus (a fluid-balance disorder), excessive thirst and urination after surgical removal of the pituitary gland, and bedwetting.

Strengths available: 100 mcg and 200 mcg tablets; 10 mcg per spray nasal spray; 100 mcg/ml nasal solution.
Dose: diabetes insipidus, (adults and children) 200-1200 mcg a day in divided doses by mouth, or adults 10-40 mcg (children 5-20 mcg) each day through the nose; bedwetting, patients aged 5-65 years, 200 mcg at bedtime by mouth (increasing to 400 mcg if needed), or 20 mcg (increased to 40 mcg) at bedtime through the nose. (Dose halved in patients with bedwetting caused by multiple sclerosis.)
Availability: NHS and private prescription.
Contains: desmopressin acetate.
Brand names: DDAVP, Desmospray, Desmotabs, Nocutil.

headache, stomach pain, stomach upset, fluid retention, low sodium levels. Nose bleeds, runny or inflamed nose with nasal preparations.

in the elderly, pregnant women, and in patients suffering from kidney disorder, heart or circulatory disease, high blood pressure, or cystic fibrosis. When treatment is for bedwetting, blood pressure and weight should be monitored regularly, fluid intake should be restricted overnight, and treatment should be discontinued during episodes of vomiting or diarrhoea.

patients with a weak heart or high blood pressure.

TRICYCLIC ANTIDEPRESSANTS, DIURETICS, chlorpromazine, carbamazepine.

Desmospray *see* desmopressin nasal spray
(Ferring Pharmaceuticals)

Desmotabs *see* desmopressin tablets
(Ferring Pharmaceuticals)

---

desogestrel *see* oral contraceptive (combined)

---

desoximetasone *see* desoxymethasone (alternative name)

---

desoxymethasone *see* topical corticosteroid oily cream/lotion

---

Destolit *see* ursodeoxycholic acid tablets
(Norgine)

Deteclo *see* demeclocycline capsules and tetracycline tablets
(Wyeth Laboratories)

Strengths available: 115.4 mg each of tetracycline and chlortetracycline, and 69.2 mg demeclocycline per tablet.

Dose: 1 tablet twice a day (up to 4 tablets a day in severe infections).

Detrunorm *see* propiverine tablets
(Schering-Plough)

Detrusitol *see* tolterodine tablets
(Pharmacia and Upjohn)

---

dexamethasone *see* corticosteroid nasal spray, dexamethasone solution/tablets, dexamethasone eye drops, Otomize, Sofradex

---

dexamethasone eye drops

Drops used as a CORTICOSTEROID for the short-term treatment of eye inflammation.

Strengths available: 0.1% single-use drops

Dose: 1-2 drops applied to the affected eye(s) up to 6 times a day (or every 30-60 minutes in severe conditions), then frequency reduced as inflammation subsides.

cataract, thinning cornea, fungal infection, rise in eye pressure.

in pregnant women and infants – do not use for extended periods.

cont.

Availability: NHS and private prescription.
Contains: dexamethasone sodium phosphate.
Brand names: Minims Dexamethasone.
Compound preparations: Maxidex, Maxitrol, Sofradex.
Other preparations: dexamethasone solution/tablets.

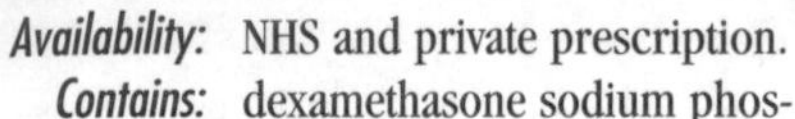

patients suffering from infected eye conditions, glaucoma, or for those who wear soft contact lenses.

 ANTIMUSCARINICS.

dexamethasone solution/tablets

A solution or tablet used as a CORTICOSTEROID to suppress inflammation and allergies. It is useful in conditions such as asthma, rheumatoid arthritis, and fluid retention in the brain.

Strengths available: 2 mg/5 ml solution; 0.5 mg or 2 mg tablets.
Dose: adults, usually 0.5-10 mg a day. Children use reduced doses.
Availability: NHS and private prescription.
Contains: dexamethasone.
Brand names: Decadron, Dexsol.
Other preparations: dexamethasone eye drops.

 patients who have untreated infections.

 live vaccines, some ANTIBIOTICS and anti-epileptics, ANTICOAGULANTS, antidiabetics, some antifungals, digoxin, cyclosporin.

 high blood sugar, thin bones, mood changes, stomach ulcers, fluid retention, potassium loss, high blood pressure, reduced growth in children.

 in pregnant women, mothers who are breastfeeding, and in patients who have had recent bowel surgery or who are suffering from inflamed veins, psychiatric disorders, thinning of the bones, stomach ulcers, tuberculosis or other infections, high blood pressure, glaucoma, epilepsy, diabetes, underactive thyroid, liver disease, stress. Withdraw gradually. Avoid contact with chicken pox for 3 months after treatment ends and seek medical attention if exposed.

dexamfetamine *see* dexamphetamine (alternative name)

dexamphetamine tablets

A tablet used as a SYMPATHOMIMETIC to stimulate the nervous system, for example, in patients who are abnormally sleepy, or to treat children who are abnormally physically active.

Strengths available: 5 mg tablets.
Dose: adults 5 mg twice a day at first increasing every 7 days by 10 mg to a maximum of 60 mg a day. Elderly patients require lower doses. Use in children as advised by specialist.
Availability: controlled drug; NHS and private prescription.

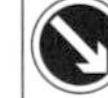 sleeplessness, restlessness, slowing of growth, mood changes, dry mouth, shaking, loss of appetite, stomach upset, dizziness, headache, fits, sweating, irregular or rapid heart beat, other heart disorders, mildly raised blood pressure, addiction, disturbance of vision, movement disorders.

Contains: dexamphetamine (dexamfetamine) sulphate.
Brand names: Dexedrine.

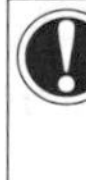
in patients with raised blood pressure, PORPHYRIA, or a history of epilepsy or movement disorders. Children must be monitored for growth disturbance. Treatment must be withdrawn gradually. Judgement and ability to drive may be affected.

alcohol, MAOIS.

children under 6 years, pregnant women, mothers who are breastfeeding, or for patients with a history of drug abuse or who are suffering from high blood pressure, abnormal movements, heart or circulation disorders, overactive thyroid gland, excitability or agitation, glaucoma.

Dexa-Rhinaspray Duo *see* corticosteroid nasal spray
(Boehringer Ingelheim)

Dexedrine *see* dexamphetamine tablets
(Medeva Pharma)

---

dexketoprofen tablets

A tablet used as a NON-STEROIDAL ANTI-INFLAMMATORY DRUG for the short-term treatment of pain due to muscle and joint disorders, dental and period pain.

Strengths available: 25 mg tablets.
Dose: adults 12.5 mg up to six times a day or 25 mg three times a day (elderly patients need lower doses at first).
Availability: NHS and private prescription.
Contains: dexketoprofen trometamol.
Brand names: Keral.

stomach upset and bleeding or ulceration, severe allergy, difficulty breathing, blood or kidney disorders, headache, dizziness, noises in the ears, sensitivity to light, vertigo. Rarely, fluid retention, liver disorders, inflamed pancreas, inflamed bowel, meningitis.

in the elderly, and in patients with heart, liver, or kidney disorders, asthma, or LUPUS.

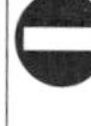
children, pregnant women, mothers who are breastfeeding, or for patients with a history of allergy to aspirin or other NSAID, blood-clotting disorders, currently active stomach ulcer or intestinal bleeding, inflamed intestines or severe heart failure.

ACE-INHIBITORS, aspirin or other non-steroidal anti-inflammatory drugs, some ANTIBIOTICS, ANTICOAGULANTS, some antidiabetic drugs, some antivirals, methotrexate, DIURETICS, lithium, tacrolimus, cyclosporin, digoxin.

Dexsol *see* dexamethasone solution
(Rosemont Pharmaceuticals)

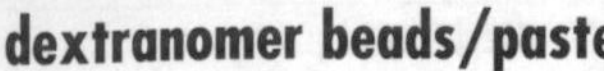

dextranomer beads/paste

Beads or a paste in sachets used as an absorbant treatment for weeping wounds including ulcers.

Dose: wash wound with saline solution and, without drying first, coat with 3 mm layer of beads or paste. Cover with appropriate dressing and repeat before the dressing is saturated.
Availability: NHS and private prescription, nurse prescription, over the counter.
Contains: dextranomer.
Brand names: Debrisan.

---

dextromoramide tablets

A tablet used as an OPIOID to control severe and prolonged pain.

Strengths available: 5 mg and 10 mg tablets.
Dose: adults up to 5 mg at first increasing to a maximum of 20 mg if required; children as advised by doctor.
Availability: controlled drug; NHS and private prescription.
Contains: dextromoramide tartrate.
Brand names: Palfium.

Not to be used for: alcoholics, women in labour, or for patients with head injury, reduced breathing ability, or at risk of non-functioning intestines.

Caution needed with: MAOIS, alcohol, sedating drugs, ritonavir.

Side effects: drowsiness, upset stomach, sweating, dizziness, breathing difficulty, low blood pressure, difficulty passing urine, dry mouth, headache, vertigo, flushing, change in heart rhythm, mood changes, rash, itching, addiction, reduced sexual desire.

Caution: in pregnant women, mothers who are breastfeeding, elderly or weakened patients, and in those suffering from breathing, kidney, or liver problems, low blood pressure, underactive thyroid, enlarged prostate, or epilepsy. (Higher doses not suitable for some of these categories.)

---

dextropoproxyphene capsules

A capsule used as an OPIOID to control pain.

Strengths available: 65 mg capsules.
Dose: 65 mg 3-4 times a day when required.
Availability: NHS and private prescription.
Contains: dextropropoxyphene hydrochloride.
Brand names: Doloxene.
Compound preparations: co-proxamol tablets.

Side effects: drowsiness, upset stomach, sweating, dizziness, breathing difficulty, low blood pressure, difficulty passing urine, dry mouth, headache, vertigo, flushing, change in heart rhythm, mood changes, rash, itching, addiction, reduced sexual desire, liver disorders, and fits with high doses.

Caution: in pregnant women, mothers who are breastfeeding, elderly or weakened patients, and in those suffering from breathing, kidney, or liver problems, low blood pressure, underactive thyroid, enlarged prostate or epilepsy. (Higher doses not suitable for some of these categories.)

 children, alcoholics, women in labour, or for patients with head injury, reduced breathing ability, PORPHYRIA, or those who have a history of drug addiction or who are suicidal or at risk of non-functioning intestines.

 MAOIS, alcohol, sedating drugs, ritonavir, ANTI-COAGULANTS, carbamazepine.

---

dextrose gel

A gel used as a quick form of glucose to treat severe low blood glucose levels in diabetics who are still conscious.

Dose: as needed when blood glucose level falls.
Availability: NHS and private prescription, over the counter.
Contains: dextrose.
Brand names: Hypostop.

DF118 *see* dihydrocodeine solution/tablets
(Martindale Pharmaceuticals)

DHC Continus *see* dihydrocodeine modified-release tablets
(Napp Pharmaceuticals)

Diabetamide *see* glibenclamide tablets
(Ashbourne Pharmaceuticals)

Diabur Test 5000

(Roche Diagnostics)
A plastic reagent strip used for the detection of glucose in the urine. This gives an approximate estimate of blood glucose levels which may be adequate for the management of Type II diabetes.

Availability: NHS and private prescription, nurse prescription, over the counter.

Diaglyk *see* gliclazide tablets
(Ashbourne Pharmaceuticals)

Diamicron *see* gliclazide tablets
(Servier Laboratories)

---

diamorphine tablets

A tablet used as an OPIOID ANALGESIC to relieve moderate to severe pain.

Strengths available: 10 mg tablets.
Dose: adults 5-10 mg every 4 hours at first increasing as required according to doctor's instructions.
Availability: controlled drug; NHS and private prescription.
Contains: diamorphine hydrochloride.

alcoholics or for patients with head injury, reduced breathing ability, PORPHYRIA, or those who have a history of drug addiction or who are suicidal or at risk of non-functioning intestines.

MAOIS, alcohol, sedating drugs, ritonavir.

drowsiness, upset stomach, sweating, dizziness, breathing difficulty, low blood pressure, difficulty passing urine, dry mouth, headache, vertigo, flushing, change in heart rhythm, mood changes, rash, itching, addiction, reduced sexual desire.

in children, pregnant women, women in labour, mothers who are breastfeeding, elderly or weakened patients, and in those suffering from breathing, kidney, or liver problems, low blood pressure, underactive thyroid, enlarged prostate or epilepsy. (Higher doses not suitable for some of these categories.)

Diamox/Diamox SR *see* acetazolamide tablets/modified-release capsules
(Wyeth Laboratories)

Dianette *see* co-cyprindiol tablets
(Schering Health Care)

Diarrest *see* oral rehydration solution, dicyclomine syrup, and codeine syrup
(Galen)
A liquid used as a combination treatment for diarrhoea, vomiting, and cramp.

Dose: adults 20 ml (children aged 4-5 years 5 ml, 6-9 years 10 ml, 10-13 years 15 ml) four times a day with water.

Diasorb *see* loperamide capsules
(Norton Healthcare)

Diastix
(Bayer Diagnostics)
A plastic reagent strip used for the detection of glucose in the urine. This gives an approximate estimate of blood glucose levels which may be adequate for the management of Type II diabetes.

Availability: NHS and private prescription, nurse prescription, over the counter.

Diazepam Rectubes *see* diazepam rectal solution
(C.P. Pharmaceuticals)

diazepam tablets/liquid/suppositories/rectal solution

A tablet, liquid, suppository, or rectal solution used as a tranquillizer for short-term treatment of anxiety, fits due to fever, muscle spasm, sleeplessness, and acute epileptic attacks. Also used as an additional treatment when withdrawing from alcohol.

Strengths available: 2 mg, 5 mg, and 10 mg tablets; 2 mg/5 ml and 5 mg/5 ml liquid; 10 mg suppositories; 2.5 mg, 5 mg, 10 mg, and 20 mg rectal solutions.

Dose: adults, usually 6-60 mg a day (in divided doses) by mouth according to condition; for sleeplessness, 5-15 mg at bedtime; children usually 1-40 mg a day by mouth; by suppository or rectal solution, usually 5-30 mg a day, depending on condition and body weight.

Availability: NHS and private prescription (5 mg/5 ml liquid not available on NHS).

Contains: diazepam.

Brand names: Diazepam Rectubes, Stesolid, Valclair, Valium (not available on NHS).

 alcohol, other sedating drugs, some antivirals and anti-epileptic medications, isoniazid, rifampicin.

 drowsiness, light-headedness, confusion, vertigo, stomach disturbances, loss of memory, aggression, headache, joint immobility, salivation changes, shaking, unsteadiness, low blood pressure, rash, changes in vision, changes in sexual desire, retention of urine, incontinence, blood changes, jaundice. Risk of addiction increases with dose and length of treatment. May impair judgement.

 in children, the elderly, pregnant women, mothers who are breastfeeding, women during labour, and in patients suffering from lung disorders, glaucoma, kidney or liver disorders, muscle weakness, PORPHYRIA, or with a history of drug or alcohol abuse. Avoid long-term use and withdraw gradually.

 patients suffering from acute lung diseases, some chronic lung diseases, severe liver disease, MYASTHENIA GRAVIS, some obsessional and psychotic disorders, or who have stopped breathing while asleep.

diazoxide tablets

A tablet used as a blood-sugar-elevating drug to treat low blood-glucose levels.

Strengths available: 50 mg tablets.

Dose: 5 mg per kilogram body weight a day in divided doses at first.

Availability: NHS and private prescription.

Contains: diazoxide.

Brand names: Eudemine.

 loss of appetite, stomach upset, fluid retention, heart rhythm disturbance, low blood pressure, abnormal movements, blood changes, abnormal hair growth. Rarely, liver or kidney disorders, headache, difficulty breathing, cataracts, blurred vision, muscular or skeletal pain.

cont.

in children, pregnant women, women in labour, and in patients with kidney disorders, gout, or heart disease.

anaesthetics, drugs that lower blood pressure, antidiabetic drugs.

Dibenyline *see* phenoxybenzamine capsules (Forley)

dibucaine *see* cinchocaine (alternative name)

diclofenac enteric-coated tablets/ dual-release capsules/modified-release capsules/modified-release tablets/suppositories/dispersible tablets

An E-C TABLET, M-R CAPSULE/TABLET, suppository, or dispersible tablet used as a NON-STEROIDAL ANTI-INFLAMMATORY DRUG to treat bone or muscular problems, arthritis, ankylosing spondylitis, and acute gout. (Diclofenac potassium also used to treat migraine in adults.)

Strengths available: 25 mg and 50 mg e-c tablets; 75 mg and 100 mg m-r capsules/ tablets; 12.5 mg, 25 mg, 50 mg, and 100 mg suppositories; 50 mg dispersible tablets. (Diclofenac potassium available only as 25 mg and 50 mg tablets.)

Dose: adults 75-150 mg a day in divided doses; children (for juvenile arthritis) use 25 mg e-c tablets or 12.5 or 50 mg suppositories only, in doses of 1-3 mg per kg body weight a day; to treat migraine using diclofenac potassium, adults, 50 mg at start of attack repeated after 2 hours and then at 4-6 hour intervals (maximum of 200 mg in 24 hours).

Availability: NHS and private prescription.

Contains: diclofenac sodium (or diclofenac potassium in Voltarol Rapid).

Brand names: Acoflam, Closteril, Dicloflex, Diclomax, Diclotard, Diclovol, Diclozip, Difenor XL, Digenac XL, Econac, Flamatak, Flamrase, Flexotard, Lofensaid, Motifene (a combination of standard-release and m-r capsules), Rheumatac Retard, Rhumalgan, Slofenac, Volraman, Volsaid Retard, Voltarol, Voltarol Rapid (diclofenac potassium).

stomach upset and bleeding or ulceration, severe allergy, difficulty breathing, blood or kidney disorders, headache, dizziness, noises in the ears, sensitivity to light, vertigo. Rarely, fluid retention, liver disorders, inflamed pancreas, inflamed bowel, meningitis. Suppositories may cause irritation around rectum.

in pregnant women, mothers who are breast-feeding, the elderly, and in patients with heart, liver, or kidney disorders, asthma, or LUPUS.

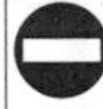
children or for patients with a history of allergy to aspirin or other NSAIDs, blood-clotting disorders, PORPHYRIA, currently active stomach ulcer or intestinal bleeding, inflamed intestines, or severe heart failure.

ACE-INHIBITORS, aspirin or other non-steroidal anti-inflammatory drugs, some ANTIBIOTICS, ANTICOAGULANTS, some antidiabetic drugs, some antivirals, methotrexate, DIURETICS, lithium, tacrolimus, cyclosporin, digoxin. ANTACIDS should not be taken at the same time as e-c tablets.

Compound preparations: Arthrotec.
Other preparations: diclofenac eye drops, diclofenac gel *see* non-steroidal anti-inflammatory drug (topical).

diclofenac eye drops

Eye drops used as a NON-STEROIDAL ANTI-INFLAMMATORY DRUG to treat inflammation and pain after eye surgery or injury.

Strengths available: 0.1% drops.
Dose: as advised by doctor.
Availability: NHS and private prescription.
Contains: diclofenac sodium.
Brand names: Voltarol Ophtha.
Other preparations: diclofenac enteric-coated tablets/dual-release capsules/modified-release capsules/modified-release tablets/suppositories/dispersible tablets, diclofenac gel *see* non-steroidal anti-inflammatory drug (topical).

mild burning sensation. Rarely, itching, reddening of the eye, sensitivity to light, inflamed cornea.

in pregnant women, mothers who are breast-feeding, and in patients with infected eye conditions.

children or for patients with a history of allergy to aspirin or non-steroidal anti-inflammatory drugs.

diclofenac gel *see* non-steroidal anti-inflammatory drug (topical)

Dicloflex/Dicloflex Retard *see* diclofenac enteric-coated tablets/modified-release tablets
(Dexcel Pharma)

Diclomax Retard *see* diclofenac modified-release capsules
(Parke Davis)

Diclotard *see* diclofenac modified-release tablets
(Galen)

Diclovol *see* diclofenac modified-release tablets
(Arun Pharmaceuticals UK)

Diclozip *see* diclofenac enteric-coated tablets
(Ashbourne Pharmaceuticals)

D

Diconal

(CeNeS)

A combination tablet used as an OPIOID and anti-sickness drug to control pain (*see* also cyclizine tablets).

Strengths available: 10 mg + 30 mg tablets.
Dose: 1 tablet every 6 hours increasing gradually to 3 tablets every 6 hours if needed.
Availability: controlled drug; NHS and private prescription.
Contains: dipipanone hydrochloride and cyclizine hydrochloride.

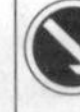
drowsiness, upset stomach, sweating, dizziness, breathing difficulty, low blood pressure, difficulty passing urine, dry mouth, headache, vertigo, flushing, change in heart rhythm, mood changes, rash, itching, addiction, reduced sexual desire, ANTIMUSCARINIC effects.

in children, pregnant women, women in labour, mothers who are breastfeeding, elderly or weakened patients, and in those suffering from breathing, kidney, or liver problems, low blood pressure, underactive thyroid, reduced ADRENAL function, diabetes, shock, low blood pressure, PHAEOCHROMOCYTOMA, enlarged prostate, or epilepsy. (Higher doses not suitable for some of these categories.)

alcoholics or for patients with head injury, reduced breathing ability, PORPHYRIA, or those who have a history of drug addiction or who are suicidal or at risk of non-functioning intestines.

MAOIS, alcohol, sedating drugs, ritonavir.

---

dicyclomine tablets/syrup

A tablet or syrup used as an anti-spasm, ANTIMUSCARINIC treatment for bowel and stomach spasm.

Strengths available: 10 mg and 20 mg tablets; 10 mg/5 ml syrup.
Dose: adults 10-20 mg three times a day; children aged 6 months-2 years 5-10 mg 3-4 times a day, aged 2-12 years 10 mg three times a day.
Availability: NHS and private prescription.
Contains: dicyclomine (dicycloverine) hydrochloride.
Brand names: Merbentyl.
Compound preparations: Diarrest, Kolanticon.

antimuscarinic effects, skin reactions, stomach upset, altered heart rhythm, difficulty passing urine, disturbed vision, dry mouth, intolerance of light, flushing, dry skin, confusion, dizziness.

in children, pregnant women, mothers who are breastfeeding, elderly patients, and those with diarrhoea or inflamed bowel, high blood pressure, abnormal heart rhythm, fever, reflux oesophagitis, or heart attack.

infants under 6 months or for patients with glaucoma, MYASTHENIA GRAVIS, enlarged prostate, or non-functioning intestines.

other antimuscarinic drugs.

---

dicycloverine *see* dicyclomine (alternative name)

Dicynene *see* ethamsylate tablets
(Sanofi Synthelabo)

didanosine tablets/enteric-coated capsules

A tablet or E-C CAPSULE used in combination with other antiviral drugs as an antiviral drug (combined with an antacid) to treat symptoms of HIV infection.

D

Strengths available: 25 mg, 100 mg, 150 mg, and 200 mg chewable or dispersible tablets; 125 mg, 200 mg, 250 mg, and 400 mg e-c capsules.
Dose: using tablets, adults 250 mg-400 mg a day (either as a single daily dose or divided into two doses), children over 3 months use reduced doses according to body weight. The dose to be taken as 2 tablets of an appropriate strength. Using e-c capsules, adults 250 mg-400 mg once a day (taken at least 2 hours after food).
Availability: NHS and private prescription.
Contains: didanosine. Tablets also contain calcium and magnesium antacids.
Brand names: Videx, Videx EC.

inflamed pancreas, weakness and numbness of hands and feet, stomach upset, blood and urine changes. Rarely, eyesight changes, liver failure, dry mouth, headache, severe allergy, diabetes.

in pregnant women, mothers who are breast-feeding, and in patients suffering from kidney or liver disorders, PHENYLKETONURIA, high uric acid levels, nerve disorders in hands and feet, or with a history of inflamed pancreas or liver disease. Your doctor may advise regular blood and urine tests, and eye checks for children.

children under 3 months, or mothers who are breastfeeding.

⇔ some ANTIBIOTICS with e-c tablets/capsules. E-c capsules not to be taken at same time as antacids.

Didronel *see* disodium etidronate tablets
(Proctor and Gamble Pharmaceuticals UK)

Didronel PMO *see* disodium etidronate tablets and calcium carbonate tablets
(Proctor and Gamble Pharmaceuticals UK)
A combination pack of the two separate tablets used to treat and prevent OSTEOPOROSIS.

Strengths available: 400 mg etidronate tablets and 1250 mg calcium carbonate tablets.
Dose: 1 etidronate tablet once a day (in the middle of a 4-hour fast) for 14 days, followed by 1 calcium carbonate tablet (dissolved in water) daily for 76 days, then the cycle repeated.

dienestrol *see* dienoestrol (alternative name)

dienoestrol *see* hormone replacement therapy – topical

diethylamine cream *see* analgesic (topical)

diethylstilbestrol *see* hormone replacement therapy – topical

D

Difenor XL *see* diclofenac modified-release tablets
(Norton Healthcare)

Differin *see* adapalene cream/gel
(Galderma (UK))

Difflam *see* non-steroidal anti-inflammatory drug (topical), benzydamine mouthwash/spray
(3M Health Care)

Diflucan *see* fluconazole capsules/suspension
(Pfizer)

diflucortolone *see* topical corticosteroid cream/oily cream/ointment

diflunisal tablets

A tablet used as an NON-STEROIDAL ANTI-INFLAMMATORY DRUG to treat pain and inflammation in arthritis and other similar disorders, and period pain.

Strengths available: 250 mg and 500 mg tablets.
Dose: usually 500-1000 mg a day (maximum of 1500 mg a day).
Availability: NHS and private prescription.
Contains: diflunisal.
Brand names: Dolobid.

ACE-INHIBITORS, aspirin or other non-steroidal anti-inflammatory drugs, some ANTIBIOTICS, ANTICOAGULANTS, some antidiabetic drugs, some antivirals, methotrexate, DIURETICS, lithium, tacrolimus, cyclosporin, aluminium hydroxide, digoxin.

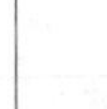
stomach upset and bleeding or ulceration, severe allergy, difficulty breathing, blood or kidney disorders, headache, dizziness, noises in the ears, sensitivity to light, vertigo. Rarely, fluid retention, liver disorders, inflamed pancreas, inflamed bowel, meningitis. Suppositories may cause irritation around rectum.

in the elderly and in patients with heart, liver, or kidney disorders, asthma, or LUPUS.

children, pregnant women, mothers who are breastfeeding, or for patients with a history of allergy to aspirin or other non-steroidal anti-inflammatory drug, blood clotting disorders, currently active stomach ulcer or intestinal bleeding, inflamed intestines, or severe heart failure.

Diftavax *see* diphtheria and tetanus vaccine
(Aventis Pasteur MSD)

Digenac XL *see* diclofenac modified-release tablets
(Genus Pharmaceuticals)

digitoxin tablets

A tablet used as a heart muscle stimulant (similar to digoxin) for heart failure and abnormal heart rhythms.

Strengths available: 100 mcg tablets.
Dose: adults 100-200 mcg a day (sometimes 100 mcg on alternate days).
Availability: NHS and private prescription.
Contains: digitoxin.

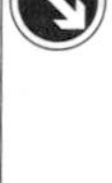 stomach upset, abdominal pain, headache, tiredness, drowsiness, confusion, visual changes, change to heart rhythm, loss of appetite, hallucinations.

 in the elderly, pregnant women, and in patients suffering from potassium deficiency, thyroid disorders, heart disorders, or recent heart attack.

 amphoteracin, mefloquine, verapamil, DIURETICS, alcohol, sedating drugs.

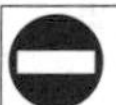 patients suffering from some types of heart disorders.

digoxin tablets/elixir

A tablet or elixir used as a heart muscle stimulant to treat heart failure and heart rhythm disturbances.

Strengths available: 62.5 mcg, 125 mcg, and 250 mcg tablets; 50 mcg/ml elixir.
Dose: adults usually 62.5-500 mcg a day (higher doses given in divided doses). Elderly patients require lower doses; children as advised by doctor.
Availability: NHS and private prescription.
Contains: digoxin.
Brand names: Lanoxin.

 stomach upset, abdominal pain, headache, tiredness, drowsiness, confusion, visual changes, change to heart rhythm, loss of appetite, hallucinations.

 in the elderly, pregnant women, and in patients suffering from potassium deficiency, kidney disorders, thyroid disorders, heart disorders, or recent heart attack.

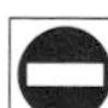 patients suffering from some types of heart disorders.

 ACE-INHIBITORS, some drugs used to treat abnormal heart rhythm, rifampicin, amphoteracin, itraconazole, anti-malarial treatments, some drugs used to treat high blood pressure or angina, DIURETICS, alcohol, sedating drugs.

D

dihydrocodeine tablets/modified-release tablets/solution

A tablet, M-R TABLET, or solution used as an OPIOID to control pain.

Strengths available: 30 mg and 40 mg tablets; 10 mg/5 ml solution.
Dose: adults usually 30 mg every 4-6 hours (occasionally higher doses) or 60-120 mg twice a day using m-r tablets; children over 4 years use reduced doses according to body weight.
Availability: NHS and private prescription.
Contains: dihydrocodeine tartrate.
Brand names: DF118 Forte, DHC Continus.
Compound preparations: co-dydramol.

children under 4 years, alcoholics, or for patients with head injury, reduced breathing ability, PORPHYRIA, or those who have a history of drug addiction or who are suicidal or at risk of non-functioning intestines.

drowsiness, upset stomach, sweating, dizziness, breathing difficulty, low blood pressure, difficulty passing urine, dry mouth, headache, vertigo, flushing, change in heart rhythm, mood changes, rash, itching, addiction, reduced sexual desire.

pregnant women, women in labour, mothers who are breastfeeding, elderly or weakened patients, and in those suffering from breathing, kidney or liver problems, low blood pressure, underactive thyroid, enlarged prostate, or epilepsy. (Higher doses not suitable for some of these categories.)

MAOIS, alcohol, sedating drugs, ritonavir.

dihydroergotamine nasal spray

A nasal spray used as an ERGOTAMINE treatment for migraine attacks.

Strengths available: 500 mcg per dose.
Dose: 1 spray in each nostril as soon as attack starts, repeated after 15 minutes if necessary. Total maximum number of sprays 4 in 24 hours or 16 in a week.
Availability: NHS and private prescription.
Contains: dihydroergotamine mesylate.
Brand names: Migranal.

azithromycin, clarithromycin, erythromycin, antiviral treatments, other drugs used to treat migraine.

stomach upset, muscular pain, abdominal pain, reduced circulation, chest pain, reduced blood supply to the heart, weak legs, inflamed nasal passages. Rarely, worsening of headache, heart attack. With excessive use, thickening of lung or abdominal tissues, gangrene, confusion.

in elderly patients and in those with liver disorders or a tendency to blood vessel disorders. Stop treatment if numbness or tingling occurs in hands or feet.

children, pregnant women, mothers who are breastfeeding, or in patients suffering from narrowed blood vessels, Raynaud's syndrome, severe high blood pressure, kidney or liver disease, some infections, overactive thyroid, PORPHYRIA, or for migraine prevention.

dihydrotachysterol solution

A solution used as a source of VITAMIN D to treat a nerve disorder caused by low calcium levels in patients with underactive parathyroid glands.

Strengths available: 0.25 mg/ml.
Dose: as directed by a doctor.
Availability: NHS and private prescription, over the counter.
Contains: dihydrotachysterol (a form of vitamin D).
Brand names: AT10.

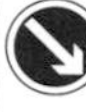
loss of appetite, raised blood calcium levels, listlessness, vertigo, stupor, nausea, urgent need to urinate, passing large volumes of pale-coloured urine, paralysis, headache, thirst.

in pregnant women. Your doctor may advise that your calcium levels should be checked regularly.

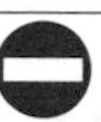
children, mothers who are breastfeeding, or for patients with nut allergy, high levels of calcium in the blood, or who have ingested excessive amounts of vitamin D.

diloxanide tablets

A tablet used to treat intestinal infections.

Strengths available: 500 mg tablets.
Dose: adults, 500 mg every 8 hours for 10 days; children use reduced doses according to body weight.
Availability: NHS and private prescription.
Contains: diloxanide furoate.

wind, vomiting, itching, rash.

pregnant women or mothers who are breast-feeding.

diltiazem modified-release tablets/long-acting capsules or tablets

An M-R TABLET or longer-acting tablet/capsule used as a CALCIUM CHANNEL BLOCKER to treat and prevent angina and high blood pressure.

Strengths available: 60 mg m-r tablets; 60 mg, 90 mg, 120 mg, 180 mg, 200 mg, 240 mg, 300 mg, and 360 mg longer-acting preparations (capsules or tablets).
Dose: using m-r tablets, initially 180 mg a day (elderly, initially 120 mg a day) increasing to a maximum of 360 mg a day in divided doses; using longer-acting products, up to 500 mg a day (depending on brand) – doses taken as either a single daily dose or divided into

stomach upset, headache, rash, slow heart rate, swollen ankles, heart conduction disorders and slow or irregular heart beat, tiredness, low blood pressure, dizziness, flushes, liver disorder, depression, sensitivity to sunlight, swollen gums, abnormal movements.

in patients suffering from liver or kidney disorders, heart failure, slow heart beat or other heart disorders. Patients using longer-acting products should remain on the same brand of diltiazem once stabilized.

cont.

two doses depending on brand.
Availability: NHS and private prescription.
Contains: diltiazem hydrochloride.
Brand names: Adizem, Angiozem, Angitil, Bi-Carzem, Calcicard, Dilzem, Optil, Slozem, Tildiem, Viazem, Zemtard, Zildil.

 children, pregnant women, mothers who are breastfeeding, or for patients suffering from very slow heart beat or heart conduction disorders.

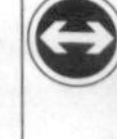 amiodarone, rifampicin, carbamazepine, phenytoin, phenobarbital, itraconazole, ALPHA-BLOCKERS, ritonavir, BETA-BLOCKERS, digoxin, cyclosporin, lithium, theophylline, aminophylline.

Dilzem SR/XL *see* diltiazem modified-release capsules
(Elan Pharma)

dimethicone *see* activated dimethicone, Asilone, Conotrane, co-simalcite suspension, Imodium Plus, Infacol, Kolanticon, Maalox Plus, Metanium, Siopel, Sprilon, Timodine, Vasogen

dimethyl sulfoxide *see* dimethyl sulphoxide (alternative name)

dimethyl sulphoxide *see* Herpid

dimeticone *see* dimethicone (alternative name)

Dimetriose capsules *see* gestrinone capsules
(Distriphar)

Dimotane *see* brompheniramine tablets/modified-release tablets/elixir
(Wyeth Laboratories)

Dimotane Plus *see* brompheniramine elixir and pseudoephedrine elixir
(Wyeth Laboratories)

Strengths available: 4 mg + 30 mg/5 ml and 2 mg + 15 mg/5 ml.
Dose: adults, 10 ml (children aged 6-12 years, 5 ml) three times a day using stronger product; children aged 2-5 years, 5 ml (aged 6-12 years, 10 ml) three times a day using weaker product.

Diocaps *see* loperamide capsules
(Berk Pharmaceuticals)

Dioctyl *see* docusate capsules
(Schwartz Pharma)

Dioderm *see* topical corticosteroid cream
(Dermal Laboratories)

Dioralyte tablets/sachets *see* oral rehydration solution
(Rhône-Poulenc Rorer)

Diovan *see* valsartan capsules
(Novartis Pharmaceuticals UK)

Dipentum *see* olsalazine capsules/tablets
(Pharmacia and Upjohn)

---

diphenhydramine *see* Caladryl

---

diphenoxylate *see* co-phenotrope tablets

---

diphtheria vaccine

Diphtheria vaccine provides active immunization against the disease by stimulating the body's production of an antitoxin. (Used only after contact with the disease.)

Strengths available: adult/adolescent strength and children's strength.

Dose: initial vaccination by three injections at 4-week intervals if no previous vaccination given. (For previously vaccinated patients one single booster dose is given.) Children's strength used for children aged 2 months-10 years; adult/adolescent strength for older patients.

Availability: NHS and private prescription.

Contains: diphtheria toxoid.

Compound preparations: diphtheria and tetanus vaccine; diphtheria, tetanus, and pertussis vaccine; diphtheria, tetanus, pertussis, and *Haemophilus influenzae* type b vaccine.

 reaction around injection site, headache, fever, general feeling of illness.

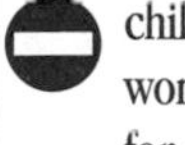 children under 2 months, adults, pregnant women, mothers who are breastfeeding, or for patients with an infection.

---

diphtheria and tetanus vaccine *see* diphtheria vaccine and tetanus vaccine

Strengths available: adult/adolescent strength and children's strength.
Dose: initial vaccination by three injections at 4-week intervals. Children's strength used for children aged 2 months-10 years; adult/adolescent strength for older patients. Children's vaccination course starts at 2 months (booster at school entry). Adults given booster after 10 years.
Brands: Diftavax.

---

diphtheria, tetanus, and pertussis vaccine *see* diphtheria vaccine, pertussis vaccine, and tetanus vaccine

Strengths available: children's strength only.
Dose: initial vaccination by three injections at 4-week intervals. Vaccination course starts at age 2 months.

---

diphtheria, tetanus, pertussis, and *Haemophilus influenzae* type b vaccine *see* diphtheria vaccine, pertussis vaccine, tetanus vaccine, and *Haemophilus influenzae* type b vaccine

Dose: as part of children's immunization schedule, three injections at 4-week intervals starting at age 2 months. May be used to complete a course started with diphtheria, tetanus, and pertussis vaccine.
Brand names: ACT-HIB DTP, Infanrix-Hib.

---

dipipanone *see* Diconal

---

dipivefrine eye drops

Eye drops used as a SYMPATHOMIMETIC treatment for glaucoma and other causes of high pressure in the eye.

Strengths available: 0.1% drops.
Dose: 1 drop into the affected eye(s) twice a day.
Availability: NHS and private prescription.
Contains: dipivefrine hydrochloride.
Brand names: Propine.

temporary stinging or redness of the eye, allergic reaction. Rarely, raised blood pressure.

in pregnant women, mothers who are breast-feeding, and in patients with narrow-angle glaucoma, or who have no lens in the eye.

children or for patients with closed-angle glaucoma or who wear soft contact lenses.

---

dipotassium clorazepate *see* potassium clorazepate (alternative name)

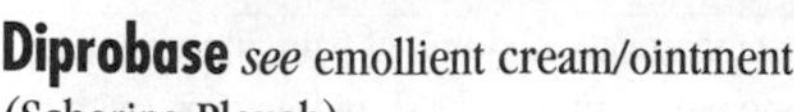
Diprobase *see* emollient cream/ointment
(Schering-Plough)

Diprobath *see* emollient bath oil
(Schering-Plough)

Diprosalic *see* topical corticosteroid ointment/scalp application and salicylic acid ointment
(Schering-Plough)

Diprosone *see* topical corticosteroid cream/ointment/lotion
(Schering-Plough)

---

dipyridamole tablets/modified-release tablets

A tablet or M-R TABLET used as an anti-platelet drug (in addition to ANTICOAGULANTS or aspirin) to prevent blood clots associated with artificial heart valves. (M-r tablets also used to prevent stroke and symptoms caused by narrowed brain blood vessels.)

Strengths available: 25 mg and 100 mg tablets; 200 mg m-r tablets.
Dose: 300-600 mg a day in 3-4 divided doses before meals; children use reduced doses according to body weight.
Availability: NHS and private prescription.
Contains: dipyridamole.
Brand names: Persantin.
Compound preparations: Asasantin Retard.

 ANTACIDS, ANTICOAGULANTS, other anti-platelet drugs.

Side effects: headache, dizziness, stomach upset, rash, low blood pressure, muscle pain, hot flushes, irregular heart beat. Rarely, rash, increased severity of heart disease, abnormal bleeding after surgery.

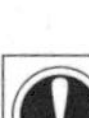 in pregnant women, mothers who are breast-feeding, and in patients suffering from rapidly worsening angina, blood clotting disorders, MYASTHENIA GRAVIS, some other heart conditions, recent heart attack, low blood pressure, migraine.

Dirythmin SA *see* dispyramide modified-release capsules
(AstraZeneca UK)

Disipal *see* orphenadrine tablets
(Sovereign Medical)

D

disodium etidronate tablets

A tablet used as a treatment for Paget's disease.

Strengths available: 200 mg tablets.
Dose: 5 mg per kg body weight a day as a single dose (in the middle of a 4-hour fast) for up to 6 months. Higher doses may be used but treatment period generally reduced. Repeat courses given only after a break of at least 3 months.
Availability: NHS and private prescription.
Contains: disodium etidronate.
Brand names: Didronel.
Compound preparations: Didronel PMO.

upset stomach, abdominal pain, increased bone pain, increased risk of fractures (with high doses), skin reactions, blood disorders, pins and needles, numbness or weakness in hands and feet, headache.

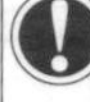
in patients suffering from kidney disorders. Your doctor will advise blood tests before starting treatment and every 3 months during treatment.

children, pregnant women, mothers who are breastfeeding, or for patients with severe kidney disease.

food, iron and mineral supplements (*see above* – do not take etidronate within 2 hours).

---

disodium phosphate dodecahydrate *see* Fleet phospho-soda solution

---

disopyramide capsules/modified-release capsules/tablets

A capsule or M-R TABLET/CAPSULE used as an anti-arrhythmic drug to treat abnormal heart rhythm.

Strengths available: 100 mg and 150 mg capsules; 250 mg m-r tablets; 150 mg m-r capsules.
Dose: 300-800 mg a day in divided doses.
Availability: NHS and private prescription.
Contains: disopyramide phosphate.
Brand names: Dirythmin SA, Isomide CR, Rythmodan.

stomach upset, low blood pressure, dry mouth, blurred vision, constipation, heart conduction defects or irregular heart beat, mental disorders, heart muscle depression, difficulty passing urine, low blood sugar, jaundice.

in the elderly, pregnant women, mothers who are breastfeeding, and in patients suffering from mild heart block, enlarged prostate, glaucoma, difficulty passing urine, low potassium levels, heart failure, kidney or liver failure.

children or for patients suffering from some types of heart block, heart muscle disease or shock, severe heart failure.

other anti-arrhythmic drugs, some ANTIBIOTICS, TRICYCLIC ANTIDEPRESSANTS, reboxetine, mizolastine, halofantrine, pimozide, sertindole, thioridazine, BETA-BLOCKERS, verapamil, DIURETICS.

Disprin CV *see* aspirin tablets
(Reckitt and Colman Products)

Disprol Paediatrics *see* paracetamol paediatric suspension
(Reckitt and Colman Products)

Distaclor *see* cefaclor capsules/modified-release tablets/syrup
(Dista Products)

Distalgesic *see* co-proxamol tablets
(Dista Products)

Distamine *see* penicillamine tablets
(Dista Products)

---

distigmine tablets

A tablet used as an ANTICHOLINESTERASE to treat MYASTHENIA GRAVIS and post-operative bladder or intestine problems.

Strengths available: 5 mg tablets.
Dose: for myasthenia gravis, adults 5 mg a day increasing to 20 mg a day if necessary (children up to 10 mg a day); for urinary retention, adults 5 mg once a day or on alternate days; to prevent complications after surgery, adults 5 mg once a day. The dose is taken half-an-hour before breakfast.
Availability: NHS and private prescription.
Contains: distigmine bromide.
Brand names: Ubretid.

 nausea, vomiting, sweating, stomach cramps, blurred vision, slow heart rate.

 in patients suffering from asthma, slow heart beat, heart disease, stomach ulcer, overactive thyroid, epilepsy, Parkinson's disease, low blood pressure, vagus nerve disorder, or who have recently suffered a heart attack.

 pregnant women or for patients suffering from bowel or urinary blockage or with weak circulation or in shock after surgery. Not to be used for patients who would be harmed by increased activity of intestines or bladder. Used for children only to treat myasthenia gravis.

---

disulfiram tablets

A tablet used as an enzyme inhibitor as an additional treatment for alcoholism.

Strengths available: 200 mg tablets.
Dose: as advised by doctor.
Availability: NHS and private prescription.
Contains: disulfiram.
Brand names: Antabuse.

 drowsiness, tiredness, nausea, bad breath, reduced sexual desire, skin allergy, liver damage, skin reactions, weakness or numbness of hands and feet. Rarely, mental disturbances.

cont.

 in patients suffering from liver, kidney, or breathing disorders, diabetes, epilepsy, drug addiction. No alcohol to be taken for 24 hours before treatment begins.

 children, pregnant women, mothers who are breastfeeding, or for patients suffering from heart failure, angina, high blood pressure, or mental disorders, or with a history of stroke.

 ANTICOAGULANTS, phenytoin, theophylline, aminophylline, sedatives, alcohol.

D

dithranol cream/ointment/paste

A cream, ointment, or paste used to treat psoriasis.

Strengths available: various strengths between 0.1% and 3.0%.

Dose: apply to the affected area and wash off after 30-60 minutes, or may be applied at bedtime and left overnight before washing off. Start treatment with lowest strength and increase only if needed.

Availability: NHS and private prescription. (Weaker strengths also available over the counter.)

Contains: dithranol.

Brand names: Dithrocream, Micanol.

Compound preparations: Psorin.

 irritation, allergy.

 stains skin and clothing.

— patients with acute or infected psoriasis. Not for application to skin folds or near eyes and sensitive areas.

Dithrocream *see* dithranol cream
(Dermal Laboratories)

Ditropan/Ditropan XL *see* oxybutynin tablets/modified-release tablets/elixir
(Sanofi Synthelabo)

Diumide-K *see* frusemide tablets and potassium chloride tablets
(ASTA Medica)

Strengths available: 40 mg + 600 mg tablets.

Dose: 1 tablet a day in the morning.

Diurexan *see* xipamide tablets
(ASTA Medica)

Dixarit *see* clonidine tablets
(Boehringer Ingelheim)

---

docosahexaenoic acid *see* Maxepa

---

docusate capsules/solution

A capsule or solution used as a softening agent and stimulant laxative to treat constipation.

Strengths available: 100 mg capsules; 50 mg/5 ml or 12.5 mg/5 ml solution.
Dose: adults up to 500 mg a day in divided doses; children 12.5 mg-25 mg three times a day according to age.
Availability: NHS and private prescription, nurse prescription, over the counter.
Contains: docusate sodium.
Brand names: Dioctyl, Docusol.
Compound preparations: co-danthrusate capsules.
Other preparations: docusate ear drops, docusate enema.

in pregnant women and mothers who are breastfeeding.

children under 6 months,or for patients with abdominal pain, nausea, vomiting, or intestinal obstruction.

liquid paraffin, other laxatives.

---

docusate ear drops

Ear drops used as a wax softener to remove ear wax.

Strengths available: 0.5% or 5% drops.
Dose: fill the ear with the solution for 2 nights before they are to be syringed.
Availability: NHS and private prescription, over the counter.
Contains: docusate sodium.
Brand names: Molcer, Waxsol.
Other preparations: docusate capsules/solution, docusate enema.

temporary irritation.

patients suffering from inflammation of the ear or perforated ear drum.

---

docusate enema

An enema (or small-volume enema) used as a bowel evacuator to treat constipation and to evacuate the bowels before surgery.

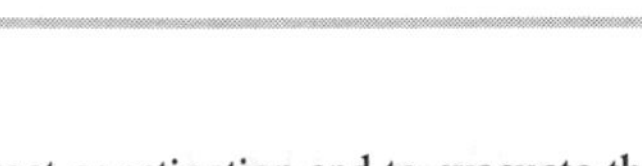

rectal irritation, diarrhoea. Rarely, rectal bleeding or liver disorder.

Strengths available: 120 mg enema or 90 mg small-volume enema.
Dose: 120 mg enema suitable for adults and children over 12 years; 90 mg small-volume

cont.

enema also suitable for children over 3 years.

Availability: NHS and private prescription, nurse prescription, over the counter.

Contains: docusate sodium.

Brand names: Fletchers' Enemette, Norgalax.

Other preparations: docusate capsules/solution, docusate ear drops.

 not for prolonged use.

 children under 3 years or for patients with abdominal pain, nausea, vomiting, haemorrhoids (piles), rectal fissures (cracks in the skin), intestinal obstruction, inflamed bowel, rectal bleeding.

↔ liquid paraffin, other laxatives.

Docusol *see* docusate solution
(Typharm)

Dolmatil *see* sulpiride tablets
(Sanofi Synthelabo)

Dolobid *see* diflunisal tablets
(Merck Sharp and Dohme)

Doloxene *see* dextropropoxyphene capsules
(Eli Lilly and Co.)

Domilium *see* domperidone tablets
(Genus Pharmaceuticals)

Domperamol *see* domperidone tablets and paracetamol tablets
(Servier Laboratories)
A combination tablet used to relieve migraine attacks.

Strengths available: 10 mg + 500 mg tablets.

Dose: 2 tablets at start of attack then repeated every 4 hours if needed (maximum of 8 tablets in 24 hours).

---

domperidone tablets/suspension/suppositories

A tablet, suspension, or suppository used as an anti-sickness drug to treat nausea, vomiting, and indigestion.

Strengths available: 10 mg tablets; 5 mg/5 ml suspension; 30 mg suppositories.

Dose: adults, 10-20 mg by mouth (or

 blood changes, rash, abnormal movements, reduction in sexual desire, enlarged breasts.

30-60 mg by suppository) every 4-8 hours for nausea and vomiting, 10-20 mg three times a day before food and at night for indigestion; children use reduced doses (as advised by doctor) only for nausea and vomiting caused by chemotherapy or radiotherapy.

in mothers who are breastfeeding.

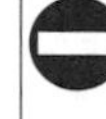
pregnant women or for routine prevention of vomiting after surgery. Not for prolonged use. Suppositories not suitable for children under 2 years.

Availability: NHS and private prescription. Also available over the counter in tablet form (dose 10 mg up to four times a day) to relieve nausea, bloating, wind, and heartburn in adults.
Contains: domperidone (domperidone maleate in tablet form).
Brand names: Domilium, Motilium.
Compound preparations: Domperamol.

D

---

donepezil tablets

A tablet used as an ANTICHOLINESTERASE treatment for Alzheimer's disease.

Strengths available: 5 mg and 10 mg tablets.
Dose: 5 mg once a day (at bedtime) at first increasing to 10 mg if necessary. Treatment initiated and supervised by a specialist.
Availability: NHS and private prescription.
Contains: donepezil hydrochloride.
Brand names: Aricept.

in patients with heart conduction disorders, asthma or other breathing disorders, difficulty passing urine, fits, or with a tendency to stomach ulcers.

stomach upset, tiredness, muscle cramps, sleeplessness, dizziness, headache, pain. Rarely, slow heart beat, heart conduction disorders, fainting, liver disorder, blood changes, loss of appetite, difficulty passing urine, fits, psychiatric disorders, stomach ulcers, intestinal bleeding.

children, pregnant women, or mothers who are breastfeeding.

NON-STEROIDAL ANTI-INFLAMMATORY DRUGS.

Doralese Tiltab *see* indoramin tablets
(SmithKline Beecham Pharmaceuticals)

---

dornase alfa nebulizer solution

A solution used for inhalation via a nebulizer to treat symptoms of cystic fibrosis.

sore throat, laryngitis, changes in the voice, chest pain, rash, eye inflammation.

Strengths available: 2.5 mg vials.
Dose: usually 2.5 mg once a day via nebulizer. Patients over 21 years may use 2.5 mg twice a day.
Availability: NHS and private prescription.

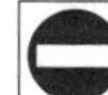
in pregnant women and mothers who are breastfeeding.

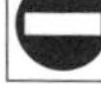
children under 5 years.

Contains: dornase alfa.
Brand names: Pulmozyme.

 not to be mixed with other drugs in the nebulizer.

dorzolamide eye drops

Eye drops used as a treatment for high pressure in the eye and for some types of glaucoma.

Strengths available: 2% drops.
Dose: if used alone, 1 drop into the affected eye three times a day; if used with a BETA-BLOCKER, 1 drop twice a day.
Availability: NHS and private prescription.
Contains: dorzolamide hydrochloride.
Brand names: Trusopt.
Compound preparations: Cosopt.

 irritation or discomfort in the eye, headache, bitter taste, eye or lid inflammation, blurred vision, nausea, tiredness, weakness, dizziness, pins and needles, rash, stones in the urine.

 in patients with closed-angle glaucoma, allergy to some antibiotics, or impaired liver function.

 children, pregnant women, mothers who are breastfeeding, or for patients with impaired kidney function or with abnormally high blood chloride levels or who wear soft contact lenses.

 leave 10 minutes between administration of other eye drops.

Dostinex *see* cabergoline tablets
(Pharmacia and Upjohn)

dosulepin *see* dothiepin (alternative name)

Dothapax *see* dothiepin capsules/tablets
(Ashbourne Pharmaceuticals)

dothiepin capsules/tablets

A capsule or tablet used as a TRICYCLIC ANTIDEPRESSANT to treat depression.

Strengths available: 25 mg capsules; 75 mg tablets.
Dose: usually 75-150 mg a day (either as a single dose at night or in divided doses through the day), and up to 225 mg in rare circumstances; elderly patients usually only up to 75 mg.
Availability: NHS and private prescription.
Contains: dothiepin (dosulepin) hydrochloride.
Brand names: Dothapax, Prepadine, Prothiaden.

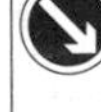 dry mouth, noises in the ears, tiredness, constipation, difficulty passing urine, blurred vision, stomach upset, palpitations, drowsiness, sleeplessness, dizziness, shaking hands, low blood pressure, weight change, sweating, fever, behavioural changes in children, confusion in the elderly, skin reactions, jaundice or blood changes, interference with sexual function, changes in heart rhythm, rash, hormone disturbances, fits, movement disorders, blood changes, breast changes in women, menstrual disorders.

children or for patients suffering from recent heart attacks, heart rhythm abnormalities, severe liver disease or elevated mood.

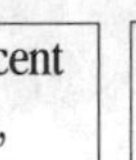
in the elderly, pregnant women, mothers who are breastfeeding, or in patients suffering from heart disease, liver and kidney disorders, thyroid disease, PHAEOCHROMOCYTOMA, epilepsy, diabetes, PORPHYRIA, glaucoma, urine retention, constipation, some other psychiatric conditions. Your doctor may advise regular blood tests.

alcohol, sedatives, MAOIS, BARBITURATES, other antidepressants, ANTIHYPERTENISVES, tranquillizers, anti-epileptic drugs, ritonavir, entacapone, selegiline, sotalol, halofantrine, drugs affecting heart rhythm, methylphenidate.

Dovonex *see* calcipotriol cream/ointment/scalp application
(Leo Pharmaceuticals)

doxazosin tablets

A tablet used as an ALPHA-BLOCKER to widen blood vessels and to treat high blood pressure and symptoms associated with enlarged prostate.

Strengths available: 1 mg, 2 mg, and 4 mg tablets.
Dose: 1 mg once a day at first increasing as needed to 16 mg a day (for blood pressure) or 8 mg a day (for prostate disorders).
Availability: NHS and private prescription.
Contains: doxazosin mesylate.
Brand names: Cardura.

low blood pressure on standing, vertigo, dizziness, headache, tiredness, weakness, fluid retention, drowsiness, nausea, inflamed nasal passages. Rarely, nose bleeds, rash, shaking, stomach upset, agitation, blurred vision, blood in the urine, liver disorders, gallstones, incontinence, impotence, severe sustained erection.

in pregnant women and in patients with liver disorders. Take extra care after the first dose because you may feel faint when standing up.

children and mothers who are breastfeeding.

anaesthetics, antidepressants, other drugs used to treat high blood pressure or angina, DIURETICS, thymoxamine, alcohol, sedating drugs.

doxepin capsules

A capsule used as a tricyclic antidepressant to treat depression.

Strengths available: 10 mg, 25 mg, 50 mg, and 75 mg capsules.
Dose: 10-100 mg three times a day or up to 100 mg as a single daily dose at bedtime.
Availability: NHS and private prescription.
Contains: doxepin hydrochloride.
Brand names: Sinequan.
Other preparations: doxepin cream.

dry mouth, noises in the ears, tiredness, constipation, difficulty passing urine, blurred vision, stomach upset, palpitations, drowsiness, sleeplessness, dizziness, shaking hands, low blood pressure, weight change, sweating, fever, behavioural changes in children, confusion in the elderly, skin reactions, jaundice or blood changes, interference with sexual function, changes in heart rhythm, rash, hormone disturbances, fits, movement disorders, blood changes, breast changes in women, menstrual disorders.

cont.

 alcohol, sedatives, MAOIS, BARBITURATES, other antidepressants, ANTIHYPERTENSIVES, tranquillizers, anti-epileptic drugs, ritonavir, entacapone, selegiline, sotalol, halofantrine, drugs affecting heart rhythm, methylphenidate.

 in the elderly, pregnant women, and in patients suffering from heart disease, liver and kidney disorders, thyroid disease, PHAEOCHROMOCYTOMA, epilepsy, diabetes, PORPHYRIA, glaucoma, urine retention, constipation, some other psychiatric conditions. Your doctor may advise regular blood tests.

 children, mothers who are breastfeeding, or for patients suffering from recent heart attacks, heart rhythm abnormalities, severe liver disease, or elevated mood.

doxepin cream

A cream used as an ANTIHISTAMINE to treat itching associated with eczema.

Strengths available: 5% cream.
Dose: apply thinly 3-4 times a day (maximum of 3 g per dose or 12 g per day).
Availability: NHS and private prescription.
Contains: doxepin hydrochloride.
Brand names: Xepin.
Other preparations: doxepin capsules.

 drowsiness, irritation or tingling at application site, rash, dry mouth and other side effects similar to doxepin capsules.

 in pregnant women, mothers who are breastfeeding, and in patients with glaucoma, difficulty passing urine, severe liver disorders, or who are in an excitable state.

 alcohol, sedatives, MAOIS, BARBITURATES, other antidepressants, ANTIHYPERTENSIVES, tranquillizers, anti-epileptic drugs, ritonavir, entacapone, selegiline, sotalol, halofantrine, drugs affecting heart rhythm.

 children under 12 years or for application to large areas.

doxycycline capsules/dispersible tablets

A capsule or dispersible tablet used as an ANTIBIOTIC to treat infections, especially chest, prostate, sinus, and pelvic infections, and acne. Also used to prevent malaria. The 20 mg capsule used in addition to dental treatment for inflammation of the gum and other tissues around the teeth.

Strengths available: 20 mg, 50 mg, and 100 mg capsules; 100 mg dispersible tablets.
Dose: usually 200 mg on the first day, then 100-200 mg a day (depending on severity and type of infection). For gum and tooth disorders, 20 mg twice a day for

 stomach upset, irritation of the oesophagus, reddening of skin, headache, disturbed vision, sensitivity to light, additional infections, pressure on the brain, reversible diabetes insipidus, liver or blood disorders, inflamed pancreas or bowel.

 in patients suffering from MYASTHENIA GRAVIS, liver or kidney disorders. Discontinue if reddening of skin occurs. Avoid use of sunlamps or excessive exposure to sunlight.

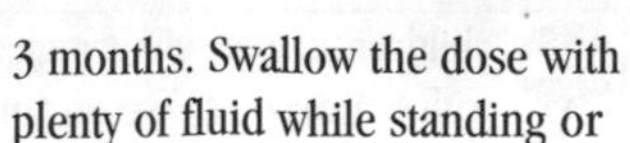

3 months. Swallow the dose with plenty of fluid while standing or sitting upright.

Availability: NHS and private prescription.
Contains: doxycycline (doxycycline hydrochloride in capsules).
Brand names: Cyclodox, Demix, Doxylar, Periostat, Vibramycin.

children under 12 years, pregnant women, mothers who are breastfeeding, or for patients suffering from LUPUS or PORPHYRIA.

ANTACIDS, iron supplements, ANTICOAGULANTS, ORAL CONTRACEPTIVES, cyclosporin.

Doxylar *see* doxycycline capsules
(Lagap Pharmaceuticals)

Dozic *see* haloperidol solution
(Rosemont Pharmaceuticals)

Drapolene *see* cetrimide cream BP
(Warner Lambert Consumer Healthcare)

Driclor *see* aluminium chloride hexahydrate solution
(Stiefel Laboratories (UK))

Droleptan *see* droperidol liquid/tablets
(Janssen-Cilag)

Dromadol XL *see* tramadol modified-release tablets
(Baker Norton Pharmaceuticals)

---

droperidol liquid/tablets

A tablet used as a sedative to calm agitated or manic patients.

Strengths available: 10 mg tablets; 1 mg/ml liquid.
Dose: adults 5-20 mg every 4-8 hours (elderly require lower doses at first); children 0.5-1.0 mg a day.
Availability: NHS and private prescription.
Contains: droperidol.
Brand names: Droleptan.

muscle spasms, restlessness, shaking hands, changes in sexual function, dry mouth, urine retention, blurred vision, heart rhythm disturbance, low blood pressure, weight change, low body temperature, breast swelling, menstrual changes, nasal congestion, nightmares, insomnia, depression, agitation, liver disorders, blood and skin changes, eye disorders, stomach upset, drowsiness, constipation, sensitivity to light. Rarely, fits or NEUROLEPTIC MALIGNANT SYNDROME.

cont.

 in pregnant women, mothers who are breastfeeding, the elderly, and in patients with heart or blood vessel disorders, infections, breathing disorders, Parkinson's disease, epilepsy, infection, kidney or liver disorders, underactive thyroid, MYASTHENIA GRAVIS, glaucoma, prostate disorders, some blood disorders.

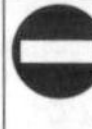 children, unconscious patients, or for patients with Parkinson's disease (or similar movement disorders), PHAEOCHROMOCYTOMA, depression, or allergy to similar drugs.

 alcohol, sedating drugs, anaesthetics, drugs that affect the heart rhythm, halofantrine, TRICYCLIC ANTIDEPRESSANTS, ritonavir.

Dumicoat
(Cox Pharmaceuticals)
A denture lacquer used as an antifungal treatment for fungal mouth infection caused by dentures.

Strengths available: 50 mg/ml solution.
Dose: apply to the upper denture (after cleaning) and allow to dry. The treatment should be repeated twice at weekly intervals.
Availability: NHS and private prescription.
Contains: miconazole.
Other preparations: miconazole cream/powder/spray/pessaries.

 in pregnant women and mothers who are breastfeeding.

 children or for patients suffering from PORPHYRIA.

 ANTICOAGULANTS, reboxetine, some antidiabetics, phenytoin, pimozide, cyclosporin, STATINS, tacrolimus.

Duofilm *see* salicylic acid collodion
(Stiefel Laboratories (UK))

Duovent
(Boehringer Ingelheim)
An aerosol or nebulizer solution used as a BRONCHODILATOR and ANTIMUSCARINIC to treat asthma and other breathing disorders such as emphysema and bronchitis.

Strengths available: 100 mcg + 40 mcg per dose (inhaler); 1.25 mg + 500 mcg per vial (nebulizer solution).
Dose: adults 1-2 puffs of inhaler 3-4 times a day; children over 6 years 1 puff of inhaler 3 times a day; nebulizer solution used for adults only (maximum of 4 vials in 24 hours).
Availability: NHS and private prescription.

 low potassium levels, shaking hands, headache, cramps, altered heart rhythm, widening of blood vessels, nervousness, severe allergic reaction, dry mouth, difficulty passing urine, constipation. glaucoma with nebulizer solution.

 in pregnant women, mothers who are breastfeeding, and in patients suffering from weak heart, irregular heart rhythm or angina, glaucoma, enlarged prostate, high blood pressure, overactive thyroid, diabetes. In asthmatics, blood potassium levels should be checked regularly. The eyes should be protected when using the nebulizer solution.

Contains: fenoterol hydrobromide and ipratropium bromide.
Other devices: Duovent Autohaler (breath-activated aerosol).

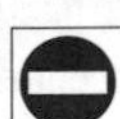 children under 6 years.

 BETA-BLOCKERS, other antimuscarinic drugs.

Duphalac Dry *see* lactulose sachets
(Solvay Healthcare)

Duphaston/Duphaston HRT *see* dydrogesterone tablets
(Solvay Healthcare)

Duragel *see* nonoxynol gel
(SSL International)

Duraphat *see* fluoride mouthwash (weekly)
(Colgate-Palmolive)

Durogesic *see* fentanyl patches
(Janssen-Cilag)

Dutonin *see* nefazodone tablets
(Bristol-Myers Squibb Pharmaceuticals)

Dyazide *see* co-triamterzide tablets
(Goldshield Healthcare)

---

dydrogesterone tablets

A tablet used as a progestogen to treat period pain, habitual and threatened abortion, endometriosis (a womb disorder), infertility, premenstrual syndrome, and as an additional treatment to oestrogen in hormone replacement.

Strengths available: 10 mg tablets.
Dose: period pain, 10 mg twice a day from the fifth to twenty-fifth day of cycle; endometriosis 10 mg 2-3 times a day from fifth to twenty-fifth day of cycle; premenstrual syndrome, 10 mg twice a day from twelfth to twenty-sixth day of cycle; hormone replacement, 10 mg

 irregular bleeding, breast discomfort, acne, headache, bloating, dizziness, skin disorder, weight change, stomach upset, changes in sexual desire, depression, sleeplessness, hair loss or growth, severe allergic reaction. Rarely, jaundice.

cont.

once or twice a day from fifteenth to twenty-eighth day of cycle.
Availability: NHS and private prescription.
Contains: dydrogesterone.
Brand names: Duphaston, Duphaston HRT.
Compound preparations: HORMONE REPLACEMENT THERAPY (COMBINED).

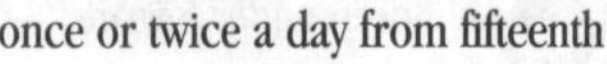

in patients suffering from high blood pressure, diabetes, heart or kidney disorders.

children, pregnant women, or for patients suffering from severe blood vessel disease, liver disorders, some forms of cancer, PORPHYRIA, undiagnosed vaginal bleeding.

cyclosporin.

Dynamin *see* isosorbide mononitrate tablets
(Berk Pharmaceuticals)

Dysman *see* mefenamic acid capsules/tablets
(Ashbourne Pharmaceuticals)

Dyspamet *see* cimetidine suspension
(Goldshield Healthcare)

Dytac *see* triamterene capsules
(Goldshield Healthcare)

Dytide *see* triamterene capsules and bendrofluazide tablets
(Goldshield Healthcare)
A capsule consisting of a combination of diuretics to treat fluid retention.

Strengths available: 50 mg + 25 mg capsules.
Dose: adults up to 3 capsules a day (2 in the morning and 1 at lunchtime) for 1 week, then reduced to 1-2 capsules a day (or every other day) for maintenance.
Contains: triamterene and benzthiazide (a similar diuretic to bendrofluazide).

Earcalm *see* acetic acid ear spray
(Stafford-Miller)

Easistix BG
(Eastern Pharmaceuticals)
A reagent strip used to detect visually blood glucose levels. Blood-glucose monitoring enables individual patients suffering from diabetes accurately to control blood glucose and manage their condition.

Availability: NHS, private prescription, over the counter.

Easistix UG

(Eastern Pharmaceuticals)

A reagent strip used for the detection of glucose in the urine. This gives an approximate estimate of blood glucose levels which may be adequate for the management of Type II diabetes.

e-c tablets/capsules/granules (enteric-coated tablets/capsules/granules)

A tablet, capsule, or granule coated to protect it from stomach acid. This allows it to pass through the stomach unaltered. Only when it reaches the intestines (where acid is no longer present) does it release its contents. This mechanism is used to deliver drugs directly to the bowel for bowel conditions, to protect drugs that might be decomposed by acid, or to ensure that drugs which might irritate the stomach are not released there. It is important not to take ANATCIDS at the same time of day as e-c preparations, because these reduce the acidity of the stomach and may lead to the contents being released there after all. Examples, diclofenac e-c tablets, budesonide e-c capsules.

Econac *see* diclofenac suppositories
(Goldshield Healthcare)

Econacort *see* econazole cream and topical corticosteroid cream
(Bristol-Myers Squibb Pharmaceuticals)

econazole cream/lotion

A cream used as an antibacterial and antifungal treatment for fungal infections of the skin, and some bacterial infections.

Strengths available: 1% cream or lotion.
Dose: apply to the affected area twice a day.
Availability: NHS and private prescription, over the counter. Cream also available on nurse prescription.
Contains: econazole nitrate.
Brand names: Ecostatin, Gyno-Pevaryl, Pevaryl.
Compound preparations: Econacort and Pevaryl TC (*see* topical corticosteroid).
Other preparations: econazole pessaries.

Side effects: rarely, skin irritation.

Caution: avoid the eyes.

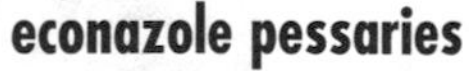

econazole pessaries

A pessary used as an antifungal and antibacterial treatment for thrush of the vulva or vagina.

Strengths available: 150 mg pessary for single use, 150 mg pessaries for repeated use.
Dose: 1 pessary inserted into the vagina at bedtime. (With pessaries formulated for repeated *cont.*

Side effects: mild irritation or burning.

use, repeat the dose for the next two nights.)

Availability: NHS and private prescription. (May be purchased over the counter for treatment of vaginal thrush only.)

Contains: econazole nitrate.

Brand names: Ecostatin, Ecostatin-1, Gyno-Pevaryl, Gyno-Pevaryl-1.

Other preparations: econazole cream, econazole twin pack (containing cream and pessaries).

Caution: when using the applicator in pregnancy.

Not to be used for: children.

Ecopace *see* captopril tablets
(Goldshield Healthcare)

Ecostatin *see* econazole cream and econazole pessaries
(Bristol-Myers Squibb Pharmaceuticals)

Edronax *see* reboxetine tablets
(Pharmacia and Upjohn)

Efalith

(Scotia Pharmaceuticals)

An anti-inflammatory ointment used to treat scaly scalp conditions.

Strengths available: 8% + 0.05% ointment.

Dose: apply thinly and evenly twice a day reducing as appropriate.

Availability: NHS and private prescription.

Contains: lithium succinate and zinc sulphate.

 irritation.

 in pregnant women, mothers who are breastfeeding, and in patients suffering from psoriasis. Avoid the eyes and mucous membranes.

 children under 12 years, women in the first 3 months of pregnancy, or for application to the breasts of mothers who are breastfeeding.

Efamast *see* gamolenic acid capsules
(Searle)

---

efavirenz capsules

A capsule used as an antiviral drug to treat HIV infections (in combination with other antivirals).

Strengths available: 50 mg, 100 mg, and 200 mg capsules.

Dose: adults 600 mg once a day; children over 3 years use reduced doses according to

body weight.
Availability: NHS and private prescription.
Contains: efavirenz.
Brand names: Sustiva.

 in pregnant women and in patients with liver or kidney disorders.

 alcohol, other sedating drugs, midazolam, grapefruit juice, BARBITURATES, ORAL CONTRACEPTIVES.

 skin disorders, mental disturbances, upset stomach, dizziness, headache, sleepiness or sleeplessness, tiredness, lack of concentration, high cholesterol or blood lipid levels, liver changes, inflamed pancreas.

 children under 3 years, mothers who are breastfeeding, or for patients with severe liver disorders or a history of mental illness or drug abuse.

E

Efcortelan *see* topical corticosteroid cream/ointment
(GlaxoWellcome UK)

Efexor/Efexor XL *see* venlafaxine tablets/modified-release capsules
(Wyeth Laboratories)

Effercitrate *see* potassium citrate mixture
(Typharm)
A tablet form of potassium citrate mixture.

Dose: adults and children over 6 years, 2 tablets (children aged 1-6 years 1 tablet) in water up to three times a day with food.

eformoterol inhalation capsules/turbohaler

A capsule for inhalation or powder inhaler used to treat airway obstruction (including night-time asthma) and to prevent symptoms induced by exercise. Used only for patients requiring long-term treatment.

Strengths available: 12 mcg capsules; powder inhalers with 6 mcg or 12 mcg per dose
Dose: 12-24 mcg twice a day using capsules or 6-12 mcg once a day (increasing to 24 mcg twice a day if needed) using powder inhaler. Additional doses of powder inhaler may be used to relieve breakthrough symptoms (up to a total daily dose of 72 mcg).
Availability: NHS and private prescription.

 shaking, nervousness, headache, irregular heartbeat, throat or eye irritation, swollen eyelids, taste disturbance, rash, sleeplessness, stomach upset, itching, difficulty breathing, severe allergy, muscle cramps, low blood potassium levels.

 in pregnant women and in patients with liver disorders, overactive thyroid, heart disorders, diabetes.

 children under 5 years (capsules) or under 12 years (powder inhaler), mothers who are breastfeeding.

 CORTICOSTEROIDS (high doses), DIURETICS, theophylline, aminophylline, SYMPATHOMIMETICS.

cont.

Contains: eformoterol (formoterol).
Brand names: Foradil, Oxis.

E45 cream/lotion/bath oil/shower gel *see* emollient cream/lotion/bath oil/shower gel

---

eicosapentaenoic acid *see* Maxepa

Elantan/Elantan LA *see* isosorbide monitrate tablets/modified-release capsules
(Schwarz Pharma)

Eldepryl *see* selegiline tablets/syrup
(Orion Pharma (UK))

Electrolade *see* oral rehydration solution
(Eastern Pharmaceuticals)

Elleste Duet/Elleste Duet Conti *see* hormone replacement therapy (combined)
(Searle)

Elleste Solo/Elleste Solo MX *see* hormone replacement therapy (oestrogen only)
(Searle)

Elocon *see* topical corticosteroid cream/ointment/scalp lotion
(Schering-Plough)

Eltroxin *see* thyroxine tablets
(Goldshield Healthcare)

Eludril *see* chlorhexidine mouthwash/spray
(Ceuta Healthcare)

Elyzol *see* metronidazole dental gel
(Cox Pharmaceuticals)

Emadine *see* emedastine eye drops
(Alcon)

Emblon *see* tamoxifen tablets
(Berk Pharmaceuticals)

Emcor/Emcor-LS *see* bisoprolol tablets
(E. Merck Pharmaceuticals)

---

emedastine eye drops

Eye drops used as an ANTIHISTAMINE treatment for hayfever.

Strengths available: 0.05% drops.
Dose: adults and children over 3 years, 1 drop into the affected eye(s) twice a day.
Availability: NHS and private prescription.
Contains: emedastine difumarate.
Brand names: Emadine.

 temporary discomfort, blurred vision, disorders of the cornea, dry or swollen eyes, headache, inflamed nasal passages, intolerance to light.

 in patients with contact lenses (leave 15 minutes before inserting lenses after using drops).

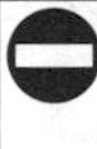 children under 3 years, pregnant women, mothers who are breastfeeding, elderly patients, or for patients with liver or kidney disorders.

 contact lenses (*see caution above*).

Emeside *see* ethosuximide capsules/syrup
(LAB)

Emflex *see* acemetacin capsules
(E. Merck Pharmaceuticals)

EMLA

(AstraZeneca UK)
A cream used as a local anaesthetic to numb the skin or genital areas before surgical procedures (such as taking blood samples or removal of genital warts).

Strengths available: 2.5% + 2.5% cream
Dose: usually applied under a covering dressing for 1-5 hours before procedure (applied for only 5-10 minutes before removal of genital warts).
Availability: NHS and private prescription.

irritation, paleness or redness of skin, fluid retention.

cont.

Contains: lignocaine, prilocaine.
Other preparations: various RECTAL CORTICOSTEROID preparations also contain similar local anaesthetics.

in patients suffering from blood disorders such as anaemia. Avoid using near the eyes or in the ear.

infants under 1 year, or for use on wounds, mucous membranes (except for genital wart removal), or areas of dermatitis.

E

emollient bar/bath preparations/cream/lotion/ointment/sachets/shower gel/spray

Preparations used to rehydrate and soften the skin, and to treat dry, scaly (and sometimes itchy) skin conditions such as eczema or psoriasis. Some preparations are added to the bath or used instead of soap. Others may be applied directly to the skin.

Dose: most products can be applied as often as necessary (but check product labels for detailed instructions).
Availability: NHS and private prescription, over the counter. Some products also available on nurse prescription (marked * in tables below).
Contains: (*see* tables below).

rarely, allergic reaction.

preparations added to the bath or used in the shower may make the bath/shower slippery – guard against slipping. Avoid the eyes.

products containing arachis oil or peanut oil should not be used for patients with peanut allergy.

Product name	*Main ingredients*	*Method of application*
Alcoderm Cream*/Lotion*	liquid paraffin	apply directly to skin
Alpha Keri Bath*	liquid paraffin, wool fat	add 10-20 ml to bath (5 ml for infants) or rub small amount on to wet skin
aqueous cream*	emulsifying ointment	apply directly to skin
Ashbourne Emollient Medicinal Bath Oil	liquid paraffin, acetylated wool alcohols	add to bath or apply to wet skin
Aveeno Bath Emollient	colloidal oatmeal	add 20-30 ml liquid to bath or apply direct to wet skin when showering
Aveeno Oilated Bath Emollient	colloidal oatmeal, mineral oil	add 1 sachet to bath (half sachet for children and less for infants) and soak for 10-15 minutes
Aveeno Cream	colloidal oatmeal	apply directly to skin

Product name	*Main ingredients*	*Method of application*
Balneum Bath Oil*	soya oil	add 20 ml to bath (10 ml for infants)
Decubal Clinic Cream	isopropyl myristate, glycerol, wool fat, dimethicone	apply directly to skin
Dermalo Bath Emollient*	wool alcohols, liquid paraffin	add 15-20 ml (children 5-10 ml) to bath and soak for 10-20 minutes, or apply to skin on sponge
Dermamist Spray*	white soft paraffin, liquid paraffin, coconut oil	sprayed on to skin after bathing (from about 20 cm distance)
Diprobase Cream*/ Ointment*	liquid paraffin, white soft paraffin	apply directly to skin
Diprobath Bath Additive*	isopropyl myristate, liquid paraffin	add 25 ml to bath (10 ml for infants)
E45 Bath Oil	cetyl dimethicone, liquid paraffin	add 15 ml to bath (5-10 ml for infants/children) and soak for 10 minutes
E45 Cream*/wash/lotion	liquid paraffin, white soft paraffin, lanolin	apply directly to skin (up to three times a day for cream)
emulsifying ointment*	white soft paraffin, liquid paraffin	use instead of soap
Epaderm Ointment*	yellow soft paraffin	apply directly to skin, add to bath, or use instead of soap
Eurax Bath Oil	acetylated wool alcohols, liquid paraffin	add 15-20 ml to bath (5-10 ml for infants/children)
50:50 Ointment*	liquid paraffin, white soft paraffin	apply directly to skin as required
Hydromol Cream*	liquid paraffin, isopropyl myristate, sodium lactate, sodium pyrrolidone carboxylate	apply directly to skin
Hydromol Emollient Bath Additive*	isopropyl myristate, liquid paraffin	add 1-3 capfuls to bath (half -2 for infants) and soak for 10-15 minutes
hydrous ointment*	wool alcohols ointment	apply directly to skin
Imuderm Bath Oil	almond oil, liquid paraffin	add 15-30 ml to bath (7.5-15 ml for children) or apply to wet skin

cont.

E

E

Product name	Main ingredients	Method of application
Infaderm Therapeutic Oil	almond oil, liquid paraffin	add 15-20 ml to bath or apply to wet skin
Keri Therapeutic Lotion*	mineral oil, lanolin oil	apply directly to skin
LactiCare Lotion*	lactic acid, sodium pyrrolidone carboxylate	apply directly to skin
Lipobase Cream*	liquid paraffin, white soft paraffin	apply directly to skin up to four times a day
liquid and white soft paraffin ointment NPF*	liquid paraffin, white soft paraffin	apply directly to skin as required
Neutrogena dermatological cream*	glycerol	apply directly to skin
Oilatum cream*	arachis (peanut) oil*	apply directly to skin
Oilatum Emollient*	acetylated wool alcohols, liquid paraffin	add 5-15 ml to bath (2.5 ml-10 ml for infants) and soak for 10-20 minutes, or apply small amount to wet skin, rinse and dry
Oilatum Fragrance Free Bath Additive*	liquid paraffin	add 1-3 capfuls to bath (half - 2 for infants)
Oilatum Shower Gel*	liquid paraffin	apply to wet skin, massage in, then rinse and dry
Ultrabase Cream*	liquid paraffin, white soft paraffin	apply directly to skin
Unguentum M Cream*	liquid paraffin, white soft paraffin	apply directly to skin
white soft paraffin*	white soft paraffin	apply directly to skin
yellow soft paraffin*	yellow soft paraffin	apply directly to skin

* *product available on nurse prescription if prescribed generically.*

Compound preparations:

Product name	Main ingredients	Used to treat	Method of application
Balneum Plus Bath Oil	soya oil, lauromacrogols	dry skin with itching	oil – add 20 ml to bath (5 ml for infants), cream – apply directly to skin twice a day

Product name	*Main ingredients*	*Used to treat*	*Method of application*
Dermol 200 Shower Emollient	benzalkonium chloride, chlorhexidine, liquid paraffin, isopropyl myristate	dry, itchy skin, including eczema and dermatitis	apply directly to skin or use instead of soap
Dermol 500 Lotion	benzalkonium chloride, liquid paraffin, chlorhexidine	dry, itchy skin, including eczema and dermatitis	apply to skin or use instead of soap
Dermol 600 Bath Emollient	benzalkonium chloride, liquid paraffin, isopropyl myristate	dry, itchy, or scaly skin	add up to 30 ml to bath (up to 15 ml for infants) and soak for 5-10 minutes
Emulsiderm Emulsion	liquid paraffin, isopropyl myristate, benzalkonium chloride	dry, itchy skin, including eczema and scaly conditions	add 7-30 ml to bath and soak for 5-10 minutes, or apply small amount directly to skin
Kamillosan Ointment	wool fat, camomile extracts	sore nipples, chapped skin, nappy rash	apply directly to skin
Oilatum Plus Bath Additive	liquid paraffin, benzalkonium chloride, triclosan	eczema at risk of infection	add 1-2 capfuls to bath (1 ml for infants over 6 months) and soak for 10-15 minutes

Emulsiderm *see* emollient bath emulsion
(Dermal Laboratories)

emulsifying ointment *see* emollient ointment

enalapril tablets

A tablet used as an ACE-INHIBITOR to treat heart failure, high blood pressure, and to prevent effects of reduced blood supply of the heart (e.g. heart attack) in patients with heart disorders.

Strengths available: 2.5 mg, 5 mg, 10 mg, and 20 mg tablets.
Dose: for heart failure 2.5 mg at first, increasing usually to 20 mg a day (may be given as 10 mg twice a day); for high blood pressure, 5 mg once a day at first, increasing to a maximum of 40 mg once a day. (Lower starting doses used in the elderly or patients with kidney disorders, or being treated with DIURETICS.)
Availability: NHS and private prescription.
Contains: enalapril maleate.

cont.

Brand names: Innovace, Pralenal.
Compound preparations: Innozide.

 in the elderly, mothers who are breastfeeding, and in patients suffering from kidney disease, auto-immune diseases (such as LUPUS), severe heart failure, or with a history of severe allergies, or in patients undergoing anaesthesia or dialysis. Your doctor may advise regular blood tests.

 chidlren, pregnant women, or for patients with some heart abnormalities, PORPHYRIA, or disorders of the blood supply to the kidney.

 skin disorders, itching, sore throat, runny nose, stomach upset, cough, blood and liver changes, kidney disorders, low blood pressure, severe allergic reaction, inflamed pancreas. Occasionally, headache, dizziness, tiredness or sleeplessness, blurred vision, noises in the ears, sweating, flushing, muscle cramp, psychological reactions, taste disturbance, difficulty breathing, fever, pins and needles, muscle or joint pain, sensitivity to sunlight, fainting, loss of appetite, bowel obstruction, inflamed membranes or blood vessels, palpitations, chest pain, stroke or heart attack, impotence, hair loss.

 DIURETICS, anaesthetics, NON-STEROIDAL ANTI-INFLAMMATORY DRUGS, potassium supplements, cyclosporin, lithium, antidiabetics.

Endekay *see* fluoride tablets/drops/mouthwash
(Manx Pharma)

Engerix B *see* hepatitis B vaccine
(SmithKline Beecham Pharmaceuticals)

Enprin *see* aspirin 75 mg enteric-coated tablets
(Galpharm International)

---

entacapone tablets

A tablet used in addition to levodopa to treat Parkinson's disease.

Strengths available: 200 mg tablets.
Dose: 200 mg with each dose of levodopa (maximum of 2000 mg a day). The dose of levodopa may need reduction.
Availability: NHS and private prescription.
Contains: entacapone.
Brand names: Comtess.

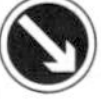 upset stomach, abdominal pain, movement disorders, anaemia, liver changes, coloured urine.

 children under 18 years, pregnant women, mothers who are breastfeeding, or for patients with liver disorders, PHAEOCHROMOCYTOMA, or a history of some muscle disorders or NEUROLEPTIC MALIGNANT SYNDROME.

 MAOIS, TRICYCLIC ANTIDEPRESSANTS, maprotiline, venlafaxine.

Entocort *see* budesonide modified-release capsules and corticosteroid enema
(AstraZeneca UK)

Epaderm *see* emollient ointment
(SSL International)

Epanutin *see* phenytoin capsules/suspension/chewable tablets
(Parke Davis)

---

ephedrine nasal drops

Nasal drops used as a SYMPATHOMIMETIC treatment for congested nose.

Strengths available: 0.5% or 1% drops.
Dose: 1-2 drops of either strength in each nostril 3-4 times a day when required.
Availability: NHS and private prescription, over the counter.
Contains: ephedrine hydrochloride.

 irritation, congestion, and less effect after excessive use.

 in infants under 3 months. Avoid excessive use.

---

ephedrine tablets/elixir

A tablet or elixir used as a SYMPATHOMIMETIC treatment for blocked or narrowed airways.

Strengths available: 15 mg tablets; 4 mg/5 ml and 15 mg/5 ml elixir.
Dose: adults 15-60 mg (children 7.5-30 mg according to age) three times a day.
Availability: NHS and private prescription.
Contains: ephedrine hydrochloride.
Brand names: CAM.
Compound preparations: Franol/Franol Plus, Haymine.

 rapid heart beat, sleeplessness, restlessness, anxiety. More rarely, irregular heart beat, shaking, dry mouth, cold hands and feet.

 in the elderly and in patients with high blood pressure, narrowed blood supply to the heart, overactive thyroid, diabetes, kidney disease, or enlarged prostate.

 MAOIS, drugs used to lower blood pressure.

Ephynal *see* vitamin E tablets
(Roche Consumer Health)

Epilim *see* sodium valproate liquid/syrup/crushable tablets/enteric-coated tablets/modified-release tablets
(Sanofi Winthrop)

Epimaz *see* carbamazepine tablets
(Norton Healthcare)

---

epinephrine *see* adrenaline (alternative name)

Epipen *see* adrenaline injection
(ALK-Abello (UK))

E

Epivir *see* lamivudine tablets/solution
(GlaxoWellcome UK)

---

epoetin alfa injection

An injection used as a hormone treatment for anaemia associated with chronic kidney failure or chemotherapy, or as a precaution before some forms of surgery.

Strengths available: 1000 unit, 2000 unit, 4000 unit, or 10,000 unit injection vials; 1000 unit, 2000 unit, 3000 unit, 4000 unit, or 10,000 unit pre-filled syringes.
Dose: as determined by doctor.
Availability: NHS and private prescription.
Contains: epoetin alfa.
Brand names: Eprex.

raised blood pressure, headache, blood clots, fits, skin reactions, influenza-like symptoms, blood disorders, severe allergic reaction, swollen eyelids.

in pregnant women, mothers who are breast-feeding, and in patients suffering from high blood pressure, reduced blood flow, some blood disorders or malignant diseases, or with a history of epilepsy or liver failure. Other forms of anaemia should be corrected, and diet or any dialysis may need correcting. Blood pressure should be monitored throughout treatment. Report any sudden stabbing headache to your doctor immediately.

patients with uncontrolled high blood pressure or (before surgery) for patients who have recently suffered a heart attack or stroke.

---

epoetin beta injection

An injection used as a hormone treatment for anaemia associated with chronic kidney failure or chemotherapy, to prevent anaemia in premature babies, or as a precaution before some forms of surgery.

Strengths available: 500 unit injection vials; 500 unit, 1000 unit, 2000 unit, 3000 unit, 4000 unit, 5000 unit, 6000 unit, or 10,000 unit prefilled syringes; (10,000 unit or 20,000 unit multidose injection pens and 50,000 unit or 100,000 unit multidose vials also

raised blood pressure, headache, blood clots, fits, skin reactions, influenza-like symptoms, blood disorders, severe allergic reaction, swollen eyelids.

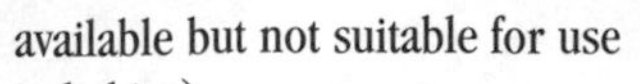

available but not suitable for use in babies).
Dose: as determined by doctor.
Availability: NHS and private prescription.
Contains: epoetin beta.
Brand names: NeoRecormon.

patients with uncontrolled high blood pressure or (before surgery) for patients who have recently suffered a heart attack or stroke. Multidose products not suitable for treating babies.

in pregnant women, mothers who are breastfeeding, and in patients suffering from high blood pressure, reduced blood flow, some blood disorders or malignant diseases, or with a history of epilepsy or liver failure. Other forms of anaemia should be corrected, and diet or any dialysis may need correcting. Blood pressure should be monitored throughout treatment. Report any sudden stabbing headache to your doctor immediately.

Epogam/Epogam paediatric *see* gamolenic acid capsules
(Searle)

Eppy *see* adrenaline eye drops
(Chauvin Pharmaceuticals)

Eprex *see* epoetin alfa injection
(Janssen-Cilag)

---

eprosartan tablets

A tablet used as an ACE-II ANTAGONIST to treat high blood pressure.

Strengths available: 300 mg, 400 mg, and 600 mg tablets.
Dose: adults 600-800 mg once a day with food; elderly patients 300 mg once a day at first.
Availability: NHS and private prescription.
Contains: eprosartan mesylate.
Brand names: Teveten.

low blood pressure, low potassium levels, inflamed nasal passages, wind, dizziness, joint pain, blood changes.

in patients with liver or kidney disorders. Your doctor may advise regular blood tests.

children, pregnant women, mothers who are breastfeeding, or for patients suffering from severe liver disorders.

anaesthetics, NON-STEROIDAL ANTI-INFLAMMATORY DRUGS, cyclosporin, DIURETICS, lithium, potassium.

Epsom salts *see* magnesium sulphate

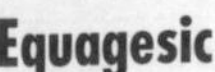

Equagesic
(Wyeth Laboratories)

A tablet used as an OPIOID ANALGESIC and muscle relaxant to control pain in muscles or bones.

Strengths available: 75 mg + 150 mg + 250 mg tablets.
Dose: adults 1-2 tablets 3-4 times a day.
Availability: controlled drug; private prescription only.
Contains: ethoheptazine citrate, meprobamate, and aspirin.

 drowsiness, dizziness, nausea, unsteadiness, rash, blood changes, low blood pressure, excitement, severe allergy, stomach bleeding, pins and needles, difficulty breathing.

 in the elderly and in patients with a history of epilepsy, or suffering from depression, suicidal behaviour, asthma, allergies, dehydration, liver or kidney disease, or heart failure.

 alcohol, other sedating drugs, phenytoin, non-steroidal anti-inflammatory drugs, some anti-diabetic drugs, ANTICOAGULANTS, methotrexate, ritonavir, CORTICOSTEROIDS, ORAL CONTRACEPTIVES, rifampicin, antidepressants, tranquillizers, uric-acid lowering agents.

 children, pregnant women, mothers who are breastfeeding, or for patients suffering from PORPHYRIA, alcoholism, stomach ulcer, blood clotting disorders, kidney failure, allergy to aspirin or NON-STEROIDAL ANTI-INFLAMMATORY DRUGS.

Equasym *see* methylphenidate tablets
(Medeva Pharma)

---

ergocalciferol *see* calciferol tablets, calcium and vitamin D tablets, vitamin D

---

ergotamine tablets/suppositories
A tablet used to treat migraine attacks,

Strengths available: 2 mg tablets.
Dose: 2 mg at start of attack, repeated after 30-60 minutes if necessary. Maximum of 6 mg in 24 hours or 12 mg in one week.
Availability: NHS and private prescription.
Contains: ergotamine tartrate.
Brand names: Lingraine (tablets dissolved under the tongue).
Compound preparations: Cafergot (with caffeine, a stimulant), Migril.
Other preparations: Cafergot suppositories (dose 1 suppository at start of attack, maximum of 2 in 24 hours or 4 in one week).

 stomach upset, muscular pain, abdominal pain, reduced circulation, chest pain, reduced blood supply to the heart, weak legs. Rarely, worsening of headache, heart attack. With excessive use, thickening of lung or abdominal tissues, gangrene, confusion.

 in elderly patients and in those with liver disorders or a tendency to blood vessel disorders. Stop treatment if numbness or tingling occurs in hands or feet.

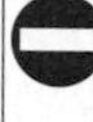 children, pregnant women, mothers who are breastfeeding, or for patients suffering from narrowed blood vessels, Raynaud's syndrome, severe high blood pressure, kidney or liver disease, some infections, overactive thyroid, PORPHYRIA or for migraine prevention.

 azithromycin, clarithromycin, erythromycin, antiviral treatments, other drugs used to treat migraine.

Ervevax *see* rubella vaccine
(SmithKline Beecham Pharmaceuticals)

Eryacne 2/4 *see* erythromycin gel
(Galderma (UK))

Erymax *see* erythromycin capsules
(Elan Pharma)

Erythrocin *see* erythromycin tablets
(Abbott Laboratories)

---

erythromycin gel/topical solution

A gel or solution used as an ANTIBIOTIC treatment for acne.

Strengths available: 2% or 4% gel; 2% solution.
Dose: apply twice a day to affected skin. With gel, start treatment with higher strength and reduce after 4 weeks if improved.
Availability: NHS and private prescription.
Contains: erythromycin.
Brand names: Eryacne, Stiemycin.
Compound preparations: Aknemycin Plus, Benzamycin, Isotrexin, Zineryt (with zinc acetate).

 irritation or dryness.

 gel forms not suitable for children.

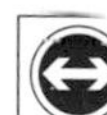 other acne treatments applied to the skin.

---

erythromycin tablets/enteric-coated tablets/capsules/enteric-coated capsules/suspension

A standard tablet/capsule, E-C TABLET/CAPSULE, or suspension used as an antibiotic, especially where the patient is allergic to penicillin, to treat infections such as chest or urine infections, acne, legionnaire's disease.

Strengths available: 250 mg e-c tablets; 125 mg/5 ml, 250 mg/5 ml, or 500 mg/5 ml suspension, (250 mg capsules or e-c capsules, and 500 mg standard tablets also available as branded products).
Dose: adults and children over 8 years, 1000-2000 mg a day in divided doses (may be doubled

for severe infections); children under 2 years 235 mg four times a day, aged 2-8 years 250 mg four times a day.

Availability: NHS and private prescription.

Contains: erythromycin, erythromycin stearate, erythromycin estolate, or erythromycin ethylsuccinate (depending on brand).

Brand names: Erymax, Erythrocin, Erythroped, Retcin, Ronmix, Tiloryth.

 stomach upset, rash. Rarely, liver and heart disturbances, hearing disorders with large doses.

 in pregnant women, mothers who are breast-feeding, and in patients with kidney or liver damage, PORPHYRIA, or who have heart rhythm abnormalities.

 liver disease (in estolate form).

 drugs altering heart rhythm, rifabutin, ANTICOAGULANTS, reboxetine, digoxin, repaglinide, carbamazepine, mizolastine, ritonavir, midazolam, tacrolimus, theophylline, aminophylline, sodium valproate, cyclosporin, pimozide, ergotamine, ANTACIDS, clozapine, sertindole.

Erythroped *see* erythromycin tablets/suspension
(Abbott Laboratories)

---

esomeprazole tablets

A tablet used as a treatment for acid reflux into the oesophagus, and for *H. pylori* eradication.

Strengths available: 20 mg and 40 mg tablets.

Dose: for reflux, usually 40 mg once a day for 4-8 weeks to heal the condition then 20 mg a day to prevent relapse (usually a further 4 weeks). Once symptoms resolved, 20 mg can be used on days when symptoms recur.

Availability: NHS and private prescription.

Contains: esomeprazole magnesium trihydrate.

Brand names: Nexium.

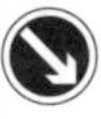 headache, upset stomach. Rarely, dizziness, dry mouth, severe allergic reaction, pins and needles, vertigo, muscle or joint disorders, fluid retention, low blood sodium levels, sweating, swollen breasts, tiredness, skin reactions, hair loss, blurred vision, sleeplessness, taste disturbance, blood and liver disorders.

 in pregnant women, patients with severe kidney or liver disorders, and in those requiring long-term treatment. Stomach cancer should be excluded before treatment.

 children, mothers who are breastfeeding, or for patients with allergy to similar drugs or some rare sugar intolerance or malabsorption states.

 diazepam, citalopram, imipramine, clomipramine, phenytoin, ketoconazole, itraconazole.

Esprit Biosensor

(Bayer Diagnostics)

A sensor disc (containing 10 test strips), used in conjunction with a Glucometer, to detect blood glucose levels. Blood-glucose monitoring enables individual patients suffering from diabetes accurately to control blood glucose and manage their condition.

Availability: NHS and private prescription, nurse prescription, over the counter.

Estracombi TTS *see* hormone replacement therapy (combined)
(Novartis Pharmaceuticals UK)

Estraderm TTS/MX *see* hormone replacement therapy (oestrogen-only)
(Novartis Pharmaceuticals UK)

estradiol *see* oestradiol (alternative name)

Estrapak 50 *see* hormone replacement therapy tablets/patches (combined)
(Novartis Pharmaceuticals UK)

Estring *see* hormone replacement therapy – topical
(Pharmacia and Upjohn)

estriol *see* oestriol (alternative name)

estrone *see* oestrone (alternative name)

estropipate tablets *see* hormone replacement therapy (oestrogen-only)

etamsylate *see* ethamsylate (alternative name)

ethambutol tablets

A tablet used (in combination with other drugs) as an antibacterial treatment for tuberculosis.

Strengths available: 100 mg and 400 mg tablets.
Dose: as advised by doctor.
Availability: NHS and private prescription.
Contains: ethambutol hydrochloride.

 visual changes, eye inflammation, rash, itching, rash, blood disorders.

 in young children, the elderly, pregnant women, mothers who are breastfeeding, and in patients suffering from kidney disorders.

 patients suffering from inflammation of the optic nerve or poor vision.

ethamsylate tablets

A tablet used as a blood-clotting agent to treat heavy periods.

Strengths available: 500 mg tablets.
Dose: 500 mg four times a day until bleeding stops. (For short-term treatment only.)
Availability: NHS and private prescription.
Contains: ethamsylate (etamsylate).
Brand names: Dicynene.

 headache, rash, nausea.

 children or for patients with PORPHYRIA.

E

Ethimil *see* verapamil tablets
(Genus Pharmaceuticals)

---

ethinylestradiol *see* ethinyloestradiol (alternative name)

---

ethinyloestradiol *see* co-cyprindiol tablets, oral contraceptive (combined), Schering PC4

---

ethoheptazine *see* Equagesic

---

ethosuximide capsules/syrup

A capsule or syrup used as an anticonvulsant to treat epilepsy.

Strengths available: 250 mg capsules; 250 mg/5 ml syrup.
Dose: adults and children over 6 years, 500 mg a day at first, increasing to 4000 mg if needed; children under 6 years use 250 mg at first (maximum of 20 mg/kg body weight).
Availability: NHS and private prescription.
Contains: ethosuximide.
Brand names: Emeside, Zarontin.

 stomach upset, dizziness, drowsiness, movement disorders, weight loss, headache, hiccups, intolerance to light, psychological disturbances, rash, liver or kidney disorders, blood changes, skin reactions, LUPUS. Rarely, swollen tongue and gums, sleep disturbance, lack of concentration, increased sexual desire, short sight, irritability, disturbed sleep, aggression, hyperactivity, vaginal bleeding.

 in pregnant women, mothers who are breast-feeding, and in patients suffering from PORPHYRIA, kidney or liver disease. Dose should be decreased gradually. Report any fever, sore throat, mouth ulcers, or bruising to your doctor immediately.

 isoniazid, antidepressants, other anti-epileptic treatments, tranquillizers and sedatives, alcohol.

---

ethyl nicotinate *see* analgesic (topical)

ethynodiol *see* oral contraceptives (progestogen-only)

etidronate *see* disodium etidronate

etodolac modified-release tablets

An M-R TABLET used as a NON-STEROIDAL ANTI-INFLAMMATORY DRUG to treat arthritis.

Strengths available: 600 mg m-r tablets.
Dose: adults 600 mg once a day.
Availability: NHS and private prescription.
Contains: etodolac.
Brand names: Lodine SR.

 stomach upset and bleeding or ulceration, severe allergy, difficulty breathing, blood or kidney disorders, headache, dizziness, noises in the ears, sensitivity to light, vertigo. Rarely, fluid retention, liver disorders, inflamed pancreas, inflamed bowel, meningitis.

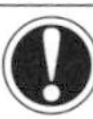 in the elderly, and in patients with heart, liver, or kidney disorders, asthma, or LUPUS.

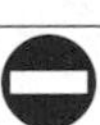 children, pregnant women, mothers who are breastfeeding, or for patients with a history of allergy to aspirin or other non-steroidal anti-inflammatory drugs, blood clotting disorders, currently active stomach ulcer or intestinal bleeding, inflamed intestines or severe heart failure.

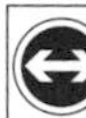 ACE-INHIBITORS, aspirin or other non-steroidal anti-inflammatory drugs, some antibiotics, digoxin, ANTICOAGULANTS, some antidiabetic drugs, some antivirals, methotrexate, DIURETICS, lithium, tacrolimus, cyclosporin.

etonogestrel implant

An implant placed under the skin and used as a progestogen contraceptive.

Strengths available: 68 mg implant.
Dose: implanted under the skin and removed within 3 years.
Availability: NHS and private prescription.
Contains: etonogestrel.
Brand names: Implanon.
Compound preparations: oral contraceptives (combined).
Other preparations: oral contraceptives (progestogen-only), norethisterone injection, medroxyprogesterone injection.

 irregular bleeding, upset stomach, dizziness, depression, skin disorders, change in appetite, weight gain, change in sexual desire, breast discomfort, headache, ovarian cyst, rarely blood clots. There appears to be a small increase in risk of breast cancer but this may be a result of earlier diagnosis through regular examinations.

 in patients suffering from heart disease, high blood pressure, disordered absorption of nutrients from the gut, diabetes, migraine, some cancers, blood lipid disorders, liver abnormalities, ovarian cysts or who have had a previous ectopic pregnancy or blood clot, or itching/ear disorders during pregnancy. Your doctor may advise regular examinations.

cont.

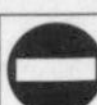 pregnant women or for patients suffering from severe heart or blood vessel disease, benign liver tumours, PORPHYRIA, undiagnosed vaginal bleeding, some womb disorders.

 BARBITURATES, phenytoin, primidone, carbamazepine, chloral hydrate, ethosuximide, rifampicin, chlorpromazine, meprobamate, griseofulvin, topiramate, modafinil, cyclosporin, nevirapine, celecoxib.

---

etynodiol *see* ethynodiol (alternative name)

E

Eucardic *see* carvedilol tablets
(Roche Products)

Eucerin *see* urea cream/lotion
(Beiersdorf UK)

Eudemine *see* diazoxide tablets
(Medeva Pharma)

Euglucon *see* glibenclamide tablets
(Hoechst Marion Roussel)

Eugynon 30 *see* oral contraceptive (combined)
(Schering Health Care)

Eumovate *see* topical corticosteroid cream/ointment
(GlaxoWellcome UK)

Eurax *see* crotamiton cream/lotion and emollient bath oil
(Novartis Consumer Health)

Eurax Hydrocortisone *see* crotamiton cream and topical corticosteroid cream
(Novartis Consumer Health)

Evista *see* raloxifene tablets
(Eli Lilly and Co.)

Evorel *see* hormone replacement therapy (oestrogen-only)
(Janssen-Cilag)

Evorel Conti/Sequi *see* hormone replacement therapy (combined)
(Janssen-Cilag)

Evorel Pak *see* hormone replacement therapy (combined)
(Janssen-Cilag)

E

ExacTech

(Medisense)

A reagent strip, used in conjunction with an ExacTech meter, to detect blood glucose levels. Blood-glucose monitoring enables individual patients suffering from diabetes accurately to control blood glucose and manage their condition.

Availability: NHS and private prescription, nurse prescription, over the counter.

Exelderm *see* sulconazole cream
(Bioglan Laboratories)

Exelon *see* rivastigmine capsules
(Novartis Pharmaceuticals UK)

Exocin *see* ofloxacin eye drops
(Allergan)

Exorex *see* coal tar lotion
(Tosara Products (UK))

Exterol

(Dermal Laboratories)

Ear drops used as a wax softener to remove ear wax.

Strengths available: 5% drops.
Dose: hold 5 drops in the ear once or twice a day for 3-4 days.
Availability: NHS and private prescription.
Contains: urea hydrogen peroxide, glycerol.

 slight fizzing, irritation.

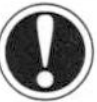 stop treatment if irritation occurs.

 patients suffering from perforated ear drum.

---

famciclovir tablets

A tablet used as an antiviral treatment for shingles and herpes infections of the genital area.

Strengths available: 125 mg, 250 mg, and 500 mg tablets.
Dose: shingles, 250 mg three times a day (or 750 mg once a day) for 7 days; for genital infections, 250 mg three times a day for 5 days for the first outbreak (125 mg twice a day for recurrent infections); to suppress genital infection, 250 mg twice a day. Patients with impaired immune system may need higher doses for longer periods.
Availability: NHS and private prescription.
Contains: famciclovir.
Brand names: Famvir.

headache, stomach upset. Rarely, dizziness, rash, hallucinations, confusion, fever, abdominal pain.

in pregnant women, mothers who are breast-feeding, and in patients with kidney disorders.

children.

famotidine tablets

A tablet used as a HISTAMINE H_2-ANTAGONIST to treat and prevent stomach ulcers, reflux of acid into the oesophagus, and Zollinger-Ellison syndrome (a condition of high acid production).

Strengths available: 20 mg and 40 mg tablets.
Dose: usually 20-40 mg once or twice a day but up to 800 mg a day in Zollinger-Ellison syndrome.
Availability: NHS and private prescription. Available over the counter for short-term treatment of adults suffering from heartburn, indigestion, or excess acid associated with food and drink, at a maximum dose of 20 mg a day.
Contains: famotidine.
Brand names: Pepcid (Pepcid AC and other brands available over the counter).

headache, dizziness, upset stomach, dry mouth, skin disorders, bowel discomfort, liver disorders, loss of appetite, tiredness. Rarely, breast swelling, severe skin disorders, inflamed pancreas, heart rhythm or conduction disorders, confusion, depression, blood disorders, severe allergic reaction, fever, muscle or joint pain, anxiety, loss of appetite, dry mouth.

in pregnant women, patients who are middle-aged or older, and in those suffering from kidney or liver disorders. Treatment may mask symptoms of stomach cancer.

children or mothers who are breastfeeding.

Famvir *see* famciclovir tablets
(SmithKline Beecham Pharmaceuticals)

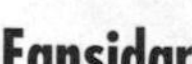

Fansidar

(Roche Products)

A tablet used (in addition to quinine) to treat malaria.

Strengths available: 25 mg + 500 mg tablets.
Dose: as advised by doctor.
Availability: NHS and private prescription.
Contains: pyrimethamine and sulfadoxine.

 newborn infants, pregnant women, mothers who are breastfeeding, or for patients suffering from severe kidney or liver disease, blood disorders, PORPHYRIA, or allergy to sulphonamide drugs.

 co-trimoxazole, trimethoprim, chloroquine, methotrexate, phenytoin.

 rash, sore throat, itching, stomach upset, folate (vitamin) deficiency. Rarely, blood changes, sleeplessness, cough, difficulty breathing, severe skin disorders, muscle or joint pain, mouth or tongue inflammation, liver disorders, inflamed pancreas or bowel, headache, depression, fits, kidney disorders, lack of co-ordination, nerve inflammation or meningitis, vertigo, noises in the ears.

 in the elderly and in patients suffering from kidney disease, asthma, or sensitivity to light. Drink plenty of non-alcoholic fluids. Your doctor may advise regular blood tests during prolonged treatment. Keep out of the sun.

Fasigyn *see* tinidazole tablets
(Pfizer)

Faverin *see* fluvoxamine tablets
(Solvay Healthcare)

---

felbinac foam/gel *see* non-steroidal anti-inflammatory drug (topical)

Feldene *see* piroxicam capsules/dispersible tablets/suppositories and non-steroidal anti-inflammatory drug (topical)
(Pfizer)

Felicium *see* fluoxetine capsules
(Opus Pharmaceuticals)

---

felodipine tablets

A tablet used as a CALCIUM-CHANNEL BLOCKER to treat high blood pressure, and to prevent angina.

Strengths available: 2.5 mg, 5 mg, and 10 mg tablets.
Dose: 5 mg once a day at first increasing to a maximum of 20 mg a day (high blood pressure) or 10 mg a day (angina). Elderly patients start with 2.5 mg dose.
Availability: NHS and private prescription.

cont.

Contains: felodipine.
Brand names: Plendil.
Compound preparations: Triapin/Triapin Mite.

swollen ankles, dizziness, tiredness, headache, flushing, palpitations, rash, mild gum swelling.

in mothers who are breastfeeding and in patients suffering from liver disorder or heart disease.

grapefruit juice, erythromycin, anti-epileptic treatments, ALPHA-BLOCKERS, ritonavir, theophylline, aminophylline.

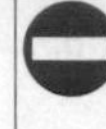
children, pregnant women, or for patients with unstable angina, some heart disorders, or within 1 month of heart attack.

F

Femapak 40/80 *see* hormone replacement therapy (combined)
(Solvay Healthcare)

Fematrix *see* hormone replacement therapy (oestrogen-only)
(Solvay Healthcare)

Femodene/ED *see* oral contraceptive (combined)
(Schering Health Care)

Femodette *see* oral contraceptive (combined)
(Schering Health Care)

Femoston 1/10, 2/10, 2/20 *see* hormone replacement therapy (combined)
(Solvay Healthcare)

Femoston-Conti *see* hormone replacement therapy (oestrogen-only)
(Solvay Healthcare)

Femseven *see* hormone replacement therapy (oestrogen-only)
(E. Merck Pharmaceuticals)

Femulen *see* oral contraceptive (progestogen-only)
(Searle)

Fenbid/Fenbid Forte *see* non-steroidal anti-inflammatory drug (topical) gel, ibuprofen modified-release capsules
(Goldshield Healthcare)

fenbufen capsules/tablets

A tablet or capsule used as a NON-STEROIDAL ANTI-INFLAMMATORY DRUG to treat pain and inflammation in rheumatic disorders or other muscle and bone problems.

Strengths available: 300 mg and 450 mg tablets; 300 mg capsules.
Dose: 300 mg in the morning and 600 mg at night, or 450 mg twice a day.
Availability: NHS and private prescription.
Contains: fenbufen.
Brand names: Lederfen.

 stomach upset and bleeding or ulceration, rash or severe skin disorder, severe allergy, breathing or lung disorders, blood or kidney disorders, headache, dizziness, noises in the ears, sensitivity to light, vertigo. Rarely, fluid retention, liver disorders, inflamed pancreas, inflamed bowel, meningitis.

 in pregnant women, the elderly, and in patients with heart, liver, or kidney disorders, asthma, or LUPUS. Stop treatment if rash develops.

 children, mothers who are breastfeeding, or for patients with a history of allergy to aspirin or other non-steroidal anti-inflammatory drugs, blood-clotting disorders, PORPHYRIA, currently active stomach ulcer or intestinal bleeding, inflamed intestines, or severe heart failure.

 ACE-INHIBITORS, aspirin or other non-steroidal anti-inflammatory drugs, some ANTIBIOTICS, ANTICOAGULANTS, some antidiabetic drugs, some antivirals, digoxin, methotrexate, DIURETICS, lithium, tacrolimus, cyclosporin.

fenchone *see* Rowatinex

fenofibrate capsules/tablets

A capsule or tablet used as a lipid-lowering drug to reduce high levels of cholesterol and other lipids in the blood.

Strengths available: 67 mg, 200 mg, and 267 mg capsules; 160 mg tablets.
Dose: adults (using capsules), usually 200 mg once a day or 67 mg three times a day (maximum four times a day); severe cases 267 mg once a day. The 160 mg tablet is equivalent to the 200 mg capsule. Children may use appropriate doses of the 67 mg capsules (according to body weight).
Availability: NHS and private prescription.
Contains: fenofibrate (or micronized fenofibrate in capsules).
Brand names: Lipantil Micro, Supralip.

 stomach upset, muscle aches, rash, itching, headache, tiredness, vertigo, dizziness, hair loss, sensitivity to light. Rarely, blood changes or impotence, liver disorders.

 in patients with kidney disease. Your doctor may advise change of diet or lifestyle, and regular blood tests for the first year.

 pregnant women, mothers who are breastfeeding, or for patients suffering from severe kidney or liver disease, or gall-bladder disorders.

 ANTICOAGULANTS, antidiabetic drugs, other drugs used to reduce cholesterol.

Fenoket *see* ketoprofen capsules
(Opus Pharmaceuticals)

fenoprofen tablets

A tablet used as a NON-STEROIDAL ANTI-INFLAMMATORY DRUG to treat pain and inflammation in rheumatic disorders and other bone or muscle problems.

Strengths available: 300 mg or 600 mg tablets.
Dose: 300-600 mg 3-4 times a day to a maximum of 3 g a day.
Availability: NHS and private prescription.
Contains: fenoprofen calcium.
Brand names: Fenopron.

stomach upset and bleeding or ulceration, severe allergy, difficulty breathing, blood or kidney disorders, headache, dizziness, noises in the ears, sensitivity to light, vertigo. Rarely, fluid retention, liver disorders, inflamed pancreas, inflamed bowel, meningitis, runny nose, sore throat, cystitis.

in pregnant women, mothers who are breast-feeding, the elderly, and in patients with heart, liver, or kidney disorders, asthma, or LUPUS.

children or for patients with a history of allergy to aspirin or other non-steroidal anti-inflammatory drugs, blood-clotting disorders, PORPHYRIA, currently active stomach ulcer or intestinal bleeding, inflamed intestines, or severe heart failure.

ACE-INHIBITORS, aspirin or other non-steroidal anti-inflammatory drugs, some antibiotics, ANTICOAGULANTS, some antidiabetic drugs, some antivirals, methotrexate, DIURETICS, lithium, tacrolimus, cyclosporin, digoxin.

Fenopron *see* fenoprofen tablets
(Typharm)

fenoterol *see* Duovent

fentanyl patches

A patch used as an OPIOID ANALGESIC to control severe chronic pain caused by cancer.

Strengths available: 25 mcg, 50 mcg, 75 mcg, or 100 mcg patches (releasing this amount each hour).
Dose: as advised by doctor. The patch is applied to non-hairy areas of chest or upper arm, and replaced every 72 hours.
Availability: controlled drug; NHS and private prescription.
Contains: fentanyl.
Brand names: Durogesic.

drowsiness, upset stomach, sweating, dizziness, breathing difficulty, low blood pressure, difficulty passing urine, dry mouth, headache, vertigo, flushing, change in heart rhythm, mood changes, rash, itching, addiction, reduced sexual desire.

 in children, pregnant women, women in labour, mothers who are breastfeeding, elderly or weakened patients, and in those suffering from breathing, kidney, or liver problems, brain tumours, low blood pressure, underactive thyroid, fever, enlarged prostate, or epilepsy. (Higher doses not suitable for some of these categories.) Avoid exposure of patch to direct heat. Dispose of used patches carefully. This is a very long-acting product and changes in dose may not produce an effect for several days.

 alcoholics or for patients with head injury, reduced breathing ability, PORPHYRIA, or those who have a history of drug addiction or who are suicidal or at risk of non-functioning intestines. Not suitable for controlling short-term pain.

MAOIS, alcohol, sedating drugs, ritonavir.

F

Fentazin *see* perphenazine tablets
(Forley)

---

fenticonazole pessaries

A pessary used as an antifungal preparation to treat vaginal thrush.

Strengths available: 200 mg and 600 mg pessaries.
Dose: 200 mg inserted into the vagina every night for 3 nights (or 600 mg for 1 night).
Availability: NHS and private prescription.
Contains: fenticonazole nitrate.
Brand names: Lomexin.

 mild irritation.

 in pregnant women and mothers who are breastfeeding.

 children.

 barrier contraceptives.

Ferraris Peak Flow Meter *see* peak flow meters
(Ferraris Medical)

Ferriprox *see* deferiprone tablets
(Swedish Orphan International)

Ferrograd *see* ferrous sulphate modified-release tablets
(Abbott Laboratories)

Ferrograd Folic *see* ferrous sulphate modified-release tablets and folic acid tablets (Abbott Laboratories)

A combination M-R TABLET used to prevent anaemia in pregnancy.

Strengths available: 325 mg + 350 mcg m-r tablets.
Dose: adults 1 a day before food.

ferrous fumarate tablets/capsules/syrup

A tablet, capsule, or syrup used as an iron supplement to treat and prevent iron deficiency.

Strengths available: 322 mg or 210 mg tablets; 305 mg capsules; 140 mg/5 ml syrup.
Dose: adults 1 x 322 mg tablet once or twice a day; 1-2 x 210 mg tablets three times a day; 1 x 305 mg capsules once or twice a day; 10-20 ml syrup twice a day. Children may use up to 5 ml syrup twice a day (depending on age and weight). Exact dose depends on level of iron deficiency (lower doses used for prevention).

 stomach upset.

 in patients with inflamed bowel, constipation, other intestinal disorders, or who have a history of stomach ulcers.

 some ANTIBIOTICS.

Availability: NHS and private prescription, over the counter.
Contains: ferrous fumarate.
Brand names: Fersaday, Fersamal, Galfer.
Compound preparations: Galfer FA, Pregaday.

ferrous gluconate tablets

A tablet used as an iron supplement to treat and prevent iron deficiency.

Strengths available: 300 mg tablets.
Dose: adults 2-6 tablets a day (in divided doses); children 1-3 tablets a day (in divided doses) according to age. Exact dose depends on level of iron deficiency (lower doses used for prevention).

 stomach upset.

 in patients with inflamed bowel, constipation, other intestinal disorders, or who have a history of stomach ulcers.

 some ANTIBIOTICS.

Availability: NHS and private prescription, over the counter.
Contains: ferrous gluconate.
Compound preparations: Ferfolic SV (with folic acid – not available on NHS).

ferrous glycine sulphate syrup

A syrup used as an iron supplement to treat and prevent iron deficiency.

Strengths available: 282 mg/5 ml syrup.
Dose: adults 5-10 ml three times a day; children 2.5-5.0 ml 1-3 times a day according to age. Exact dose depends on level of iron deficiency (lower doses used for prevention).
Availability: NHS and private prescription, over the counter.
Contains: ferrous glycine sulphate.
Brand names: Plesmet.

 stomach upset.

 in patients with inflamed bowel, constipation, other intestinal disorders, or who have a history of stomach ulcers.

 some ANTIBIOTICS.

F

ferrous sulphate tablets/modified-release tablets/modified-release capsules

A tablet or M-R TABLET/CAPSULE used as an iron supplement to treat and prevent iron deficiency.

Strengths available: 200 mg tablets; 160 mg and 325 mg m-r tablets; 150 mg m-r capsules.
Dose: adults 200 mg 1-3 times a day using standard tablets or 150-325 mg a day using m-r tablets/capsules. Children over 1 year may use 1 x 150 mg m-r capsule (opened to release contents) once a day, and children over 6 years may use 1 x 160 mg m-r tablet once a day. Exact dose depends on level of iron deficiency (lower doses used for prevention).
Availability: NHS and private prescription, over the counter.
Contains: ferrous sulphate.
Brand names: Feospan (not available on NHS), Ferrograd, Slow-Fe.
Compound preparations: Fefol (with folic acid – not available on NHS), Ferrograd Folic, Slow-Fe Folic.

 stomach upset.

 in patients with inflamed bowel, constipation, other intestinal disorders, or who have a history of stomach ulcers.

 some ANTIBIOTICS.

Fersaday *see* ferrous fumarate tablets
(Goldshield Healthcare)

Fersamal *see* ferrous fumarate tablets/syrup

fexofenadine tablets

A tablet used as an ANTIHISTAMINE to treat symptoms of hayfever or persistent itchy skin conditions.

 rarely, drowsiness, dizziness, headache, agitation, stomach upset, dry mouth.

Strengths available: 120 mg and 180 mg tablets.
Dose: adults, for hayfever 120 mg (for itchy skin conditions 180 mg) once a day.

cont.

Availability: NHS and private prescription.
Contains: fexofenadine hydrochloride.
Brand names: Telfast.

 in pregnant women and in patients suffering from kidney disease.

 some antidepressants, ritonavir, alcohol, sedatives.

 children under 12 years or mothers who are breastfeeding.

50:50 Ointment *see* liquid and white soft paraffin ointment NPF
(The Boots Company)

Filair/Filair Forte *see* beclomethasone inhaler
(3M Health Care)

finasteride 1 mg tablets

A tablet used to increase hair growth and prevent further loss of hair in male baldness.

Strengths available: 1 mg tablets.
Dose: 1 mg once a day starting when hair thinning has become apparent.
Availability: private prescription only.
Contains: finasteride
Brand names: Propecia.
Other preparations: finasterid 5 mg tablets.

 children or women.

 decreased sexual desire and performance.

 in patients suffering from prostate cancer or difficulty passing urine. Your doctor may advise regular tests before and during treatment. Female partners of patients being treated who are (or who may become) pregnant should not handle the tablets and avoid exposure to semen by using a condom. Improvement in symptoms will not be apparent until 3-6 months after starting treatment.

finasteride 5 mg tablets

A tablet used to treat enlarged prostate gland.

Strengths available: 5 mg tablets.
Dose: 5 mg once a day.
Availability: NHS and private prescription.
Contains: finasteride.
Brand names: Proscar.
Other preparations: finasteride 1 mg tablets.

 impotence, decreased sexual desire and function, breast tenderness and swelling, severe allergic reaction.

 children or women.

 in patients suffering from prostate cancer or difficulty passing urine. Your doctor may advise regular tests before and during treatment. Female partners of patients being treated who are (or who may become) pregnant should not handle the tablets and avoid exposure to semen by using a condom. Improvement may not be seen for some months.

FinePoint Lancets
(Lifescan)
Diabetics who need to test their blood regularly can use lancets to pierce the skin, either with or without the use of a finger-pricking device.

Lancet width and length: 25G/0.5 mm (Type A).
Availability: NHS and private prescription, over the counter.
Compatible finger-pricking devices: Autoclix, Hypolance, Penlet II Plus, Soft Touch.

Fisonair *see* sodium cromoglycate inhaler
(Rhône-Poulenc Rorer)

Flagyl *see* metronidazole tablets/suspension/suppositories
(Distriphar)

Flamatak MR/SR *see* diclofenac modified-release tablets
(Cox Pharmaceuticals)

Flamatrol *see* piroxicam capsules
(Berk Pharmaceuticals)

Flamazine *see* silver sulphadiazine cream
(Smith and Nephew Healthcare)

Flamrase/Flamrase SR *see* diclofenac enteric-coated tablets/modified-release tablets
(Berk Pharmaceuticals)

---

flavoxate tablets
A tablet used as an antispasmodic treatment for incontinence, abnormally frequent or urgent urination, bedwetting, painful urination, and bladder spasm after catheter inserted.

Strengths available: 200 mg tablets.
Dose: 200 mg three times a day.
Availability: NHS and private prescription.
Contains: flavoxate hydrochloride.
Brand names: Urispas.

ANTIMUSCARINIC effects, headache, skin reactions, stomach upset, altered heart rhythm, difficulty passing urine, disturbed vision, dry mouth, intolerance of light, flushing, dry skin, confusion, dizziness.

in pregnant women, mothers who are breastfeeding, elderly patients, and those with liver or kidney disease, PORPHYRIA, overactive thyroid, nerve disorders, heart disease, reflux oesophagitis, or enlarged prostate.

cont.

 children under 12 years or for patients with glaucoma, MYASTHENIA GRAVIS, non-functioning or obstructed/inflamed intestines, or obstructed outlet to the bladder.

flecainide tablets

A tablet used as an anti-arrhythmic treatment for abnormal heart rhythm.

Strengths available: 50 mg and 100 mg tablets.
Dose: 50-100 mg twice a day at first, increasing to 300-400 mg a day if necessary, and reducing to minimum necessary to keep symptoms under control.
Availability: NHS and private prescription.
Contains: flecainide acetate.
Brand names: Tambocor.

 other anti-arrhythmic drugs, antidepressants, quinine, halofantrine, ritonavir, BETA-BLOCKERS, verapamil, DIURETICS.

 dizziness, disturbed vision. Rarely, stomach upset, itchy rash, loss of memory, fits, confusion, hallucinations, depression, abnormal movements, unsteadiness, liver disturbance, sensitivity to light, tingling, weakness or numbness of hands and feet, lung disorders.

 in pregnant women, mothers who are breastfeeding, the elderly, and in patients fitted with pacemakers or who suffer from kidney or liver problems, some heart disorders.

 children or for patients suffering from heart failure or some other heart disorders.

Fleet enema

(E. C .De Witt and Co.)

A solution used as an enema to treat constipation and to empty the bowels before surgery, examinations, etc.

Dose: adults and children over 12 years, 1 enema given rectally as required; children aged 3-12 years reduced dose according to body weight.
Availability: NHS and private prescription, nurse prescription, over the counter.
Contains: sodium acid phosphate, sodium phosphate.
Other preparations: Fletchers' phosphate enema.

 irritation.

 in elderly or weak patients and in patients on restricted sodium intake.

 children under 3 years or for patients with heart failure, immediate stomach or intestinal disorder, or where absorption from the intestines is increased.

Fleet phospho-soda solution

(E. C. De Witt and Co.)

A solution used to empty the bowels before surgery, examinations, etc.

Dose: adults, the contents of 1 bottle diluted with 120 ml water and

 nausea, vomiting, bloating, abdominal cramp.

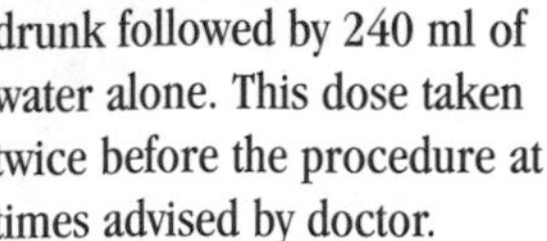

drunk followed by 240 ml of water alone. This dose taken twice before the procedure at times advised by doctor.

Availability: NHS and private prescription, over the counter.

Contains: sodium dihydrogen phosphate dihydrate, disodium phosphate dodecahydrate.

 in pregnant women, mothers who are breast-feeding, unconscious patients, and in those with heart or kidney disease, colostomy, inflamed bowel, diabetes, or whose diet is restricted in sodium. Drink plenty of clear fluids.

 children or for patients with blocked or perforated bowel, non-functioning intestines, kidney or heart failure, or some other stomach or intestinal disorders.

 some medicines used to treat high blood pressure or angina, antidiabetics, diuretics, lithium, medications taken regularly (e.g. oral contraceptives, anti-epileptics).

F

Fletchers' arachis oil retention enema *see* arachis oil enema
(Pharmax)

Fletchers' enemette *see* docusate enema
(Pharmax)

Fletchers' phosphate enema

(Pharmax)

A solution used as an enema to treat constipation and to empty the bowels before surgery, examinations, etc.

Dose: adults and children over 12 years, 1 enema given rectally as required; children aged 3-12 years treated only on advice of a doctor.

Availability: NHS and private prescription, nurse prescription (if prescribed generically), over the counter.

Contains: sodium acid phosphate, sodium phosphate.

Other preparations: Fleet enema.

 irritation.

 in elderly or weak patients, and in patients on restricted sodium intake.

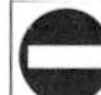 children under 3 years, or for patients with heart failure, immediate stomach or intestinal disorder, or where absorption from the intestines is increased.

Flexin *see* indomethacin modified-release tablets
(Napp Pharmaceuticals)

Flexotard MR *see* diclofenac modified-release tablets
(Pharmacia and Upjohn)

Flixonase *see* corticosteroid nasal spray
(Allen and Hanburys)

Flixotide *see* fluticasone inhaler
(Allen and Hanburys)

Flomax MR *see* tamsulosin capsules
(Yamanouchi Pharma)

Florinef *see* fludrocortisone tablets
(Bristol-Myers Squibb Pharmaceuticals)

Floxapen *see* flucloxacillin capsules/syrup
(Beecham Research Laboratories)

Fluanxol *see* flupenthixol tablets
(Lundbeck)

Fluarix *see* influenza vaccine
(SmithKline Beecham Pharmaceuticals)

Fluclomix *see* flucloxacillin capsules
(Ashbourne Pharmaceuticals)

flucloxacillin *see* co-fluampicil capsules/solution/syrup, flucloxacillin capsules/suspension

flucloxacillin capsules/solution/syrup

A capsule or suspension used as a penicillin ANTIBIOTIC for skin, soft tissue, chest, and other infections.

Strengths available: 250 mg and 500 mg capsules;125 mg/5 ml solution; 125 mg/5 ml and 250 mg/5 ml syrup.

Dose: adults 250-500 mg every 6 hours (half-an-hour before food); children 62.5-250 mg every 6 hours according to age.

Availability: NHS and private prescription.

severe allergic reaction (including rash, fever, joint pain, difficulty breathing, anaemia, and kidney disorder), upset stomach. Rarely, jaundice and other liver disorders, blood changes, pins and needles.

in patients with kidney disorders or a history of allergies.

Contains: flucloxacillin sodium (capsules and solution), flucloxacillin magnesium (syrup).
Brand names: Floxapen, Fluclomix, Flucloxin, Ladropen.
Compound preparations: co-fluampicil capsules.

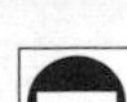 patients allergic to penicillin antibiotics.

 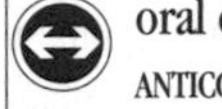 oral contraceptives (combined), ANTICOAGULANTS, methotrexate.

Flucloxin *see* flucloxacillin capsules/suspension (OPD Pharmaceuticals)

---

fluconazole capsules/suspension

A capsule or suspension used as an antifungal treatment for vaginal or oral thrush, and general fungal infections.

Strengths available: 50 mg, 150 mg, and 200 mg capsules; 50 mg/5 ml and 200 mg/5 ml suspension.
Dose: adults, 150 mg as a single dose for vaginal thrush and male genital infections; 50-100 mg a day for most other infections (up to 400 mg a day in patients with impaired immune system). Children use reduced doses according to age and weight.
Availability: NHS and private prescription. Available over the counter only to treat vaginal thrush.
Contains: fluconazole.
Brand names: Diflucan.

 upset stomach. Rarely, liver disorders, headache, rash, severe allergic reaction, severe skin disorders.

 in patients suffering from kidney disorders or at risk of developing liver disease. Women must use adequate contraception (*see also* caution below).

 pregnant women, mothers who are breast-feeding, or for patients with liver disease. Not suitable for treating genital infections in children under 16 years.

 rifampicin, rifabutin, ANTICOAGULANTS, reboxetine, some antidiabetics, phenytoin, mizolastine, pimozide, antivirals, midazolam, cyclosporin, STATINS, oral contraceptives, tacrolimus, theophylline, aminophylline.

---

fludrocortisone tablets

A tablet used as a CORTICOSTEROID replacement treatment in Addison's disease and ADRENAL disorders.

Strengths available: 100 mcg tablets.
Dose: adults 50-300 mcg a day; children use reduced doses according to body weight.
Availability: NHS and private prescription.
Contains: fludrocortisone acetate.
Brand names: Florinef.

cont.

high blood sugar, thin bones, mood changes, stomach ulcers, fluid retention, potassium loss, high blood pressure, menstrual irregularity, hairiness, increased likelihood of infection, euphoria, depression, sleeplessness, aggravation of schizophrenia and epilepsy, eye disorders, thinning of skin, acne, bruising, blood changes, stomach upset, inflamed pancreas, muscle abnormality, suppression of the adrenal glands, ulcerated or infected oesophagus, general feeling of being unwell, hiccups, reduced growth in children.

in pregnant women, mothers who are breastfeeding, and in patients who have had recent bowel surgery or who are suffering from inflamed veins, psychiatric disorders, thinning of the bones, stomach ulcers, tuberculosis or other infections, high blood pressure, glaucoma, epilepsy, diabetes, underactive thyroid, liver disease, stress. Withdraw gradually. Avoid contact with chicken pox for 3 months after treatment ends and seek medical attention if exposed.

children or for patients who have untreated infections.

live vaccines, some ANTIBIOTICS and anti-epileptics, ANTICOAGULANTS, antidiabetics, some antifungals, digoxin, cyclosporin.

---

fludroxycortide *see* flurandrenolone (alternative name)

---

flumetasone *see* flumethasone (alternative name)

---

flumethasone *see* Locorten-Vioform

---

flunisolide nasal spray *see* corticosteroid nasal spray

---

flunitrazepam tablets

A tablet used as a sedative for the short-term treatment of sleeplessness, or to bring on sleep at unusual times.

Strengths available: 1 mg tablets.
Dose: 0.5-2.0 mg at bedtime (elderly maximum 1 mg).
Availability: private prescription only.
Contains: flunitrazepam.
Brand names: Rohypnol.

drowsiness, light-headedness, confusion, vertigo, stomach disturbances, loss of memory, aggression, headache, joint immobility, salivation changes, shaking, unsteadiness, low blood pressure, rash, changes in vision, changes in sexual desire, retention of urine, incontinence, blood changes, jaundice. Risk of addiction increases with dose and length of treatment. May impair judgement.

in elderly or weak patients, pregnant women, mothers who are breastfeeding, and in patients suffering from lung disorders, kidney or liver disorders, muscle weakness, PORPHYRIA, or with a history of drug or alcohol abuse, or personality disorder. Avoid long-term use, and withdraw gradually.

 children or for patients suffering from acute lung diseases, some chronic lung diseases, severe liver disease, MYASTHENIA GRAVIS, some obsessional and psychotic disorders, or who have stopped breathing while asleep.

 alcohol, other sedating drugs, some antivirals and anti-epileptic medications.

fluocinolone *see* topical corticosteroid cream/gel/ointment

fluocinonide *see* topical corticosteroid cream/ointment

fluocortolone *see* topical corticosteroid cream/ointment, rectal corticosteroid

Fluor-a-day *see* fluoride tablets
(Dental Health Products)

fluoride tablets/drops/mouthwashes/dental gel

A tablet, drops, mouthwash, or dental gel used as a fluoride supplement to prevent tooth decay.

Strengths available: 1.1 mg and 2.2 mg tablets; 0.55 mg/0.15 ml drops; 0.05% daily mouthwash; 0.2% or 2% weekly mouthwash; 0.4% dental gel.

Dose: dose of tablets and drops depends on fluoride content of drinking water – consult a dentist or pharmacist for advice; mouthwashes are used for 1 minute to rinse the mouth, either weekly or daily, depending on preparation (dilute the 2% weekly strength before use); the dental gel is used to brush tooth surfaces once a day

Availability: NHS and private prescription, over the counter.

Contains: sodium fluoride (tablets, drops, and mouthwashes), stannous fluoride (dental gel).

Brand names: Duraphat, En-De-Kay, Fluor-a-day, FluoriGard, FluoriGard Gelkam.

 discoloration of teeth.

 in young children.

 children under 6 months. Mouthwashes not suitable for children under 6 or 8 years (depending on brand). Dental gel not suitable for children under 3 years.

FluoriGard *see* fluoride tablets/mouthwash/dental gel
(Colgate-Palmolive)

F

fluorometholone eye drops

Eye drops used as a CORTICOSTEROID treatment for inflammation of the eye where no infection is present.

Strengths available: 0.1% drops.
Dose: 1-2 drops into the affected eye(s) 2-4 times a day.
Availability: NHS and private prescription.
Contains: fluorometholone.
Brand names: FML.

 rise in eye pressure, thinning of cornea, cataract, eye infection.

 avoid prolonged use in pregnant women or infants, and in patients with glaucoma.

 patients suffering from eye infections or who wear soft contact lenses.

F

fluoxetine capsules/liquid

A capsule or liquid used to treat depression, bulimia nervosa (an eating disorder), some premenstrual disorders, or obsessive-compulsive disorder.

Strengths available: 20 mg or 60 mg capsules; 20 mg/5 ml liquid.
Dose: adults usually 20 mg a day (or up to 60 mg for some conditions).
Availability: NHS and private prescription.
Contains: fluoxetine hydrochloride.
Brand names: Felicium, Prozac.

 stomach upset, loss of appetite and weight, dry mouth, nervousness, drowsiness, sweating, shaking, headache, sleeplessness, dizziness, weakness, fits, change in sexual function, movement disorders, low blood sodium levels, psychiatric disorders, change in blood sugar levels, severe allergic reaction, fever, NEUROLEPTIC MALIGNANT SYNDROME, liver disorders. Also possibly abnormal bleeding, blood changes, bruising, brain blood supply disorders, inflamed pancreas, hair loss, violent behaviour.

 children, mothers who are breastfeeding, or for patients with elevated mood.

 ANTICOAGULANTS, other antidepressants, anti-epileptic treatments, clozapine, haloperidol, zotepine, sertindole, ritonavir, sumatriptan, lithium, alcohol, sedating drugs, drugs used for Parkinson's disease.

 in pregnant women and in patients with epilepsy, liver or kidney disorders, or a history of heart disease, blood clotting disorders, or some psychiatric conditions. Treatment should be withdrawn slowly.

flupenthixol tablets

A tablet used as a sedative for the short-term treatment of depression (with or without anxiety), and schizophrenia (or similar disorders) in higher doses.

Strengths available: 0.5 mg, 1 mg, and 3 mg tablets.
Dose: for depression, adults 1 mg in the morning at first increasing to maximum of 3 mg if necessary, (elderly patients 0.5 mg at first and maximum of 2 mg); for schizophrenia and similar disorders, adults 3-9 mg twice a day at first,

 excitement, restlessness, sleeplessness. Rarely, shaking hands, disturbance of vision, headache, Parkinson-like movements. With high doses, side effects as for chlorpromazine.

adjusted according to response (maximum 18 mg a day).

Availability: NHS and private prescription.
Contains: flupenthixol (flupentixol).
Brand names: Depixol, Fluanxol.
Other preparations: flupenthixol injection (used to treat schizophrenia and other psychological disorders).

anaesthetics, antidepressants, anti-epileptics, halofantrine, ritonavir, OPIOID ANALGESICS, pimozide, amiodarone, disopyramide, quinidine, procainamide.

in pregnant women and in patients with Parkinson's disease, heart or circulation disorders, confusion in the elderly, PORPHYRIA, liver or kidney disease. With high doses, cautions as for chlorpromazine.

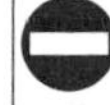

children, mothers who are breastfeeding, excitable or overactive patients, or for those with severe depression. High doses not to be used in patients suffering from porphyria. For high doses, *see* chlorpromazine.

flupentixol *see* flupenthixol (alternative name)

fluphenazine tablets

A tablet used as a sedative to treat schizophrenia, behavioural problems, anxiety, agitation, excitement, and other similar disorders.

Strengths available: 1 mg, 2.5 mg, and 5 mg tablets.
Dose: adults 2-10 mg a day (in divided doses) according to condition, and up to a maximum of 20 mg a day (10 mg in elderly).
Availability: NHS and private prescription.
Contains: fluphenazine hydrochloride.
Brand names: Moditen.
Compound preparations: Motipress, Motival.

alcohol, sedatives, antidepressants, some antidiabetic drugs, anaesthetics, drugs affecting heart rhythm, anti-epileptic medications, ritonavir, halofantrine, sotalol, lithium.

movement disorders, muscle spasms, restlessness, shaking, dry mouth, heart rhythm disturbance, low blood pressure, weight gain, blurred vision, impotence, low body temperature, breast swelling, menstrual changes, blood, liver, eye, and skin changes, drowsiness, apathy, nightmares, sleeplessness, depression, blocked nose, difficulty passing water. Rarely, fits.

in pregnant women, mothers who are breastfeeding, the elderly, and in patients suffering from heart, lung, or circulation disorders, epilepsy, Parkinson's disease, thyroid disorders, infections, MYASTHENIA GRAVIS, kidney or liver disease, glaucoma, enlarged prostate, or some blood disorders. Should be withdrawn gradually.

children, unconscious patients, or for those suffering from depression, poor circulation in the brain, weak heart, blood or bone marrow disorders, severe kidney or liver impairment, or PHAEOCHROMOCYTOMA.

flurandrenolone cream/ointment/tape *see* topical corticosteroid

flurazepam capsules

A capsule used for the short-term treatment of severe sleeplessness.

Strengths available: 15 mg and 30 mg capsules.
Dose: adults 15-30 mg at bedtime, (elderly patients 15 mg only).
Availability: private prescription only.
Contains: flurazepam hydrochloride.
Brand names: Dalmane.

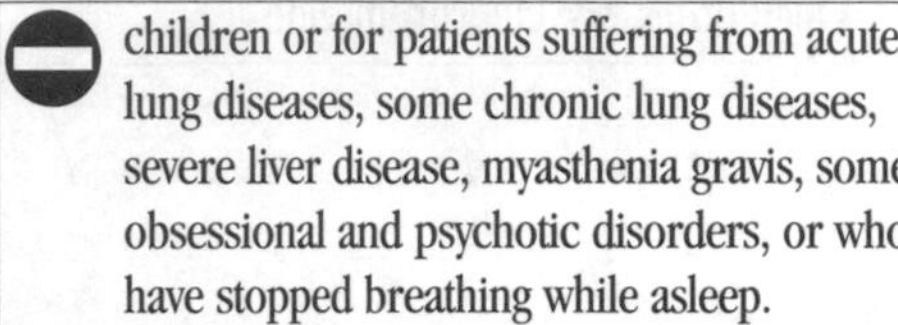
children or for patients suffering from acute lung diseases, some chronic lung diseases, severe liver disease, myasthenia gravis, some obsessional and psychotic disorders, or who have stopped breathing while asleep.

 alcohol, other sedating drugs, some antivirals and anti-epileptic medications.

 drowsiness, light-headedness, confusion, vertigo, stomach disturbances, loss of memory, aggression, headache, joint immobility, salivation changes, shaking, unsteadiness, low blood pressure, rash, changes in vision, changes in sexual desire, retention of urine, incontinence, blood changes, jaundice. Risk of addiction increases with dose and length of treatment. May impair judgement.

 in elderly or weak patients, pregnant women, mothers who are breastfeeding, and in patients suffering from lung disorders, kidney or liver disorders, muscle weakness, PORPHYRIA, or with a history of drug or alcohol abuse, or personality disorder. Avoid long-term use and withdraw gradually.

flurbiprofen eye drops

A solution used as a NON-STEROIDAL ANTI-INFLAMMATORY DRUG to prevent closing of the pupil during eye surgery, and to treat inflammation after glaucoma operations when CORTICOSTEROIDS cannot be used.

Strengths available: 0.03% solution in single-use vials.
Dose: as advised by doctor.
Availability: NHS and private prescription.
Contains: flurbiprofen sodium.
Brand names: Ocufen.
Other preparations: flurbiprofen throat lozenges, flurbiprofen suppositories/tablets/M-R TABLETS.

flurbiprofen throat lozenges

A lozenge used as a NON-STEROIDAL ANTI-INFLAMMATORY DRUG to treat sore throats.

Strengths available: 8.75 mg lozenges.
Dose: adults, 1 lozenge dissolved in the mouth every 3-6 hours (maximum of 5 in 24 hours).
Availability: NHS and private prescription.
Contains: flurbiprofen.
Brand names: Strefen.
Other preparations: flurbiprofen eye drops, flurbiprofen suppositories/tablets/M-R TABLETS.

 stomach upset and bleeding or ulceration, mouth ulcers, rash, severe allergy, difficulty breathing, blood or kidney disorders, headache, dizziness, noises in the ears, sensitivity to light, vertigo. Rarely, fluid retention, liver disorders, inflamed pancreas, inflamed bowel, meningitis.

 in the elderly, pregnant women, and in patients with heart, liver, or kidney disorders, high blood pressure, asthma or LUPUS.

 children under 12 years or for patients with a history of allergy to aspirin or other NSAIDs, blood-clotting disorders, currently active stomach ulcer or intestinal bleeding, inflamed intestines, or severe heart failure.

 ACE-INHIBITORS, aspirin or other non-steroidal anti-inflammatory drugs, some ANTIBIOTICS, ANTICOAGULANTS, some antidiabetic drugs, some antivirals, methotrexate, DIURETICS, lithium, tacrolimus, cyclosporin, aluminium hydroxide.

flurbiprofen suppositories/tablets/m-r capsules

A suppository, tablet, or M-R CAPSULE used as a NON-STEROIDAL ANTI-INFLAMMATORY DRUG to treat mild to moderate pain as a result of surgery, rheumatic disorders, other muscle and bone problems, and period pain.

Strengths available: 100 mg suppositories, 50 mg and 100 mg tablets; 200 mg m-r capsules.
Dose: adults usually 150 mg-200 mg each day (either by suppository or orally) with a maximum of 300 mg a day. For period pain use an initial dose of 100 mg then 50-100 mg every 4-6 hours (maximum 300 mg in 24 hours).
Availability: NHS and private prescription.
Contains: flurbiprofen.
Brand names: Froben, Froben SR.
Other preparations: flurbiprofen eye drops, flurbiprofen lozenges.

 ACE-INHIBITORS, aspirin or other non-steroidal anti-inflammatory drugs, some ANTIBIOTICS, ANTICOAGULANTS, some antidiabetic drugs, some antivirals, methotrexate, DIURETICS, lithium, digoxin, tacrolimus, cyclosporin, aluminium hydroxide.

 stomach upset and bleeding or ulceration, rash, severe allergy, difficulty breathing, blood or kidney disorders, headache, dizziness, noises in the ears, sensitivity to light, vertigo. Rarely, fluid retention, liver disorders, inflamed pancreas, inflamed bowel, meningitis. Suppositories may cause irritation around rectum.

 in the elderly, pregnant women, mothers who are breastfeeding, and in patients with heart, liver, or kidney disorders, high blood pressure, asthma, or LUPUS.

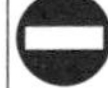 children or for patients with a history of allergy to aspirin or other non-steroidal anti-inflammatory drugs, blood-clotting disorders, currently active stomach ulcer or intestinal bleeding, inflamed intestines or severe heart failure. Suppositories not to be used for patients with inflammation of the anus or rectum.

fluticasone cream/ointment *see* topical corticosteroid cream/ointment

fluticasone inhaler/nebulizer solution

An aerosol (or other inhalation device) used as a CORTICOSTEROID to prevent asthma.

Strengths available: 25 mcg, 50 mcg, 100 mcg, 250 mcg, and 500 mcg per dose. Other strengths available in alternative devices, *see* below.
Dose: using aerosol or similar device, adults usually 100-250 mcg twice a day; children

cont.

4-16 years 50-100 mcg twice a day. Dose adjusted according to response. (Adult dose may be increased to 1000 mcg twice a day in severe cases.) Using nebulizer solution, adults 500-2000 mcg twice a day (children aged 4-16 years up to 1000 mcg twice a day only). Must be used regularly for maximum benefit.

Availability: NHS and private prescription.
Contains: fluticasone propionate.
Brand names: Flixotide.
Compound preparations: Seretide.
Other devices: Flixotide accuhaler (breath-activated dry powder inhalation device), Flixotide diskhaler (disks of powder for inhalation), Flixotide Evohaler (CFC-free aerosol).

hoarseness, thrush in the mouth and throat, difficulty breathing. High doses may give rise to general corticosteroid side effects (*see* prednisolone tablets) or glaucoma. Rarely, rash, swollen hands or feet, or severe allergic reaction.

in pregnant women, patients transferring from corticosteroids taken by mouth, and in patients suffering from tuberculosis of the lung or undergoing stressful events (such as infection or surgery).

products over 100 mcg per dose are not recommended for children. No product (any strength) recommended for children under 4 years.

(with high doses, ANTICOAGULANTS).

---

fluticasone nasal spray *see* corticosteroid nasal spray

---

fluvastatin capsules/modified-release tablets

A capsule used as a STATIN to reduce cholesterol and other lipid levels in patients who do not respond to dietary changes.

Strengths available: 20 mg and 40 mg capsules; 84.24 mg M-R TABLETS.
Dose: adults aged 18 years and over, usually 20-40 mg once a day (in the evening), occasionally increased to 40 mg twice a day.
Availability: NHS and private prescription.
Contains: fluvastatin sodium.
Brand names: Lescol.

sleeplessness, muscle pain and inflammation, headache, stomach upset, liver changes. Report any unexplained muscle pain to your doctor.

in patients with liver disorders. Your doctor may advise regular blood tests. Women of childbearing age should use adequate contraception during treatment and for 1 month afterwards.

children under 18 years, pregnant women, mothers who are breastfeeding, or for patients with current liver disease.

itraconazole, cyclosporin, other lipid-lowering drugs.

Fluvirin *see* influenza vaccine
(Medeva Pharma)

fluvoxamine tablets

A tablet used as an antidepressant to treat depression.

Strengths available: 50 mg and 100 mg tablets.
Dose: adults, 100 mg in the evening at first, increasing if necessary to a maximum of 300 mg a day. (Doses over 100 mg given in divided doses through the day.)
Availability: NHS and private prescription.
Contains: fluvoxamine maleate.
Brand names: Faverin.

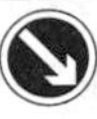 stomach upset, loss of appetite and weight, dry mouth, nervousness, drowsiness, sweating, shaking, headache, sleeplessness, dizziness, weakness, fits, change in sexual function, movement disorders, low blood sodium levels, psychiatric disorders, discoloured skin.

 in pregnant women, mothers who are breast-feeding, and in patients with epilepsy, liver or kidney disorders, or a history of heart disease, blood-clotting disorders, or some psychiatric conditions. Treatment should be withdrawn slowly.

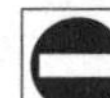 children or for patients with elevated mood.

ANTICOAGULANTS, other antidepressants, anti-epileptic treatments, clozapine, ritonavir, sumatriptan, zolmitriptan, lithium, alcohol, sedatives, theophylline, aminophylline.

FML *see* fluorometholone eye drops (Allergan)

---

folic acid syrup/tablets

A syrup or tablet used to treat megaloblastic anaemia (anaemia with large red blood cells), and to treat or prevent other folate deficiencies. In pregnancy, it is used to prevent neural tube defects (such as spina bifida) in the foetus.

Strengths available: 2.5 mg/5 ml and 0.4 mg/5 ml syrup; 5 mg and 0.4 mg tablets.
Dose: adults usually 5 mg a day (rarely up to 15 mg a day); children under 1 year use reduced doses according to weight. To prevent neural tube defects in pregnancy, usually 0.4 mg a day for the first 12 weeks (or 5 mg a day if used in a woman who already has a neural tube defect).
Availability: NHS and private prescription. 0.4 mg tablets and 0.4 mg/5 ml syrup also available on nurse prescription and over the counter.
Contains: folic acid.
Brand names: Folicare, Lexpec, Preconceive.
Compound preparations: Ferrograd Folic, Ketovite, Lexpec with iron, Lexpec with iron M (higher strength of folic acid), Pregaday, Slow Fe Folic.

nausea, constipation, discoloration of teeth with syrup.

your doctor may advise additional supplements of vitamin B_{12}.

phenobarbital, phenytoin, primidone.

Folicare *see* folic acid syrup
(Rosemont Pharmaceuticals)

follicle-stimulating hormone *see* follitropin alfa/beta injection, human menopausal gonadotrophin injection, urofollitrophin injection

follitropin alfa/beta injection

An injection used to treat infertility through failure of ovulation in women, and to stimulate the ovaries for *in vitro* fertilization.

F

Strengths available: 37.5 units, 75 units, and 150 units follitropin alfa; 50 units, 100 units, 150 units, 200 units, 300 units, and 600 units follitropin beta.
Dose: as advised by doctor.
Availability: NHS and private prescription.
Contains: follitropin alfa or follitropin beta (follicle-stimulating hormone, or FSH).
Brand names: Gonal-F (alfa), Puregon (beta).
Compound preparations: human menopausal gonadotrophin injection.

 skin reaction around injection site, overstimulation of ovaries, multiple pregnancies.

 in patients with ADRENAL or thyroid disorders, or high levels of prolactin (a hormone) in the blood. Hormone or brain disorders must be treated before using this drug.

— children, pregnant women, mothers who are breastfeeding, or for patients with some brain, ovary, uterus, or breast cancers, ovarian cysts, or undiagnosed vaginal bleeding.

Foradil *see* eformoterol capsules
(Novartis Pharmaceuticals UK)

formaldehyde gel

A gel used as a skin softener to treat verrucas.

Strengths available: 0.75% gel.
Dose: apply twice a day and cover, rubbing down with a pumice stone between treatments.
Availability: NHS and private prescription, over the counter.
Contains: formaldehyde.
Brand names: Veracur.
Other preparations: formaldehyde solution.

 irritation.

 do not apply to healthy skin.

 patients with diabetes or poor circulation, or to treat warts on the face or anal/genital areas.

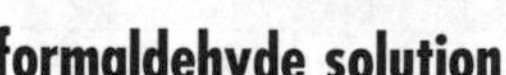

formaldehyde solution

A solution used as a soak to treat verrucas.

Strengths available: 3% formaldehyde lotion BP in water.
Dose: soak the affected area for 15-20 minutes at night.
Availability: NHS and private prescription, over the counter.
Contains: formaldehyde.
Other preparations: formaldehyde gel.

irritation.

do not apply to healthy skin.

patients with diabetes or poor circulation, or to treat warts on the face or anal/genital areas.

F

---

formoterol *see* eformoterol (alternative name)

Fortagesic *see* pentazocine tablets and paracetamol tablets
(Sanofi Winthrop)
A tablet used to treat muscle, joint, and bone pain.

Strengths available: 15 mg + 500 mg tablets.
Dose: adults, 2 tablets up to four times a day (children aged 7-12 years 1 tablet every 3-4 hours, maximum 4 in 24 hours).
Availability: private prescription only.

Fortipine LA *see* nifedipine modified-release tablets
(Goldshield Healthcare)

Fortovase *see* saquinavir capsules
(Roche Products)

Fosamax *see* alendronate tablets
(Merck Sharp and Dohme)

---

fosinopril tablets

A tablet used as an ACE-INHIBITOR to treat high blood pressure and (in combination with a DIURETIC) heart failure.

Strengths available: 10 mg and 20 mg tablets.
Dose: 10 mg once a day at first, increasing if necessary to a maximum of 40 mg a day. (In patients with high blood pressure, any diuretic is discontinued before starting this drug, and reintroduced later if needed.)
Availability: NHS and private prescription.

cont.

Contains: fosinopril sodium.
Brand names: Staril.

rash, itching, sore throat, runny nose, stomach upset, cough, blood and liver changes, kidney disorders, low blood pressure, severe allergic reaction, inflamed pancreas. Occasionally, headache, dizziness, tiredness, taste disturbance, fever, pins and needles, muscle or joint pain, sensitivity to sunlight, inflamed membranes or blood vessels, chest pain.

in the elderly, mothers who are breastfeeding, and in patients suffering from kidney disease, auto-immune diseases (such as LUPUS), severe heart failure, or with a history of severe allergies, or in patients undergoing anaesthesia or dialysis. Your doctor may advise regular blood tests.

children, pregnant women, or for patients with some heart abnormalities, disorders of the blood supply to the kidney. Not to be taken on the same day as dialysis.

DIURETICS, anaesthetics, NON-STEROIDAL ANTI-INFLAMMATORY DRUGS, potassium supplements, cyclosporin, lithium, antidiabetics.

framycetin dressings

A sterile, impregnated gauze dressing used for burns, wounds, ulcers, and other infected areas.

Strengths available: 1% dressing.
Availability: NHS and private prescription.
Contains: framycetin sulphate.
Brand names: Sofra-Tulle.
Compound preparations: Sofradex (for eyes/ears).
Other preparations: framycetin eye drops/ointment.

possible ear damage if large areas treated. May induce allergy to framycetin at a later date.

in children, the elderly, and in patients with kidney damage or those with large areas of skin being treated.

framycetin eye drops/ointment

Eye drops or eye ointment used as an ANTIBIOTIC treatment for conjunctivitis, styes, or eyelid infections.

Strengths available: 0.5% eye drops; 0.5% eye ointment.
Dose: for drops, apply 1-2 drops into the affected eye(s) every 1-2 hours, reducing as infection is controlled; for ointment, apply 2-3 times a day (or use drops during the day and ointment at night).
Availability: NHS and private prescription.
Contains: framycetin sulphate.
Brand names: Soframycin.
Compound preparations: Sofradex.
Other preparations: framycetin dressings.

frangula *see* Normacol Plus

Franol/Franol-Plus *see* theophylline tablets and ephedrine tablets
(Sanofi Winthrop)

Strengths available: 120 mg + 11 mg tablets (Franol), or 120 mg +15 mg tablets (Franol-Plus).
Dose: 1 tablet (of either strength) three times a day and at bedtime.

Frisium *see* clobazam tablets
(Hoechst Marion Roussel)

Froben/Froben-SR *see* flurbiprofen suppositories/tablets/modified-release tablets
(Knoll)

F

Froop *see* frusemide tablets
(Ashbourne Pharmaceuticals)

Froop-Co *see* co-amilofruse tablets
(Ashbourne Pharmaceuticals)

Fru-Co *see* co-amilofruse tablets
(Baker Norton Pharmaceuticals)

---

fructose *see* oral rehydration solution

Frumil/Frumil-LS/Frumil Forte *see* co-amilofruse tablets
(Distriphar)

---

frusemide tablets/oral solution

A tablet or liquid used as a DIURETIC to treat fluid retention and reduction in urination caused by kidney failure.

Strengths available: 20 mg, 40 mg, and 500 mg tablets; 1 mg/ml, 4 mg/ml, 8 mg/ml, and 10 mg/ml oral solution.
Dose: for oedema, initially 40 mg a day increasing if necessary, and reducing to 20-40 mg on alternate days for maintenance (children use reduced doses); for kidney failure, 250 mg a day at first, increasing to 2 g if necessary.

low blood potassium, magnesium, or sodium, stomach upset, rash, cramps, blood changes, breast enlargement, gout, high blood sugar. Rarely, sensitivity to light.

in pregnant women, mothers who are breast-feeding, and in patients suffering from kidney or liver damage, diabetes, gout, enlarged prostate, or impaired urination.

cont.

Availability: NHS and private prescription.
Contains: frusemide (furosemide).
Brand names: Froop 40, Frusid, Frusol, Lasix.
Compound preparations: co-amilofruse, Diumide-K, Frusene, Lasikal, Lasilactone.

 children or for patients suffering from cirrhosis of the liver or kidney failure where urine production is absent.

 ANTIHYPERTENSIVES, NON-STEROIDAL ANTI-INFLAMMATORY DRUGS, drugs affecting heart rhythm, some ANTIBIOTICS, antidiabetics, halofantrine, pimozide, digoxin, lithium.

Frusene *see* frusemide tablets and triamterene capsules
(Orion Pharma (UK))
A tablet used to treat heart failure and fluid retention in the heart, liver, or abdomen.

Strengths available: 40 mg + 50 mg tablets.
Dose: adults, usually ½ tablet to 2 tablets a day (maximum of 6 a day).

Frusid *see* frusemide tablets
(DDSA Pharmaceuticals)

Frusol *see* frusemide solution
(Rosemont Pharmaceuticals)

FSH *see* follicle-stimulating hormone

Fucibet *see* fusidic acid cream and topical corticosteroid cream
(Leo Pharmaceuticals)

Fucidin *see* fusidic acid cream/ointment/gel/dressings/suspension/tablets
(Leo Pharmaceuticals)

Fucidin-H *see* fusidic acid cream/ointment and topical corticosteroid cream/ointment
(Leo Pharmaceuticals)

Fucithalmic *see* fusidic acid eye drops
(Leo Pharmaceuticals)

Full Marks *see* phenothrin liquid/lotion/mousse
(SSL International)

Fungilin *see* amphoteracin lozenges/suspension
(Bristol-Myers Squibb Pharmaceuticals)

Furadantin *see* nitrofurantoin tablets
(Goldshield Healthcare)

---

furosemide *see* frusemide (alternative name)

---

fusafungine spray

A spray used as an anti-inflammatory and ANTIBIOTIC treatment for infection and inflammation of the nose, mouth, and throat. (Also for infections of the upper respiratory passages.)

Caution: treatment should be withdrawn after 7 days if no improvement.

Strengths available: 500 mcg per dose.
Dose: adults, 1 spray into each nostril or into the mouth every 4 hours; children, 1 spray every 6 hours.
Availability: private prescription. Also available on NHS if for infection and inflammation of the nose, mouth, or throat.
Contains: fusafungine.
Brand names: Locabiotal.

---

fusidic acid cream/ointment/gel/dressings

A cream, ointment, gel, or impregnated dressing used as an antibacterial treatment for skin infections.

Side effects: rarely, allergy.

Strengths available: 2% cream, ointment, gel, and dressing.
Dose: apply the cream/ointment/gel 3-4 times a day (or less often if covered with a dressing).
Availability: NHS and private prescription.
Contains: fusidic acid.
Brand names: Fucidin.
Other preparations: fusidic acid eye drops, fusidic acid tablets/suspension.
Compound preparations: Fucibet and Fucidin-H (*see* topical corticosteroids).

---

fusidic eye drops

Eye drops used as an antibacterial treatment for conjunctivitis.

temporary irritation, allergy.

Strengths available: 1% drops.
Dose: 1 drop twice a day into the affected eye(s).
Availability: NHS and private prescription.

cont.

Contains: fusidic acid.
Brand names: Fucithalmic.
Other preparations: fusidic acid cream/gel/ointment/dressing, fusidic acid tablets/suspension.

---

fusidic acid tablets/suspension

A tablet or suspension used as an ANTIBIOTIC to treat rare infections, such as bone or heart infections.

Strengths available: 250 mg tablets; 250 mg/5 ml suspension.
Dose: adults, 2 tablets or 15 ml suspension three times a day (or 4 tablets three times a day for severe infections); children aged 1-5 years, 5 ml suspension (aged 5-12 years 10 ml) three times a day; children under 1 year use reduced doses according to body weight.
Availability: NHS and private prescription.
Contains: sodium fusidate (tablets), fusidic acid (suspension).
Brand names: Fucidin.
Other preparations: fusidic acid cream/gel/ointment/dressing, fusidic acid eye drops.

Side effects: stomach upset, jaundice, rash, kidney disorders, blood disorders.

Caution: your doctor may advise regular checks on your liver function.

Fybogel *see* ispaghula husk
(Reckitt and Colman Products)

Fybogel-Mebeverine *see* ispaghula husk and mebeverine tablets
(Reckitt and Colman Products)
Granules used to treat irritable bowel syndrome.

Strengths available: 3.5 g + 135 mg per sachet.
Dose: adults 1 sachet 2-3 times a day before meals.

Fybozest Orange *see* ispaghula husk
(Reckitt and Colman Products)

---

gabapentin capsules/tablets

A capsule or tablet used (in addition to other drugs) as an anticonvulsant to treat epilepsy, and to treat pain caused by dysfunction of the nervous system.

Strengths available: 100 mg, 300 mg, and 400 mg capsules; 600 mg and 800 mg tablets.

drowsiness, weakness, dizziness, lack of co-ordination, headache, shaking, stomach upset, inflamed nasal passages, poor eyesight, involuntary eye movements, double vision, weight gain, loss of memory, nervousness, cough, pins and needles, joint or muscle pain, discoloured skin, liver or blood disorders, inflamed pancreas.

Dose: adults, 300 mg once a day at first increasing to a maximum of 2400 mg a day (in divided doses) for epilepsy, or 1800 mg a day for nerve pain. Children use reduced doses (according to body weight) to treat epilepsy.
Availability: NHS and private prescription.
Contains: gabapentin.
Brand names: Neurontin.

 in pregnant women, mothers who are breast-feeding, the elderly, and in patients suffering from diabetes, kidney disorders, or who are on dialysis. Withdraw gradually.

 children under 6 years (for epilepsy) or under 18 years (for nerve pain).

 alcohol, sedatives.

Gabitril *see* tiagabine tablets
(Sanofi Winthrop)

---

galantamine tablets

A tablet used to treat Alzheimer's disease.

Strengths available: 4 mg, 8 mg, and 12 mg tablets.
Dose: adults, 4 mg twice a day at first increasing gradually to a maximum of 12 mg twice a day if needed.
Availability: NHS and private prescription.
Contains: galantamine.
Brand names: Reminyl.

 weight loss, stomach upset, loss of appetite, falls, urine infection, dizziness, drowsiness, confusion, sleeplessness, inflamed nasal passages, shaking, slow heart rate, fainting.

 in pregnant women and in patients suffering from liver disorders, severe asthma, other breathing disorders, or those at risk of stomach ulcers.

 some antidepressants, quinidine, ketoconazole, erythromycin, ritonavir, ANTIMUSCARINIC drugs, BETA-BLOCKERS, digoxin, alcohol, sedating drugs.

 children, mothers who are breastfeeding, or for patients with kidney or severe liver disorders, blocked intestines, or who are recovering from intestinal surgery.

Galcodine/Galcodine paediatric *see* codeine linctus/codeine linctus paediatric
(Galen)

Galenamet *see* cimetidine tablets
(Galen)

Galenamox *see* amoxycillin capsules/suspension
(Galen)

G

Galenphol/Galenphol paediatric/Galenphol strong *see* pholcodine linctus/paediatric linctus/strong linctus
(Galen)

Galfer *see* ferrous fumarate capsules/syrup
(Galen)

Galfer FA *see* ferrous fumarate capsules and folic acid tablets
(Galen)
A combination capsule used to prevent anaemia and folic acid deficiency in pregnancy.

Strengths available: 305 mg + 350 mcg capsules.
Dose: adults 1 capsule a day before food.

Galpseud *see* pseudoephedrine linctus/tablets
(Galen)

Galpseud Plus *see* pseudoephedrine linctus and chlorpheniramine syrup
(Galen)
A combination product used to treat hayfever.

Strengths available: 30 mg + 2 mg per 5 ml linctus.
Dose: adults 10 ml (children aged 2-6 years 2.5 ml, aged 6-12 years 5 ml) three times a day.

Gamanil *see* lofepramine tablets
(E. Merck Pharmaceuticals)

---

gamma globulin *see* human normal immunoglobulin injection

Gammabulin *see* human normal immunoglobulin injection
(Hyland-Immuno)

---

gamolenic acid capsules
An oil-filled capsule used to relieve the symptoms of eczema, and to treat breast pain in women.

Strengths available: 40 mg or 80 mg capsules (to be swallowed whole); 80 mg paediatric capsules (which can be

nausea, headache, indigestion, Rarely, rash, itching, and abdominal pain. May unmask undiagnosed epilepsy.

emptied on to food).

Dose: for eczema, adults 160-240 mg twice a day (children aged 1-12 years, 80-160 mg twice a day); for breast pain, 240-320 mg a day (in one dose or divided into two doses) reducing or discontinuing when pain relieved (usually 8-12 weeks).

Availability: NHS and private prescription.

Contains: gamolenic acid.

Brand names: Efamast (for breast pain), Epogam and Epogam Paediatric (for eczema).

 in pregnant women and in patients with a history of epilepsy or being treated with drugs that may cause fits.

 children under 1 year.

 drugs that may cause fits.

---

ganciclovir capsules

A capsule used as an antiviral treatment for inflamed retina of the eye due to cytomegalovirus in patients without fully functioning immune systems (e.g. after transplant or in HIV infection).

Strengths available: 250 mg and 500 mg capsules.

Dose: adults, 1000 mg three times a day or 500 mg six times a day with food; children under 12 as advised by doctor.

Availability: NHS and private prescription.

Contains: ganciclovir.

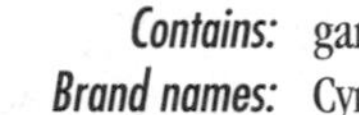

Brand names: Cymevene.

 in patients with kidney damage or with a history of blood disorders. Your doctor will advise regular blood tests. Adequate contraception must be used in women until 90 days after treatment ends.

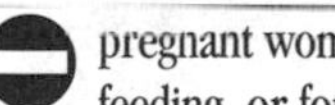 pregnant women, mothers who are breast-feeding, or for patients with allergy to aciclovir, or some blood disorders.

 blood changes, stomach upset, loss of appetite, rash, headache, itching, fever, liver disorder. Rarely, fluid retention, infections, stomach upset or bleeding, tiredness, mouth ulcers, difficulty swallowing or breathing, chest pain, irregular heart rhythm, high or low blood pressure, migraine, confusion, psychological disorders, drowsiness, dizziness, abnormal or unsteady movements, pins and needles, coma, breast pain, increased frequency of passing urine, inability to make sperm, weak or painful muscles, eye pain, hair loss, acne, sweating, blood clots, widened blood vessels, disturbed taste, vision, or hearing.

 drugs that suppress the bone marrow or stop cells reproducing, didanosine, zidovudine, alcohol, sedating drugs.

Ganda

(Chauvin Pharmaceuticals)

Eye drops used as a SYMPATHOMIMETIC drug to treat glaucoma.

Strengths available: 1% + 0.2% or 3% + 0.5% eye drops.

Dose: 1 drop into the affected eye(s) once or twice a day.

 pain in the eye, headache, redness, skin reaction, dark pigmentation, increased eye pressure, dropping of the upper eyelid, inflamed cornea.

cont.

Availability: NHS and private prescription.
Contains: guanethidine monosulphate and adrenaline.

 your doctor may advise that the eye should be checked every 6 months if treatment is prolonged.

 MAOIS.

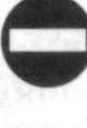 patients suffering from narrow-angle glaucoma or absence of the lens.

Garamycin *see* gentamicin eye drops
(Schering-Plough)

Gastrobid Continus *see* metoclopramide modified-release tablets
(Napp Pharmaceuticals)

Gastrocote *see* alginate liquid/tablets
(SSL International)

Gastroflux *see* metoclopramide tablets
(Ashbourne Pharmaceuticals)

Gaviscon/Gaviscon Advance *see* alginate liquid/tablets/sachets
(Reckitt and Colman Products)

---

gelatin *see* Orabase, Orahesive

Gelcosal *see* coal tar and salicylic acid ointment BP
(Quinoderm)

Gelcotar *see* coal tar solution/gel
(Quinoderm)

Gelkam *see* fluoride dental gel
(Colgate-Palmolive)

GelTears *see* carbomer eye drops
(Chauvin Pharmaceuticals)

---

gemfibrozil capsules/tablets

A capsule or tablet used as a lipid-lowering treatment for raised blood lipid levels (cholesterol and triglycerides).

Strengths available: 300 mg capsules; 600 mg tablets.
Dose: usually 600 mg twice a day (range of 900-1500 mg a day).
Availability: NHS and private prescription.
Contains: gemfibrozil.
Brand names: Lopid.

pregnant women, women who are breast-feeding, alcoholics, or for patients suffering from gallstones or liver disease.

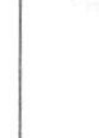
stomach upset, skin disorders, severe allergic reaction, impotence, headache, dizziness, painful extremities, muscle disorders, blurred vision, jaundice, inflamed pancreas, abnormal heart rhythm, swollen larynx.

in patients with kidney damage. Your doctor may advise regular blood tests before and during treatment.

ANTICOAGULANTS, antidiabetic treatments, STATINS.

Genotropin *see* somatropin injection
(Pharmacia and Upjohn)

---

gentamicin eye/ear drops

Drops used as an ANTIBIOTIC to treat infections of the outer ear or eye.

Strengths available: 0.3% drops.
Dose: 2-4 drops into the ear 3-4 times a day and at night, or 1-2 drops into the affected eye(s) 3-4 times a day.
Availability: NHS and private prescription.
Contains: gentamicin sulphate.
Brand names: Garamycin, Genticin, Minims Gentamicin (single-use containers).
Compound preparations: Gentisone-HC (with hydrocortisone, *see* topical corticosteroid)

additional infection, temporary irritation, inducement of allergy. (Blurred vision with eye drops.)

in pregnant women and mothers who are breastfeeding.

ear drops not for use in patients suffering from perforated ear drum.

Gentamicin Minims *see* gentamicin eye drops
(Chauvin Pharmaceuticals)

---

gentian mixture

An acid or alkaline mixture used as a tonic to improve appetite.

Dose: 10 ml three times a day before meals.

cont.

Availability: NHS and private prescription, over the counter.

children.

Contains: gentian infusion and hydrochloric acid (in gentian mixture acid); sodium bicarbonate and gentian infusion (in gentian mixture alkaline).

---

gentian violet *see* crystal violet paint BP 1980

Genticin *see* gentamicin eye/ear drops
(Roche Products)

Gentisone-HC *see* gentamicin ear drops
(Roche Products)
A combined ANTIBIOTIC and CORTICOSTEROID used to treat inflammation of the outer ear due to eczema.

Dose: 2-4 drops into the ear 3-4 times a day and at night.

---

gestodene *see* oral contraceptive (combined)

Gestone *see* progesterone injection
(Ferring Pharmaceuticals)

---

gestrinone capsules
A capsule used to treat endometriosis (a womb and menstrual disorder).

Strengths available: 2.5 mg capsules.
Dose: 2.5 mg twice a week on days 1 and 4 of the cycle then on the same two days each week for the rest of the treatment (usually 6 months).
Availability: NHS and private prescription.
Contains: gestrinone.
Brand names: Dimetriose.

vaginal bleeding (spotting), acne, weight gain, stomach upset, cramp, depression, voice changes, hair growth, liver disorders, change in sexual desire, flushing, fluid retention, smaller breasts, nervousness, reduced appetite.

in patients suffering from diabetes, high blood cholesterol (or lipids) or heart, liver or kidney disease. Ensure adequate contraception (barrier methods must be used).

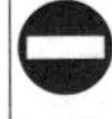
children, pregnant women, mothers who are breastfeeding, or for patients with severe heart, liver, or kidney disorders, blood vessel disease, or disturbance of metabolism.

ORAL CONTRACEPTIVES.

Glandosane *see* saliva (artificial) spray
(Fresenius Kabi)

Glau-Opt *see* timolol eye drops
(Opus Pharmaceuticals)

---

glibenclamide tablets

A tablet used as an antidiabetic drug to treat diabetes.

Strengths available: 2.5 mg and 5 mg tablets.
Dose: adults, 5 mg (elderly patients 2.5 mg) a day at first, increasing if needed to a maximum of 15 mg a day. The dose is taken with breakfast.
Availability: NHS and private prescription.
Contains: glibenclamide.
Brand names: Daonil, Diabetamide, Euglucon, Semi-Daonil.

children, pregnant women, mothers who are breastfeeding, during surgery, or for patients suffering from juvenile diabetes, hormone disorders, stress, infections, PORPHYRIA, severe illness, or severe liver or kidney disorders.

allergy (including skin rash, fever, and jaundice), stomach upset, headache. Rarely, blood disorders.

in the elderly and in patients suffering from kidney or liver disorders.

ACE-INHIBITORS, alcohol, ANABOLIC STEROIDS, NON-STEROIDAL ANTI-INFLAMMATORY DRUGS, some ANTIBIOTICS, ANTICOAGULANTS, MAOIS, fluconazole, miconazole, some tranquillizers, BETA-BLOCKERS, nifedipine, CORTICOSTEROIDS, DIURETICS, some drugs used to lower blood cholesterol or lipids, lithium, ORAL CONTRACEPTIVES, testosterone, cimetidine, sulphinpyrazone.

Glibenese *see* glipizide tablets
(Pfizer)

---

gliclazide tablets

A tablet used as an antidiabetic drug to treat diabetes.

Strengths available: 80 mg tablets.
Dose: adults, 40-80 mg a day at first increasing if needed to a maximum of 320 mg a day. The dose is taken with breakfast or doses above 160 mg are divided into two and taken with main meals.
Availability: NHS and private prescription.
Contains: gliclazide.
Brand names: Diaglyk, Diamicron, Vivazide.

allergy (including skin rash, fever, and jaundice), stomach upset, headache. Rarely, blood disorders.

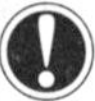
in the elderly and in patients suffering from kidney or liver disorders.

children, pregnant women, mothers who are breastfeeding, during surgery, or for patients suffering from juvenile diabetes, hormone disorders, stress, infections, PORPHYRIA, severe illness, or severe liver or kidney disorders.

cont.

 ACE-INHIBITORS, alcohol, ANABOLIC STEROIDS, NON-STEROIDAL ANTI-INFLAMMATORY DRUGS, some ANTIBIOTICS, ANTICOAGULANTS, MAOIS, fluconazole, miconazole, some tranquillizers, BETA-BLOCKERS, nifedipine, CORTICOSTEROIDS, DIURETICS, some drugs used to lower blood cholesterol or lipids, lithium, ORAL CONTRACEPTIVES, testosterone, cimetidine, sulphinpyrazone.

glimepiride tablets

A tablet used as an antidiabetic drug to treat diabetes.

Strengths available: 1 mg, 2 mg, 3 mg, and 4 mg tablets.
Dose: adults, 1 mg a day at first increasing if needed to a maximum of 6 mg a day. The dose is taken before or with breakfast.
Availability: NHS and private prescription.
Contains: glimepiride.
Brand names: Amaryl.

 children, pregnant women, mothers who are breastfeeding, during surgery, or for patients suffering from juvenile diabetes, severe liver or kidney disorders, hormone disorders, stress, infections, PORPHYRIA, severe illness, or severe liver or kidney disorders.

 allergy (including skin rash, fever, and jaundice), stomach upset, headache, liver disorders, blood vessel inflammation, lowered blood sodium levels. Rarely, blood disorders.

 in the elderly and in patients suffering from kidney or liver disorders. Your doctor will advise regular blood and liver tests.

 ACE-INHIBITORS, alcohol, ANABOLIC STEROIDS, NON-STEROIDAL ANTI-INFLAMMATORY DRUGS, some ANTIBIOTICS, ANTICOAGULANTS, MAOIS, fluconazole, miconazole, some tranquillizers, BETA-BLOCKERS, nifedipine, CORTICOSTEROIDS, DIURETICS, some drugs used to lower blood cholesterol or lipids, lithium, ORAL CONTRACEPTIVES, testosterone, cimetidine, sulphinpyrazone.

glipizide tablets

A tablet used as an antidiabetic drug to treat diabetes.

Strengths available: 2.5 mg or 5 mg tablets.
Dose: adults, 2.5-5.0 mg a day at first increasing if needed to a maximum of 20 mg a day. The dose is taken with breakfast or doses above 15 mg are divided and taken with main meals.
Availability: NHS and private prescription.
Contains: glipizide.
Brand names: Glibenese, Minodiab.

 children, pregnant women, mothers who are breastfeeding, during surgery, or for patients suffering from juvenile diabetes, hormone disorders, stress, infections, PORPHYRIA, severe illness, or severe liver or kidney disorders.

allergy (including skin rash, fever, and jaundice), stomach upset, headache, dizziness, drowsiness, confusion, tiredness, shaking, disturbance of vision, liver or blood disorders, metabolic reactions, low blood sodium levels, PORPHYRIA. Rarely, blood disorders.

in the elderly and in patients suffering from kidney or liver disorders.

 other sedating drugs, ACE-INHIBITORS, alcohol, ANABOLIC STEROIDS, NON-STEROIDAL ANTI-INFLAMMATORY DRUGS, some ANTIBIOTICS, ANTICOAGULANTS, MAOIS, fluconazole, miconazole, some tranquillizers, BETA-BLOCKERS, nifedipine, CORTICOSTEROIDS, DIURETICS, some drugs used to lower blood cholesterol or lipids, lithium, ORAL CONTRACEPTIVES, testosterone, cimetidine, sulphinpyrazone.

gliquidone tablets

A tablet used as an antidiabetic drug to treat diabetes.

Strengths available: 30 mg tablets.
Dose: adults, 15 mg a day at first increasing if needed to a maximum of 180 mg a day (maximum single dose 60 mg). The dose is taken with breakfast or doses above 60 mg are divided and taken with main meals.
Availability: NHS and private prescription.
Contains: gliquidone.
Brand names: Glurenorm.

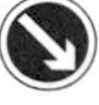 allergy (including skin rash, fever, and jaundice), stomach upset, headache. Rarely, blood disorders.

 in the elderly and in patients suffering from kidney or liver disorders.

 children, pregnant women, mothers who are breastfeeding, during surgery, or for patients suffering from juvenile diabetes, hormone disorders, stress, infections, PORPHYRIA, severe illness, or severe liver or kidney disorders.

 other sedating drugs, ACE-INHIBITORS, alcohol, ANABOLIC STEROIDS, NON-STEROIDAL ANTI-INFLAMMATORY DRUGS, some ANTIBIOTICS, ANTICOAGULANTS, MAOIS, fluconazole, miconazole, some tranquillizers, BETA-BLOCKERS, nifedipine, CORTICOSTEROIDS, DIURETICS, some drugs used to lower blood cholesterol or lipids, lithium, ORAL CONTRACEPTIVES, testosterone, cimetidine, sulphinpyrazone.

Glucagon *see* glucagon injection
(Novo Nordisk Pharmaceuticals)

---

glucagon injection

An injection administered by the subcutaneous, intramuscular, or intravenous route to treat severe low blood glucose levels (e.g. in diabetics when too much insulin has been used). A similar effect can be achieved in conscious patients by giving sugar by mouth.

Strengths available: 1 mg (1 unit) per injection.
Dose: adults and children, 0.5-1.0 mg immediately.
Availability: NHS and private prescription.
Contains: glucagon hydrochloride.
Brand names: Glucagen.

 upset stomach, low blood potassium levels, allergy.

 in pregnant women and mothers who are breastfeeding. If a suitable response is not seen within 20 minutes of the dose, further treatment is needed urgently. The injection must be prepared before use by dissolving a powder in the accompanying solution.

 patients with PHAEOCHROMOCYTOMA or some types of cancer affecting the pancreas. Not effective for patients with long-standing low blood-glucose levels or who have not eaten recently or have poorly functioning ADRENAL glands.

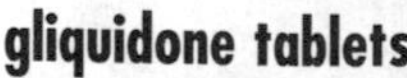

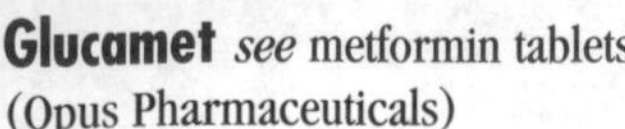

Glucamet *see* metformin tablets
(Opus Pharmaceuticals)

Glucobay *see* acarbose tablets
(Bayer Pharma Business Group)

Glucolet Finger Pricking Device *see* Ames Lancets, Baylet Lancets, FinePoint lancets, B-D Microfine+ Lancets, Milward Steri-Let/Steri-Let Ultra-Fine Lancets, Monolet Lancets, Monolet Extra Lancets, Unilet SuperLite Lancets, Unilet Universal ComforTouch Lancets, Vitrex Soft Lancets
(Bayer Diagnostics)

Availability: private prescription, over the counter.

Glucophage *see* metformin tablets
(Lipha Pharmaceuticals)

---

glucose *see* oral rehydration solution

Glucostix

(Bayer Diagnostics)

A plastic reagent strip used either visually or – more accurately – in conjunction with the Glucometer GX meter to detect blood glucose levels. Blood-glucose monitoring enables individual patients suffering from diabetes accurately to control blood glucose and manage their condition.

Availability: NHS and private prescription, nurse prescription, over the counter.

Glucotide

(Bayer Diagnostics)

A plastic reagent strip used in conjunction with the Glucometer 4 meter to detect blood glucose levels. Blood-glucose monitoring enables individual patients suffering from diabetes accurately to control blood glucose and manage their condition.

Availability: NHS and private prescription, nurse prescription, over the counter.

Gluco Tip (Fine) Lancets

(A. Menarini Diagnostics)

Diabetics who need to test their blood regularly can use lancets to pierce the skin, either with or without the use of a finger-pricking device.

Lancet width and length: 26G/0.45 mm (Type A).

Availability: NHS and private prescription, over the counter.

Glucotrend/Glucotrend Plus

(Roche Diagnostics)

A reagent strip used in conjunction with Glucotrend, Glucotrend 2, and Glucotrend Premium meters to detect blood glucose levels. Blood-glucose monitoring enables individual patients suffering from diabetes accurately to control blood glucose and manage their condition.

Availability: NHS and private prescription, nurse prescription, over the counter.

Glurenorm *see* gliquidone tablets
(Sanofi Winthrop)

---

glutaraldehyde solution

A solution used as a anti-viral, skin-drying agent to treat warts.

Strengths available: 10% solution.
Dose: apply the solution to the wart twice a day and rub down hard skin.
Availability: NHS and private prescription, over the counter.
Contains: glutaraldehyde.
Brand names: Glutarol.

 rash, irritation, or brown-staining of skin.

 avoid accidental application to healthy skin.

 warts on the face or anal or genital areas.

Glutarol *see* glutaraldehyde solution
(Dermal Laboratories)

---

glycerin *see* glycerol (alternative name)

---

glycerol *see* Audax, Exterol, glycerol suppositories, magnesium sulphate paste BP, sodium citrate enema, thymol glycerin compound BP 1988

---

glycerol suppositories BP

A suppository used as a stimulant laxative to treat constipation.

Strengths available: 1g, 2g, and 4g suppositories.
Dose: use 1 suppository when necessary (infants 1g, children 2g, and adults 4g). Moisten with water before insertion into the rectum.
Availability: NHS and private prescription, nurse prescription, over the counter.
Contains: glycerol (glycerin).

---

glyceryl trinitrate tablets/modified-release tablets/buccal tablets/patch/spray/ 2% ointment

A tablet, M-R TABLET, buccal tablet, patch, spray, or ointment used as a NITRATE to treat and prevent angina. The buccal tablets are also used to treat heart failure.

headache, flushing, dizziness, low blood pressure on standing, rapid or slow heart rate. Patients on long-acting or patch forms may find the effect wears off (in which case your doctor may advise a 'treatment-free' period each day).

in patients suffering from severe liver or kidney damage, underactive thyroid gland, history of heart attack, malnutrition, low body temperature.

children, or for patients suffering from allergy to nitrates, low blood pressure, reduced blood volume, some heart conditions, severe anaemia, head injury or brain haemorrhage, closed-angle glaucoma.

sildenafil. Drugs that dry the mouth (such as ANTIMUSCARINICS) may affect performance of tablet forms.

Strengths available: 300 mcg, 500 mcg, and 600 mcg tablets; 2.6 mg and 6.4 mg m-r tablets; 1 mg, 2 mg, 3 mg, and 5 mg buccal tablets; 400 mcg per dose spray; 2% ointment; 5 mg, 10 mg, and 15 mg-per-24 hours patch.

Dose: for adults with angina attack the following doses when required: standard tablets (held under the tongue) 300-1000 mcg; buccal tablets (held between top lip and gum) 1-3 mg; 1-2 sprays under the tongue. To prevent angina: m-r tablets (swallowed whole) 2.6-12.8 mg three times a day; buccal tablets (held between top lip and gum) 1-5 mg three times a day; patches (applied to chest or upper arm) 5-15 mg replaced at 24-hour intervals; usually 1-2 inches of ointment applied to chest, arm, or thigh (without rubbing in and secured with tape) every 3-4 hours or as needed. To treat heart failure (using buccal tablets only), 5-10 mg three times a day.

Availability: NHS and private prescription, over the counter.

Contains: glyceryl trinitrate.

Brand names: Coro-Nitro, Deponit, Glytrin, GTN, Minitran, Nitro-Dur, Nitrolingual, Nitromin, Percutol, Suscard, Sustac, Transiderm-Nitro.

---

glycine *see* Cicatrin, Titralac

Glytrin *see* glyceryl trinitrate spray
(Sanofi Winthrop)

Gonal-F *see* follitopin alfa injection
(Serono Laboratories (UK))

Gopten *see* trandolapril capsules
(Knoll)

---

goserelin injection

An implant used as a hormone treatment for endometriosis or pre-thinning of the womb lining before surgery. Also used as part of *in-vitro* fertilization treatment to desensitize the pituitary gland.

Strengths available: 3.6 mg implant.
Dose: 1 implant inserted beneath the skin of the abdomen every 28 days. Used for up to 6 months in endometriosis, up to 3 months before surgery, and as advised by doctor in *in-vitro* fertilization techniques.
Availability: NHS and private prescription.
Contains: goserelin acetate.
Brand names: Zoladex.

 hot flushes, emotional upsets, changes in size of breasts, loss of sexual desire, sweating, rash, reduced bone density, headache, dry vagina, skin reactions, asthma, severe allergy, joint pain, vision disturbances, pins and needles, ovarian cysts, temporary changes in blood pressure, changes in head and body hair, fluid retention, weight change, bleeding on withdrawal of treatment.

 in patients at risk of OSTEOPOROSIS or who have ovarian cysts. Your doctor will advise you to use non-hormonal methods of contraception.

 children, pregnant women, mothers who are breastfeeding, or for patients with undiagnosed vaginal bleeding. Not to be used for more than 6 months.

---

gramicidin *see* Graneodin, Neosporin, Sofradex, topical corticosteroid

---

granisetron tablets

A tablet used to treat nausea and vomiting caused by radiotherapy or other cancer treatments.

Strengths available: 1 mg and 2 mg tablets.
Dose: adults, 1-2 mg when treatment starts followed by 2 mg a day (either as one single dose or divided into two) while treatment continues; children, reduced doses according to body weight.
Availability: NHS and private prescription.
Contains: granisetron hydrochloride.
Brand names: Kytril.

 constipation, headache, liver changes, rash.

 in pregnant women and in patients with partially blocked intestines.

 mothers who are breastfeeding.

Graneodin *see* also neomycin cream
(Bristol-Myers Squibb Pharmaceuticals)
An ANTIBIOTIC combination cream used to treat superficial skin infections.

Dose: apply 2-4 times a day. Usually used only for a maximum of 7 days.
Contains: neomycin, gramicidin.

Gregoderm *see* neomycin cream, nystatin ointment, topical corticosteroid ointment
(Unigreg)

---

griseofulvin tablets

A tablet used as an antifungal treatment for infections of the nails, skin, hair, and scalp where skin treatments are not appropriate.

Strengths available: 125 mg and 500 mg tablets.
Dose: adults, 500-1000 mg a day (reducing higher doses when response occurs). May be taken as a single daily dose or divided through the day. Children use reduced doses according to age and weight.
Availability: NHS and private prescription.
Contains: griseofulvin.
Brand names: Grisovin.

 drowsiness, stomach upset, headache, dizziness, blood changes, skin reactions, confusion, numbness of hands or feet, lack of co-ordination, allergies, sensitivity to light. Rarely, precipitation of LUPUS.

 in mothers who are breastfeeding and in patients on prolonged treatment. Women must use adequate non-hormonal contraception during treatment and for one month afterwards. Men must not father children during treatment or for six months afterwards.

 ANTICOAGULANTS, anti-epileptic treatments, ORAL CONTRACEPTIVES, alcohol, sedating drugs.

 pregnant women or for patients with liver disease, PORPHYRIA, lupus.

Grisovin *see* griseofulvin tablets
(GlaxoWellcome UK)

---

growth hormone *see* somatropin

GTN *see* glyceryl trinitrate tablets
(Martindale Pharmaceuticals)

---

guanethidine *see* Ganda

Guarem *see* guar gum sachets
(Shire Pharmaceuticals)

guar gum sachets

Dispersible granules used as a bulking agent to treat diabetes and dumping syndrome (abnormal reactions after eating).

Strengths available: 5 g sachets.
Dose: 1 sachet dispersed in 200 ml of liquid (or stirred into food and eaten with 200 ml liquid) three times a day (immediately before each meal).
Availability: NHS and private prescription, over the counter.
Contains: guar gum.
Brand names: Guarem.

 wind, swollen abdomen, diarrhoea.

 glucose levels should be checked in diabetics. Do not take immediately before going to bed. Take sufficient fluid with this product.

 children or for patients suffering from a blocked intestine or disorder of the oesophagus.

 other anti-diabetic treatments.

Gynefix

(F.P. Sales)
A copper-bearing intra-uterine device used to prevent pregnancy.

Dose: inserted into the womb by a specially trained doctor and replaced after 5 years.
Availability: NHS and private prescription.
Contains: copper wire.

 children, pregnant women, or for patients suffering from allergy to copper, abnormal uterus, severe genital infections, acute pelvic inflammatory disease, womb disease, abnormal vaginal bleeding, or some other disorders of the genital or urine systems, or with a history of ectopic pregnancies, or who have undergone surgery to the fallopian tubes.

 pelvic infection, pain, abnormal bleeding, perforation of the uterus. On insertion, persistent low heart rate, asthma attack, epileptic attack.

 in patients suffering from anaemia, heavy periods, diabetes, epilepsy, or who have had inflammatory heart conditions or pelvic inflammatory diseases or who are at risk from sexually transmitted diseases. Patients should be checked 3 months after insertion and then annually,

 ANTICOAGULANTS.

Gyno-Daktarin *see* miconazole cream and miconazole pessaries
(Janssen-Cilag)

Gynol II *see* nonoxynol cream/gel
(Janssen-Cilag)

Gyno-Pevaryl/Gyno-Pevaryl-1 *see* ecostatin cream and ecostatin pessaries
(Janssen-Cilag)

Haelan *see* topical corticosteroid cream/ointment/tape
(Typharm)

Haemophilus influenzae type b vaccine

A vaccine used to provide active immunization against diseases caused by *Haemophilus influenzae* type b (e.g. meningitis).

Dose: infants under 13 months, three doses (by injection) at 1-month intervals; children over 13 months and adults who require protection but who have not previously received the vaccine, single dose only.
Availability: NHS and private prescription.
Contains: capsular polysaccharide of *Haemophilus influenzae* type b.
Brand names: ACT-HIB, HibTITER.
Compound preparations: diphtheria, tetanus, pertussis, and *Haemophilus influenzae* type b vaccine.

Side effects: fever, headache, tiredness, loss of appetite, stomach upset, rash, fits, skin disorders, irritability, prolonged crying, poor oxygen supply to the legs (giving bluish colour), severe allergic reaction.

Not to be used for: infants under 2 months, patients with feverish illness, pregnant women, or mothers who are breastfeeding. Not normally required over the age of 4 years.

Halciderm *see* topical corticosteroid cream
(Bristol-Myers Squibb Pharmaceuticals)

---

halcinonide *see* topical corticosteroid cream

Haldol *see* haloperidol solution/tablets
(Janssen-Cilag)

Half Beta-Prograne *see* propranolol modified-release capsules
(Tillomed Laboratories)

Half-Inderal LA *see* propranolol modified-release capsules
(Zeneca Pharma)

Half Securon SR *see* verapamil modified-release tablets
(Knoll)

Half Sinemet-CR *see* co-careldopa tablets
(DuPont Pharmaceuticals)

halibut-liver oil capsules *see* vitamins A and D capsules

haloperidol tablets/capsules/solution

A capsule, tablet, or solution used as a sedative to treat psychiatric disorders (such as schizophrenia), severe anxiety, persistent hiccups, and movement disorders.

Strengths available: 1.5 mg, 5 mg, 10 mg, and 20 mg tablets; 0.5 mg capsules; 1 mg/ml sugar-free liquid; 2 mg/ml liquid.

Dose: for psychiatric disorders, adults 1.5 mg-3 mg 2-3 times a day at first increasing as needed (maximum of 120 mg a day in severe cases) then reduced for maintenance; children use reduced doses according to age and weight; elderly patients start with half adult dose). For severe anxiety, (adults only) 0.5 mg twice a day. For hiccups (adults only) 1.5 mg three times a day adjusted as necessary. For movement disorders, 0.5-1.5 mg three times a day (maximum 10 mg a day).

Availability: NHS and private prescription.

Contains: haloperidol.

Brand names: Dozic, Haldol, Serenace.

movement disorders, muscle spasms, restlessness, shaking, dry mouth, heart rhythm disturbance, low blood pressure, weight change, blurred vision, impotence, low body temperature, breast swelling, menstrual changes, blood, liver, eye, and skin changes, drowsiness, apathy, nightmares, sleeplessness, depression, blocked nose, difficulty passing water. Rarely, fits, sensitivity to sunlight.

in pregnant women, mothers who are breastfeeding, the elderly, and in patients suffering from heart, lung, or circulation disorders, epilepsy, thyroid disorders, infections, MYASTHENIA GRAVIS, kidney or liver disease, glaucoma, enlarged prostate, or some blood disorders. Should be withdrawn gradually.

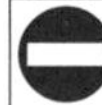
unconscious patients, or for those suffering from severe kidney or liver impairment, bone marrow depression, Parkinson's disease (or similar disorders), or PHAEOCHROMOCYTOMA.

alcohol, sedatives, ANTIDEPRESSANTS, some antidiabetic drugs, anaesthetics, anti-epileptic medications, drugs affecting heart rhythm, ritonavir, halofantrine, sotalol, lithium, rifampicin, nefazodone.

Harmogen *see* hormone replacement therapy (oestrogen-only)
(Pharmacia and Upjohn)

Havrix Junior/Monodose *see* hepatitis A vaccine
(SmithKline Beecham Pharmaceuticals)

Hay-Crom *see* sodium cromoglycate eye drops
(Baker Norton Pharmaceuticals)

Haymine *see* chlorpheniramine tablets and ephedrine tablets
(Pharmax)
Used for allergic reactions.

Strengths available: 10 mg + 15 mg tablets.
Dose: adults 1 tablet each morning (and 1 at night if needed).

H-B Vax *see* hepatitis B vaccine
(Aventis Pasteur MSD)

HCG *see* human chorionic gonadotrophin

Heliclear *see H. pylori* eradication
(Wyeth Laboratories)

Heminevrin *see* clomethiazole capsules/syrup
(AstraZeneca UK)

---

heparinoid cream/gel

A cream or gel used as an anti-inflammatory agent to treat superficial inflammation of veins (due to blood clot) and bruising.

Strengths available: 0.3% cream or gel.
Dose: adults and children over 5 years, apply up to four times a day.

Not to be used for: children under 5 years, or on open wounds or mucous membranes.

Availability: NHS and private prescription, over the counter.
Contains: heparinoid (mucopolysaccharide polysulphate).
Brand names: Hirudoid.
Compound preparations: Anacal, Lasonil (with hyaluronidase), Movelat (*see* topical corticosteroid).

hepatitis A vaccine

An injection used to provide active immunization against hepatitis A.

Strengths available: adult- and children's-strength vaccinations available.
Dose: one injection followed by a booster 6-12 months later.
Availability: NHS and private prescription.
Contains: inactivated hepatitis A virus.
Brand names: Avaxim, Havrix Monodose, Vaqta.
Compound preparations: Hepatyrix, Twinrix.

 soreness, reddening, and hardening of the skin at the injection site, fever, tiredness, headache, diarrhoea, rash, muscle or joint pain, nausea, loss of appetite, general feeling of being unwell, temporary mild liver changes.

 in pregnant women, mothers who are breast-feeding, and in patients on dialysis or suffering from infection, liver disorders, or changed immunity.

 children under 1 or 2 years (depending on brand) or for patients suffering from feverish infections.

hepatitis B vaccine

An injection used as a vaccine to provide active immunization against hepatitis B.

Dose: an initial dose of 1 ml for adults (children 0.5 ml) by injection followed by two more (after 1 and 2 months, or 1 and 6 months, or 7 and 21 days), then a booster at 12 months. Children's dose applies to ages 16 or 18 and under (depending on product).
Availability: NHS and private prescription.
Contains: hepatitis B antigen.
Brand names: Engerix B, HB-Vax II.
Compound preparations: Twinrix.

 mild fever, nausea, dizziness, general feeling of being unwell, temporary soreness, reddening, or hardening of skin at injection site.

 in pregnant women, mothers who are breast-feeding, and in patients with reduced immunity, severe heart or breathing disorders, or who undergo dialysis.

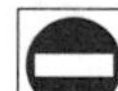 patients suffering from feverish illness.

Hepatyrix *see* hepatitis A vaccine and typhoid vaccine

(SmithKline Beecham Pharmaceuticals)

Dose: adults and children over 15 years, 1 single dose, with booster for hepatitis A after 12 months (using this or hepatitis A vaccine) and booster for typhoid every 3 years with typhoid vaccine if needed.

Herpid

(Yamanouchi Pharma)

A solution used as an anti-viral treatment for shingles and cold sores.

Strengths available: 5% solution.
Dose: apply four times a day for 4 days.
Availability: NHS and private prescription.
Contains: idoxuridine in dimethyl sulphoxide (sulfoxide).

 in mothers who are breastfeeding. Avoid contact with the eyes, mucous membranes, and fabrics.

 children under 12 years, pregnant women, and patients suffering from certain allergic skin conditions. Not to be used in the mouth.

hexachlorophane powder

A powder used to prevent infections in newborn infants, and to treat recurring skin infections.

Strengths available: 0.33% powder.
Dose: adults, apply to affected area once a day; infants, dust the affected area at each nappy change.
Availability: NHS and private prescription, over the counter.
Contains: hexachlorophane (hexachlorophene).
Brand names: Ster-Zac.

 allergy, rarely, sensitivity to sunlight.

children under 2 years (except on advice of doctor or midwife), pregnant women, or on burns or wounds.

hexachlorophene *see* hexachlorophane (alternative name)

hexamine hippurate tablets

A tablet used as an antibacterial agent for the long-term treatment and prevention of urine infections.

Strengths available: 1 g tablets.
Dose: adults, 1 g 2-3 times a day; children aged 6-12 years, 0.5 g twice a day.
Availability: NHS and private prescription, over the counter.
Contains: hexamine hippurate (methenamine hippurate).
Brand names: Hiprex.

 stomach upset, rash, bladder irritation.

 in pregnant women.

 children under 6 years or for patients suffering from dehydration, severe kidney disorders, or chemical imbalance.

 potassium citrate mixture or other drugs that make the urine less acidic, sulphadiazine, sulphametopyrazine, co-trimoxazole.

hexetidine mouthwash

A mouthwash used as an antiseptic rinse to treat thrush, ulcers, bad breath, inflammation of the mouth or gums, sore throat, and before/after dental surgery.

Strengths available: 0.1% solution.
Dose: adults and children over 6 years, use 15 ml to rinse the mouth or gargle 2-3 times a day.
Availability: NHS and private prescription, over the counter.
Contains: hexetidine.
Brand names: Oraldene

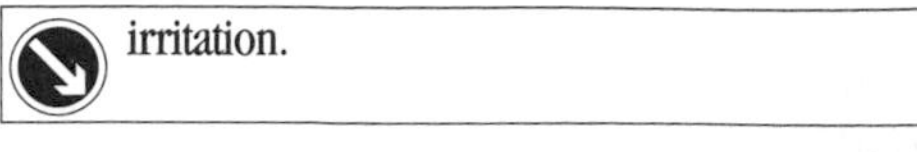
irritation.

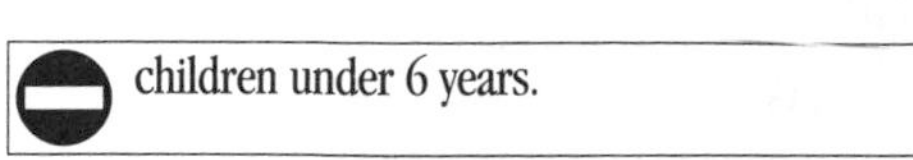
children under 6 years.

Hexopal *see* inositol nicotinate tablets/suspension
(Sanofi Winthrop)

---

hexyl nicotinate *see* analgesic (topical)

Hibiscrub *see* chlorhexidine solution
(SSL International)

Hibisol *see* chlorhexidine solution
(SSL International)

HibTITER *see Haemophilus influenzae* type B vaccine
(Wyeth Laboratories)

Hioxyl *see* hydrogen peroxide cream
(Quinoderm)

Hiprex *see* hexamine hippurate tablets
(3M Health Care)

Hirudoid *see* heparinoid cream/gel
(Sankyo Pharma UK)

---

histamine H_2-antagonist (blocker)

A drug that works on the stomach to reduce acid production by blocking the histamine pathway. Example, ranitidine tablets.

Hivid *see* zalcitabine tablets
(Roche Products)

---

homatropine eye drops

Eye drops used as an ANTIMUSCARINIC preparation to widen the pupil of the eye and to treat inflammation of the interior of the eye.

Strengths available: 1% or 2% drops; 2% single-use drops.
Dose: as advised by doctor.
Availability: NHS and private prescription.
Contains: homatropine hydrobromide.
Brand names: Minims Homatropine (single-use drops).

 disturbance of vision, temporary stinging, raised pressure inside the eye. With prolonged treatment, irritation, redness, inflammation or fluid retention in the eye.

 in the very young and the elderly (*see* above) and in long-sighted patients. Patients should not drive for 1-2 hours after treatment.

 patients with narrow-angle glaucoma.

---

hormone replacement therapy (combined)

A tablet or patch used as an oestrogen and progestogen for hormone replacement during and after the menopause to alleviate menopausal symptoms. This type of HRT is suitable for women who have not had a hysterectomy (i.e. who still have a womb). Some products are used additionally to prevent thinning of the bones (marked * in table opposite).

Dose: *see* table below. Patches are applied to non-hairy areas of skin below the waist. Treatment generally starts between days 1 and 5 of the menstrual cycle (if periods are still occurring) but check product pack for exact details.
Availability: NHS and private prescription.
Contains: (*see* table opposite).

 enlarged breasts, fluid retention, abdominal pain, upset stomach, vaginal bleeding, weight gain, headache, dizziness, rash, changes in sexual desire, depression, migraine, cramp. Rarely, liver changes, jaundice, raised blood pressure, blood clots. Contact lenses may irritate. Patch treatments may cause irritation at the patch site. There is a slightly increased risk of breast and womb cancer – your doctor will advise regular checks.

  in patients suffering from high blood pressure, diabetes, asthma, epilepsy, womb diseases, gall bladder disorder, migraine, multiple sclerosis, PORPHYRIA, LUPUS, liver disorders, some ear disorders, or a history or increased risk of breast disorders (including cancer) and blood clots. Your doctor may advise you to have regular examinations. Treatment generally discontinued 6 weeks before general surgery.

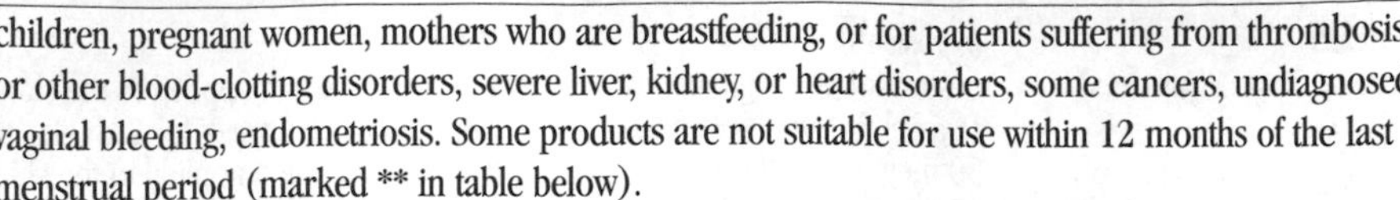

children, pregnant women, mothers who are breastfeeding, or for patients suffering from thrombosis or other blood-clotting disorders, severe liver, kidney, or heart disorders, some cancers, undiagnosed vaginal bleeding, endometriosis. Some products are not suitable for use within 12 months of the last menstrual period (marked ** in table below).

ACE-INHIBITORS, ANTICOAGULANTS, ANTIDEPRESSANTS, BARBITURATES, carbamazepine, cyclosporin, some anti-epileptic treatments, BETA-BLOCKERS.

Product	*Ingredients*	*Dose*
Adgyn Combi (tablets)	oestradiol 2 mg tablets and oestradiol 2 mg + norethisterone 1 mg tablets	1 tablet a day (in the sequence indicated by the pack)
Climagest (tablets)	oestradiol valerate 1 mg or 2 mg tablets and oestradiol valerate 1 mg or 2 mg + norethisterone 1 mg tablets	1 tablet a day (in the sequence indicated by the pack)
Climesse* ** (tablets)	oestradiol valerate 2 mg + norethisterone 700 mcg	1 tablet a day
Cyclo-Progynova (tablets)	oestradiol 1 mg or 2 mg* tablets and oestradiol 1 mg or 2 mg* + levonorgestrel 250 mcg or 500 mcg tablets	1 tablet a day (in the sequence indicated by the pack) for 3 weeks followed by 1 week without treatment before beginning cycle again.
Elleste-Duet (tablets)	oestradiol 1 mg or 2 mg* tablets and oestradiol 1 mg or 2 mg* + norethisterone 1 mg tablets	1 tablet a day (in the sequence indicated by the pack)
Elleste-Duet Conti* ** (tablets)	oestradiol 2 mg + norethisterone 1 mg	1 tablet a day
Estracombi* (patches)	oestradiol 50 mcg (Estraderm) patches and oestradiol 50 mcg + norethisterone 250 mcg (Estragest)patches	1 Estraderm patch applied to the skin and replaced twice a week for 2 weeks, then 1 Estragest patch applied to the skin and replaced twice a week for 2 weeks (and the cycle repeated)
Estrapak 50* (tablets and patches)	oestradiol 50 mcg patches and norethisterone 1 mg tablets	1 patch applied to the skin and replaced twice a week, with 1 tablet added to the treatment each day from days 15-26 of each 28-day cycle
Evorel Conti* (patches)	oestradiol 50 mcg + norethisterone 170 mcg	1 patch applied to the skin and replaced twice a week
Evorel Pak* (patches and tablets)	oestradiol 50 mcg patches and norethisterone 1 mg tablets	1 patch applied to the skin and replaced twice a week, with 1 tablet added to the treatment each day from days 15-26 of each 28-day cycle. Patch dose increased to 2 patches twice a week if necessary.

cont.

Product	Ingredients	Dose
Evorel Sequi* (patches)	oestradiol 50 mcg patches (Evorel 50) and oestradiol 50 mcg + norethisterone 170 mcg patches (Evorel Conti)	1 Evorel 50 patch applied to the skin and replaced twice a week for 2 weeks, then 1 Evorel Conti patch applied to the skin and replaced twice a week for 2 weeks (and the cycle repeated)
Femapak (patches and tablets)	oestradiol 40 mg or 80 mg* patches (Fematrix 40 or 80*) anddydrogesterone 10 mg tablets (Duphaston)	1 patch applied to the skin and replaced twice a week with 1 tablet added to the treatment each day from days 15-28 of each 28-day cycle.
Femoston 1/10, 2/10*, or 2/20* (tablets)	oestradiol 1 mg or 2 mg tablets and oestradiol 1 mg or 2 mg + dydrogesterone 10 mg or 20 mg tablets	1 tablet a day (in the sequence indicated by the pack)
Femoston Conti * ** (tablets)	oestradiol 1 mg + dydrogesterone 5 mg	1 tablet a day
Kliofem * ** (tablets)	oestradiol 2 mg + norethisterone 1 mg	1 tablet a day
Kliovance (tablets)**	oestradiol 1 mg + norethisterone 500 mcg	1 tablet a day
Nuvelle * (tablets)	oestradiol 2 mg tablets and oestradiol 2 mg + levonorgestrel 75 mcg tablets	1 tablet a day (in the sequence indicated by the pack)
Nuvelle Continuous* ** (tablets)	oestradiol 2 mg + norethisterone 1 mg	1 tablet a day
Nuvelle TS (patches)	oestradiol 80 mcg patches (Phase I) and oestradiol 50 mcg + levonorgestrel 20 mcg patches (Phase II)	1 Phase I patch applied to the skin and replaced twice a week for 2 weeks, then 1 Phase II patch applied to the skin and replaced twice a week for 2 weeks (and the cycle repeated)
Premique* ** (tablets)	conjugated oestrogen 625 mcg + medroxyprogesterone 5 mg	1 tablet a day
Premique Cycle* (tablets)	conjugated oestrogen 625 mcg tablets and conjugated oestrogen 625 mcg + medroxyprogesterone 10 mg tablets	1 tablet a day (in the sequence indicated by the pack)
Prempak-C* (tablets)	conjugated oestrogens 0.625 mg or 1.25 mg tablets and conjugated oestrogen 0.625 mg or 1.25 mg + norgestrel 150 mcg tablets	1 tablet a day (in the sequence indicated by the pack)
Tridestra (tablets)	oestradiol valerate 2 mg tablets and oestradiol 2 mg + medroxyprogesterone 20 mg tablets	1 tablet a day (in the sequence indicated by the pack)

Product	*Ingredients*	*Dose*
Trisequens* and Trisequens Forte* (tablets)	oestradiol 2 mg or 4 mg + norethisterone 1 mg	1 tablet a day (in the sequence indicated by the pack)

** Products used to treat menopausal symptoms and thinning of bones.*
***Not suitable for use within 12 months of the last menstrual period.*

hormone replacement therapy (oestrogen only)

A tablet, implant, gel, or patch used as an oestrogen for hormone replacement during and after the menopause to alleviate menopausal symptoms. Some products are used additionally to prevent thinning of the bones (marked * in table below). The Ovestin brand is used only for vaginal or urinary symptoms associated with hormone deficiency.

Dose: *see* table below. Patches are applied to non-hairy areas of skin below the waist.
Availability: NHS and private prescription.
Contains: (*see* table below).

 enlarged breasts, fluid retention, abdominal pain, upset stomach, vaginal bleeding, weight gain, headache, dizziness, rash, changes in sexual desire, depression, migraine, cramp. Rarely liver changes, jaundice, raised blood pressure, blood clots. Contact lenses may irritate. Patch treatments may cause irritation at the patch site. There is a slightly increased risk of breast and womb cancer – your doctor will advise regular checks.

 in patients suffering from high blood pressure, diabetes, asthma, epilepsy, womb diseases, gall bladder disorder, migraine, multiple sclerosis, PORPHYRIA, LUPUS, liver disorders, some ear disorders, or a history or increased risk of breast disorders (including cancer) and blood clots. Your doctor may advise you to have regular examinations and to take additional progestogen treatment at regular intervals if you still have an intact womb. Treatment generally discontinued 6 weeks before general surgery.

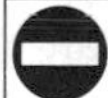 children, pregnant women, mothers who are breastfeeding, or for patients suffering from thrombosis or other blood-clotting disorders, severe liver, kidney, or heart disorders, some cancers, undiagnosed vaginal bleeding, endometriosis, or women with an intact womb (unless progestogen also taken *see* cautions above).

 ACE-INHIBITORS, ANTICOAGULANTS, ANTIDEPRESSANTS, BARBITURATES, carbamazepine, cyclosporin, some anti-epileptic treatments, BETA-BLOCKERS.

Product	*Ingredients*	*Dose*
Adgyn Estro (tablets)	oestradiol 2 mg	2 mg a day
Climaval (tablets)	oestradiol valerate 1 mg or 2 mg	1-2 mg a day
Dermestril (patches)	oestradiol 25 mcg, 50 mcg, or 100 mcg	1 patch applied to the skin and replaced every 3-4 days
Elleste-Solo (tablets)	oestradiol 1 mg or 2 mg	1-2 mg a day

cont.

Product	*Ingredients*	*Dose*
Elleste-Solo MX (patches)	oestradiol 40 mg or 80 mg*	1 patch applied to the skin and replaced twice a week
Estraderm-MX (patches)	oestradiol 25 mcg, 50 mcg*, 75 mg*, or 100 mcg	1 patch applied to the skin and replaced twice a week
Estraderm-TTS (patches)	oestradiol 25 mcg, 50 mcg*, or 100 mcg	1 patch applied to the skin and replaced twice a week
oestradiol (estradiol) implant*	oestradiol 25 mg, 50 mg, or 100 mg	25-100 mcg implant inserted under the skin every 4-8 months
ethinyloestradiol (ethinylestradiol) tablets	ethinyloestradiol 10 mcg or 50 mcg	10-20 mcg a day
Evorel (patches)	oestradiol 25 mcg, 50 mcg*, 75 mg*, or 100 mcg*	1 patch applied to the skin and replaced twice a week
Fematrix (patches)	oestradiol 40 mg or 80 mg*	1 patch applied to the skin and replaced twice a week
Femseven* (patches)	oestradiol 50 mcg, 75 mg, or 100 mcg	1 patch applied to the skin and replaced once a week
Harmogen* (tablets)	estropipate 1.5 mg	1.5 mg once a day, increased to 3 mg if necessary for menopausal symptoms
Hormonin* (tablets)	oestradiol 600 mcg, oestriol 270 mcg, and oestrone 1.4 mg per tablet	1-2 a day. May be used continuously or for 3 weeks followed by 1 week without treatment before continuing.
Menorest (patches)	oestradiol 37.5 mcg, 50 mcg*, or 75 mcg*	1 patch applied to the skin and replaced every 3-4 days
Oestrogel* (gel in pump)	oestradiol 0.75 mg per measure	2 measures applied to skin on arms, shoulders, or inner thighs once a day, increased to 4 measures a day if necessary for menopausal symptoms
Ovestin (tablets)**	oestriol 1 mg	0.5-3 mg once a day for up to 1 month, then 0.5-1 mg once a day until symptoms improve.
Premarin* (tablets)	conjugated oestrogens (0.625 mg or 1.25 mg)	0.625-1.25 mg a day.
Progynova (tablets)	oestradiol valerate 1 mg or 2 mg*	1-2 mg a day
Progynova TS/Forte (patches)	oestradiol 50 mcg or 100 mcg	1 patch applied to the skin and replaced once a week. May be used continuously or for 3 weeks followed by 1 week without treatment before continuing.
Sandrena (gel in sachets)	oestradiol 0.5 mg or 1 mg	0.5-1.5 mg applied to lower trunk or thighs once a day

Product	Ingredients	Dose
Zumenon (tablets)	oestradiol 1 mg or 2 mg*	1-2 mg a day

** Products used to treat menopausal symptoms and thinning of bones.*
***Used only to treat vaginal and urinary symptoms due to hormone deficiency.*

hormone replacement therapy (topical)

A cream, vaginal tablet, or pessary used as an oestrogen treatment for inflammation of the vagina or disorders of the vulva in women after the menopause. Also used before vaginal surgery.

Dose: *see* table below. The dose is applied directly into the vagina, and treatment should be withdrawn every few months to reassess whether it is still needed.
Availability: NHS and private prescription.
Contains: (*see* table below).

irritation of the vagina or vulva. Rarely enlarged breasts, fluid retention, abdominal pain, upset stomach, vaginal bleeding, weight gain, headache, dizziness, rash, changes in sexual desire, depression, migraine, cramp, liver changes, jaundice, raised blood pressure, and blood clots. Contact lenses may irritate. There is a slightly increased risk of breast and womb cancer – your doctor will advise regular checks.

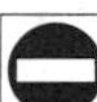
children, pregnant women, mothers who are breastfeeding, or for patients suffering from thrombosis or other blood-clotting disorders, severe liver, kidney, or heart disorders, some cancers, undiagnosed vaginal bleeding, endometriosis. Patients with allergy to peanuts should not use products containing arachis (peanut) oil*.

ACE-INHIBITORS, ANTICOAGULANTS, ANTIDEPRESSANTS, BARBITURATES, carbamazepine, cyclosporin, some anti-epileptic treatments, BETA-BLOCKERS.

in patients suffering from high blood pressure, diabetes, asthma, epilepsy, womb diseases, gall bladder disorder, migraine, multiple sclerosis, PORPHYRIA, LUPUS, liver disorders, some ear disorders, or a history or increased risk of breast disorders (including cancer) and blood clots. Your doctor may advise you to have regular examinations and to take additional progestogen treatment at regular intervals if you still have an intact womb. Some products are not suitable for use in women who rely on barrier contraceptives (*see* table). Treatment generally discontinued 6 weeks before general surgery.

Product	Ingredients	Dose	Effect on barrier contraceptives (condoms and diaphragms)
Estring (vaginal ring)	oestradiol	Inserted into the vagina and replaced after 3 months. (Maximum of 2 years continuous treatment.)	Unknown
Ortho-Dienoestrol (cream with applicator)	dienoestrol (dienestrol). Also: arachis oil*	1-2 applicatorsful a day for 1-2 weeks, then reduce to half dose for 1-2 weeks, then maintain at 1 applicatorful 1-3 weeks.	Known to cause damage

cont.

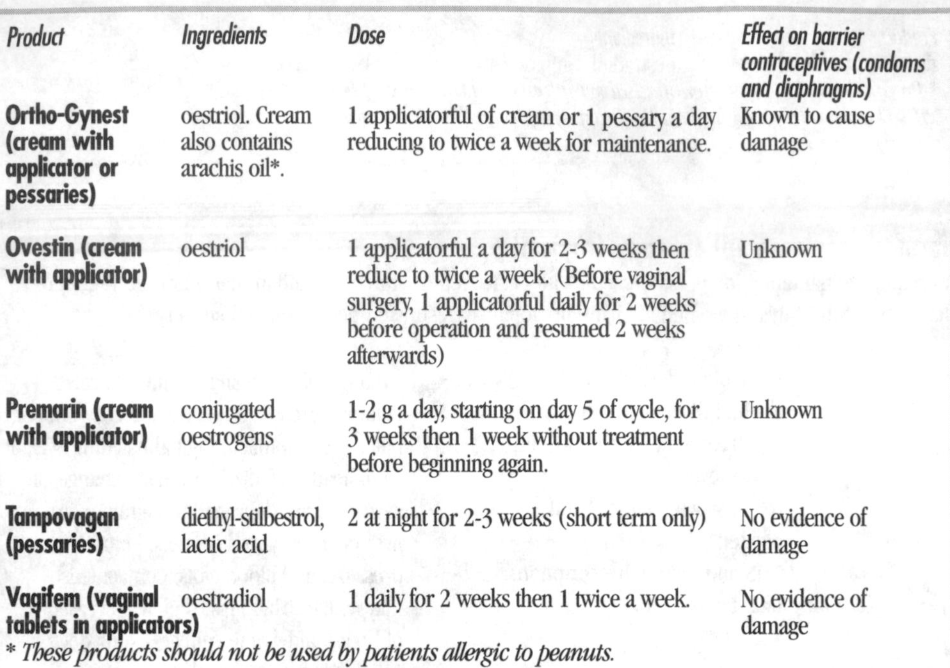

Product	*Ingredients*	*Dose*	*Effect on barrier contraceptives (condoms and diaphragms)*
Ortho-Gynest (cream with applicator or pessaries)	oestriol. Cream also contains arachis oil*.	1 applicatorful of cream or 1 pessary a day reducing to twice a week for maintenance.	Known to cause damage
Ovestin (cream with applicator)	oestriol	1 applicatorful a day for 2-3 weeks then reduce to twice a week. (Before vaginal surgery, 1 applicatorful daily for 2 weeks before operation and resumed 2 weeks afterwards)	Unknown
Premarin (cream with applicator)	conjugated oestrogens	1-2 g a day, starting on day 5 of cycle, for 3 weeks then 1 week without treatment before beginning again.	Unknown
Tampovagan (pessaries)	diethyl-stilbestrol, lactic acid	2 at night for 2-3 weeks (short term only)	No evidence of damage
Vagifem (vaginal tablets in applicators)	oestradiol	1 daily for 2 weeks then 1 twice a week.	No evidence of damage

* *These products should not be used by patients allergic to peanuts.*

Hormonin *see* hormone replacement therapy (oestrogen-only)
(Shire Pharmaceuticals)

H. pylori eradication

A combination of ANTIBIOTICS and ulcer-healing drugs used to eradicate the *Helicobacter pylori* organism which may be the cause of many stomach ulcers.

Dose: adults, any one of the following courses of treatment may be used:
omeprazole 20 mg (or lansoprazole 30 mg, or pantoprazole 40 mg, or esomeprazole 20 mg, or rabeprazole 20 mg) twice a day, clarithromycin 500 mg twice a day, and amoxycillin 1000 mg twice a day for 7 days;
omeprazole 20 mg (or lansoprazole 30 mg or pantoprazole 40 mg) twice a day, clarithromycin 500 mg twice a day, and metronidazole 400 mg twice a day for 7 days;
amoxycillin 1 g (or metronidazole 400 mg) twice a day, ranitidine bismuth citrate 400 mg twice a day, and clarithromycin 500 mg twice a day for 7 days;
omeprazole 20 mg twice a day, amoxycillin 500 mg three times a day, and metronidazole 400 mg three times a day for 7 days;
lansoprazole 30 mg (or ranitidine bismuth citrate 400 mg) twice a day, amoxycillin 1000 mg twice a day, and metronidazole 400 mg twice a day for 7 days;
omeprazole 20 mg twice a day, clarithromycin 250 mg twice a day, and tinidazole 500 mg twice a day for 7 days.

Availability: NHS and private prescription.

Side effects, cautions, etc. *see* individual drug entries.

Compound packs: Heliclear (containing lansoprazole, clarithromycin, and amoxycillin as separate items).

Humaject *see* insulin

Humalog *see* insulin

Human Actrapid *see* insulin

human chorionic gonadotrophin *see* chorionic gonadotrophin

Human Insulatard *see* insulin

human menopausal gonadotrophin injection

An injection used to treat infertility through failure of ovulation in women, and to stimulate the ovaries for *in vitro* fertilization. Some brands also used to treat low sperm count and underdeveloped sex organs in males.

Strengths available: 75 unit + 75 unit injections.
Dose: as advised by doctor.
Availability: NHS and private prescription.
Contains: follicle-stimulating hormone (FSH) and luteinizing hormone (LH) – this combination also known as menotrophin.
Brand names: Menogon, Menopur, Pergonal.

 skin reaction around injection site, over-stimulation of ovaries, multiple pregnancies.

 in patients with ADRENAL or thyroid disorders, or high levels of prolactin (a hormone) in the blood. Hormone or brain disorders must be treated before using this drug.

 children, pregnant women, mothers who are breastfeeding, or for patients with some brain, ovary, uterus, or breast cancers, prostate or testicular cancer, ovarian cysts, or undiagnosed vaginal bleeding.

Human Mixtard *see* insulin

Human Monotard *see* insulin

human normal immunoglobulin injection

An injection prepared from human blood that contains antibodies effective against diseases such as measles and rubella. It is used in patients who are not immune but who have had contact with the

cont.

disease or are at risk of infection and who cannot receive the usual vaccine (e.g. pregnant women who have been in contact with rubella).

Dose: as advised by doctor.
Availability: NHS and private prescription.
Contains: human normal immunoglobulin (gamma globulin).
Brand names: Gammabulin, Kabiglobulin.

general feeling of being unwell, chills, fever. Rarely, shock and severe allergy.

in patients with a history of reaction to blood products, or who already have immunoglobulin antibodies in the blood.

live virus vaccines.

Human Ultratard *see* insulin

Human Velosulin *see* insulin

Humapen *see* insulin injection devices
(Eli Lilly and Co.)

Humatrope *see* somatropin injection
(Eli Lilly and Co.)

Humulin *see* insulin
(Eli Lilly and Co.)

---

hyaluronidase *see* Lasonil

Hydergine *see* co-dergocrine tablets
(Novartis Pharmaceuticals UK)

---

hydralazine tablets

A tablet used to widen blood vessels and to treat high blood pressure and (with NITRATES) heart failure.

Strengths available: 25 mg and 50 mg tablets.
Dose: for high blood pressure, 25-50 mg twice a day; for heart failure, 25 mg 3-4 times a day at first increasing to 50-75 mg four times a day.
Availability: NHS and private prescription.
Contains: hydralazine hydrochloride.
Brand names: Apresoline.

blood changes, stomach upset, rash, sensitivity to light, loss of appetite, impotence, fast or irregular heart beat, flushing, fluid retention, headache, fever, nerve inflammation, muscle or joint pain, increased tears, congested nose, inflamed pancreas, dizziness, difficulty breathing, anxiety, liver and urine abnormalities, and LUPUS-like symptoms after long periods of treatment.

in pregnant women, mothers who are breastfeeding, and in patients suffering from heart or circulation disorder, liver or kidney disease. Treatment should be withdrawn gradually.

children, women in the first 6 months of pregnancy, or for patients with very fast heart rate, some heart diseases, PORPHYRIA or lupus.

anaesthetics.

Hydrex *see* chlorhexidine solution
(Adams Healthcare)

---

hydrochloric acid *see* gentian mixture (acid)

---

hydrochlorothiazide tablets

A tablet used as a DIURETIC to treat fluid retention and high blood pressure.

Strengths available: 25 mg and 50 mg tablets.
Dose: adults, to treat fluid retention 25-75 mg daily, to treat high blood pressure 25-50 mg daily; elderly patients, start with lower dose (12.5 mg); children, lower doses used according to doctor's advice.
Availability: NHS and private prescription.
Contains: hydrochlorothiazide.
Brand names: HydroSaluric.
Compound preparations: Accuretic, Carace Plus, Co-amilozide, Co-betaloc, Co-triamterzide, Cozaar Comp, Co-zidocapt, Innozide, Kalten, Moducren, Monozide, Secadrex, Zestoretic.

low potassium levels, rash, sensitivity to light, blood changes, gout, tiredness, stomach upset, low blood pressure, dizziness, vertigo, abnormal skin sensations, headache, yellow vision, jaundice, kidney and pancreas disorders.

in pregnant women and in patients suffering from diabetes, liver or kidney disease, chemical imbalance, LUPUS, or gout. Your doctor may advise that a potassium supplement is needed.

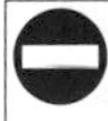
mothers who are breastfeeding, patients with allergies to similar drugs, or for patients suffering from severe kidney or liver failure, raised calcium levels, Addison's disease, or failure to produce urine.

lithium, digoxin, ANTIHYPERTENSIVES, drugs that cause drowsiness, ACE-INHIBITORS, CORTICOSTEROIDS, antidiabetics, NON-STEROIDAL ANTI-INFLAMMATORY DRUGS, drugs that alter heart rhythm, carbamazepine, pimozide.

---

hydrocortisone *see* Actinac, corticosteroid enema/internal foam, Gentisone-HC, hydrocortisone eye drops/eye ointment, hydrocortisone pellets, hydrocortisone tablets, Neo-Cortef, Otosporin, rectal corticosteroid, topical corticosteroid

---

hydrocortisone cream/ointment *see* topical corticosteroid cream/ointment

---

hydrocortisone eye drops/eye ointment

Eye drops or an eye ointment used as a CORTICOSTEROID for the short-term treatment of eye inflammation when no infection is present.

Strengths available: 1% eye drops; 0.5% eye ointment.
Dose: usually 1-2 drops in the affected eye(s) 4-6 times a day, or the ointment used 3-4 times a day.
Availability: NHS and private prescription.
Contains: hydrocortisone acetate.
Compound preparations: Neo-Cortef.

rise in eye pressure, thinning of cornea, cataract, eye infection.

avoid prolonged use in pregnant women or infants.

patients suffering from eye infections, glaucoma, corneal ulcer, or who wear contact lenses.

---

hydrocortisone foam aerosol *see* corticosteroid enema/internal foam

---

hydrocortisone pellets

A pellet used as a CORTICOSTEROID to treat mouth ulcers.

Strengths available: 2.5 mg pellets.
Dose: 1 pellet dissolved in the mouth (in contact with the ulcer) four times a day.
Availability: NHS and private prescription, over the counter.
Contains: hydrocortisone sodium succinate.
Brand names: Corlan.

rarely, worsening of mouth infection.

in pregnant women, diabetics, and in patients with recurrent mouth infection. To be used to treat children under 12 years only on advice of a doctor.

patients with untreated mouth infection or ulcers caused by trauma.

---

hydrocortisone tablets

A tablet used as a CORTICOSTEROID to replace hydrocortisone lacking due to ADRENAL gland malfunction.

Strengths available: 10 mg or 20 mg tablets.
Dose: adults, usually 20-30 mg a day. Children 10-30 mg a day.
Availability: NHS and private prescription.
Contains: hydrocortisone.
Brand names: Hydrocortone.

high blood sugar, thin bones, mood changes, stomach ulcers, fluid retention, potassium loss, high blood pressure, menstrual irregularity, hairiness, increased likelihood of infection, euphoria, depression, sleeplessness, aggravation of schizophrenia and epilepsy, eye disorders, thinning of skin, acne, bruising, blood changes, stomach upset, inflamed pancreas, muscle abnormality, suppression of the ADRENAL glands, ulcerated or infected oesophagus, general feeling of being unwell, hiccups, reduced growth in children.

in pregnant women, mothers who are breast-feeding, and in patients who have had recent bowel surgery or who are suffering from inflamed veins, psychiatric disorders, thinning of the bones, stomach ulcers, tuberculosis or other infections, high blood pressure, glaucoma, epilepsy, diabetes, underactive thyroid, liver disease, stress. Withdraw gradually. Avoid contact with chicken pox for 3 months after treatment ends and seek medical attention if exposed.

patients who have untreated infections.

live vaccines, some ANTIBIOTICS and anti-epileptics, ANTICOAGULANTS, antidiabetics, some antifungals, digoxin, cyclosporin.

Hydrocortone *see* hydrocortisone tablets (Merck Sharp and Dohme)

hydroflumethiazide *see* co-flumactone tablets

hydrogen peroxide cream/solution

A cream or solution used as a disinfectant to treat minor wounds, infections, leg ulcers, and bed sores.

avoid the eyes and normal skin. Use care if treating large or deep wounds.

iodine, potassium permanganate.

Strengths available: 6% or 3% solution; 1% or 1.5% cream.
Dose: the solution used as needed to cleanse the skin. The cream applied 2-3 times a day for up to 3 weeks.
Availability: NHS and private prescription, over the counter.
Contains: hydrogen peroxide.
Brand names: Crystacide, Hioxyl.

hydrogen peroxide mouthwash

A mouthwash used for oral hygiene to treat ulcerated gums and other mouth disorders.

Strengths available: 6% solution (requires dilution before use) or 1.5% solution (ready to use).
Dose: rinse mouth for 1-3 minutes 2-4 times a day (after meals and at bedtime). Dilute 15 ml of 6% solution in half a tumblerful of water before use. Use 10 ml of the 1.5% solution without dilution.
Availability: NHS and private prescription, over the counter.
Contains: hydrogen peroxide.
Brand names: Peroxyl (1.5%).

Hydromol *see* emollient cream/bath oil
(Quinoderm)

hydromorphone capsules/modified-release capsules

A capsule or M-R CAPSULE used as an OPIOID ANALGESIC to relieve severe pain.

Strengths available: 1.3 mg or 2.6 mg capsules; 2 mg, 4 mg, 8 mg, 16 mg, or 24 mg m-r capsules.
Dose: adults 1 x 1.3 mg capsule every 4 hours or 4 mg m-r capsules every 12 hours at first increased as required according to doctor's instructions. Capsules and m-r capsules may be swallowed whole or emptied on to food.
Availability: controlled drug; NHS and private prescription.
Contains: hydromorphone hydrochloride.
Brand names: Palladone.

 drowsiness, upset stomach, sweating, dizziness, breathing difficulty, low blood pressure, difficulty passing urine, dry mouth, headache, vertigo, flushing, change in heart rhythm, mood changes, rash, itching, addiction, reduced sexual desire.

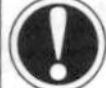 in pregnant women, women in labour, mothers who are breastfeeding, elderly or weakened patients, and in those suffering from breathing, kidney, or liver problems, low blood pressure, underactive thyroid, enlarged prostate, or epilepsy. (Higher doses not suitable for some of these categories.)

 children under 12 years, alcoholics, or for patients with head injury, reduced breathing ability, PORPHYRIA, or those who have a history of drug addiction or who are suicidal or at risk of non-functioning intestines.

 MAOIS, alcohol, sedating drugs, ritonavir.

Hydrosaluric *see* hydrochlorothiazide tablets
(Merck Sharp and Dohme)

hydrotalcite *see* co-simalcite suspension

hydrous ointment BP *see* emollient cream

hydroxocobalamin injection

An injection used as a vitamin B_{12} supplement to treat various anaemias, Leber's disease, and poor eyesight caused by tobacco.

Strengths available: 1000 mcg per injection.
Dose: as advised by doctor.
Availability: NHS (when prescribed as a generic) and private prescription.
Contains: hydroxocobalamin (vitamin B_{12}).

Brand names: Cobalin-H, Neo-Cytamen.

 itching, skin disorders, fever, hot flushes, nausea, dizziness, low blood potassium levels. Rarely, severe allergy.

 CHLORAMPHENICOL.

hydroxyapatite tablets/granules

Tablets or granules used as a calcium-phosphorus supplement to treat OSTEOPOROSIS, rickets, osteomalacia (a bone disorder), and given to mothers who are breastfeeding.

Strengths available: 830 mg tablets; 3320 mg sachets of granules.
Dose: 4-8 tablets or 1-2 sachets a day (in divided doses) with meals.
Availability: NHS and private prescription, over the counter.
Contains: hydroxyapatite compound.
Brand names: Ossopan.

 mild stomach upset.

 in patients suffering from kidney disorders, severe immobility, sarcoidosis, or with a history of kidney stones.

 patients with high levels of calcium in the blood or urine, some tumours, overactive parathyroid glands.

H

hydroxychloroquine tablets

A tablet used as an anti-arthritic drug to treat rheumatoid arthritis, LUPUS, and skin conditions made worse by sunlight.

Strengths available: 200 mg tablets.
Dose: as advised by doctor.
Availability: NHS and private prescription.
Contains: hydroxychloroquine sulphate.
Brand names: Plaquenil.

 headache, fits, stomach upset, skin disorders, hair loss, eye disorders, blood disorders, loss of hair or hair pigment, allergy.

 in mothers who are breastfeeding and in patients suffering from PORPHYRIA, kidney or liver disease, severe stomach or intestinal disorder, nervous or blood disorders, MYASTHENIA GRAVIS, psoriasis, or with a history of epilepsy. The eyes should be tested before and during prolonged treatment.

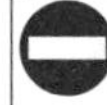 pregnant women or for patients suffering from maculopathy (eye disease).

hydroxyethylcellulose *see* Artificial Tears Minims

hydroxyprogesterone injection

An injection used as a progestogen treatment to prevent abortion in pregnant women where this is habitual.

Strengths available: 250 mg or 500 mg injections.
Dose: 250-500 mg injected once a week during the first half of pregnancy.
Availability: NHS and private prescription.
Contains: hydroxyprogesterone hexanoate (hydroxyprogesterone caproate).
Brand names: Proluton Depot.

occasionally, skin reaction at site of injection, coughing, difficulty breathing, circulation or liver disorder.

in diabetic patients. The pregnancy must be carefully monitored.

women with a history of liver cancer or skin disorders associated with pregnancy.

cyclosporin.

hydroxyzine syrup/tablets

A tablet or syrup used as an ANTIHISTAMINE to treat anxiety and itching.

Strengths available: 10 mg and 25 mg tablets; 10 mg/5 ml syrup.
Dose: for anxiety (adults only) 50-100 mg four times a day; for itching, adults 25 mg at night at first increasing if needed to 25 mg four times a day; children over 6 months 5-100 mg a day (in divided doses) according to patient's age and severity of condition.
Availability: NHS and private prescription.
Contains: hydroxyzine hydrochloride.
Brand names: Atarax, Ucerax (tablets not allowed on NHS).

drowsiness, reduced reactions, dizziness, excitation, movement disorders (with high doses), headache, ANTIMUSCARINIC effects. Rarely, heart rhythm disturbances, severe allergic reaction, skin disorders, noises in the ears, sensitivity to sunlight, confusion, depression, fits, shaking, sweating, muscle pain, pins and needles, liver disorders, hair loss, sleep disturbances.

in the elderly and in patients suffering from enlarged prostate, liver or kidney disorders, difficulty passing urine, epilepsy, glaucoma, stomach ulcer causing blockage, or stomach obstruction. To be used to treat children only for itching.

infants under 6 months, pregnant women, mothers who are breastfeeding, or for patients suffering from PORPHYRIA.

sedating drugs, alcohol, ANTIDEPRESSANTS.

Hygroton *see* chlorthalidone tablets
(Alliance Pharmaceuticals)

hyoscine butylbromide tablets

A tablet used as an ANTIMUSCARINIC treatment for bowel spasm or painful periods.

Strengths available: 10 mg tablets.
Dose: adults, 20 mg four times a day; children 6-12 years (for bowel spasm), 10 mg three times a day
Availability: NHS and private prescription, over the counter.
Contains: hyoscine butylbromide.
Brand names: Buscopan.

 antimuscarinic effects, skin reactions, stomach upset, altered heart rhythm, difficulty passing urine, disturbed vision, dry mouth, intolerance of light, flushing, dry skin, confusion, dizziness.

 in children, elderly patients, and in those with diarrhoea or inflamed bowel, high blood pressure, abnormal heart rhythm, fever, reflux oesophagitis, or heart attack.

 patients with glaucoma, MYASTHENIA GRAVIS, PORPHYRIA, enlarged prostate, or non-functioning intestines.

 other antimuscarinic drugs.

hyoscine patches

A patch used as an ANTIMUSCARINIC drug to prevent travel sickness.

Strengths available: 1.5 mg patch.
Dose: adults and children over 10 years, 1 patch applied to the skin behind the ear 5-6 hours before travelling and replaced after 72 hours if still travelling. (Put replacement patch behind the other ear.)
Availability: NHS and private prescription.
Contains: hyoscine.
Brand names: Scopoderm.
Other preparations: tablet forms of hyoscine available over the counter (e.g. Joy-rides, Kwells).

 drowsiness, dry mouth, dizziness, blurred vision, difficulty passing urine.

 in the elderly, pregnant women, and in patients suffering from heart or circulation disorders, blocked intestines, liver or kidney disease, PORPHYRIA, difficulty passing urine.

 children under 10 years, mothers who are breastfeeding, or for patients suffering from glaucoma.

 alcohol, other sedating drugs, other antimuscarinic drugs.

Hypoguard Supreme

(Hypoguard)

A plastic reagent strip used, either visually or, more accurately, in conjunction with the Hypoguard Supreme meter to detect blood glucose levels. Blood-glucose monitoring enables individual patients suffering from diabetes accurately to control blood glucose and manage their condition.

Availability: NHS and private prescription, nurse prescription, over the counter.

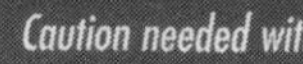

Hypolance Finger Pricking Device *see* Baylet Lancets, B-D Micro-Fine+ Lancets, Cleanlet Fine Lancets, FinePoint Lancets, Milward Steri-Let/Steri-Let Ultra-Fine Lancets, Monolet Lancets, Monolet Extra Lancets, Unilet G SuperLite Lancets, Unilet GP Lancets, Unilet Universal ComforTouch Lancets, Vitrex Soft Lancets
(Hypoguard)

Availability: private prescription, over the counter.

Hypolar Retard *see* nifedipine modified-release tablets
(Lagap Pharmaceuticals)

Hypostop *see* dextrose gel
(Bio Diagnostics)

Hypotears *see* polyvinyl alcohol eye drops
(CIBA Vision Ophthalmics)

I

Hypovase *see* prazosin tablets
(Invicta Pharmaceuticals)

---

hypromellose eye drops/single-dose units

Eye drops used to treat tear deficiency.

Strengths available: 0.3%, 0.5%, and 1% eye drops; 0.32% single-use drops.
Dose: used as needed for relief.
Availability: NHS and private prescription, over the counter.
Contains: hypromellose.
Brand names: Artelac SDU, Isopto Alkaline, Isopto Plain, Moisture-eyes.
Compound preparations: Isopto Carbachol, Isopto Carpine, Isopto Frin, Maxidex, Maxitrol, Ilube (with acetylcysteine, used 3-4 times a day) – also used to treat abnormal mucous production, Tears Naturale (with dextran).

Hypurin *see* insulin

Hytrin/Hytrin BPH *see* terazosin tablets
(Abbott Laboratories)

Ibugel/Ibugel Forte *see* non-steroidal anti-inflammatory drug (topical)
(Dermal Laboratories)

Ibuleve/Ibuleve Maximum Strength *see* non-steroidal anti-inflammatory drug (topical)
(Dendron)

Ibumousse *see* non-steroidal anti-inflammatory drug (topical)
(Dermal Laboratories)

---

ibuprofen cream/gel/mousse/spray *see* non-steroidal anti-inflammatory drug (topical)
cream/gel/mousse/spray

---

ibuprofen tablets/modified-release tablets/modified-release capsules/suspension/granules

A tablet, M-R TABLET, M-R CAPSULE, suspension (or syrup), or granules used as a NON-STEROIDAL ANTI-INFLAMMATORY DRUG to treat pain and inflammation caused by rheumatic disorders, muscle and joint disorders, and other pain (such as migraine, period pain), and fever and pain in children.

Strengths available: 200 mg, 400 mg, and 800 mg tablets; 800 mg m-r tablets; 300 mg m-r capsules; 100 mg/5 ml suspension or syrup; 600 mg granules per sachet.

Dose: adults, 1200-2400 mg a day in divided doses after food; children, usually 50-200 mg 3-4 times a day (according to age), but higher doses sometimes used in juvenile arthritis.

Availability: NHS and private prescription. Lower-strength preparations available over the counter.

Contains: ibuprofen.

Brand names: Arthrofen, Brufen, Fenbid, Motrin.

Compound preparations: Codafen.

stomach upset and bleeding or ulceration, severe allergy, difficulty breathing, blood or kidney disorders, headache, dizziness, noises in the ears, sensitivity to light, vertigo. Rarely, fluid retention, liver disorders, inflamed pancreas, inflamed bowel, meningitis.

in pregnant women, mothers who are breast-feeding, the elderly, and in patients with heart, liver, or kidney disorders, blood-clotting disorders, asthma, LUPUS, or a history of stomach ulcers.

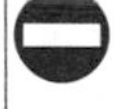

patients with a history of allergy to aspirin or other NSAID, currently active stomach ulcer, or intestinal bleeding.

ACE-INHIBITORS, aspirin or other non-steroidal anti-inflammatory drugs, some ANTIBIOTICS, ANTICOAGULANTS, some antidiabetic drugs, some antivirals, methotrexate, DIURETICS, lithium, digoxin, tacrolimus, cyclosporin.

Ibuspray *see* non-steroidal anti-inflammatory drug (topical) spray
(Dermal Laboratories)

---

ichthammol *see* ichthammol ointment BP 1980, zinc paste and ichthammol bandage

---

ichthammol ointment BP 1980

An ointment used to treat eczema.

irritation.

Dose: apply 1-3 times a day.
Availability: NHS and private prescription, over the counter.
Contains: ichthammol, yellow soft paraffin, wool fat.
Compound preparations: zinc and ichthammol cream BP (with zinc cream), zinc paste and ichthammol bandage.

Ichthopaste *see* zinc paste and ichthammol bandage
(Smith and Nephew Healthcare)

Icthaband *see* zinc paste and ichthammol bandage
(SSL International)

---

idoxuridine *see* Herpid

Ikorel *see* nicorandil tablets
(Rhône-Poulenc Rorer)

Ilube *see* hypromellose eye drops
(Alcon)

Imazin XL/Forte *see* isosorbide mononitrate modified-release tablets and aspirin 75 mg tablets
(Napp Pharmaceuticals)

Strengths available: 60 mg + 75 mg or 60 mg + 150 mg tablets.
Dose: 1-2 of lower-strength (Imazin XL) or 1 higher-strength tablet (Imazin XL Forte) each morning.

Imdur *see* isosorbide mononitrate modified-release tablets
(AstraZeneca UK)

---

imidapril tablets

A tablet used as an ACE-INHIBITOR to treat high blood pressure.

Strengths available: 5 mg, 10 mg, and 20 mg tablets.
Dose: adults, 5 mg (elderly patients 2.5 mg) at first increasing if needed to maximum of 20 mg

a day (elderly 10 mg).

Availability: NHS and private prescription.
Contains: imidapril hydrochloride.
Brand names: Tanatril.

in the elderly and in patients suffering from kidney or liver disease, some heart abnormalities, low blood sodium, psoriasis, auto-immune diseases (such as LUPUS), severe heart failure, or with a history of severe allergies, or in patients undergoing anaesthesia or dialysis. Your doctor may advise regular blood tests.

children, pregnant women, mothers who are breastfeeding, or for patients with disorders of the blood supply to the kidney.

rash, itching, sore throat, runny nose, stomach upset, cough, blood and liver changes, kidney disorders, low blood pressure, severe allergic reaction, inflamed pancreas. Occasionally, headache, dizziness, tiredness, taste disturbance, dry mouth, inflamed tongue, abdominal pain, bowel obstruction, breathing disorders, sleep disturbance, depression, confusion, blurred vision, noises in the ears, impotence, fever, pins and needles, muscle or joint pain, sensitivity to sunlight, inflamed membranes or blood vessels.

DIURETICS, anaesthetics, NON-STEROIDAL ANTI-INFLAMMATORY DRUGS, potassium supplements, cyclosporin, lithium, antidiabetics.

Imigran *see* sumatriptan tablets/nasal spray
(GlaxoWellcome UK)

Imigran Subject *see* sumatriptan injection
(GlaxoWellcome UK)

---

imipramine syrup/tablets

A tablet or syrup used as a TRICYCLIC ANTIDEPRESSANT to treat depression, and night-time bedwetting in children.

Strengths available: 10 mg and 25 mg tablets; 25 mg/5ml syrup.
Dose: adults (depression) up to 75 mg a day (in divided doses) at first increasing to 200 mg if needed (maximum of 300 mg in hospital patients); elderly patients 10 mg a day at first increasing to maximum of 50 mg a day; children over 7 years (for bedwetting) 25-75 mg at bedtime (according to age) for a maximum of 3 months.
Availability: NHS and private prescription.
Contains: imipramine hydrochloride.
Brand names: Tofranil.

dry mouth, noises in the ears, tiredness, constipation, difficulty passing urine, blurred vision, stomach upset, palpitations, drowsiness, sleeplessness, dizziness, shaking hands, low blood pressure, weight change, sweating, fever, behavioural changes in children, confusion in the elderly, skin reactions, jaundice or blood changes, interference with sexual function, changes in heart rhythm, rash, hormone disturbances, fits, movement disorders, blood changes, breast changes in women, menstrual disorders.

in the elderly, pregnant women, mothers who are breastfeeding, and in patients suffering from heart disease, liver and kidney disorders, thyroid disease, PHAEOCHROMOCYTOMA, epilepsy, diabetes, PORPHYRIA, glaucoma, urine retention, constipation, some other psychiatric conditions. Your doctor may advise regular blood tests.

cont.

 children under 7 years or for patients suffering from recent heart attack, heart rhythm abnormalities, severe liver disease, or elevated mood.

 alcohol, sedatives, MAOIS, BARBITURATES, other ANTIDEPRESSANTS, ANTIHYPERTENSIVES, tranquillizers, anti-epileptic drugs, ritonavir, entacapone, selegiline, sotalol, halofantrine, drugs affecting heart rhythm, methylphenidate.

---

imiquimod cream

A cream in sachets used as a treatment for warts on the external genital areas and around the anus.

Strengths available: 5% cream.
Dose: apply the cream thinly three times a week at bedtime for up to 16 weeks. Wash off after 6-10 hours. Wash off the cream before sexual contact.
Availability: NHS and private prescription.
Contains: imiquimod.
Brand names: Aldara.

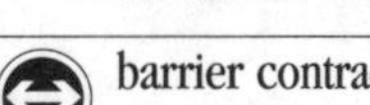 barrier contraceptives (effect unknown).

 itching, pain, redness, or broken skin at the site of application. Also fluid retention, ulceration, and scabbing. Risk of tightening of the foreskin in uncircumcised men.

 in pregnant women, mothers who are breast-feeding, the elderly, and in uncircumcised men.

 children or for treating internal warts. Not to be applied to broken or normal skin.

---

immunoglobulin *see* human normal immunoglobulin injection

Immunoprin *see* azathioprine tablets
(Ashbourne Pharmaceuticals)

Imodium *see* loperamide capsules/liquid
(Janssen-Cilag)

Implanon *see* etonogestrel implant
(Organon Laboratories)

Imuderm *see* emollient bath oil
(Goldshield Healthcare)

Imunovir *see* inosine pranobex tablets
(Ardern Healthcare)

Imuran *see* azathioprine tablets
(GlaxoWellcome UK)

Inadine *see* povidone iodine dressing
(Johnson and Johnson Medical)

---

indapamide tablets/modified-release tablets

A tablet or M-R TABLET used as a DIURETIC to treat high blood pressure.

Strengths available: 2.5 mg tablets, 1.5 mg m-r tablets.
Dose: 2.5 mg (standard tablet) or 1.5 mg (m-r tablet) in the morning.
Availability: NHS and private prescription.
Contains: indapamide.
Brand names: Natrilix, Natrilix SR, Nindaxa.

 low potassium levels, upset stomach, headache, dizziness, tiredness, muscle cramps, rash, loss of appetite. Rarely, low blood pressure on standing, high blood-glucose levels, pins and needles, blood changes, sensitivity to light, kidney disorders, impotence, visual disturbance, palpitations.

 in the elderly, pregnant women, mothers who are breastfeeding, and in patients suffering from severe kidney or liver disease, gout, overactive parathyroid glands, or who have high levels of ADRENAL hormones.

 children or for patients suffering from severe liver failure or who have recently suffered a stroke.

 digoxin, drugs affecting heart rhythm, laxatives, lithium, NON-STEROIDAL ANTI-INFLAMMATORY DRUGS, some antidiabetics, carbamazepine, some other drugs used to lower blood pressure, halofantrine, pimozide, cyclosporin.

Inderal/Inderal LA *see* propranolol tablets/modified-release capsules
(Zeneca Pharma)

Inderetic *see* propranolol modified-release capsules and bendrofluazide tablets
(Zeneca Pharma)

Strengths available: 80 mg + 2.5 mg capsules.
Dose: adults 1 capsule twice a day.

Inderex *see* propranolol modified-release capsules and bendrofluazide tablets
(Zeneca Pharma)

Strengths available: 160 mg + 5 mg M-R CAPSULES.
Dose: adults 1 each day.

---

indinavir capsules

A capsule used, in combination with other drugs, as an antiviral treatment for HIV infection.

Strengths available: 200 mg, 333 mg, and 400 mg capsules.
Dose: adults 800 mg every 8 hours (1 hour before or 2 hours after food). Dose reduced to 600 mg if also taking ketoconazole/itraconazole or in patients with liver disorders.
Availability: NHS and private prescription.
Contains: indinavir.
Brand names: Crixivan.

 rifabutin, rifampicin, ketoconazole, itraconazole, pimozide, alprazolam, midazolam, ergotamine, simvastatin, sildenafil.

 upset stomach, headache, dizziness, sleeplessness, dry mouth, taste disturbance, muscle pain, pins and needles, skin disorders (including rash, pigmentation, and dryness), weakness, itching, hair loss, kidney disorders (including stones), pain or difficulty passing urine, liver disorders, blood changes, disturbance of metabolism.

 in pregnant women and in patients with liver disorders, diabetes, or blood-clotting disorders. Drink plenty of fluids.

 children or mothers who are breastfeeding.

I

Indocid/Indocid-R *see* indomethacin capsules/suppositories/modified-release capsules (Merck Sharp and Dohme)

indometacin *see* indomethacin (alternative name)

indomethacin capsules/modified-release capsule/modified-release tablet/suspension/suppository

A capsule, M-R CAPSULE, M-R TABLET, suspension, or suppository used as a NON-STEROIDAL ANTI-INFLAMMATORY DRUG to treat pain and inflammation caused by rheumatic disorders, muscle and joint disorders, gout, and other pain (such as period pain).

Strengths available: 25 mg and 50 mg capsules; 25 mg, 50 mg, and 75 mg m-r tablets; 75 mg m-r capsules; 25 mg/5ml suspension; 100 mg suppositories.
Dose: adults 50-200 mg a day by mouth in divided doses after food (maximum of 75 mg a day in period pain); 100 mg at night (or twice a day) by suppository. Total combined treatments must not exceed 200 mg a day.
Availability: NHS and private prescription.
Contains: indomethacin (indometacin).

 stomach upset and bleeding or ulceration, severe allergy, difficulty breathing, blood or kidney disorders, headache, dizziness, noises in the ears, sensitivity to light, vertigo. Rarely, fluid retention, liver disorders, inflamed pancreas, inflamed bowel, meningitis, confusion, sleeplessness, fits, mental disturbance, depression, blood disorders, fainting, eye disorders, high blood pressure, high blood-glucose levels, tingling or numbness in hands and feet, narrowed intestines. Suppositories may cause irritation or bleeding.

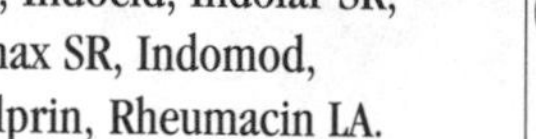

Brand names: Flexin, Indocid, Indolar SR, Indomax SR, Indomod, Pardelprin, Rheumacin LA.

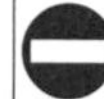 patients with a history of allergy to aspirin or other non-steroidal anti-inflammatory drugs, currently active stomach ulcer or intestinal bleeding, or those with polyps in the nose that are linked to sudden swelling of membranes. Patients with piles or inflamed lower bowel should not use suppositories.

 in pregnant women, mothers who are breast-feeding, the elderly, and in patients with heart, liver, or kidney disorders, epilepsy, Parkinson's disease, mental disorders, blood-clotting disorders, asthma, LUPUS, or a history of stomach ulcers. Your doctor may advise regular eye and blood tests during prolonged treatment.

 ACE-INHIBITORS, aspirin or other non-steroidal anti-inflammatory drugs, some ANTIBIOTICS, ANTICOAGULANTS, some antidiabetic drugs, some antivirals, methotrexate, DIURETICS, lithium, tacrolimus, digoxin, cyclosporin.

Indolar SR *see* indomethacin modified-release capsules
(Lagap Pharmaceuticals)

Indomax 75 SR *see* indomethacin modified-release capsules
(Ashbourne Pharmaceuticals)

Indomod *see* indomethacin modified-release capsules
(Pharmacia and Upjohn)

---

indoramin tablets

A tablet used as an ALPHA-BLOCKER to treat high blood pressure and urine obstruction caused by prostate disease.

Strengths available: 20 mg, 25 mg, and 50 mg tablets.

Dose: adults for high blood pressure, 25 mg twice a day at first increasing gradually to a maximum of 200 mg a day (in 2-3 divided doses); for prostate disease, usually 20 mg twice a day increasing to maximum of 100 mg a day (20 mg once a day at night may be sufficient in elderly patients).

Availability: NHS and private prescription.

 drowsiness, dry mouth, blocked nose, weight gain, inability to ejaculate, dizziness, depression, shaking hands.

 in pregnant women, mothers who are breast-feeding, and in patients suffering from kidney or liver disorders, Parkinson's disease, epilepsy, recently diagnosed heart failure (additional treatment needed), or who have a history of depression.

 children or for patients with established heart failure.

 alcohol, sedatives, MAOIS, anaesthetics, ANTIDEPRESSANTS, other drugs used to lower blood pressure, DIURETICS, thymoxamine.

cont.

Contains: indoramin.
Brand names: Baratol, Doralese.

Infacol
(Pharmax)
A liquid supplied with a dropper for administration, and used as an anti-wind preparation to treat colic and griping pain in infants.

Strengths available: 40 mg/ml liquid.
Dose: infants 0.5-1.0 ml before feeds.
Availability: NHS and private prescription, over the counter.
Contains: activated dimethicone (dimeticone).
Other brand names: (other brands available over the counter, e.g. Dentinox Colic Drops, Woodward's Colic Drops).

Infaderm Therapeutic Oil *see* emollient bath oil
(Goldshield Healthcare)

Infanrix *see* diphtheria, tetanus, and pertussis vaccine
(SmithKline Beecham Pharmaceuticals)

Infanrix-Hib *see* diphtheria, tetanus, pertussis, and *Haemophilus influenzae* type B vaccine
(SmithKline Beecham Pharmaceuticals)

influenza vaccine
An inactivated vaccine administered by injection, and recommended for elderly patients and others at high risk (such as asthmatics and diabetics).

Dose: adults and children over 3 years, 0.5 ml by injection; children 6 months-3 years usually given half adult dose. Children under 13 years who have not been previously immunized are given a second dose after 4 weeks. Otherwise, the vaccination is repeated annually (usually in October-November each year).
Availability: NHS and private prescription.
Contains: influenza vaccine.
Brand names: Begrivac, Fluarix, Fluvirin, Influvac.

influenza-like symptoms, skin reaction at injection site, headache, fever, tiredness, general feeling of illness. Rarely, inflammation of brain or spinal cord.

in pregnant women.

children under 6 months or for patients suffering from feverish illness or with allergy to eggs or chicken.

warfarin, phenytoin, theophylline, aminophylline.

Influvac *see* influenza vaccine
(Solvay Healthcare)

Innovace *see* enalapril tablets
(Merck Sharp and Dohme)

Innozide *see* enalapril tablets and hydrochlorothiazide tablets
(Merck Sharp and Dohme)

Strengths available: 20 mg + 12.5 mg tablets.
Dose: adults 1-2 tablets a day.

---

inosine pranobex tablets

A tablet used as an antiviral treatment for herpes infections of the skin or genital organs, as an additional treatment for genital warts, and to treat some types of brain inflammation.

Strengths available: 500 mg tablets.
Dose: adults, for herpes infections 1000 mg four times a day; for genital warts 1000 mg three times a day; for brain inflammation as advised by doctor.
Availability: NHS and private prescription.
Contains: inosine pranobex.
Brand names: Imunovir.

 increased levels of uric acid in the blood and urine.

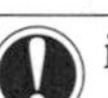 in patients suffering from kidney disorders, gout, or raised uric acid levels.

 children or pregnant women.

---

inositol nicotinate tablets/suspension

A tablet or suspension used to widen blood vessels and treat Raynaud's disease (a condition caused by spasm of the blood vessels) and intermittent claudication (difficulty walking caused by circulation disorders).

Strengths available: 500 mg and 750 mg tablets; 1000 mg/5 ml suspension.
Dose: adults, 1000 mg 3-4 times a day or 1500 mg twice a day.
Availability: NHS and private prescription, over the counter.
Contains: inositol nicotinate.
Brand names: Hexopal.
Compound preparations: Ketovite.

 rarely, flushing, dizziness, nausea, vomiting, low blood pressure on standing, headache, pins and needles, rash, fluid retention.

 in pregnant women.

 children.

Instillagel

(Clinimed)

A gel supplied in a syringe and used as an antiseptic and anaesthetic to lubricate the urethra during procedures such as catheterization.

Strengths available: 2% + 0.25% gel
Dose: 6-11 ml introduced into the urethra before procedure.
Availability: NHS and private prescription, nurse prescription (if prescribed generically).
Contains: lignocaine hydrochloride, chlorhexidine gluconate.
Other preparations: some RECTAL CORTICOSTEROID preparations contain similar local anaesthetics.

Insulatard *see* insulin

---

insulin

An injectable liquid used to treat diabetes.

Dose: usually by subcutaneous injection (self-administered by patient) but occasionally intramuscular or intravenous depending on type of insulin) according to patient's requirements.
Availability: NHS and private prescription.
Contains: (*see* table below)

allergy at injection site, alteration in fat at injection site. Low blood sugar if too much insulin given.

in patients transferring from other types of insulin, in pregnant women, and in patients suffering from infection, emotional distress, liver or kidney disease, or requiring surgery.

ACE-INHIBITORS, alcohol, anabolic steroids, alcohol, MAOIS, BETA-BLOCKERS, nifedipine, some lipid-lowering agents, octreotide, lithium, ORAL CONTRACEPTIVES, testosterone.

Humaject *see* Humulin I, M1, M2, M3, M4, S
(Eli Lilly and Co.)

Humalog
(Eli Lilly and Co.)

Ingredients: insulin lispro.
Duration of action: very rapidly acting.

Humalog Mix 25
(Eli Lilly and Co.)

Ingredients: insulin lispro, insulin lispro protamine suspension.
Duration of action: biphasic (mixed effect).

Humalog Mix 50 Turbo
(Eli Lilly and Co.)

Ingredients: insulin lispro, insulin lispro protamine.
Duration of action: biphasic (mixed effect).

Human Actrapid
(Novo Nordisk Pharmaceuticals)

Ingredients: human neutral insulin.
Duration of action: short acting.

Human Insulatard/Human Insulatard ge
(Novo Nordisk Pharmaceuticals)

Ingredients: human isophane insulin.
Duration of action: intermediate acting.

Human Mixtard/Human Mixtard ge
(Novo Nordisk Pharmaceuticals)

Ingredients: human neutral insulin, human isophane insulin.
Duration of action: biphasic (mixed effect).

Human Monotard
(Novo Nordisk Pharmaceuticals)

Ingredients: human insulin zinc suspension.
Duration of action: intermediate acting.

Human Ultratard
(Novo Nordisk Pharmaceuticals)

Ingredients: human insulin zinc suspension (crystalline).
Duration of action: long acting.

Human Velosulin
(Novo Nordisk Pharmaceuticals)

Ingredients: human neutral soluble insulin.
Duration of action: short acting.

Humulin I
(Eli Lilly and Co.)

Ingredients: human isophane insulin.
Duration of action: intermediate acting.

cont.

Humulin Lente
(Eli Lilly and Co.)

Ingredients: human insulin zinc suspension (mixed).
Duration of action: intermediate acting.

Humulin M1, M2, M3, M4, M5
(Eli Lilly and Co.)

Ingredients: human neutral insulin, human isophane insulin.
Duration of action: biphasic (mixed effect).

Humulin S
(Eli Lilly and Co.)

Ingredients: human neutral insulin.
Duration of action: short acting.

Humulin Zn
(Eli Lilly and Co.)

Ingredients: human insulin zinc suspension (crystalline).
Duration of action: intermediate acting.

Hypurin Bovine Isophane
(C.P. Pharmaceuticals)

Ingredients: beef isophane insulin.
Duration of action: intermediate acting

Hypurin Bovine Lente
(C.P. Pharmaceuticals)

Ingredients: beef insulin zinc suspension.
Duration of action: long acting.

Hypurin Bovine Neutral
(C.P. Pharmaceuticals)

Ingredients: beef neutral insulin.
Duration of action: short acting.

Hypurin Bovine PZI
(C.P. Pharmaceuticals)

Ingredients: beef protamine zinc insulin.
Duration of action: long acting.

Hypurin Porcine 30/70
(C.P. Pharmaceuticals)

Ingredients: pork neutral insulin, pork isophane insulin.
Duration of action: biphasic (mixed effect).

Hypurin Porcine Isophane
(C.P. Pharmaceuticals)

Ingredients: pork isophane insulin.
Duration of action: intermediate acting.

Hypurin Porcine Neutral
(C.P. Pharmaceuticals)

Ingredients: pork neutral insulin.
Duration of action: short acting.

Insuman Basal
(Hoechst Marion Roussel)

Ingredients: human isophane insulin.
Duration of action: intermediate acting.

Insuman Comb 25
(Hoechst Marion Roussel)

Ingredients: human neutral insulin, human isophane insulin.
Duration of action: biphasic (mixed effect).

Insuman Rapid
(Hoechst Marion Roussel)

Ingredients: human neutral insulin.
Duration of action: short acting.

Lantus
(Aventis)

Ingredients: insulin glargine.
Duration of action: very long acting.

Lentard mc
(Novo Nordisk Pharmaceuticals)

Ingredients: beef and pork insulin zinc suspensions (mixed).
Duration of action: intermediate acting.

cont.

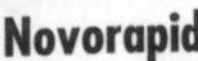

Novorapid
(Novo Nordisk Pharmaceuticals)

Ingredients: insulin aspart.
Duration of action: very rapid acting.

Pork Actrapid
(Novo Nordisk Pharmaceuticals)

Ingredients: pork neutral insulin.
Duration of action: short acting.

Pork Insulatard
(Novo Nordisk Pharmaceuticals)

Ingredients: pork isophane insulin.
Duration of action: intermediate acting.

Pork Mixtard
(Novo Nordisk Pharmaceuticals)

Ingredients: pork neutral insulin, pork isophane insulin.
Duration of action: biphasic (mixed effect).

insulin injection devices

Insulin may be injected by drawing up the liquid into a syringe or by inserting a pre-filled cartridge of insulin into a pen device. The following brands are all prescribable on the NHS:

Single-use syringes with needle attached (in sizes 0.3 ml, 0.5 ml, 1 ml):
B-D Microfine +
Monoject (0.5 ml and 1 ml only)
Omnikan (0.5 ml and 1 ml only)
Unifine

Pen devices for use with cartridges of insulin:

Pen	*Type of insulin suitable*	*Compatible needles*	*Availability*
Autopen	1.5 ml or 3 ml cartridges of Lilly insulins, 3 ml cartridges of Novo Nordisk insulins	Microfine+, Novofine, Unifine Pentip	NHS, private prescription, over the counter
B-D Ultra Pen	1.5 ml or 3 ml cartridges of Lilly insulins, 1.5 ml cartridges of Novo Nordisk insulins	Microfine+, Novofine, Unifine Pentip	NHS, private prescription, over the counter
Novopen 3	3 ml cartridges of Novo Nordisk insulins	Novofine recommended	NHS, private prescription, over the counter
Optipen Pro 1	3 ml cartridges of Insuman	Penfine needles	Free from Hoechst Marion Roussel

Pen	*Type of insulin suitable*	*Compatible needles*	*Availability*
Humapen	3 ml cartridges of Lilly insulins	Microfine+ recommended	Free from Eli Lilly and Co.

Needles available:

Needle	*Sizes available*	*Also compatible with:*	*Availability*
B-D Microfine+	12.7 mm x 29G, 8 mm x 31G, 5 mm x 31G	Humaject pre-filled pens	NHS, private prescription, over the counter
Novofine	12 mm x 28G, 8 mm x 30G, 6 mm x 30G, 6 mm x 31G	Actrapid, Human Insulatard, Human Mixtard, and Novorapid pre-filled pens	NHS, private prescription, over the counter
Unifine Pentip	8 mm x 30G, 12 mm x 29G		NHS, private prescription, over the counter
Penfine			Private prescription, over the counter

A needle-clipping device is also available on NHS prescription and nurse prescription:
B-D Safe Clip

Insuman *see* insulin

Intal *see* sodium cromoglycate inhaler, nebulizer solution, spincaps
(Rhône-Poulenc Rorer)

Intralgin *see* analgesic (topical)
(3M Health Care)

Invirase *see* saquinavir capsules
(Roche Products)

---

iodine oral solution (aqueous)

A solution used (in addition to carbimazole or propylthiouracil) to treat overactive thyroid before surgery.

Strengths available: 130 mg/ml solution.
Dose: 0.1-0.3 ml three times a day, diluted in milk or water, for 10-14 days.
Availability: NHS and private prescription, over the counter.
Contains: iodine and potassium iodide.

symptoms of a cold, excess tear production, headache, inflammation of eye or larynx, pain in salivary glands, rash, bronchitis. With prolonged treatment, depression, sleeplessness, impotence, goitre in breastfed babies if mothers treated.

cont.

 in pregnant women and children.

 mothers who are breastfeeding, or for long-term use.

Iodoflex *see* cadexomer iodine dressing
(Smith and Nephew Healthcare)

Iodosorb *see* cadexomer iodine ointment/sachets
(Smith and Nephew Healthcare)

Ionamin *see* phentermine capsules
Cambridge Healthcare

Ionil T *see* coal tar shampoo and salicylic acid lotion
(Galderma (UK))
Used to treat scalp psoriasis and other scaly scalp disorders.

Dose: adults and children over 12 years, apply once or twice a week.

Iopidine *see* apraclonidine eye drops
(Alcon)

---

ipecacuanha *see* ammonia and ipecacuanha mixture BP

---

ipratropium inhaler/powder capsule/nebulizer solution

An inhaler, powder capsule (for inhalation), or nebulizer solution used as an ANTIMUSCARINIC preparation to relieve blocked airways, especially as a result of bronchitis.

Strengths available: 20 mcg and 40 mcg per dose inhaler; 250 mcg and 500 mcg per vial nebulizer solution.

Dose: adults, by inhaler or inhaled powder from capsule, adults 20-40 mcg (occasionally 80 mcg) 3-4 times a day, by nebulizer 100-500 mcg up to four times a day. Children under 6 years, 20 mcg (aged 6-12 years 20-40 mcg) three times a day by inhaler. Children aged 3-14 years, 100-500 mcg by nebulizer three times a day.

 dry mouth, constipation, difficulty passing urine.

 in pregnant women and in patients suffering from enlarged prostate or glaucoma.

 children under 3 years (nebulizer solution) or under 6 years (inhaler) or under 12 years (powder capsules).

 other antimuscarinic drugs.

Availability: NHS and private prescription.
Contains: ipratropium bromide.
Brand names: Atrovent, Respontin, Steri-Neb ipratropium, Tropiovent.
Other devices: Atrovent Aerocaps (capsules of powder for inhalation), Atrovent Autohaler (breath-activated inhaler).
Compound preparations: Combivcnt, Duovent.

ipratropium nasal spray

A nasal spray used as an ANTIMUSCARINIC treatment for nasal discharge associated with rhinitis (inflamed nasal passages).

Strengths available: 0.03% nasal spray (21 mcg per dose).
Dose: adults 2 sprays in each nostril 2-3 times a day.
Availability: NHS and private prescription.
Contains: ipratropium bromide.
Brand names: Rinatec.

 dry nose, irritation, nose bleeds.

 in pregnant women, mothers who are breast-feeding, and in patients with glaucoma.

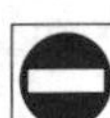 children under 12 years.

irbesartan tablets

A tablet used as an ACE-II ANTAGONIST to treat high blood pressure.

Strengths available: 75 mg, 150 mg, and 300 mg tablets.
Dose: initially 150 mg once a day (75 mg in elderly patients and those on dialysis) increasing if necessary to 300 mg once a day.
Availability: NHS and private prescription.
Contains: irbesartan.
Brand names: Aprovel.

 low blood pressure, high potassium levels, severe allergic reaction, flushing, blood changes, headache, dizziness, muscle or joint pain.

 in patients with heart, liver, or kidney disorders. Your doctor may advise regular blood tests.

 children, pregnant women, or for mothers who are breastfeeding.

 anaesthetics, NON-STEROIDAL ANTI-INFLAMMATORY DRUGS, cyclosporin, DIURETICS, lithium, potassium.

iron sorbitol injection

An injection used as an iron supplement to treat iron-deficiency anaemia.

Dose: as advised by doctor.
Availability: NHS and private prescription.
Contains: iron sorbitol.
Brand names: Jectofer.

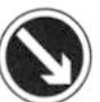 upset stomach, blood in urine, skin reaction at site of injection, disturbance of taste, dizziness, flushing, headache, muscle pain, itchy allergic rash, low blood pressure, irregular heart rhythm, severe allergy.

cont.

 children under 3 kg, women in early pregnancy, or for patients with liver or kidney disorders, heart abnormalities or irregular heart rhythm, urine infection, leukaemia, or anaemia that is not due to iron deficiency.

 in elderly, underweight, or weak patients, and in those suffering from asthma, red blood cell disorders, or with a history of allergies or problems with iron storage.

 iron preparations taken by mouth, CHLORAMPHENICOL.

Irriclens *see* saline solution (sterile)
(Convatec)

Isib *see* isosorbide mononitrate tablets
(Ashbourne Pharmaceuticals)

Isib 50/60 XL *see* isosorbide mononitrate modified-release capsules
(Ashbourne Pharmaceuticals)

I

Ismo/Ismo-retard *see* isosorbide mononitrate tablets/modified-release tablets
(Roche Products)

---

isocarboxazid tablets

A tablet used as an MAOI to treat depression.

Strengths available: 10 mg tablets.
Dose: adults, 30 mg a day (in one single dose or divided throughout the day) increasing if necessary to 60 mg a day for 4-6 weeks, then reduced to 10-20 mg a day for maintenance; elderly patients 5-10 mg a day.
Availability: NHS and private prescription.
Contains: isocarboxazid.

 severe high blood pressure reactions with certain foods and medicines, sleeplessness, low blood pressure on standing, dizziness, drowsiness, weakness, dry mouth, constipation, stomach upset, blurred vision, difficulty passing urine, fluid retention, rash, weight gain, confusion, agitation, shaking, excitement, abnormal heart rhythm, sweating, fits, blood changes, psychiatric disorders, pins and needles, nerve inflammation, sexual disturbances, headache, abnormal muscle or eye movements, liver disorders.

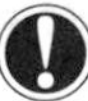 in pregnant women, mothers who are breast-feeding, the elderly, and in patients suffering from diabetes, epilepsy, heart or circulatory disorders, blood disorders, agitation, PORPHYRIA, or those currently undergoing electroconvulsive therapy or surgery. Treatment should be withdrawn gradually.

 children or for patients suffering from liver disease, PHAEOCHROMOCYTOMA, or those who are currently excitable or who have disorders of the blood supply to the brain.

alcohol, sedating drugs, apraclonidine, brimonidine, pethidine and other opioids, SYMPATHOMIMETICS, other ANTIDEPRESSANTS, antidiabetics, anti-epileptic treatments, drugs used to lower blood pressure, oxypertine, clozapine, buspirone, levodopa, selegiline, entacapone, some drugs used to treat migraine, tetrabenazine, sedatives. The following foods should be avoided (until 14 days after treatment ends): cheese, meat extracts, broad beans, bananas, Marmite, yeast extracts, wine, beer, other alcohol, pickled herrings, vegetable proteins.

Isocard *see* isosorbide dinitrate transdermal spray
(Eastern Pharmaceuticals)

Isodur XL *see* isosorbide mononitrate modified-release capsules
(Galen)

Isogel *see* ispaghula husk
(Pfizer Consumer Healthcare)

Isoket Retard *see* isosorbide dinitrate modified-release tablets
(Schwarz Pharma)

---

isometheptene *see* Midrid

Isomide CR *see* disopyramide modified-release capsules
(Tillomed Laboratories)

---

isoniazid tablets

A tablet used in combination with other drugs to treat and prevent tuberculosis.

Strengths available: 50 mg and 100 mg tablets.
Dose: adults, usually 300 mg once a day; children use reduced doses according to body weight.
Availability: NHS and private prescription.
Contains: isoniazid.
Compound preparations: Rifater, Rifinah, Rimactazid.

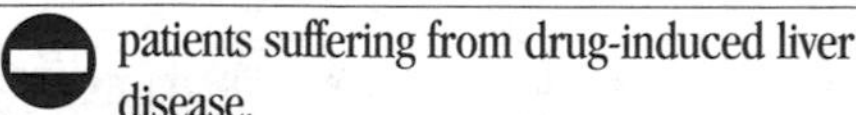
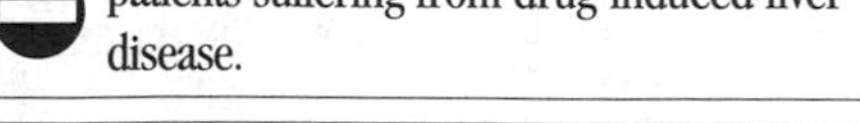
patients suffering from drug-induced liver disease.

nausea, vomiting, nerve inflammation (high doses), fits, mental disturbances, blood changes, liver disorder, fever, LUPUS-like symptoms, skin disorders, high blood-glucose levels, breast swelling.

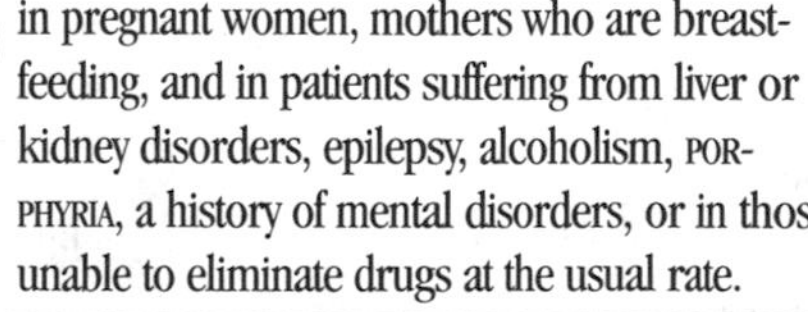
in pregnant women, mothers who are breast-feeding, and in patients suffering from liver or kidney disorders, epilepsy, alcoholism, PORPHYRIA, a history of mental disorders, or in those unable to eliminate drugs at the usual rate.

anti-epileptic treatments, theophylline, aminophylline.

I

isopropyl alcohol *see* Hibisol, Manusept

---

isopropyl myristate *see* emollient preparations

Isopto Alkaline *see* hypromellose eye drops
(Alcon)

Isopto atropine *see* atropine eye drops and hypromellose eye drops
(Alcon)

Isopto carbachol

(Alcon)
Eye drops used as a cholinergic and lubricant treatment for glaucoma.

Dose: 2 drops into the eye up to four times a day.
Availability: NHS and private prescription.
Contains: carbachol, hypromellose.

headache, discomfort in the eye, blurred vision, short sight, other changes in the eye. Rarely, low blood pressure, slow heart beat, breathing difficulties, increased saliva or tears, sweating, upset stomach, urgent need to pass urine.

in patients with dark-coloured or damaged eyes, and in those suffering from heart disease, high blood pressure, asthma, stomach ulcers, difficulty passing urine, or Parkinson's disease. Patients are advised not to drive because vision may be impaired in poor light (e.g. at night).

children or for patients with some eye disorders (e.g. iritis, uveitis, some forms of glaucoma), or those wearing soft contact lenses.

soft contact lenses.

Isopto carpine *see* pilocarpine eye drops and hypromellose eye drops
(Alcon)

Strengths available: 0.5%, 1%, 2%, 3%, or 4% pilocarpine with 0.5% hypromellose.
Dose: apply up to four times a day.

Isopto frin

(Alcon)
Eye drops used as a SYMPATHOMIMETIC and lubricant to treat temporary redness of the eye caused by minor irritations.

Dose: 1-2 drops into the affected eye(s) up to four times a day.
Availability: NHS and private prescription, over the counter.

Contains: phenylephrine hydrochloride, hypromellose.

 in infants and in patients suffering from some types of glaucoma.

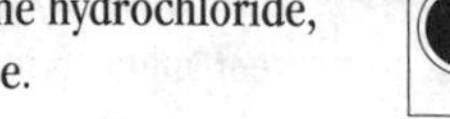

patients wearing soft contact lenses.

 soft contact lenses (*see* above).

Isopto plain *see* hypromellose eye drops
(Alcon)

Isordil *see* isosorbide dinitrate tablets
(Shire Pharmaceuticals)

---

isosorbide dinitrate tablets/modified-release tablets or capsules/sublingual tablet/transdermal spray/sublingual spray

A tablet, M-R TABLET, M-R CAPSULE, sublingual tablet, transdermal spray, or sublingual spray used as a NITRATE to prevent and treat angina and to treat heart failure.

Strengths available: 10 mg, 20 mg, and 30 mg tablets; 20 mg or 40 mg m-r tablets; 20 mg or 40 mg m-r capsules; 5 mg sublingual tablets or 1.25 mg per dose sublingual spray (for use under the tongue); 30 mg per dose transdermal spray (for use on the skin).

Dose: to treat an immediate angina attack (or prevent an anticipated one) 1.25-3.75 mg as sublingual spray or 5-10 mg as sublingual tablets; for long-term prevention of angina, 30-120 mg a day in divided doses by mouth or 30-120 mg a day (in divided doses) by spray application to the skin of the chest; for heart failure 40-160 mg a day by mouth in divided doses. Maximum dose by mouth 240 mg a day.

Availability: NHS and private prescription, over the counter.

Contains: isosorbide dinitrate.

Brand names: Angitak, Cedocard Retard, Isocard, Isoket Retard, Isordil, Sorbid SA.

 headache, flushing, dizziness, low blood pressure on standing, rapid or slow heart rate. Patients on long-acting preparations may find the effect wears off (in which case your doctor may advise a treatment-free period each day).

 in patients suffering from severe liver or kidney damage, underactive thyroid gland, history of heart attack, malnutrition, low body temperature.

 children or for patients suffering from allergy to nitrates, low blood pressure, reduced blood volume, some heart conditions, severe anaemia, head injury or brain haemorrhage, closed-angle glaucoma.

 sildenafil. Drugs that dry the mouth (such as ANTIMUSCARINICS) may affect performance of sublingual products.

I

isosorbide mononitrate tablets/modified-release tablets/modified-release capsules

A tablet, M-R TABLET, or M-R CAPSULE used as a NITRATE to prevent angina and as an additional treatment for heart failure.

Strengths available: 10 mg, 20 mg, and 40 mg tablets; 25 mg, 40 mg, 50 mg, or 60 mg m-r tablets; 25 mg, 50 mg, or 60 mg m-r capsules.
Dose: to prevent angina, 40-80 mg a day in divided doses at first (20 mg if nitrates not previously used), then up to 120 mg a day if needed.
Availability: NHS and private prescription, over the counter.
Contains: isosorbide mononitrate.
Brand names: Angeze, Chemydur 60XL, Dynamin, Elantan, Imdur, Isib, Ismo, Isodur, Isotard, Ketanodur, MCR-50, Modisal, Monit, Mono-Cedocard, Monodur, Monomax SR, Monosorb XL.
Compound preparations: Imazin XL.

headache, flushing, dizziness, low blood pressure on standing, rapid or slow heart rate. Patients on long-acting preparations may find the effect wears off (in which case your doctor may advise a treatment-free period each day).

in patients suffering from severe liver or kidney damage, underactive thyroid gland, history of heart attack, malnutrition, low body temperature.

children or for patients suffering from allergy to nitrates, low blood pressure, reduced blood volume, some heart conditions, severe anaemia, head injury or brain haemorrhage, closed-angle glaucoma.

sildenafil.

Isotard *see* isosorbide mononitrate modified-release tablets (Galen)

isotretinoin gel

A gel used to treat acne.

Strengths available: 0.05% gel.
Dose: apply sparingly once or twice a day for a minimum of 6-8 weeks.
Availability: NHS and private prescription.
Contains: isotretinoin.
Brand names: Isotrex.
Compound preparations: Isotrexin.
Other preparations: isotretinoin capsules.

irritation, reddening or dryness of skin, itching, crusting or peeling, increased sensitivity to sunlight, temporary change in skin colour, severe acne, swollen or irritated eyes.

on sensitive areas of skin and the angles of the nose. Women of childbearing age must use adequate contraception.

children, pregnant women, mothers who are breastfeeding, or for patients with a family history of skin cancer. Not for application to mouth, eyes, mucous membranes, damaged or sunburned skin, areas of eczema. Avoid exposure to sunlight and do not use sun-lamps/sunbeds.

products that cause the skin to peel (e.g. benzoyl peroxide and some cosmetic products).

isotretinoin capsules

A capsule used to treat severe acne.

Strengths available: 5 mg or 20 mg capsules.
Dose: as advised by doctor. Treatment usually lasts for 12-16 weeks. Repeat treatments not recommended.
Availability: NHS and private prescription (hospital specialist only).
Contains: isotretinoin.
Brand names: Roaccutane.
Other preparations: isotretinoin gel.

dry and fragile skin and mucous membranes, dry eyes or nose, nosebleeds, tiredness, hair loss, liver disorders, fits, nausea, headache, sweating, drowsiness, irregular periods, rarely blood or urine changes, blood vessel inflammation, bone changes, hair growth, eye and ear disorders, muscle or joint pain, psychological disturbance, increased pigment in face, enlarged lymph glands, inflamed bowel, infections, high pressure in the brain.

in patients with diabetes, dry eyes, or a history of depression. Women must use adequate contraception during treatment and for at least 4 weeks afterwards. Your doctor will advise regular blood tests. Do not donate blood during treatment or for at least 1 month afterwards. Do not have legs or other body hair waxed (or any similar harsh skin treatment) while on this medication or for 6 months afterwards. Night vision may be impaired.

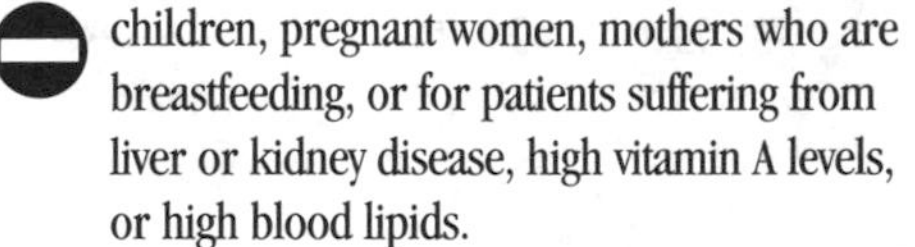
children, pregnant women, mothers who are breastfeeding, or for patients suffering from liver or kidney disease, high vitamin A levels, or high blood lipids.

vitamin A, tetracycline ANTIBIOTICS, contact lenses (due to dry eyes), sedatives, alcohol.

Isotrex *see* isotretinoin gel
(Stiefel Laboratories (UK))

Isotrexin *see* isotretinoin gel and erythromycin gel
(Stiefel Laboratories (UK))

Strengths available: 0.05% + 2% gel.
Dose: as for isotretinoin gel.

---

ispaghula husk

Granules or effervescent granules used as a bulking agent or lipid-lowering agent to treat constipation, diverticular disease, spastic and irritable colon, and high levels of cholesterol in the blood, which have not responded to changes in diet.

Dose: adults, usually 3.5 g (in at least 150 ml water) twice a day; children 2.5-5.0 ml measure in water twice a day.
Availability: NHS and private prescription, nurse prescription, over the counter.

Side effects: wind, bloating, obstructed intestines.

cont.

Contains: ispaghula husk.
Brand names: Fybogel, Fybozest, Isogel, Konsyl, Regulan.
Compound preparations: Fybogel-Mebeverine, Manevac.

in elderly, weak, or diabetic patients, and in those with narrowed or poorly functioning intestines. Drink plenty of fluids.

children (except for intestinal conditions) or for patients with blocked intestines, difficulty swallowing, or relaxed bowel.

---

isradipine tablets

A tablet used as a CALCIUM CHANNEL BLOCKER to treat high blood pressure.

Strengths available: 2.5 mg tablets.
Dose: adults, 2.5 mg twice a day at first increasing to maximum of 10 mg twice a day if needed. (Reduced doses for elderly patients.)
Availability: NHS and private prescription.
Contains: isradipine.
Brand names: Prescal.

weight gain, rapid or irregular heart beat, fluid retention, headache, flushing, dizziness, tiredness, abdominal pain, skin rash, liver changes, worsening of angina.

in pregnant women, mothers who are breast-feeding, and in patients suffering from liver or kidney disorders, diabetes, or some rare heart conditions.

grapefruit juice, drugs affecting heart rhythm, rifampicin, some anti-epileptic treatments, ALPHA-BLOCKERS, ritonavir, theophylline, aminophylline.

children or for patients with certain heart disorders or who have recently suffered a heart attack.

Istin *see* amlodipine tablets
(Pfizer)

---

itraconazole capsules/liquid

A capsule or liquid used as an antifungal treatment for skin, vaginal, or mouth infections.

Strengths available: 100 mg capsules; 10 mg/ml liquid.
Dose: adults, usually 100-200 mg a day (but differs for patients with poor immune system). Length of course depends on condition. For vaginal thrush, 200 mg twice a day for 1 day.
Availability: NHS and private prescription.
Contains: itraconzole.
Brand names: Sporanox.

headache, upset stomach, dizziness, liver disorders, rash, irregular periods, severe allergy, numbness in hands or feet. With prolonged use, fluid retention, hair loss, low blood potassium levels.

in patients with liver or kidney disorders, AIDS, or low numbers of white blood cells. Women must use adequate contraception until the next menstrual period after treatment ends.

children, elderly patients, pregnant women (unless condition is life-threatening), or for mothers who are breastfeeding.

rifampicin, ANTICOAGULANTS, rifabutin, reboxetine, repaglinide, phenytoin, mizolastine, sertindole, pimozide, indinavir, ritonavir, saquinavir, midazolam, CALCIUM CHANNEL BLOCKERS, digoxin, cyclosporin, STATINS, ORAL CONTRACEPTIVES, tacrolimus.

Jectofer *see* iron sorbitol injection
(AstraZeneca UK)

Jelonet *see* paraffin gauze dressing
(Smith and Nephew Healthcare)

Jomethid XL *see* ketoprofen modified-release tablets
(Cox Pharmaceuticals)

K-Y jelly

(Johnson and Johnson Medical)
A non-irritating jelly used to provide additional vaginal lubrication.

Dose: apply a little jelly to the vagina as needed.
Availability: NHS and private prescription, over the counter.

Kabiglobulin *see* human normal immunoglobulin injection
(Pharmacia and Upjohn)

Kalspare *see* chlorthalidone tablets and triamterene capsules
(Dominion Pharma)

Strengths available: 50 mg + 50 mg tablets.
Dose: adults 1-2 tablets each morning.

Kalten *see* atenolol tablets, hydrochlorothiazide tablets, and amiloride tablets
(Zeneca Pharma)

Strengths available: 50 mg + 25 mg + 2.5 mg capsules.
Dose: adults 1-2 each day.

J

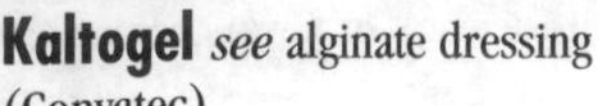

Kaltogel *see* alginate dressing
(Convatec)

Kaltostat *see* alginate dressing
(Convatec)

Kamillosan *see* emollient ointment
(Goldshield Healthcare)

Kaodene *see* kaolin mixture BP and codeine syrup
(Sovereign Medical)
Used to relieve the symptoms of simple diarrhoea.

Strengths available: 1.5 g + 5 mg in 5 ml.
Dose: adults 20 ml (children over 5 years 10 ml) 3-4 times a day.
Availability: private prescription, over the counter.

---

kaolin mixture BP

A mixture used as an adsorbent to treat diarrhoea.

Strengths available: 20% mixture (1 g/5 ml).
Dose: adults 10-20 ml every 4 hours.
Availability: NHS and private prescription, over the counter.
Contains: kaolin.
Compound preparations: Kaodene, kaolin and morphine mixture BP (with morphine).

Side effects: blocked intestines.

Not to be used for: patients with blocked intestines.

Kapake *see* co-codamol tablets/sachets
(Galen)

Kaplon *see* captopril tablets
(Berk Pharmaceuticals)

Kay-Cee-L *see* potassium chloride syrup
(Geistlich Sons)

Keflex *see* cephalexin capsules/suspension/tablets
(Eli Lilly and Co.)

Keftid *see* cefaclor capsules/suspension
(Galen)

Kelfizine W *see* sulfametopyrazine tablets
(Pharmacia and Upjohn)

Kemadrin *see* procyclidine tablets
(GlaxoWellcome UK)

Kenalog *see* triamcinolone injection
(Bristol-Myers Squibb Pharmaceuticals)

Keppra *see* levetiracetam tablets
(UCB Pharma)

Keral *see* dexketoprofen tablets
(A. Menarini Pharmaceuticals)

Keri Therapeutic Lotion *see* emollient lotion
(Bristol-Myers Squibb Pharmaceuticals)

Kerlone *see* betaxolol tablets
(Sanofi Synthelabo)

Ketanodur *see* isosorbide mononitrate modified-release tablets
(Necessity Supplies)

Ketil *see* ketoprofen capsules and ketoprofen gel
(Tillomed Laboratories)

Ketocid *see* ketoprofen modified-release capsules
(Trinity Pharmaceuticals)

---

ketoconazole cream/shampoo

A cream or shampoo used as an anti-fungal treatment for fungus infections of the skin (such as thrush), dandruff, or scaly scalp disorders.

Strengths available: 2% shampoo; 2% cream.
Dose: apply cream to the affected area once or twice a day; apply the shampoo usually twice a week for 2-4 weeks, then once every 1-2 weeks to prevent recurrence.
Availability: private prescription. Some brands also available over the counter. Shampoo also allowed on NHS prescription. Cream allowed on NHS prescription only for certain scaly scalp disorders and pityriasis versicolor.
Contains: ketoconazole.
Brand names: Daktarin Gold, Nizoral.
Other preparations: ketoconazole tablets.

Side effects: occasionally, irritation or allergy.

---

ketoconazole tablets

A tablet used as an anti-fungal treatment for severe fungal infections, including persistent vaginal thrush, and to prevent fungal infection in patients with a weak immune system.

Strengths available: 200 mg tablets.
Dose: adults 200-400 mg (elderly 200 mg) once a day with food until at least 1 week after symptoms have gone. (Used for 5 days only for vaginal thrush.) Children use reduced doses according to body weight.
Availability: NHS and private prescription.
Contains: ketoconazole.
Brand names: Nizoral.
Other preparations: ketoconazole shampoo/cream.

Side effects: liver disorders, severe allergy, stomach upset, itching, rash, headache, blood changes. Rarely, breast enlargement, pins and needles, intolerance to light, hair loss, low level of sperm production.

in elderly patients. Your doctor may advise regular liver checks.

pregnant women, mothers who are breast-feeding, or for patients with liver disorders.

rifampicin, rifabutin, ANTICOAGULANTS, reboxetine, repaglinide, phenytoin, mizolastine, sertindole, pimozide, antiviral treatments, midazolam, cyclosporin, STATINS, ORAL CONTRACEPTIVES, sildenafil, tacrolimus, theophylline, aminophylline.

---

ketoprofen capsules/modified-release capsules/suppositories/modified-release tablets

A capsule, M-R CAPSULE/TABLET or suppository used as a NON-STEROIDAL ANTI-INFLAMMATORY DRUG to treat pain and inflammation in rheumatoid arthritis, other muscle, bone, and joint disorders, after bone surgery, painful periods, and gout.

Strengths available: 50 mg and 100 mg capsules; 100 mg, 150 mg, and 200 mg m-r capsules; 200 mg m-r

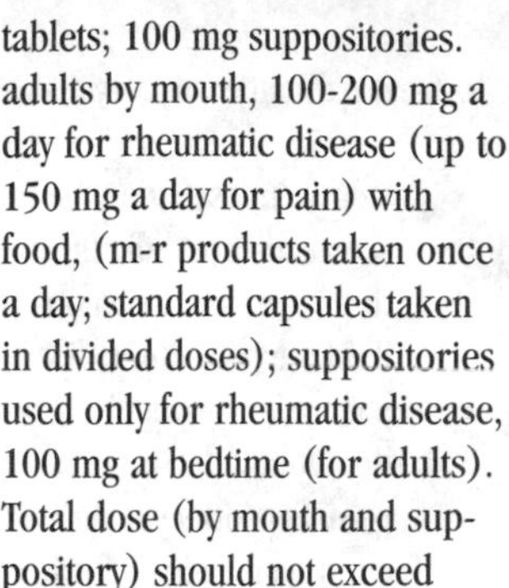

tablets; 100 mg suppositories.

Dose: adults by mouth, 100-200 mg a day for rheumatic disease (up to 150 mg a day for pain) with food, (m-r products taken once a day; standard capsules taken in divided doses); suppositories used only for rheumatic disease, 100 mg at bedtime (for adults). Total dose (by mouth and suppository) should not exceed 200 mg a day.

Availability: NHS and private prescription.

Contains: ketoprofen.

Brand names: Fenoket, Jomethid XL, Ketil, Ketocid, Ketotard XL, Ketovail, Ketozip XL 200, Ketpron XL, Larafen CR, Orudis, Oruvail.

Other preparations: ketoprofen gel [*see* non-steroidal anti-inflammatory drugs (topical)].

 stomach upset and bleeding or ulceration, rash, severe allergy, difficulty breathing, blood or kidney disorders, headache, dizziness, noises in the ears, sensitivity to light, vertigo. Rarely, fluid retention, liver disorders, inflamed pancreas, inflamed bowel, meningitis. Suppositories may cause irritation around rectum.

 in the elderly, pregnant women, mothers who are breastfeeding, and in patients with heart, liver, or kidney disorders, high blood pressure, asthma or LUPUS.

 children or for patients with a history of allergy to aspirin or other non-steroidal anti-inflammatory drugs, severe kidney disorders, blood-clotting disorders, currently active stomach ulcer or intestinal bleeding, inflamed intestines, or severe heart failure. Suppositories not to be used for patients with inflammation of the anus or rectum.

 ACE-INHIBITORS, aspirin or other non-steroidal anti-inflammatory drugs, some ANTIBIOTICS, ANTICOAGULANTS, some antidiabetic drugs, some antivirals, methotrexate, DIURETICS, lithium, tacrolimus, cyclosporin, digoxin, aluminium hydroxide.

K

---

ketoprofen gel *see* non-steroidal anti-inflammatory drugs (topical)

---

ketorolac trometamol eye drops

Eye drops used to prevent and treat inflammation after eye surgery.

Strengths available: 0.5% eye drops.

Dose: 1 drop three times a day for up to 3 weeks, starting a day before operation.

Availability: NHS and private prescription.

Contains: ketorolac trometamol.

Brand names: Acular.

 ANTICOAGULANTS, anti-platelet drugs (which prevent blood clots).

 temporary burning or stinging, irritation, blurred vision.

 in patients with blood-coagulation disorders or a history of stomach ulcers.

 children, pregnant women, mothers who are breastfeeding, or for patients with allergy to aspirin or other NON-STEROIDAL ANTI-INFLAMMATORY DRUGS, or who wear soft contact lenses.

---

ketorolac tablets

A tablet used as a NON-STEROIDAL ANTI-INFLAMMATORY DRUG to treat pain after surgery.

Strengths available: 10 mg tablets.
Dose: adults, 10 mg every 4-6 hours for up to 7 days (maximum of 40 mg per day); elderly patients 10 mg every 6-8 hours.
Availability: NHS and private prescription.
Contains: ketorolac trometamol.
Brand names: Toradol.

in the elderly and in patients with a low body weight, heart failure, liver disorders, high blood pressure, reduced blood volume, kidney disorders.

ACE-INHIBITORS, aspirin or other non-steroidal anti-inflammatory drugs, some ANTIBIOTICS, ANTICOAGULANTS, some antidiabetic drugs, some antivirals, methotrexate, DIURETICS, lithium, tacrolimus, cyclosporin, aluminium hydroxide, oxpentifylline, alcohol, sedatives.

stomach upset and bleeding or ulceration, severe allergy, difficulty breathing, blood disorders, skin reactions, headache, dizziness, fluid retention, liver disorders, inflamed pancreas, meningitis, drowsiness, sweating, dry mouth, thirst, mental changes, muscle pain, fits, kidney or urine disorders, bruising, chest pain, pale or flushed skin, high blood pressure, slow or irregular heart rate, abnormal bleeding.

children under 16 years, pregnant women, mothers who are breastfeeding, or for patients with moderate to severe kidney disorders, dehydration, bleeding in the brain, or with a history of allergy to aspirin or other NSAIDs, asthma, nasal polyps, blood-clotting disorders, stomach ulcer or intestinal bleeding.

Ketostix

(Bayer Diagnostics)

A plastic reagent strip used to test for the presence of ketones in the urine. Raised ketone levels indicate an imbalance in the metabolism of fat in the body, such as occurs when a patient is suffering from diabetes.

Availability: NHS and private prescription, nurse prescription, over the counter.

Ketotard XL *see* ketoprofen modified-release capsules

(Galen)

ketotifen tablets/capsules/elixir

A tablet, capsule, or elixir used as an ANTIHISTAMINE to prevent asthma and to treat allergies such as hayfever and conjunctivitis.

Strengths available: 1 mg tablets; 1 mg capsules; 1 mg/5 ml elixir.
Dose: adults, usually 1-2 mg twice a day (children over 2 years, 1 mg twice a day) with food.
Availability: NHS and private prescription.

drowsiness, reduced reaction, dizziness, dry mouth, weight gain.

Contains: ketotifen hydrogen fumarate.
Brand names: Zaditen.

 alcohol, sedatives, antidiabetics taken by mouth, MAOIS, TRICYCLIC ANTIDEPRESSANTS, ritonavir.

 when used to prevent asthma, continue previous preventive treatment for 2-4 weeks after starting this medication and withdraw slowly when treatment ends.

 children under 2 years, pregnant women, or for mothers who are breastfeeding.

Ketovail *see* ketoprofen modified-release capsules
(Approved Prescriptions Services)

Ketovite tablets/liquid

(Paines and Byrne)
A tablet and liquid used as a multivitamin supplement in artificial diets.

Dose: 1 tablet three times a day together with 5 ml liquid once a day.
Availability: NHS and private prescription. (Liquid also available over the counter.)
Contains: tablets: acetomenaphtone, vitamins B_1, B_2, B_3, B_5, B_6, C, E, H, inositol, folic acid. Liquid: vitamins A, B_{12}, D, choline.

Ketozip *see* ketoprofen modified-release capsules
(Ashbourne Pharmaceuticals)

Ketpron XL *see* ketoprofen modified-release capsules
(Goldshield Healthcare)

Ketur Test

(Roche Diagnostics)
A plastic reagent strip used to test for the presence of ketones in the urine. Raised ketone levels indicate an imbalance in the metabolism of fat in the body, such as occurs when a patient is suffering from diabetes.

Availability: NHS and private prescription, nurse prescription, over the counter.

Kinidin Durules *see* quinidine modified-release tablets
(AstraZeneca UK)

Klaricid/Klaricid XL *see* clarithromycin tablets/modified-release tablets/sachets/suspension
(Abbott Laboratories)

Klean-Prep

(Norgine)

A powder used as a strong laxative to clean the bowel before surgery or diagnostic procedures.

Dose: 1 sachet dissolved in 1 litre of water and consumed at the rate of 250 ml every 10-15 minutes until no further solid matter is passed (or until 4 litres has been drunk).

Availability: NHS and private prescription, over the counter.

Contains: macrogol, sodium sulphate, sodium bicarbonate, sodium chloride, potassium chloride. (Also contains aspartame.)

nausea, bloating, abdominal pain, vomiting, irritated anus.

in pregnant women and in patients with swallowing disorders, diabetes, kidney disorders, heart disease, ulcerated bowel, or reflux oesophagitis.

children or for patients weighing under 20 kg, or who have active ulceration of bowel or stomach, heart failure, perforated or obstructed bowel, non-functional or inflamed bowel.

all other medications (take at least 1 hour before using this preparation).

Kliofem *see* hormone replacement therapy tablets (combined)
(Novo Nordisk Pharmaceuticals)

Kliovance *see* hormone replacement therapy tablets (combined)
(Novo Nordisk Pharmaceuticals)

Kloref tablets

(Cox Pharmaceuticals)

An effervescent tablet used as a potassium supplement to treat potassium deficiency.

Strengths available: equivalent to 500 mg potassium chloride.

Dose: adults 1-2 tablets in water three times a day increasing if necessary; children as advised by doctor.

Availability: NHS and private prescription, over the counter.

Contains: betaine hydrochloride, potassium benzoate, potassium bicarbonate, potassium chloride.

nausea and vomiting, obstruction and ulceration of the bowel or oesophagus.

in the elderly and in patients suffering from kidney disorders, narrowed or ulcerated intestines, or who have a history of stomach ulcers.

patients with severe kidney failure or high chloride or acid levels in the blood.

some DIURETICS, ACE-INHIBITORS, cyclosporin.

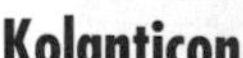

Kolanticon

(Peckforton Pharmaceuticals)

A gel used as an antacid, anti-spasm, and antimuscarinic treatment for bowel or stomach spasm, acidity, wind, and stomach ulcers.

Dose: adults, 10-20 ml every 4 hours when required.
Availability: NHS and private prescription, over the counter.
Contains: dicyclomine hydrochloride, aluminium hydroxide, magnesium oxide, activated dimethicone.

antimuscarinic effects, skin reactions, stomach upset, altered heart rhythm, difficulty passing urine, disturbed vision, dry mouth, intolerance of light, flushing, dry skin, confusion, dizziness.

in the elderly patients and in patients suffering from diarrhoea or inflamed bowel, high blood pressure, abnormal heart rhythm, fever, reflux oesophagitis, or heart attack.

children or for patients suffering from glaucoma, myasthenia gravis, enlarged prostate, or non-functioning intestines.

other antimuscarinic drugs, e-c tablets/capsules, some antibiotics.

Konakion *see* phytomenadione tablets/oral solution
(Roche Products)

Konsyl *see* ispaghula husk
(Eastern Pharmaceuticals)

Kytril *see* granisetron tablets
(SmithKline Beecham Pharmaceuticals)

---

labetolol tablets

A tablet used as a beta-blocker to treat high blood pressure (including high blood pressure with angina, in pregnancy, and after heart attack).

Strengths available: 50 mg, 100 mg, 200 mg, and 400 mg tablets.
Dose: 100 mg twice a day with food at first, increasing as needed every 14 days to a maximum of 2400 mg a day in 3-4 divided doses; elderly patients 50 mg twice a day at first.
Availability: NHS and private prescription.
Contains: labetolol hydrochloride.
Brand names: Trandate.

low blood pressure on standing, headache, tingling scalp, difficulty passing urine, stomach pain, nausea, vomiting, liver damage, tiredness, wheezing, rash.

in pregnant women, mothers who are breast-feeding, the elderly, and in patients suffering from diabetes, kidney or liver disorders, myasthenia gravis, or with a history of allergies. May need to be withdrawn before surgery. Withdraw gradually.

cont.

L

 children or for patients suffering from heart block or failure, asthma, PHAEOCHROMOCYTOMA, or a history of breathing disorders.

 general anaesthetics, CALCIUM-CHANNEL BLOCKERS, ALPHA-BLOCKERS, clonidine, ANTIHYPERTENSIVES, amiodarone, antidiabetics, thymoxamine, theophylline, aminophylline.

lacidipine tablets

A tablet used as a CALCIUM-CHANNEL BLOCKER to treat high blood pressure.

Strengths available: 2 mg or 4 mg tablets.
Dose: adults, 2 mg once a day at first, increasing at 3-4-week intervals to 4 mg, then 6 mg a day if needed.
Availability: NHS and private prescription.
Contains: lacidipine.
Brand names: Motens.

 headache, dizziness, flushing, fluid retention, increased frequency of urination, stomach upset, muscle cramp, rash, palpitations, chest pain (withdraw immediately), weakness, swollen gums.

 in patients suffering from liver disease and some heart disorders.

 grapefruit juice, amiodarone, anti-epileptic treatments, itraconazole, ALPHA-BLOCKERS, ritonavir, BETA-BLOCKERS, theophylline, aminophylline.

 children, pregnant women, mothers who are breastfeeding, or for patients suffering from narrowed aortic heart valve.

Lacri-Lube *see* liquid paraffin eye ointment
(Allergan)

LactiCare *see* emollient lotion
(Stiefel Laboratories (UK))

lactic acid *see* Calmurid-HC, Cuplex, Duofilm, emollient, hormone replacement therapy – topical, Salactol, Salatac

Lactugal *see* lactulose solution
(Intrapharm Laboratories)

lactulose sachets/solution

A solution or sachet used as a laxative to treat constipation, or brain disease due to liver problems.

Strengths available: 3.35 g/5 ml solution; 10 g per sachet.
Dose: for constipation, children aged 0-1 year 2.5 ml solution, aged 1-5 years 5 ml solution, aged 5-10 years 10 ml solution or half a sachet; adults usually 15 ml solution or 1 sachet (all taken twice a day). For liver disorders, adults 30-50 ml solution or 2-3

sachets three times a day. Sachets can be emptied on to tongue and swallowed with fluid, sprinkled on to food, or mixed into a drink.

Availability: NHS and private prescription, nurse prescription, over the counter.

Contains: lactulose.

Brand names: Duphalac (not available on NHS), Duphalac Dry, Lactugal, Lemlax, Regulose.

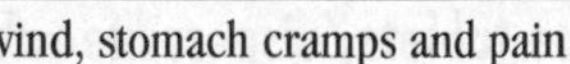
wind, stomach cramps and pain.

in patients sensitive to lactose. May take up to 48 hours to have effect in constipation.

patients suffering from galactosaemia (an inherited disorder) or blocked intestine.

Ladropen *see* flucloxacillin capsules
(Berk Pharmaceuticals)

Lamictal *see* lamotrigine tablets/dispersible tablets
(GlaxoWellcome UK)

Lamisil *see* terbinafine cream/tablets
(Novartis Pharmaceuticals UK)

---

lamivudine tablets/solution

A tablet or solution used as an antiviral to treat HIV infection (in combination with other drugs) or hepatitis B infection.

Strengths available: 100 mg and 150 mg tablets; 25 mg/5 ml and 50 mg/5 ml solution.

Dose: for HIV infection, adults 150 mg twice a day (children use reduced doses according to body weight); for hepatitis B infections, adults and children over 16 years 100 mg once a day.

Availability: NHS and private prescription.

Contains: lamivudine.

Brand names: Epivir, Zeffix.

Compound preparations: Combivir.

stomach upset, abdominal pain, tiredness, headache, sleeplessness, fever, cough, rash, hair loss, muscle or bone pain, numbness in hands or feet, inflamed pancreas, blood changes, nasal symptoms.

in pregnant women and in patients with kidney or liver disorders.

mothers who are breastfeeding, pregnant women in the first 3 months of pregnancy, or for children under 16 years (except in HIV infection).

trimethoprim, co-trimoxazole.

L

lamotrigine tablets/dispersible tablets

A tablet or dispersible tablet used as an anti-epileptic treatment for epilepsy.

Strengths available: 25 mg, 50 mg, 100 mg, and 200 mg tablets; 5 mg, 25 mg, and 100 mg dispersible tablets.
Dose: adults 25 mg once a day for the first 2 weeks, then 50 mg once a day for the next 2 weeks, increasing usually to 100-200 mg a day (maximum of 500 mg a day). Dose may need adjustment if other anti-epileptic treatments are also taken. Children treated only in combination with other drugs (dose as advised by doctor).
Availability: NHS and private prescription.
Contains: lamotrigine.
Brand names: Lamictal.

skin reactions, severe allergy, double or blurred vision, dizziness, drowsiness, headache, stomach upset, confusion, irritability, aggression, weakness, shaking, sleeplessness, fever, tiredness, influenza-like symptoms, liver disorder, enlarged lymph glands, blood changes, sensitivity to sunlight, inflamed eyes, lack of co-ordination, agitation.

in the elderly, pregnant women, mothers who are breastfeeding, and in patients suffering from rash, fever, influenza, drowsiness, kidney disorders, or worsening of symptoms. Must be withdrawn gradually. Your doctor may advise regular check-ups. Tell your doctor immediately if influenza-like symptoms or a rash develops.

alcohol, sedatives, other anti-epileptic treatments.

children under 2 years or for patients suffering from liver damage.

L

Lamprene *see* clofazimine capsules
(Alliance Pharmaceuticals)

lanolin/lanolin oil *see* emollient preparations

Lanoxin/Lanoxin PG *see* digoxin elixir/tablets
(GlaxoWellcome UK)

lansoprazole capsules/suspension

A capsule or suspension used to treat stomach ulcers (and to treat or prevent those caused by NON-STEROIDAL ANTI-INFLAMMATORY DRUGS), to treat acid reflux into the oesophagus and other acid-related indigestion symptoms, and for *H. PYLORI* ERADICATION.

Strengths available: 15 mg or 30 mg capsules; 30 mg per sachet suspension.
Dose: for reflux, usually 30 mg once a day for 4-8 weeks to heal the condition, then 15-30 mg a day to prevent relapse; for ulcers, 30 mg once a day for 4-8 weeks (then continuing with 15 mg once a day for duodenal ulcers); for ulcers caused by non-steroidal anti-inflammatory drugs, 15-30 mg once a day for 4-8 weeks; for acid-related indigestion, 15-30 mg once a day in the morning for 2-4 weeks; for other conditions

of excess acid (such as Zollinger-Ellison syndrome), up to 120 mg a day (in divided doses) may be required.

Availability: NHS and private prescription.
Contains: lansoprazole.
Brand names: Zoton.
Compound preparations: Heliclear (*see H. pylori* eradication).

children or pregnant women.

headache, upset stomach, skin irritation. Rarely, blood changes, swollen hands and feet, depression, joint pain, itching, severe allergy, tiredness, dry mouth, skin reactions, hair loss, blurred vision, sensitivity to sunlight, pins and needles, kidney and liver disorders, bruising, vertigo, hallucinations, sleeplessness, taste disturbance, confusion, swollen breasts, and impotence.

in mothers who are breastfeeding and in patients aged over 45 years or with liver disorders. Stomach cancer should be excluded before treatment.

ANTICOAGULANTS, ORAL CONTRACEPTIVES, phenytoin, digoxin, carbamazepine.

Lantus *see* insulin

Larafen CR *see* ketoprofen modified-release capsules
(Lagap Pharmaceuticals)

Largactil *see* chlorpromazine syrup/tablets
(Distriphar (UK))

Lariam *see* mefloquine tablets
(Roche Products)

Lasikal *see* frusemide tablets and potassium chloride tablets
(Borg Medicare)

Strengths available: 20 mg + 750 mg M-R TABLETS.
Dose: adults up to 4 a day.

Lasilactone *see* frusemide tablets and spironolactone tablets
(Borg Medicare)

Strengths available: 20 mg + 50 mg capsules.
Dose: adults 1-4 a day.

Lasix *see* frusemide tablets/solution
(Borg Medicare)

Lasonil *see* heparinoid gel
(Bayer Consumer Care)

Lasoride *see* co-amilofruse tablets
(Borg Medicare)

---

latanoprost eye drops

Eye drops used to treat glaucoma and high pressure inside the eye for patients for whom other treatments are unsuitable or have failed.

Strengths available: 50 mcg/ml drops.
Dose: 1 drop into the affected eye(s) once a day (in the evening).
Availability: NHS and private prescription.
Contains: latanoprost.
Brand names: Xalatan.

 irritation, ulceration or reddening of the eye, brown colour in the eye, inflammation or fluid retention inside the eye, changes to eyelashes, darkened eyelids, worsening of asthma, difficulty breathing.

 in patients suffering from asthma, some types of glaucoma, or who have no lens in the eye. Report any change in eye colour to your doctor (treatment may need to be withdrawn). Leave at least 5 minutes between use of this and other eye drops.

 children, pregnant women, mothers who are breastfeeding, or for patients wearing contact lenses.

 some other eye drops (*see* above).

---

lauromacrogols *see* Anacal, emollient preparations

Laxoberal *see* sodium picosulphate liquid
(Boehringer Ingelheim)

---

lecithin *see* Psoriderm cream/lotion

Lederfen *see* fenbufen capsules/tablets
(Wyeth Laboratories)

Ledermycin *see* demeclocycline capsules
(Wyeth Laboratories)

Lederspan *see* triamcinolone injection
(Wyeth Laboratories)

leflunomide tablets

A tablet used as a disease-modifying agent to treat severe rheumatoid arthritis.

Strengths available: 10 mg, 20 mg, and 100 mg tablets.
Dose: adults 100 mg once a day for 3 days then reduced to 10-20 mg once a day.
Availability: NHS and private prescription (specialist supervision).
Contains: leflunomide.
Brand names: Arava.

upset stomach, loss of appetite, abdominal pain, disorders of the mouth, weight loss, increased blood pressure, dizziness, weakness, headache, pins and needless, inflamed or ruptured tendons, hair loss, dry skin, eczema, skin disorders, itching, blood disorders, taste disturbances, anxiety, liver disorders, high lipid levels in the blood, severe allergic reaction, low potassium or phosphate levels.

children under 18 years, pregnant women, mothers who are breastfeeding, or for patients with liver disorders, serious kidney disorders, low protein levels, mouth ulcers, serious infection, reduced bone-marrow function, blood disorders, or poorly functioning immune system.

in patients suffering from kidney disorders or with a history of tuberculosis. Women must use effective contraception during treatment and for 2 years afterwards. Men who are treated should not father children for at least 3 months after treatment ends. Your doctor will advise regular check-ups and blood tests.

vaccines, other similar drugs, alcohol, methotrexate, phenytoin, warfarin, tolbutamide.

L

Lemlax *see* lactulose solution
(Co-Pharma)

Lentard *see* insulin

Lentizol *see* amitriptyline modified-release capsules
(Parke Davis and Co.)

lercanidipine tablets

A tablet used as a CALCIUM-CHANNEL BLOCKER to treat high blood pressure.

Strengths available: 10 mg tablets.
Dose: 10 mg once a day increasing to 20 mg if necessary. Take at least

swollen hands and feet, irregular heart rhythm, flushing, dizziness, headache, weakness, stomach upset, low blood pressure, muscle pain, drowsiness, rash, increased urine production.

cont.

15 minutes before food.
Availability: NHS and private prescription.
Contains: lercanidipine hydrochloride.
Brand names: Zanidip.

 grapefruit juice, amiodarone, anti-epileptic treatments, itraconazole, ALPHA-BLOCKERS, ritonavir, BETA-BLOCKERS, theophylline, aminophylline, alcohol, sedatives.

 in patients with kidney, liver, or some heart disorders.

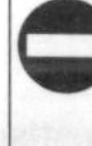 children, pregnant women, mothers who are breastfeeding, or for patients with narrowed aortic heart valve, unstable angina, untreated heart failure, or within 1 month of heart attack.

Lescol/Lescol XL *see* fluvastatin capsules
(Novartis Pharmaceuticals UK)

Leucovorin *see* calcium folinate tablets
(Wyeth Laboratories)

---

leuprorelin injection

An injection used to treat endometriosis in women and to reduce fibroids or thin the uterus lining before surgery.

Strengths available: 3.75 mg injection.
Dose: for endometriosis, 3.75 mg injected every month (for maximum 6 months) beginning during the first 5 days of period; to thin the uterus lining, 3.75 mg injected 5-6 weeks before surgery, beginning during days 3-5 of period; for fibroids, for endometriosis, 3.75 mg injected every month (usually for 3-4 months, maximum 6 months).
Availability: NHS and private prescription.
Contains: leuprorelin acetate.
Brand names: Prostap SR.

 hot flushes, headache, emotional upset, dryness of the vagina, tender breasts, nausea, dizziness, tiredness, sleep disturbance, sweating, decreased bone density, itching, skin rash, joint pain, changes in vision, pins and needles, swollen face, change in hair, weight change, blood changes, palpitations, high blood pressure.

 in patients with bone disorders (or a family history of OSTEOPOROSIS), or who habitually drink alcohol, smoke, or take other drugs that decrease bone density. Use an effective barrier contraceptive throughout treatment.

 children, pregnant women, mothers who are breastfeeding, or for patients at risk from osteoporosis, or who have undiagnosed vaginal bleeding.

---

levacetylmethadol solution

A solution used to treat addiction to OPIOID ANALGESICS in patients already stabilized on methadone.

Strengths available: 10 mg/ml solution.

Dose: as advised by doctor. Doses given every 48-72 hours (three times a week).
Availability: NHS and private prescription (specialist use).
Contains: levacetylmethadol hydrochloride.
Brand names: OrLAAM.

 children under 15 years, pregnant women, mothers who are breastfeeding, or for patients with severe kidney or liver disorders, some heart rhythm abnormalities, PORPHYRIA, or who are at risk of non-functioning intestines.

 MAOIS, alcohol, sedating drugs, other opioids, drugs affecting heart rhythm, ANTIDEPRESSANTS, mizolastine, chloroquine, hydroxychloroquine, quinine, chlorpromazine, haloperidol, pimozide, thioridazine, sotalol, DIURETICS, ORAL CONTRACEPTIVES, ritonavir.

 drowsiness, upset stomach, sweating, dizziness, breathing difficulty, low blood pressure, difficulty passing urine, dry mouth, headache, vertigo, flushing, change in heart rhythm, mood changes, rash, itching, addiction, reduced sexual desire.

 in children, pregnant women, women in labour, mothers who are breastfeeding, elderly or weakened patients, and in those suffering from breathing, kidney, or liver problems, low blood pressure, head injury, reduced breathing ability, underactive thyroid, enlarged prostate, epilepsy, or who are suicidal. (Higher doses not suitable for some of these categories.) Patients using modified-release preparations should continue with the same brand of product when dose is stabilized. Patients under 18 years must be monitored.

levetiracetam tablets

A tablet used (in addition to other anti-epileptic drugs) to treat epilepsy.

Strengths available: 250 mg, 500 mg, and 1000 mg tablets.
Dose: adults and children over 16 years, 500 mg twice a day at first, increasing if necessary to a maximum of 1500 mg twice a day.
Availability: NHS and private prescription.
Contains: levetiracetam.
Brand names: Keppra.

 alcohol, sedating drugs.

 drowsiness, weakness, dizziness, stomach upset, rash, depression, double vision, headache, loss of appetite, loss of memory, unsteadiness, fits, emotional disorder, sleeplessness, nervousness, shaking, vertigo.

 in pregnant women and in patients with kidney or severe liver disorders. Treatment should be withdrawn slowly.

 children under 16 years or for mothers who are breastfeeding.

levobunolol eye drops

Eye drops used as a BETA-BLOCKER to treat glaucoma and high pressure inside the eye. Some of the preparation may be absorbed into the body (*see* side-effects, cautions etc. for propranolol tablets).

Strengths available: 0.5% drops and single-use drops.
Dose: 1 drop into the affected eye(s) once or twice a day.

cont.

L

Availability: NHS and private prescription.
Contains: levobunolol hydrochloride.
Brand names: Betagan.

 eye irritation or redness, headache, dizziness, dry eyes, disorders of the cornea, other effects due to beta-blockers (*see* propranolol tablets).

 children, pregnant women, or for patients suffering from heart block or failure, asthma, PHAEOCHROMOCYTOMA, or with a history of breathing disorders.

 in mothers who are breastfeeding, the elderly, and in patients with diabetes or breathing problems, kidney or liver disorders, MYASTHENIA GRAVIS, or with a history of allergies.

 general anaesthetics, calcium-channel blockers, ALPHA-BLOCKERS, clonidine, ANTIHYPERTENSIVES, amiodarone, antidiabetics, thymoxamine, theophylline, aminophylline.

levocabastine eye drops/nasal spray

Eye drops or a nasal spray used as an ANTIHISTAMINE to treat allergic rhinitis (such as hayfever) and conjunctivitis caused by allergy.

Strengths available: 0.05% eye drops; 0.05% nasal spray.
Dose: for allergic conjunctivitis, adults and children over 9 years, apply the eye drops twice a day (maximum four times a day) for up to 4 weeks each year in total; for allergic rhinitis, adults and children over 9 years, 2 sprays of nasal spray in each nostril twice a day (maximum four times a day) for up to 4 weeks each year in total.
Availability: NHS and private prescription. (Also available over the counter for the treatment of hayfever.)
Contains: levocabastine hydrochloride.
Brand names: Livostin. (Livostin Direct available over the counter.)

 eye drops: irritation, headache, swelling around eyes, blurred vision, drowsiness, difficulty breathing, itchy skin rash. Nasal spray: irritation, drowsiness, headache, tiredness.

 in pregnant women.

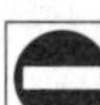 children under 9 years. Patients with kidney failure should not use the nasal spray.

 alcohol, sedatives.

levodopa tablets

A tablet used as an anti-parkinson drug to treat Parkinson's disease.

Strengths available: 500 mg tablets.
Dose: 125-500 mg a day (in divided doses) at first, increasing as needed.
Availability: NHS and private prescription.
Contains: levodopa.

 stomach upset, sleeplessness, low blood pressure on standing, dizziness, rapid or irregular heart beat, agitation, red colour in urine or faeces, abnormal movements, mental disorders, depression, drowsiness, sweating, flushing, headache, bleeding in the stomach or intestines, numbness in hands and feet, taste disturbance, liver changes, rash, itching. A condition similar to NEUROLEPTIC MALIGNANT SYNDROME on stopping treatment.

Compound preparations: co-beneldopa, co-careldopa.

 children or for patients with some types of glaucoma.

 anaesthetics, MAOIS, alcohol, sedating drugs.

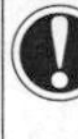 in pregnant women, mothers who are breast-feeding, and in patients suffering from heart or breathing disorders, stomach ulcers, diabetes, glaucoma, skin cancer, mental disorders, osteomalacia (softening and bending of bones). Your doctor may advise regular check-ups. Must be withdrawn gradually.

---

levofloxacin tablets

A tablet used as an ANTIBIOTIC to treat chest, sinus, urine, skin, and soft tissue infections.

Strengths available: 250 mg and 500 mg tablets.
Dose: adults, 250 mg-500 mg once or twice a day depending on condition. Course usually lasts 7-14 days.
Availability: NHS and private prescription.
Contains: levofloxacin.
Brand names: Tavanic.

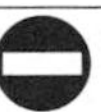 children, pregnant women, or for mothers who are breastfeeding.

 ANTICOAGULANTS, cyclosporin, NON-STEROIDAL ANTI-INFLAMMATORY DRUGS, glibenclamide, theophylline, aminophylline, ANTACIDS, iron, cimetidine, sucralfate, alcohol, sedating drugs.

 allergy, stomach upset, headache, dizziness, sleep disorders, skin disorders. Rarely, loss of appetite, blood changes, drowsiness, fits, confusion, depression, hallucinations, pins and needles, sensitivity to light, muscle and joint disorders, inflamed lungs, distortion of the senses, liver and kidney disorders, weakness, shaking, anxiety, rapid heart beat, low blood pressure, low blood glucose levels.

 in patients suffering from kidney disease or with a history of epilepsy or nervous system disorders. Avoid excessive exposure to sunlight. Report any pain or inflammation in the limbs to your doctor.

---

levomepromazine *see* methotrimeprazine (alternative name)

Levonelle-2 *see* levonorgestrel tablets
(Schering Health Care)

---

levonorgestrel 750 mcg tablets

A tablet used as a progestogen contraceptive in an emergency within 72 hours of intercourse.

Strengths available: 750 mcg tablets.
Dose: 1 tablet as soon as possible after intercourse (up to 72 hours afterwards), then 1 more tablet 12 hours later.
Availability: NHS and private prescription.
Contains: levonorgestrel.
Brand names: Levonelle-2.

irregular bleeding, upset stomach, dizziness, breast discomfort, headache, tiredness.

cont.

Compound preparations: Schering PC4, HORMONE REPLACEMENT THERAPY (combined), ORAL CONTRACEPTIVE (COMBINED), ORAL CONTRACEPTIVE (PROGESTOGEN ONLY).

Other preparations: Mirena.

in patients suffering from heart disease, high blood pressure, disordered absorption of nutrients from the gut, diabetes, migraine, some cancers, liver abnormalities, ovarian cysts, or who have had a previous ectopic pregnancy or blood clot. If vomiting occurs consult your doctor. Barrier contraceptives must be used until the next period.

BARBITURATES, phenytoin, primidone, carbamazepine, chloral hydrate, ethosuximide, rifampicin, chlorpromazine, meprobamate, griseofulvin, topiramate, modafinil, cyclosporin, nevirapine, celecoxib.

children, pregnant women, men, or for women suffering from severe heart or blood vessel disease, some liver disorders, PORPHYRIA, undiagnosed vaginal bleeding, breast cancer, some womb disorders.

---

levothyroxine *see* thyroxine (alternative name)

Lexotan *see* bromazepam tablets
(Roche Products)

Lexpec *see* folic acid solution
(Rosemont Pharmaceuticals)

L

LH *see* luteinizing hormone

Librium *see* chlordiazepoxide capsules
(ICN Pharmaceuticals)

Lidifen *see* ibuprofen tablets
(Berk Pharmaceuticals)

---

lidocaine *see* lignocaine (alternative name)

---

lignocaine *see* Anodesyn, lignocaine ointment, methylprednisolone injection, RECTAL CORTICOSTEROID preparations

---

lignocaine ointment/gel

An ointment used to numb the skin or mucous membranes.

Strengths available: 5% ointment; 2% gel.
Dose: as advised by your doctor.
Availability: NHS and private prescription, nurse prescription, over the counter.
Contains: lignocaine (lidocaine).
Brand names: Xylocaine.
Compound preparations: Anodesyn, Emla, Instillagel, some RECTAL CORTICOSTEROID preparations. (Compound preparations are not available on nurse prescription and some are not available over the counter.)

rarely, allergic reaction.

in pregnant women and in patients suffering from epilepsy, heart conduction disorders, slow heart beat, poor liver function, or severe shock.

drugs used to control heart rhythm.

Li-liquid *see* lithium syrup
(Rosemont Pharmaceuticals)

Lingraine *see* ergotamine tablets
(Sanofi Winthrop)

Lioresal *see* baclofen tablets/liquid
(Novartis Pharmaceuticals UK)

liothyronine tablets

A tablet used as a thyroid hormone to treat severe thyroid deficiency.

Strengths available: 20 mcg tablets.
Dose: adults, 20 mcg a day at first, increased to 60 mcg a day (in 2-3 divided doses); elderly patients and children take 5 mcg a day at first and increase gradually.
Availability: NHS and private prescription.
Contains: liothyronine sodium.
Brand names: Tertroxin.

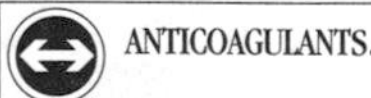
ANTICOAGULANTS.

abnormal heart rhythm, chest pain, rapid heart rate, muscle cramp or weakness, headache, shaking, restlessness, flushing, excitability, sweating, upset stomach, fever, intolerance of heat, rapid weight loss.

in the elderly, pregnant women, mothers who are breastfeeding, and in patients suffering from diabetes, disorders of the pituitary gland, or poor ADRENAL function.

patients suffering from excessive levels of thyroid hormones, heart or circulation problems, or where effort causes anginal chest pain.

Lipantil Micro *see* fenofibrate capsules
(Fournier Pharmaceuticals)

Liparol 400XL *see* bezafibrate modified-release tablets
(Ashbourne Pharmaceuticals)

---

lipase *see* pancreatin capsules

Lipitor *see* atorvastatin tablets
(Parke Davis and Co.)

Lipobase *see* emollient cream
(Yamanouchi Pharma)

Lipobay *see* cerivastatin tablets
(Bayer Pharma Business Group)

Lipostat *see* pravastatin tablets
(Bristol-Myers Squibb Pharmaceuticals)

---

liquid and white soft paraffin ointment NPF *see* emollient ointment

---

liquid paraffin *see* emollient preparations, liquid paraffin emulsion, liquid paraffin eye ointment, liquid paraffin and magnesium hydroxide emulsion, Metanium, proflavine cream BPC, simple eye ointment, white soft paraffin and liquid paraffin ointment NPF

---

liquid paraffin emulsion BP

An emulsion used as a laxative to treat constipation.

Dose: 10-30 ml at night when required.
Availability: NHS and private prescription, over the counter.
Contains: liquid paraffin.
Compound preparations: liquid paraffin and magnesium hydroxide emulsion BP.

Side effects: seepage of paraffin from rectum, rectal irritation, lung disorders, inadequate absorption of some vitamins.

Not to be used for: children under 3 years. Not for prolonged use.

---

liquid paraffin eye ointment

An ointment used to lubricate the eyes in dry eye conditions.

Dose: applied as required.
Availability: NHS and private prescription, over the counter.

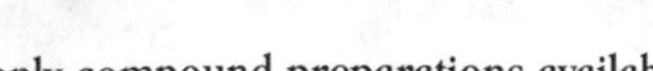

Contains: (only compound preparations available).
Compound preparations: Lacri-lube (with white soft paraffin and wool alcohols), Lubri-Tears (with white soft paraffin and wool fat).

liquid paraffin and magnesium hydroxide emulsion BP

An emulsion used as a laxative to treat constipation.

Dose: adults 5-20 ml when required.
Availability: NHS and private prescription, over the counter.
Contains: liquid paraffin, magnesium hydroxide.
Brand names: MilPar (not available on NHS).

 colic.

 in the elderly and in patients who are weak or suffering from kidney or liver damage.

 children or for sudden, severe symptoms.

Liquifilm Tears *see* polyvinyl alcohol eye drops
(Allergan)

lisinopril tablets

A tablet used, in addition to other drugs, as an ACE-INHIBITOR to treat heart failure, high blood pressure (including that due to kidney disease), diabetic kidney disease, and as a treatment after heart attack.

Strengths available: 2.5 mg, 5 mg, 10 mg, and 20 mg tablets.
Dose: usually 2.5 mg a day at first increasing to 5-40 mg a day depending on condition.
Availability: NHS and private prescription.
Contains: lisinopril.
Brand names: Carace, Zestril.
Compound preparations: Carace Plus, Zestoretic.

 DIURETICS, anaesthetics, NON-STEROIDAL ANTI-INFLAMMATORY DRUGS, potassium supplements, cyclosporin, lithium, antidiabetics.

rash, itching, sore throat, runny nose, stomach upset, cough, blood and liver changes, kidney disorders, low blood pressure, severe allergic reaction, inflamed pancreas. Occasionally, headache, dizziness, tiredness, taste disturbance, fever, pins and needles, sensitivity to sunlight, inflamed membranes or blood vessels, rapid heart beat, stroke, heart attack, dry mouth, confusion, psychological changes, hair loss, sweating, weakness, impotence.

 in the elderly, mothers who are breastfeeding, and in patients suffering from kidney disease, auto-immune diseases (such as LUPUS), severe heart failure, or with a history of severe allergies, or in patients undergoing anaesthesia or dialysis. Your doctor may advise regular blood tests.

 children, pregnant women, or for patients with some heart abnormalities or disorders of the blood supply to the kidney. Not to be taken on the same day as dialysis.

Liskonum *see* lithium modified-release tablets
(SmithKline Beecham Pharmaceuticals)

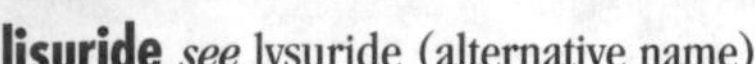

lisuride *see* lysuride (alternative name)

Litarex *see* lithium modified-release tablets
(Cox Pharmaceuticals)

---

lithium succinate *see* Efalith

---

lithium tablets/modified-release tablets/solution

A tablet, M-R TABLET, or solution used to treat and prevent mania, recurrent depression, aggressive or self-injuring behaviour, and bipolar disorder (where the mood swings from mania to depression).

Strengths available: for lithium carbonate: 250 mg standard tablets; 200 mg, 400 mg, and 450 mg m-r tablets. For lithium citrate: 564 mg m-r tablets; 509 mg/5 ml, 520 mg/5 ml, or 1018 mg/5 ml solution.
Dose: as advised by doctor (usually by result of blood test).
Availability: NHS and private prescription.
Contains: lithium citrate or lithium carbonate.
Brand names: Camcolit, Li-Liquid, Liskonum, Litarex, Lithonate, Priadel.

upset stomach, shaking hands, muscular weakness, brain and heart disturbances, weight gain, fluid retention, overactive or underactive thyroid gland, thirst, frequent urination, skin reactions.

in pregnant women, the elderly, and in patients suffering from MYASTHENIA GRAVIS or who are due to undergo surgery. Once stabilized on treatment, patients should continue with the same brand of medication. Drink plenty of fluids and avoid changes to dietary sodium content.

children, mothers who are breastfeeding, or for patients suffering from kidney or heart disease, Addison's disease, underactive thyroid gland, or disturbed sodium balance in the body.

DIURETICS, ACE-INHIBITORS, NON-STEROIDAL ANTI-INFLAMMATORY DRUGS, ANTACIDS, metronidazole, some ANTIDEPRESSANTS, methyldopa.

Lithonate *see* lithium modified-release tablets
(Approved Prescriptions Services)

Livial *see* tibolone tablets
(Organon Laboratories)

Livostin *see* levocabastine eye drops/nasal spray
(CIBA Vision Ophthalmics)

Locabiotal *see* fusafungine spray
(Servier Laboratories)

Loceryl *see* amorolfine cream/lacquer
(Galderma (UK))

Locoid/Locoid-C/Locoid Crelo/Locoid Lipocream *see* topical corticosteroid cream/ointment/lotion/scalp application
(Cercle Rouge)

Locorten-Vioform

(Novartis Pharmaceuticals UK)
Drops used as an antibacterial and CORTICOSTEROID treatment for inflammation of the outer ear when accompanied by infection.

Dose: adults and children over 2 years, 2-3 drops into the affected ear(s) twice a day for 7-10 days.
Availability: NHS and private prescription.
Contains: clioquinol, flumethasone (flumetasone) pivalate.

 irritation, hair discoloration.

 in pregnant women and mothers who are breastfeeding.

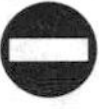 children under 2 years or for patients suffering from perforated ear drum or simple ear infection. Not for prolonged use.

Lodine *see* etodolac modified-release tablets
(Shire Pharmaceuticals)

lodoxamide eye drops

Eye drops used as an anti-allergy treatment for allergic conjunctivitis (eye inflammation).

Strengths available: 0.1% drops.
Dose: adults and children over 4 years apply four times a day.
Availability: NHS and private prescription.
Contains: lodoxamide trometamol.
Brand names: Alomide.

 temporary irritation, burning, stinging, itching, or watering of the eye. Occasionally, dizziness and flushing.

 in pregnant women and mothers who are breastfeeding.

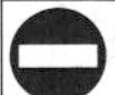 children under 4 years or for patients who wear soft contact lenses.

Loestrin 20/30 *see* oral contraceptive (combined)
(Parke Davis and Co.)

Lofensaid/Lofensaid Retard *see* diclofenac enteric-coated tablets/modified-release tablets (Opus Pharmaceuticals)

lofepramine tablets/suspension

A tablet used as a TRICYCLIC ANTIDEPRESSANT to treat depression.

Strengths available: 70 mg tablets; 70 mg/5 ml suspension.
Dose: 70-210 mg a day in divided doses. (Lower doses sometimes suitable for elderly patients.)
Availability: NHS and private prescription.
Contains: lofepramine hydrochloride.
Brand names: Gamanil, Lomont.

children or for patients suffering from recent heart attacks, heart rhythm abnormalities, liver disease, severe kidney disorders, or elevated mood.

alcohol, sedatives, MAOIS, BARBITURATES, other antidepressants, ANTIHYPERTENSIVES, tranquillizers, anti-epileptic drugs, ritonavir, entacapone, selegiline, sotalol, halofantrine, drugs affecting heart rhythm, methylphenidate, thyroxine.

dry mouth, noises in the ears, tiredness, constipation, difficulty passing urine, blurred vision, stomach upset, palpitations, drowsiness, sleeplessness, dizziness, shaking hands, low blood pressure, weight change, sweating, fever, behavioural changes in children, confusion in the elderly, skin reactions, liver disorders, blood changes, interference with sexual function, changes in heart rhythm, rash, hormone disturbances, fits, movement disorders, blood changes, breast changes in women, menstrual disorders.

in the elderly, pregnant women, mothers who are breastfeeding, and in patients suffering from heart disease, kidney disorders, thyroid disease, PHAEOCHROMOCYTOMA, epilepsy, diabetes, PORPHYRIA, glaucoma, urine retention, constipation, some other psychiatric conditions. Your doctor may advise regular blood tests.

lofexidine tablets

A tablet used to control the symptoms of withdrawal from OPIOID drugs.

Strengths available: 200 mcg tablets.
Dose: adults, 200 mcg twice a day at first increasing if necessary by 200-300 mcg a day to a maximum of 2400 mcg a day. Treatment should be maintained for 7-10 days (or longer if opioids still being used) then withdrawn over the next 2-4 days.
Availability: NHS and private prescription.
Contains: lofexidine hydrochloride.
Brand names: Britlofex.

drowsiness, dry nose and mouth, low blood pressure, (high blood pressure when withdrawn), slow heart beat.

in pregnant women, mothers who are breastfeeding, and in patients suffering from very weak heart, slow heart rate, kidney disorders, disorders of blood vessels in the brain, recent heart attack, or with a history of depression.

children.

alcohol, sedatives.

Logynon/Logynon ED *see* oral contraceptive (combined)
(Schering Health Care)

---

lomefloxacin eye drops

Eye drops used as an ANTIBIOTIC to treat bacterial eye infections.

Strengths available: 0.3% eye drops.
Dose: apply into the affected eye(s) every 5 minutes for 5 doses, then reduce to twice a day for 7-9 days.
Availability: NHS and private prescription.
Contains: lomefloxacin hydrochloride.
Brand names: Okacyn.

temporary irritation or burning.

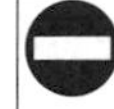
pregnant women, mothers who are breast-feeding, or for patients wearing contact lenses.

Lomexin *see* fenticonazole pessaries
(Dominion Pharma)

Lomont *see* lofepramine suspension
(Rosemont Pharmaceuticals)

Lomotil *see* co-phenotrope tablets
(Goldshield Healthcare)

Loniten *see* minoxidil tablets
(Pharmacia and Upjohn)

Loperagen *see* loperamide capsules
(Goldshield Healthcare)

---

loperamide capsules/tablets/liquid

A capsule, tablet, or liquid used to treat acute diarrhoea in adults and children over 4 years (in conjunction with ORAL REHYDRATION products) and adults only for chronic (long-term) diarrhoea.

Strengths available: 2 mg capsules and tablets; 1 mg/5 ml liquid.
Dose: acute diarrhoea, adults 4 mg at first then 2 mg after each loose bowel motion to a maximum of 16 mg a day for up to 5 days, children aged 4-8 years 1 mg 3-4 times a day for up to 3 days, children aged 9-12 years 2 mg four times a day for up to 5 days. For chronic diarrhoea, adults 4-

skin reactions, stomach cramps and bloating, constipation, dizziness, drowsiness, non-functioning bowel, dry mouth.

cont.

L

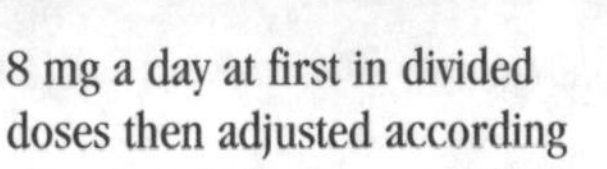

8 mg a day at first in divided doses then adjusted according to response (maximum 16 mg a day).

Availability: NHS and private prescription. Also available over the counter for adults with acute diarrhoea.

Contains: loperamide hydrochloride.

Brand names: Diasorb, Diocaps, Imodium, Loperagen, Norimode. Other brands available over the counter.

Compound preparations: Imodium Plus (with dimethicone) – not suitable for children.

Caution: in pregnant women, mothers who are breast-feeding, and in patients suffering from acute dysentery or liver disorders.

Not to be used for: children under 4 years or for patients suffering from swollen abdomen, currently inflamed bowel, or where the bowel is non-functional (or where a slow bowel function must be avoided).

Caution needed with: alcohol, sedating drugs.

Lopid *see* gemfibrozil capsules/tablets
(Parke Davis and Co.)

---

loprazolam tablets

A tablet used as a sleeping tablet for the short-term treatment of sleeplessness.

Strengths available: 1 mg tablets.

Dose: adults, 1-2 mg at bedtime; elderly or weak patients, 0.5-1.0 mg at bedtime.

Availability: NHS and private prescription.

Contains: loprazolam mesylate.

drowsiness, light-headedness, confusion, vertigo, stomach disturbances, loss of memory, aggression, headache, joint immo-bility, salivation changes, shaking, unsteadiness, low blood pressure, rash, changes in vision, changes in sexual desire, retention of urine, incontinence, blood changes, jaundice. Risk of addiction increases with dose and length of treatment. May impair judgement.

in elderly or weak patients, pregnant women, mothers who are breastfeeding, and in patients suffering from lung disorders, kidney or liver disorders, muscle weakness, PORPHYRIA, or with a history of drug or alcohol abuse, or personality disorder. Avoid long-term use and withdraw gradually.

children, or for patients suffering from acute lung diseases, some chronic lung diseases, severe liver disease, MYASTHENIA GRAVIS, some obsessional and psychotic disorders, or who have stopped breathing while asleep.

Caution needed with: alcohol, other sedating drugs, ritonavir, phenytoin.

Lopresor/Lopresor SR *see* metoprolol tablets/modified-release tablets
(Novartis Pharmaceuticals UK)

---

loratadine tablets/syrup

A tablet or syrup used as an ANTIHISTAMINE treatment to relieve the symptoms of allergies such as hayfever or skin reactions.

Strengths available: 10 mg tablets; 5 mg/5 ml syrup.
Dose: adults and children over 6 years, 10 mg once a day; children 2-5 years (or less than 30 kg in weight), 5 mg once a day.
Availability: NHS and private prescription, over the counter.
Contains: loratadine.
Brand names: Clarityn. (Other brands available over the counter.)

 rarely, drowsiness, dizziness, headache, agitation, stomach upset, dry mouth.

 in patients suffering from kidney disease.

 children under 2 years, pregnant women, or mothers who are breastfeeding.

 some ANTIDEPRESSANTS, ritonavir, alcohol, sedating drugs.

lorazepam tablets

A tablet used as a sedative for the short-term treatment of anxiety or sleeplessness.

Strengths available: 1 mg and 2.5 mg tablets.
Dose: for anxiety, adults 1-4 mg (elderly or weak patients 0.5-2.0 mg) a day in divided doses; for sleeplessness, adults 1-2 mg at night.
Availability: NHS and private prescription.
Contains: lorazepam.
Brand names: Ativan (not available on NHS).

 drowsiness, light-headedness, confusion, vertigo, stomach disturbances, loss of memory, aggression, headache, joint immobility, salivation changes, shaking, unsteadiness, low blood pressure, rash, changes in vision, changes in sexual desire, retention of urine, incontinence, blood changes, jaundice. Risk of addiction increases with dose and length of treatment. May impair judgement.

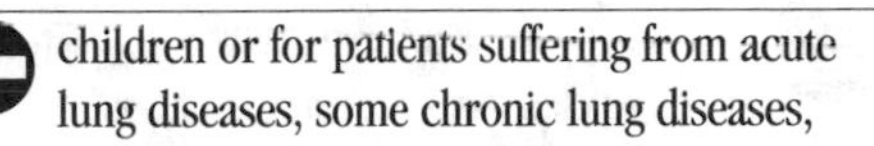 children or for patients suffering from acute lung diseases, some chronic lung diseases, severe liver disease, MYASTHENIA GRAVIS, some obsessional and psychotic disorders, or who have stopped breathing while asleep.

 in the elderly, pregnant women, mothers who are breastfeeding, women during labour, and in patients suffering from lung disorders, glaucoma, kidney or liver disorders, muscle weakness, PORPHYRIA, or with a history of drug or alcohol abuse. Avoid long-term use and withdraw gradually.

alcohol, other sedating drugs, phenytoin, ritonavir, rifampicin.

L

lormetazepam tablets

A tablet used as a sedative for the short-term treatment of sleeplessness.

Strengths available: 0.5 mg and 1 mg tablets.
Dose: adults, 1 mg (elderly and weak patients 0.5 mg) at bedtime.
Availability: NHS and private prescription.
Contains: lormetazepam.

 drowsiness, light-headedness, confusion, vertigo, stomach disturbances, loss of memory, aggression, headache, joint immobility, salivation changes, shaking, unsteadiness, low blood pressure, rash, changes in vision, changes in sexual desire, retention of urine, incontinence, blood changes, jaundice. Risk of addiction increases with dose and length of treatment. May impair judgement.

cont.

 in elderly or weak patients, pregnant women, mothers who are breastfeeding, and in patients suffering from lung disorders, kidney or liver disorders, muscle weakness, PORPHYRIA, or with a history of drug or alcohol abuse, or personality disorder. Avoid long-term use and withdraw gradually.

 children or for patients suffering from acute lung diseases, some chronic lung diseases, severe liver disease, MYASTHENIA GRAVIS, some obsessional and psychotic disorders, or who have stopped breathing while asleep.

 alcohol, other sedating drugs, ritonavir, phenytoin.

losartan tablets

A tablet used as an ANTIHYPERTENSIVE to treat high blood pressure.

Strengths available: 25 mg or 50 mg tablets.
Dose: adults, usually 50 mg (elderly 25 mg) once a day increasing if necessary to a maximum of 100 mg a day.
Availability: NHS and private prescription.
Contains: losartan potassium.
Brand names: Cozaar.
Compound preparations: Cozaar-Comp.

 low blood pressure, high potassium levels, severe allergic reaction, headache, dizziness, muscle or joint pain, diarrhoea, migraine, taste disturbance, dizziness, rash and itching, liver disorders, anaemia.

 in patients with liver or kidney disorders. Your doctor may advise regular blood tests.

 children, pregnant women, or mothers who are breastfeeding.

 anaesthetics, NON-STEROIDAL ANTI-INFLAMMATORY DRUGS, cyclosporin, DIURETICS, potassium.

L

Losec *see* omeprazole capsules/tablets
(AstraZeneca UK)

Lotriderm *see* clotrimazole cream and topical corticosteroid cream
(Dominion Pharma)

Loxapac *see* loxapine capsules
(Wyeth Laboratories)

loxapine capsules

A capsule used to treat mental disorders.

Strengths available: 10 mg, 25 mg, and 50 mg capsules.
Dose: adults, 20-50 mg a day (in two divided doses) at first, increasing to a maximum of 250 mg a day (in 2-4 divided doses) if needed, then reduced to maintenance of

20-100 mg a day.
Availability: NHS and private prescription.
Contains: loxapine succinate.
Brand names: Loxapac.

in pregnant women, mothers who are breast-feeding, the elderly, and in patients suffering from heart, lung, or circulation disorders, epilepsy, Parkinson's disease, thyroid disorders, infections, MYASTHENIA GRAVIS, kidney or liver disease, glaucoma, enlarged prostate, or some blood disorders. Should be withdrawn gradually.

alcohol, sedatives, ANTIDEPRESSANTS, anaesthetics, anti-epileptic medications, drugs affecting heart rhythm, ritonavir, halofantrine, lithium.

stomach upset, movement disorders, muscle spasms, restlessness, shaking, flushing, headache, pins and needles, extreme thirst, dry mouth, heart rhythm disturbance, low blood pressure, weight change, blurred vision, impotence, low or high body temperature, breast swelling, menstrual changes, blood, liver, eye, and skin changes, drowsiness, apathy, difficulty breathing, nightmares, sleeplessness, depression, blocked nose, difficulty passing water. Rarely, fits.

unconscious patients, or for those suffering from severe kidney or liver impairment, bone marrow depression, PORPHYRIA, or PHAEOCHROMOCYTOMA.

Luborant *see* saliva (artificial) spray
(Antigen Pharmaceuticals)

Lubri-Tears *see* liquid paraffin eye ointment
(Alcon)

Ludiomil *see* maprotiline tablets
(Novartis Pharmaceuticals UK)

---

lupus

An abbreviated name for various lupus diseases, especially systemic lupus erythematosus, thought to be an auto-immune reaction causing an allergy-like rash resulting in thickened areas of skin. Other lupus conditions cause similar skin reactions.

Lustral *see* sertraline tablets
(Invicta Pharmaceuticals)

---

luteinizing hormone *see* human menopausal gonadotrophin injection

---

Lyclear *see* permethrin cream/creme rinse
(Warner Lambert Consumer Healthcare)

---

lymecycline capsules

A capsule used as a tetracycline ANTIBIOTIC to treat acne and other infections such as bronchitis.

Strengths available: 408 mg capsules (equivalent to 300 mg tetracycline).
Dose: for general infections, adults 408 mg twice a day (up to 1632 mg a day in severe infections); for acne, adults 408 mg once a day for at least 8 weeks.
Availability: NHS and private prescription.
Contains: lymecycline.
Brand names: Tetralysal 300.

stomach upset, irritation of the oesophagus, reddening of skin, headache, disturbed vision, sensitivity to light, additional infections, pressure on the brain, reversible diabetes insipidus, liver disorders, inflamed pancreas or bowel.

in patients suffering from liver or kidney disorders. Discontinue if reddening of skin occurs.

children under 12 years, pregnant women, mothers who are breastfeeding, or for patients suffering from LUPUS.

milk, ANTACIDS, iron supplements, ANTICOAGULANTS, ORAL CONTRACEPTIVES.

---

lysine aspirin *see* Migramax

Lysovir *see* amantadine capsules
(Alliance Pharmaceuticals)

---

lysuride tablets

A tablet used as a hormone blocker to treat Parkinson's disease.

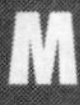

Strengths available: 200 mcg tablets.
Dose: 200 mcg at bedtime at first increasing slowly to a maximum of 5000 mcg a day (in three divided doses) after food.
Availability: NHS and private prescription.
Contains: lysuride maleate (lisuride).

low blood pressure, upset stomach, dizziness, headache, tiredness, general feeling of being unwell, drowsiness, skin disorders, abdominal pain, mental disorders (including hallucinations), Raynaud's phenomenon (numbness and tingling in hands and feet).

in pregnant women and in patients suffering from PORPHYRIA or with a history of mental disturbance or tumour of the pituitary gland.

children or for patients suffering from severe circulation disorders (including heart circulation).

alcohol, sedatives.

---

m-r tablets/capsules/granules

M-r (or modified-release) preparations have been adapted to ensure the contents are not released immediately after swallowing. The ingredients are usually released gradually over a long period of time to give sustained effect. Example, carbamazepine modified-release tablets. Some preparations are designed to release the contents only when they reach the bowel, where they need to work. Example, budesonide m-r capsules. Enteric coating is another way of modifying the release of a drug, *see* e-c tablets/capsules.

Maalox/Maalox Plus/Maalox TC *see* aluminium hydroxide gel/tablets and magnesium hydroxide mixture
(Rhône-Poulenc Rorer)

Dose: adult doses to be taken four times a day after meals or when required: Maalox, 10-20 ml suspension; Maalox TC, 5-15 ml suspension or 1-3 tablets; Maalox Plus, 5-10 ml.
Contains: aluminium hydroxide, magnesium hydroxide, dimethicone.

Macrobid *see* nitrofurantoin capsules
(Goldshield Healthcare)

Macrodantin *see* nitrofurantoin modified-release capsules
(Goldshield Healthcare)

---

macrogol *see* Hypotears, Klean-Prep, Movicol

Madopar/Madopar CR *see* co-beneldopa capsules
(Roche Products)

Magnapen *see* co-fluampicil capsules/suspension
(C.P. Pharmaceuticals)

---

magnesium alginate *see* alginate liquid/tablets/infant sachets

---

magnesium carbonate *see* alginate liquid/tablets, magnesium carbonate aromatic mixture, magnesium citrate powder, magnesium trisilicate mixture BP/magnesium trisilicate compound oral powder BP

---

magnesium carbonate aromatic mixture BP
A mixture used as an ANTACID to treat indigestion.

Dose: adults, 10 ml three times a day in water.
Availability: NHS and private prescription,

 diarrhoea, belching.

 in patients suffering from kidney damage.

over the counter.
Contains: magnesium carbonate, sodium bicarbonate, aromatic cardamom tincture.

 children or for patients with low phosphate levels in the blood.

 E-C TABLETS/CAPSULES, some ANTIBIOTICS.

---

magnesium citrate powder

An effervescent powder in a sachet used as a laxative to induce the total emptying of the bowels before X-ray or bowel surgery.

Dose: each sachet dissolved in 200 ml hot water and drunk 30 minutes later. For adults, one dose taken at 8 a.m. and one at 2-4 p.m. on the day before the procedure. (Elderly or weak patients, and children over 10 years, half adult dose; children aged 5-9 years one-third adult dose.)
Availability: NHS and private prescription, over the counter.
Contains: magnesium carbonate, citric acid.
Brand names: Citramag.

 nausea, vomiting, bloating, abdominal cramp.

 in pregnant women, mothers who are breast-feeding, unconscious patients, and in those with heart or kidney disease, inflamed bowel, or diabetes. Drink plenty of clear fluids.

 children under 5 years or for patients with blocked or perforated bowel, non-functioning intestines, heart failure, or some other stomach or intestinal disorders.

---

magnesium hydroxide mixture BP

A mixture used as a laxative to treat constipation.

Dose: adults 25-50 ml when required.
Availability: NHS and private prescription, nurse prescription, over the counter.
Contains: hydrated magnesium oxide.
Compound preparations: liquid paraffin and magnesium hydroxide emulsion, Maalox/Maalox TC, Maalox Plus, Mucaine, Mucogel.

 colic.

 in the elderly and in patients who are weak or suffering from kidney or liver damage.

 sudden, severe symptoms.

 E-C TABLETS/CAPSULES, some ANTIBIOTICS.

---

magnesium oxide *see* Asilone, Kolanticon, magnesium hydroxide mixture BP

---

magnesium sulphate (Epsom salts)

A laxative used to evacuate the bowels quickly.

Dose: adults 5-10 g in water on an empty stomach.
Availability: NHS and private prescription, over the counter.

Contains: magnesium sulphate.
Compound preparations: Andrews Liver Salts (not available on NHS – also contains citric acid and sodium bicarbonate), Picolax.

 colic.

 in the elderly and in patients who are weak or suffering from kidney or liver damage.

 sudden, severe symptoms.

---

magnesium sulphate paste BP

A paste used to treat carbuncles and boils.

Dose: apply under a dressing.
Availability: NHS and private prescription, nurse prescription, over the counter.
Contains: magnesium sulphate, glycerol, phenol.

stir before use.

---

magnesium trisilicate *see* alginate liquid/tablets, magnesium trisilicate compound tablets BP, magnesium trisilicate mixture BP/magnesium trisilicate compound oral powder BP, Pyrogastrone

---

magnesium trisilicate mixture BP/magnesium trisilicate compound oral powder BP

A liquid or powder used as an ANTACID to treat acidity and indigestion.

Dose: adults, 10 ml mixture three times a day in water or 1-5 g powder in liquid when required.
Availability: NHS and private prescription, over the counter.
Contains: magnesium trisilicate, magnesium carbonate, sodium bicarbonate.

 diarrhoea.

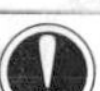 in patients suffering from kidney disorders.

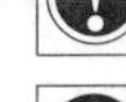 patients with low phosphate levels in the blood.

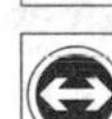 E-C TABLETS/CAPSULES, some ANTIBIOTICS, iron preparations.

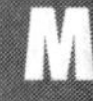

---

magnesium trisilicate compound tablets BP

A tablet used as an ANTACID to treat acidity and indigestion.

Dose: adults 1-2 tablets chewed when required.
Availability: NHS and private prescription, over the counter.
Contains: magnesium trisilicate, aluminium hydroxide.

 diarrhoea.

 in patients suffering from kidney disorders.

 patients with low phosphate levels in the blood.

 E-C TABLETS/CAPSULES, some ANTIBIOTICS, iron preparations.

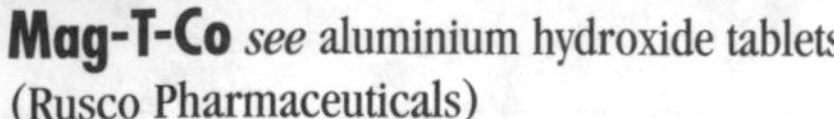

Mag-T-Co *see* aluminium hydroxide tablets
(Rusco Pharmaceuticals)

Malarone *see* also proguanil tablets and atovaquone suspension
(GlaxoWellcome UK)
A tablet used to treat malaria which is thought to be resistant to other drugs.

Strengths available: 100 mg + 250 mg tablets.
Dose: adults and children over 40 kg in weight, 4 tablets (children weighing 11-20 kg 1 tablet; children weighing 21-30 kg, 2 tablets; children weighing 31-40 kg 3 tablets) once a day for 3 days.

---

malathion liquid/shampoo

A liquid or shampoo used to treat scabies, head lice, and pubic lice.

 irritation.

 avoid contact with the eyes.

infants under 6 months (except on advice of a doctor). Not for use on broken or infected skin. Not to be used more than once a week for 3 weeks. Alcoholic liquids not to be used for head lice in patients with severe eczema, asthma, or for scabies or pubic lice, or for small children.

Strengths available: 0.5% liquid (either alcoholic or water based); 1% cream shampoo.
Dose: the liquid applied to the dry scalp and hair roots and allowed to dry naturally then washed off after 12 hours (for lice) or 24 hours (for scabies). The shampoo applied to wet hair and rinsed after 5 minutes, repeated immediately, and then the procedure repeated twice at intervals of 3 days. In scabies, the lotion should be applied to the body excluding the head and neck (but for small children, elderly patients, or those with weak immune systems or in whom treatment has failed, it may be necessary to apply to the face, scalp, neck, and ears).
Availability: NHS and private prescription, over the counter. Liquid also available on nurse prescription.
Contains: malathion.
Brand names: Derbac-M, Prioderm, Quellada M, Suleo-M. (Prioderm Shampoo not available on NHS.)

---

malic acid *see* Aserbine, saliva (artificial)

Maloprim *see* also pyrimethamine tablets and dapsone tablets
(GlaxoWellcome UK)
A tablet used to prevent malaria.

Strengths available: 12.5 mg + 100 mg tablets.

Dose: adults, 1 tablet (children aged 1-5 years one-quarter of a tablet; aged 6-11 years half a tablet) once a week starting 1 week before entering the affected area and continuing for 4 weeks after leaving.

Manerix *see* moclobemide tablets
(Roche Products)

Manevac

(Galen)
Granules used as a bulking agent and stimulant laxative to treat constipation.

Dose: adults, 5-10 ml (or 1-2 sachets) with water or a warm drink at night (in severe cases up to four doses per day may be taken for up to 3 days); children over 5 years, 5 ml (or 1 sachet) once a day.

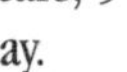

Availability: NHS and private prescription, nurse prescription (if prescribed generically), over the counter.

Contains: senna, ispaghula.

wind, bloating, diarrhoea, abdominal cramp.

the dose should not be taken immediately before going to bed.

children under 5 years or for patients with obstructed bowel.

---

mannitol *see* alginate sachets

Manusept *see* triclosan liquid
(SSL International)

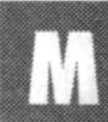

MAOI (mono-amine oxidase inhibitor)

An ANTIDEPRESSANT that may interact with some foods (such as cheese, pickled herrings, broad bean pods, fermented soya bean products, and meat/yeast extracts) and other drugs. Example, isocarboxazid tablets.

---

maprotiline tablets

A tablet used as an ANTIDEPRESSANT to treat depression.

Strengths available: 10 mg, 25 mg, 50 mg, and 75 mg tablets.

Dose: adults 25-75 mg (elderly patients 25 mg) a day at first, either in a single dose at night or in divided doses. Increased as needed to a maximum of 150 mg a day.

Availability: NHS and private prescription.

Contains: maprotiline hydrochloride.

cont.

Brand names: Ludiomil.

in the elderly, pregnant women, mothers who are breastfeeding, and in patients suffering from heart disease, liver and kidney disorders, thyroid disease, PHAEOCHROMOCYTOMA, diabetes, PORPHYRIA, glaucoma, urine retention, constipation, some other psychiatric conditions, or with a history of epilepsy. Your doctor may advise regular blood tests.

alcohol, sedatives, MAOIS, BARBITURATES, other ANTIDEPRESSANTS, ANTIHYPERTENSIVES, tranquillizers, anti-epileptic drugs, ritonavir, entacapone, selegiline, sotalol, halofantrine, drugs affecting heart rhythm, methylphenidate.

dry mouth, noises in the ears, tiredness, constipation, difficulty passing urine, blurred vision, stomach upset, palpitations, drowsiness, sleeplessness, dizziness, shaking hands, low blood pressure, weight change, sweating, fever, behavioural changes in children, confusion in the elderly, skin reactions, jaundice or blood changes, interference with sexual function, changes in heart rhythm, rash, hormone disturbances, fits, movement disorders, blood changes, breast changes in women, menstrual disorders.

children or for patients suffering from recent heart attacks, heart rhythm abnormalities, severe liver disease, or elevated mood.

Marevan *see* warfarin tablets
(Goldshield Healthcare)

Marvelon *see* oral contraceptive (combined)
(Organon Laboratories)

Masnoderm *see* clotrimazole cream
(Dominion Pharma)

M

Maxalt/Maxalt Melt *see* rizatriptan tablets/wafers
(Merck Sharp and Dohme)

Maxepa

(Seven Seas Health Care)
A capsule or liquid used (in addition to dietary measures) as a lipid-lowering agent to treat high triglyceride levels in the blood.

Dose: adults 5 capsules or 5 ml liquid twice a day with food.
Availability: NHS and private prescription, over the counter.
Contains: eicosapentaenoic acid, docosahexaenoic acid (omega-3 marine triglycerides), vitamin A, vitamin D.

nausea, wind. May aggravate high cholesterol levels.

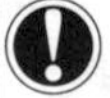
in patients suffering from bleeding disorders, diabetes, high cholesterol levels, or asthma due to NON-STEROIDAL ANTI-INFLAMMATORY DRUGS.

children.

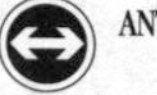
ANTICOAGULANTS.

Maxidex
(Alcon)
Drops used as a CORTICOSTEROID and lubricant for the short-term treatment of eye inflammation.

Dose: apply 4-6 times a day (or every 30-60 minutes in severe conditions), then frequency reduced as inflammation subsides.
Availability: NHS and private prescription.
Contains: dexamethasone, hypromellose.
Compound preparations: Maxitrol.
Other preparations: dexamethasone tablets, hypromellose eye drops.

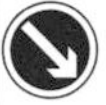 cataract, thinning cornea, fungal infection, rise in eye pressure.

 in pregnant women and infants – do not use for extended periods.

 patients suffering from infected eye conditions, glaucoma, or for patients who wear soft contact lenses.

Maxitrol
(Alcon)
Eye drops or ointment used as a CORTICOSTEROID, ANTIBIOTIC, and lubricant for the short-term treatment of infected inflammation of the eye.

Dose: 1-2 drops 4-6 times a day or the ointment applied 3-4 times a day.
Availability: NHS and private prescription.
Contains: dexamethasone, neomycin sulphate, hypromellose, polymyxin B sulphate.

 cataract, thinning cornea, fungal infection, rise in eye pressure.

 in pregnant women and infants – do not use for extended periods.

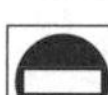 patients suffering from infected eye conditions, glaucoma, or for patients who wear soft contact lenses.

Maxivent *see* salbutamol inhaler/nebulizer solution
(Ashbourne Pharmaceuticals)

Maxolon/Maxolon SR *see* metoclopramide tablets/modified-release tablets/syrup
(Shire Pharmaceuticals)

Maxtrex *see* methotrexate tablets
(Pharmacia and Upjohn)

MCR-50 *see* isosorbide mononitrate modified-release capsules
(Pharmacia and Upjohn)

measles vaccine

Measles vaccine has been replaced by a combined measles/mumps/rubella vaccine for all children who are eligible – *see* MMR vaccine.

mebendazole tablets/suspension

A tablet or suspension used as a vermicide to treat worms.

stomach upset, abdominal pain, rash, itching, severe allergic reaction.

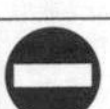
in mothers who are breastfeeding.

children under 2 years or pregnant women.

Strengths available: 100 mg tablets; 100 mg/5 ml suspension.
Dose: for adults and children over 2 years with threadworm, 100 mg as a single dose, repeated if necessary after 2-3 weeks; for adults and children over 2 years with other types of worm, 100 mg twice a day for 3 days.
Availability: NHS and private prescription, nurse prescription. (Also available over the counter for treatment of threadworm only.)
Contains: mebendazole.
Brand names: Pripsen tablets, Vermox. (Other brands available over the counter.)

mebeverine tablets/modified-release capsules/liquid

A tablet, M-R CAPSULE, or liquid used as an anti-spasm treatment for bowel spasm disorders such as irritable bowel syndrome.

in pregnant women, mothers who are breastfeeding, and in patients suffering from blocked intestines or PORPHYRIA.

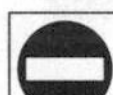
children under 10 years.

Strengths available: 135 mg tablets, 200 mg m-r capsules, 50 mg/5 ml liquid.
Dose: adults 135-150 mg (as tablet or liquid) three times a day, (taken 20 minutes before meals) or 200 mg (m-r capsule) twice a day (taken 20 minutes before food); children over 10 years may use adult dose of standard tablets or liquid (not m-r capsules).
Availability: NHS and private prescription. (Standard tablets available over the counter in strengths 135 mg or 100 mg for relief of irritable bowel symptoms.)
Contains: mebeverine hydrochloride (tablets and m-r capsules), mebeverine embonate (liquid).
Brand names: Colofac. (Other brands available over the counter.)
Compound preparations: Fybogel-Mebeverine.

mecysteine *see* methyl cysteine (alternative name)

Medic-Aid Personal Best *see* peak flow meter

M

Medicaid *see* cetrimide cream
(Eastern Pharmaceuticals)

MediSense G2

(Medisense)
A reagent strip, used in conjunction with MediSense Card, MediSense Pen, and Precision QID meters, to detect blood glucose levels. Blood-glucose monitoring enables individual patients suffering from diabetes accurately to control blood glucose and manage their condition.

Availability: NHS and private prescription, nurse prescription, over the counter.

MediSense Optium

(Medisense)
An electrode used in conjunction with a MediSense Optium Sensor to detect blood glucose levels. Blood-glucose monitoring enables individual patients suffering from diabetes accurately to control blood glucose and manage their condition.

Availability: NHS and private prescription, nurse prescription, over the counter.

Medi-Test Glucose

(BHR Pharmaceuticals)
A plastic reagent strip used for the detection of glucose in the urine. This gives an approximate estimate of blood glucose levels which may be adequate for the management of Type II diabetes.

Availability: NHS and private prescription, nurse prescription, over the counter.

Medi-Test Glycaemie C

(BHR Pharmaceuticals)
A reagent strip used either visually or, more accurately, in conjunction with the Glycotronic C meter to detect blood glucose levels. Blood-glucose monitoring enables individual patients suffering from diabetes accurately to control blood glucose and manage their condition.

Availability: NHS, private prescription, nurse prescription, over the counter.

Medi-Test Protein 2

(BHR Pharmaceuticals)
A strip used as an indicator for the detection of protein in the urine. Protein in the urine may indicate damage to or disease of the kidneys.

Availability: NHS and private prescription, nurse prescription, over the counter.

Medocodene *see* co-codamol capsules
(Schwarz Pharma)

Medrone *see* methylprednisolone tablets
(Pharmacia and Upjohn)

---

medroxyprogesterone tablets

A tablet used as a progestogen treatment for abnormal bleeding of the uterus, absence of periods, endometriosis, and other hormone-dependent disorders.

Strengths available: 2.5 mg, 5 mg, or 10 mg tablets.
Dose: 2.5-10 mg a day according to condition. Sometimes taken in cycles for 5-10 days at a time.
Availability: NHS and private prescription.
Contains: medroxyprogesterone acetate.
Brand names: Adgyn Medro, Provera.
Other preparations: medroxyprogesterone injection.

 children, pregnant women, or for patients suffering from some cancers, liver disease, undiagnosed vaginal bleeding, or PORPHYRIA.

 cyclosporin, alcohol, sedating drugs.

 stomach upset, disorders of the skin and mucous membranes, depression, sleeplessness, drowsiness, hair loss or growth, jaundice, severe allergic reaction, breast pain, milk production, abnormal menstrual bleeding, weight gain, fluid retention, changes in sexual desire.

 in mothers who are breastfeeding and in patients suffering from diabetes, high blood pressure, epilepsy, migraine, asthma, heart or kidney disease, or who have a history of depression.

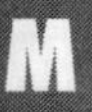

medroxyprogesterone injection

An injection used as a progestogen contraceptive.

Strengths available: 150 mg injection.
Dose: 150 mg injected and repeated every 12 weeks for continued effect.
Availability: NHS and private prescription.
Contains: medroxyprogesterone acetate.
Brand names: Depo-Provera.
Other preparations: etonogestrel implant, medroxy-progesterone tablets, norethis-terone injection.

 irregular bleeding, upset stomach, dizziness, depression, skin disorders, change in appetite, weight gain, change in sexual desire, breast discomfort, headache, ovarian cyst, rarely blood clots. There appears to be a small increase in risk of breast cancer but this may result from earlier diagnosis through regular examinations.

 in patients suffering from heart disease, high blood pressure, disordered absorption of nutrients from the gut, diabetes, migraine, some cancers, blood lipid disorders, liver abnormalities, ovarian cysts, or who have had a previous ectopic pregnancy or blood clot, or itching/ear disorders during pregnancy. Your doctor may advise regular examinations.

pregnant women or for patients suffering from severe heart or blood vessel disease, benign liver tumours, PORPHYRIA, undiagnosed vaginal bleeding, some womb disorders.

BARBITURATES, phenytoin, primidone, carbamazepine, chloral hydrate, ethosuximide, rifampicin, chlorpromazine, meprobamate, griseofulvin, topiramate, modafinil, cyclosporin, nevirapine, celecoxib.

mefenamic acid tablets/capsules/suspension

A tablet, capsule, or suspension used as a NON-STEROIDAL ANTI-INFLAMMATORY DRUG to relieve pain in rheumatoid arthritis, osteoarthritis, and related conditions, and to treat period pain.

Strengths available: 250 mg capsules, 500 mg tablets, 50 mg/5ml suspension.
Dose: adults, 500 mg three times a day after food; children use reduced doses for a maximum of 7 days (except in juvenile arthritis).
Availability: NHS and private prescription.
Contains: mefenamic acid.
Brand names: Dysman, Ponstan.

stomach upset and bleeding or ulceration, drowsiness, rash, severe allergy, difficulty breathing, blood or kidney disorders, headache, dizziness, noises in the ears, sensitivity to light, vertigo. Rarely, fluid retention, liver disorders, inflamed pancreas, inflamed bowel, meningitis, and fits with overdoses.

in the elderly, pregnant women, mothers who are breastfeeding, and in patients with heart, liver, or kidney disorders, high blood pressure, asthma, PORPHYRIA or LUPUS.

ACE-INHIBITORS, aspirin or other non-steroidal anti-inflammatory drugs, some ANTIBIOTICS, ANTICOAGULANTS, some antidiabetic drugs, some antivirals, methotrexate, DIURETICS, lithium, tacrolimus, cyclosporin, digoxin, alcohol, sedating drugs.

infants under 6 months or for patients with a history of allergy to aspirin or other NSAIDs, severe kidney disorders, blood-clotting disorders, currently active stomach ulcer or intestinal bleeding, inflamed intestines, or severe heart failure.

M

mefloquine tablets

A tablet used to treat and prevent malaria.

Strengths available: 250 mg tablets.
Dose: to prevent malaria, adults 1 tablet (children take lower doses according to body weight) once a week for at least 6 weeks, starting 1-3 weeks before entering malarious area and continuing for 4 weeks after leaving. Maximum use 12 months. For treatment of malaria, as advised by doctor.
Availability: NHS and private prescription. (Not generally prescribed on NHS for prevention of malaria.)
Contains: mefloquine hydrochloride.

dizziness, upset stomach, loss of appetite, headache, skin changes, psychological changes, disturbed balance, fits, drowsiness, sleep disorders, abdominal or joint pain, pins and needles, shaking, disturbance of vision, muscle pain or weakness, noises in the ears, blood changes, high or low blood pressure, rash, itching, hair loss, weakness, tiredness, fever, liver disorders.

cont.

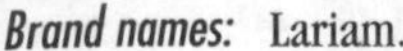

Brand names: Lariam.

in pregnant women, mothers who are breast-feeding, and in patients suffering from heart conduction disorders, epilepsy, kidney or liver disorders. Women of child-bearing age should use adequate contraception while taking this medication and for 3 months afterwards.

some drugs affecting heart rhythm, anti-epileptic treatments, halofantrine, pimozide, typhoid vaccine, quinine, chloroquine, alcohol, sedating drugs.

children under 3 months (or less than 5 kg in weight), women in the first 3 months of pregnancy, or for patients with severe liver damage, a history of mental disorder, or who are allergic to quinine.

Melgisorb *see* alginate dressing
(Molnlycke Health Care)

Melleril *see* thioridazine tablets/suspension/syrup
(Novartis Pharmaceuticals UK)

---

meloxicam tablets/suppositories

A tablet or suppository used as a NON-STEROIDAL ANTI-INFLAMMATORY DRUG to relieve pain and inflammation in rheumatic disease, osteoarthritis, and other joint disorders.

Strengths available: 7.5 mg and 15 mg tablets; 7.5 mg suppositories.
Dose: 7.5-15 mg each day.
Availability: NHS and private prescription.
Contains: meloxicam.
Brand names: Mobic.

stomach upset and bleeding or ulceration, rash, severe allergy, difficulty breathing, blood or kidney disorders, headache, dizziness, noises in the ears, sensitivity to light, vertigo. Rarely, fluid retention, liver disorders, inflamed pancreas, inflamed bowel, meningitis.

in the elderly, pregnant women, mothers who are breastfeeding, and in patients with heart, liver, or kidney disorders, high blood pressure, asthma, or LUPUS.

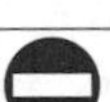

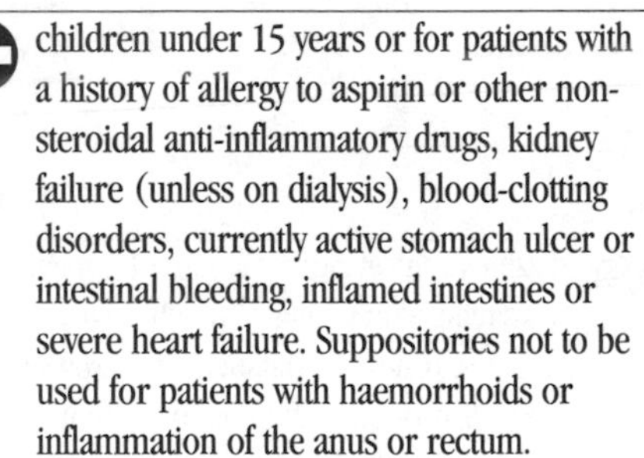

children under 15 years or for patients with a history of allergy to aspirin or other non-steroidal anti-inflammatory drugs, kidney failure (unless on dialysis), blood-clotting disorders, currently active stomach ulcer or intestinal bleeding, inflamed intestines or severe heart failure. Suppositories not to be used for patients with haemorrhoids or inflammation of the anus or rectum.

ACE-INHIBITORS, aspirin or other non-steroidal anti-inflammatory drugs, some ANTIBIOTICS, digoxin, ANTICOAGULANTS, some antidiabetic drugs, some antivirals, methotrexate, DIURETICS, lithium, tacrolimus, cyclosporin.

---

menadiol tablets

A tablet used as a vitamin K supplement to treat patients with bleeding (or likely to bleed) owing to low levels of clotting factors in the blood (e.g. in jaundice caused by bile obstruction).

Strengths available: 10 mg tablets.

M

Dose: adults, usually 10 mg a day (or up to 40 mg if necessary); children, usually 5-20 mg a day..
Availability: NHS and private prescription, over the counter.
Contains: menadiol sodium phosphate (a form of vitamin K).

in patients with vitamin E deficiency or suffering from anaemia or jaundice caused by medication.

young infants and women in late pregnancy.

ANTICOAGULANTS.

Mengivac *see* meningitis vaccine (A + C)
(Aventis Pasteur MSD)

Meningitec *see* meningitis vaccine (C)
(Wyeth Laboratories)

---

meningitis vaccine (A + C)

A vaccination used to provide active immunization against meningitis A and meningitis C.

Dose: adults and children, 1 injection of 0.5 ml.
Availability: NHS and private prescription.
Contains: meningitis A and C vaccine.
Brand names: AC Vax, Mengivac (A + C).

mild fever, discomfort at the site of the injection.

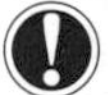
in pregnant women and mothers who are breastfeeding.

children under 18 months or under 2 months (depending on brand used) or for patients suffering from infections or fever.

drugs that suppress the immune system.

---

meningitis vaccine (C)

A vaccine used to provide long-term protection against meningitis C.

Dose: adults and children over 1 year, one single injection of 0.5 ml; younger children receive two or three doses (according to age) at intervals of 1 month.
Availability: NHS and private prescription.
Contains: meningococcal group C conjugate vaccine.
Brand names: Meningitec, Menjugate, Neisvac-C, (some brands not recommended for children under 1 year).
Compound preparations: meningitis vaccine (A + C)

redness or swelling at injection site, fever, headache, irritability.

in patients with suppressed immunity or some blood disorders.

children under 2 months, patients with a fever, or for those allergic to diphtheria toxoid.

Menjugate *see* meningitis vaccine (C)
(Chiron UK)

Menogon *see* human menopausal gonadotrophin injection
(Ferring Pharmaceuticals)

Menopur *see* human menopausal gonadotrophin injection
(Ferring Pharmaceuticals)

Menorest *see* hormone replacement therapy patches (oestrogen-only)
(Rhône-Poulenc Rorer)

---

menotrophin *see* human menopausal gonadotrophin injection

---

menthol *see* analgesic (topical), Denorex, Rowachol

---

menthone *see* Rowachol

---

meprobamate tablets

A tablet used as a tranquillizer for the short-term treatment of anxiety.

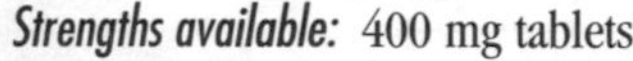

Strengths available: 400 mg tablets.
Dose: adults, 400 mg 3-4 times a day.
Availability: controlled drug; NHS and private prescription.
Contains: meprobamate.
Compound preparations: Equagesic.

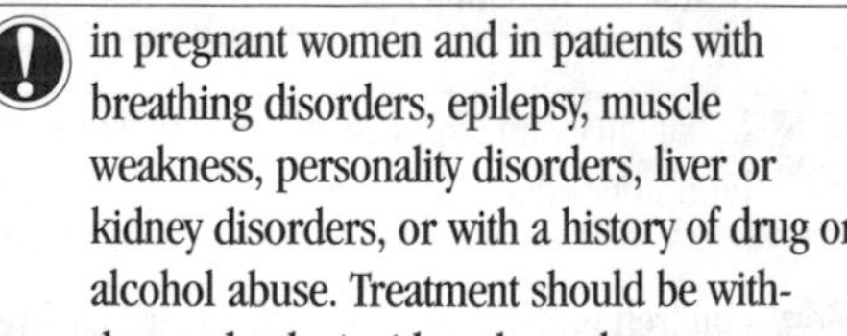

in pregnant women and in patients with breathing disorders, epilepsy, muscle weakness, personality disorders, liver or kidney disorders, or with a history of drug or alcohol abuse. Treatment should be withdrawn slowly. Avoid prolonged use.

drowsiness, light-headedness, confusion, vertigo, stomach disturbances, loss of memory, pins and needles, weakness, headache, excitement, aggression, headache, joint immobility, salivation changes, shaking, unsteadiness, low blood pressure, rash, changes in vision, changes in sexual desire, retention of urine, incontinence, blood changes, jaundice. Risk of addiction increases with dose and length of treatment. May impair judgement.

alcohol, sedating drugs, ritonavir.

children, mothers who are breastfeeding, or for patients suffering from severe breathing difficulty or PORPHYRIA.

M

meptazinol tablets

A tablet used as an OPIOID ANALGESIC to relieve pain.

Strengths available: 200 mg tablets.
Dose: adults, 200 mg every 3-6 hours.
Availability: NHS and private prescription.
Contains: meptazinol.
Brand names: Meptid.

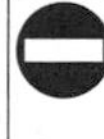

children, alcoholics, or for patients with head injury, reduced breathing ability, PORPHYRIA, or those who have a history of drug addiction or who are suicidal or at risk of non-functioning intestines.

MAOIS, alcohol, sedating drugs, ritonavir.

drowsiness, upset stomach, sweating, dizziness, breathing difficulty, low blood pressure, difficulty passing urine, dry mouth, headache, vertigo, flushing, change in heart rhythm, mood changes, rash, itching, addiction, reduced sexual desire.

in children, pregnant women, women in labour, mothers who are breastfeeding, elderly or weakened patients, and in those suffering from breathing, kidney, or liver problems, low blood pressure, underactive thyroid, enlarged prostate or epilepsy. (Higher doses not suitable for some of these categories.)

Meptid *see* meptazinol tablets
(Shire Pharmaceuticals)

Merbentyl *see* dicyclomine tablets/syrup
(Distriphar)

---

mercaptamine *see* cysteamine (alternative name)

Mercilon *see* oral contraceptive (combined)
(Organon Laboratories)

Merocaine *see* cetylpyridinium chloride lozenges
(SSL International)

Merocets *see* cetylpyridinium chloride lozenges
(SSL International)

---

mesalazine enteric-coated tablets/modified-release tablets/suppositories/enema/m-r granules

An E-C or M-R TABLET, suppository, enema, or sachet of m-r granules used to treat ulcerative colitis and to maintain patients in remission.

Strengths available: 250 mg and 400 mg e-c tablets; 1000 mg per dose enemas; 1000 mg or 2000 mg retention enemas; 250 mg, 500 mg, and 1000 mg suppositories; 250 mg and 500 mg M-R TABLETS; 1000 mg sachets.
Dose: adults up to 3000 mg a day (as e-c tablets or suppositories), 4000 mg a day (as M-R TABLETS or granules), 2000 mg a day (as enema).
Availability: NHS and private prescription.
Contains: mesalazine.
Brand names: Asacol, Pentasa, Salofalk.

 children or for patients suffering from severe kidney or liver disorders, blood clotting abnormalities, or who are allergic to salicylates (such as aspirin).

 stomach upset, headache, blood changes, worsening of colitis, rash, abdominal pain, allergic disorders affecting lungs or heart, symptoms similar to LUPUS, kidney or liver disorders, inflamed pancreas.

 in pregnant women, mothers who are breast-feeding, the elderly, and in patients suffering from kidney disorders. Report any unexplained bleeding, bruising, sore throat, fever, or general illness to your doctor who may advise blood tests. Patients stabilized on tablet forms of mesalazine should continue with the same brand of medication.

 ANTICOAGULANTS, some antidiabetic treatments, methotrexate, lactulose, products that decrease the acidity of the motions. ANTACIDS should not be taken at the same time as e-c tablets.

mesterolone tablets

A tablet used as a male sex hormone to treat low hormone levels and infertility in men.

Strengths available: 25 mg tablets.
Dose: 25 mg 3-4 times a day for several months, then 50-75 mg a day.
Availability: NHS and private prescription.
Contains: mesterolone.
Brand names: Pro-Viron.

 in the elderly, boys before puberty, and in patients with heart, liver, or kidney disorders, high blood pressure, heart disease, epilepsy, migraine, bone cancer. Your doctor may advise regular examination of the prostate.

 liver disorders, painful persistent erection, prostate abnormalities, headache, depression, stomach upset or bleeding, changes in sexual desire, swollen breasts, anxiety, weakness, chemical disturbances in the body, pins and needles, increased bone growth, hair growth or loss, acne, sexual development.

 children, women, or for men with breast, prostate, or liver cancer, high levels of calcium in the blood, or some types of kidney disorders.

Mestinon *see* pyridostigmine tablets
(ICN Pharmaceuticals)

mestranol *see* oral contraceptive tablets (combined)

Metanium

(Roche Consumer Health)

An ointment used as a barrier to treat nappy rash and similar skin disorders.

Dose: apply as needed.
Availability: NHS and private prescription, nurse prescription, over the counter.
Contains: titanium dioxide, titanium peroxide, titanium salicylate, dimethicone, light liquid paraffin, white soft paraffin, benzoin tincture.

Meted *see* salicylic acid shampoo
(DermaPharm)

Metenix *see* metolazone tablets
(Borg Medicare)

---

metformin tablets

A tablet used as an antidiabetic to treat diabetes.

Strengths available: 500 mg and 850 mg tablets.
Dose: 500 mg every 8 hours or 850 mg twice a day with meals at first increasing gradually if needed to a maximum of 3000 mg a day.
Availability: NHS and private prescription.
Contains: metformin hydrochloride.
Brand names: Glucamet, Glucophage, Orabet.

upset stomach, acidosis (a metabolic disorder), decreased vitamin B_{12} absorption.

in the elderly.

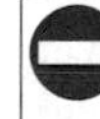
children, pregnant women, mothers who are breastfeeding, or for patients suffering from liver or kidney disorders, heart failure, stress, infection, dehydration, alcoholism, heart attack.

NON-STEROIDAL ANTI-INFLAMMATORY DRUGS, ACE-INHIBITORS, alcohol, anabolic steroids, MAOIS, diazoxide, BETA-BLOCKERS, nifedipine, CORTICOSTEROIDS, DIURETICS, some lipid-lowerers, lithium, ORAL CONTRACEPTIVES, orlistat, testosterone, cimetidine.

---

methadone mixture

A mixture used as an opioid to treat opioid addiction.

Strengths available: 1 mg/ml mixture.
Dose: 10-20 mg a day at first increased as needed. (Usual dose 40-60 mg a day.)
Availability: controlled drug; NHS and private prescription.

cont.

Contains: methadone hydrochloride.
Brand names: Methadose, Physeptone, Pinadone.
Other preparations: methadone linctus (weaker product used to treat severe cough), methadone tablets.

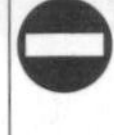 children, non-dependent adults, alcoholics, or patients with head injury, reduced breathing ability, PORPHYRIA, or those who have a history of drug addiction or who are suicidal or at risk of non-functioning intestines.

 MAOIS, alcohol, sedating drugs, ritonavir, zidovudine.

 drowsiness, upset stomach, sweating, dizziness, breathing difficulty, low blood pressure, difficulty passing urine, dry mouth, headache, vertigo, flushing, change in heart rhythm, mood changes, rash, itching, addiction, reduced sexual desire.

 in pregnant women, women in labour, mothers who are breastfeeding, elderly or weakened patients, and in those suffering from breathing, kidney, or liver problems, low blood pressure, underactive thyroid, enlarged prostate, or epilepsy. (Higher doses not suitable for some of these categories.)

---

methadone tablets

A tablet used as an OPIOID ANALGESIC to treat severe pain.

Strengths available: 5 mg tablets.
Dose: 5-10 mg every 6-8 hours adjusted according to response.
Availability: controlled drug; NHS and private prescription.
Contains: methadone hydrochloride.
Brand names: Physeptone.
Other preparations: methadone mixture.

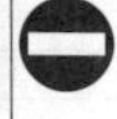 children, alcoholics, or for patients with head injury, reduced breathing ability, PORPHYRIA, or those who have a history of drug addiction or who are suicidal or at risk of non-functioning intestines.

 drowsiness, upset stomach, sweating, dizziness, breathing difficulty, low blood pressure, difficulty passing urine, dry mouth, headache, vertigo, flushing, change in heart rhythm, mood changes, rash, itching, addiction, reduced sexual desire.

 in pregnant women, women in labour, mothers who are breastfeeding, elderly or weakened patients, and in those suffering from breathing, kidney, or liver problems, low blood pressure, underactive thyroid, enlarged prostate, or epilepsy. (Higher doses not suitable for some of these categories.)

 MAOIS, alcohol, sedating drugs, ritonavir, zidovudine.

Methadose *see* methadone mixture
(Rosemont Pharmaceuticals)

---

methenamine *see* hexamine (alternative name)

---

methionine *see* co-methiamol tablets

M

methocarbamol tablets

A tablet used as a muscle relaxant to treat skeletal muscle spasm.

Strengths available: 750 mg tablets.
Dose: adults, 1500 mg (elderly 750 mg or less) four times a day reducing to 750 mg three times a day where appropriate.
Availability: NHS and private prescription.
Contains: methocarbamol.
Brand names: Robaxin.

drowsiness, allergy, tiredness, dizziness, light-headedness, restlessness, anxiety, confusion, fits, rash, severe allergic reaction, nausea.

in pregnant women, mothers who are breast-feeding, and in patients suffering from kidney or liver disease.

children or for patients in a coma or suffering from brain damage, epilepsy, or MYASTHENIA GRAVIS.

alcohol, sedatives.

methotrexate tablets

A tablet used to treat rheumatoid arthritis and severe psoriasis.

Strengths available: 2.5 mg and 10 mg tablets.
Dose: as advised by doctor (usually 7.5-25 mg once a week).
Availability: NHS and private prescription.
Contains: methotrexate.
Brand names: Maxtrex.

stomach pain, liver and bone marrow disorder, lung or mucous membrane inflammation, skin disorders, infections.

in the elderly and in patients suffering from blood, stomach, or intestinal disorders, mental illness, poorly functioning immune system, liver or kidney disorders, or PORPHYRIA. Your doctor may advise regular tests. Men and women should avoid conception for 6 months after treatment ends. Report any infections, cough, breathing disorders, or sore throat to your doctor.

children, pregnant women, mothers who are breastfeeding, or for patients suffering from severe kidney or liver disorders, infections, or serious blood disorders.

aspirin, NON-STEROIDAL ANTI-INFLAMMATORY DRUGS, co-trimoxazole, trimethoprim, cyclosporin, acitretin, alcohol, sulfadiazine, sulfametopyrazine, folic acid, some vaccines, phenytoin, penicillin ANTIBIOTICS.

methotrimeprazine tablets

A tablet used as a sedative to treat schizophrenia and other mental disorders, and to treat severe pain accompanied by restlessness, distress, or vomiting.

Strengths available: 25 mg tablets.
Dose: for mental disorders, 25-200 mg a day (in divided doses) at first increasing as needed to a maxi-

movement disorders, muscle spasms, restlessness, shaking, dry mouth, heart rhythm disturbance, low blood pressure (especially in the elderly), weight gain, blurred vision, impotence, low body temperature, breast swelling, menstrual changes, blood, liver, eye, and skin changes, drowsiness, apathy, nightmares, sleeplessness, depression, blocked nose, difficulty passing urine. Rarely, fits.

cont.

M

mum of 1000 mg a day; for pain, 12.5-50 mg every 4-8 hours.

Availability: NHS and private prescription.

Contains: methotrimeprazine (levomepromazine) maleate.

Brand names: Nozinan.

 alcohol, sedatives, ANTIDEPRESSANTS, some antidiabetic drugs, anaesthetics, anti-epileptic medications, drugs affecting heart rhythm, ritonavir, halofantrine, sotalol, propranolol, lithium.

 in pregnant women, mothers who are breast-feeding, the elderly, and in patients suffering from heart, lung, or circulation disorders, epilepsy, Parkinson's disease, thyroid disorders, infections, MYASTHENIA GRAVIS, kidney or liver disease, glaucoma, enlarged prostate, or some blood disorders. Should be withdrawn gradually.

 children, unconscious patients, or for patients suffering from severe kidney or liver impairment, bone marrow depression, or PHAEOCHROMOCYTOMA.

---

methyl salicylate *see* analgesic (topical), Monphytol

---

methyl undecenoate *see* Monphytol

---

methylcellulose tablets

A tablet used as an adsorbent and bulking agent to treat constipation, diarrhoea, ulcerative colitis, diverticular disease, obesity, and to control the bowel in colostomy patients.

Strengths available: 500 mg tablets.

Dose: adult dose for constipation, diarrhoea, or colostomy control 3-6 tablets night and morning (with at least 300 ml liquid when treating constipation and with minimal liquid when treating diarrhoea or controlling colostomy); for obesity, adults 3 tablets with liquid 30 minutes before a meal or when hungry.

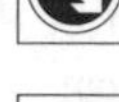 wind, bloating, obstructed intestines.

 in pregnant women, elderly or weak patients, or those with narrowed or poorly functioning intestines.

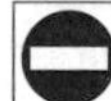 children or for patients with blocked intestines, difficulty swallowing, or relaxed bowel.

Availability: NHS and private prescription, nurse prescription, over the counter.

Contains: methylcellulose 450.

Brand names: Celevac.

---

methyl cysteine tablets

A tablet used to thin mucus and treat bronchitis or phlegm.

Strengths available: 100 mg tablets.

Dose: for treatment, adults 100-200 mg 3-4 times a day at first then reduced to 200 mg twice a day after 6 weeks; children over 5 years, 100 mg three times a day. For pre-

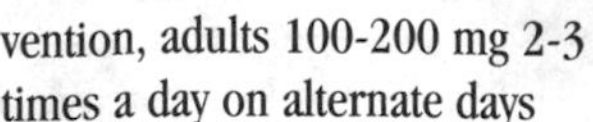

vention, adults 100-200 mg 2-3 times a day on alternate days (winter months only).

Availability: private prescription, over the counter.

Contains: methylcysteine (mecysteine) hydrochloride.

Brand names: Visclair.

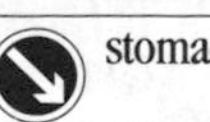 stomach upset.

 children under 5 years.

methyldopa tablets

A tablet used to treat high blood pressure.

Strengths available: 125 mg, 250 mg, and 500 mg tablets.

Dose: adults, 250 mg 2-3 times a day increasing slowly to a maximum of 3000 mg a day if required; elderly patients 125 mg twice a day at first, and maximum 2000 mg a day.

Availability: NHS and private prescription.

Contains: methyldopa.

Brand names: Aldomet.

 drowsiness, dry or inflamed mouth, inflamed salivary glands, slow heart rate, worsening of angina, low blood pressure on standing, headache, dizziness, weakness, muscle or joint pain, pins and needles, blocked nose, depression, tiredness, stomach upset, blood disorders, rash, diarrhoea, fluid retention, liver disorders, inflamed pancreas, symptoms of LUPUS, nightmares, mental disorders, movement disorders, disorders of sexual desire or function, bone marrow disorders, fever, heart inflammation, swollen breasts, absence of menstrual periods, high prolactin levels.

 patients suffering from PHAEOCHROMOCYTOMA, PORPHYRIA, current liver disease, or depression.

 alcohol, sedatives, anaesthetics, MAOIS, lithium.

 in patients suffering from kidney disease or with a history of depression or liver disease or undergoing general anaesthetic. Your doctor may advise regular blood tests.

methylphenidate tablets

A tablet used as a stimulant to treat children with attention-deficit disorder.

Strengths available: 5 mg, 10 mg, and 20 mg tablets.

Dose: children over 6 years, 5 mg once or twice a day at first increasing as necessary at weekly intervals to a maximum of 60 mg a day in divided doses.

 sleeplessness, restlessness, slowing of growth, mood changes, dry mouth, shaking, loss of appetite, stomach upset, dizziness, headache, fits, sweating, irregular or rapid heart beat, other heart disorders, mildly raised blood pressure, addiction, disturbance of vision, movement disorders, skin disorders, fever, joint pain, hair loss, blood disorders.

 in patients with raised blood pressure, PORPHYRIA, some emotional or mental disorders, or a history of epilepsy or movement disorders. Children must be monitored for growth disturbance, and regular blood tests are advised. Treatment must be withdrawn gradually. Judgement and ability to drive may be affected.

cont.

Availability: controlled drug; NHS and private prescription.
Contains: methylphenidate hydrochloride.
Brand names: Equasym, Ritalin, Tranquilyn.

 alcohol, MAOIS, TRICYCLIC ANTIDEPRESSANTS, some drugs used to lower blood pressure.

children under 6 years, pregnant women, mothers who are breastfeeding, or for patients with a history of drug abuse or who are suffering from high blood pressure, abnormal movements, heart or circulation disorders, overactive thyroid gland, excitability or agitation, glaucoma.

methylphenobarbital *see* methylphenobarbitone (alternative name)

methylphenobarbitone tablets

A tablet used as a BARBITURATE to treat epilepsy.

Strengths available: 30 mg, 60 mg, and 200 mg tablets.
Dose: adults, 100-600 mg a day. (Children use reduced doses according to weight.)
Availability: controlled drug; NHS and private prescription.
Contains: methylphenobarbitone (methylphenobarbital).
Brand names: Prominal.

 tolerance, addiction, drowsiness, skin reactions, hangover, dizziness, allergies, headache, confusion, excitement, lack of co-ordination, breathing difficulties, blood disorder.

 in children, elderly or weak patients, pregnant women, mothers who are breastfeeding, and in patients with kidney, liver, or lung disease. Treatment should be withdrawn gradually.

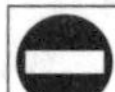 patients with a history of alcohol or drug abuse or suffering from PORPHYRIA.

 ANTICOAGULANTS, ANTIDEPRESSANTS, other anti-epileptic medications, griseofulvin, alcohol, sedatives, some antivirals, some drugs used to treat high blood pressure and angina, cyclosporin, CORTICOSTEROIDS, thyroxine, ORAL CONTRACEPTIVES, tibolone, theophylline, aminophylline.

M

methylprednisolone injection

An injection used as a CORTICOSTEROID to treat inflammation and allergies, such as hayfever, asthma, rheumatoid arthritis, and some skin disorders.

Strengths available: 40 mg/ml injection.
Dose: as advised by doctor.
Availability: NHS and private prescription.
Contains: methylprednisolone acetate.
Brand names: Depo-Medrone.

 high blood sugar, thin bones, mood changes, stomach ulcers, fluid retention, potassium loss, high blood pressure, menstrual irregularity, hairiness, increased likelihood of infection, euphoria, depression, sleeplessness, aggravation of schizophrenia and epilepsy, eye disorders, thinning of skin, acne, bruising, blood changes, stomach upset, inflamed pancreas, muscle abnormality, suppression of the ADRENAL glands, ulcerated or infected oesophagus, general feeling of being unwell, hiccups, reduced growth in children.

Compound preparations: Depo-Medrone with Lidocaine (with lignocaine, a local anaesthetic).

 patients who have untreated infections.

 live vaccines, some ANTIBIOTICS and anti-epileptics, ANTICOAGULANTS, antidiabetics, some antifungals, digoxin, cyclosporin.

 in pregnant women, mothers who are breast-feeding, and in patients who have had recent bowel surgery or who are suffering from inflamed veins, psychiatric disorders, thinning of the bones, stomach ulcers, tuberculosis or other infections, high blood pressure, glaucoma, epilepsy, diabetes, underactive thyroid, liver disease, stress. Withdraw gradually. Avoid contact with chicken pox for 3 months after treatment ends and seek medical attention if exposed.

methylprednisolone tablets

A tablet used as a CORTICOSTEROID to suppress inflammation and allergies. It is useful in conditions such as asthma, rheumatoid arthritis, and fluid retention in the brain.

Strengths available: 2 mg, 4 mg, 16 mg, and 100 mg tablets.
Dose: adults, usually 2-40 mg each day. Children's doses determined by doctor.
Availability: NHS and private prescription.
Contains: methylprednisolone.
Brand names: Medrone.

 in pregnant women, mothers who are breast-feeding, and in patients who have had recent bowel surgery or who are suffering from inflamed veins, psychiatric disorders, thinning of the bones, stomach ulcers, tuberculosis or other infections, high blood pressure, glaucoma, epilepsy, diabetes, underactive thyroid, liver disease, stress. Withdraw gradually. Avoid contact with chicken pox for 3 months after treatment ends and seek medical attention if exposed.

 high blood sugar, thin bones, mood changes, stomach ulcers, fluid retention, potassium loss, high blood pressure, menstrual irregularity, hairiness, increased likelihood of infection, euphoria, depression, sleeplessness, aggravation of schizophrenia and epilepsy, eye disorders, thinning of skin, acne, bruising, blood changes, stomach upset, inflamed pancreas, muscle abnormality, suppression of the ADRENAL glands, ulcerated or infected oesophagus, general feeling of being unwell, hiccups, reduced growth in children.

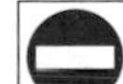 patients who have untreated infections.

 live vaccines, some ANTIBIOTICS and anti-epileptics, ANTICOAGULANTS, antidiabetics, some antifungals, digoxin, cyclosporin.

methysergide tablets

A tablet used as an anti-spasmodic treatment for migraine, severe headache, and diarrhoea associated with carcinoid disease.

Strengths available: 1 mg tablets.
Dose: for migraine and headache, adults 1 mg at night increasing to 1-2 mg three times a day with

 stomach upset, drowsiness, dizziness, lassitude, fluid retention, arterial spasm, thickened membranes in the abdomen (discontinue treatment), leg cramps, weight gain, rash, hair loss, mental disturbances, sleeplessness, pins and needles, low blood pressure on standing, rapid heart beat.

cont.

food; for diarrhoea, adults 12-20 mg a day under hospital supervision.
Availability: NHS and private prescription.
Contains: methysergide maleate.
Brand names: Deseril.

 in patients with a history of stomach ulcers. Treatment should be withdrawn gradually (and withdrawn periodically for assessment).

 children, pregnant women, mothers who are breastfeeding, undernourished patients, or for patients suffering from severe high blood pressure, collagen disorders, heart or circulation disease, liver or kidney disease, weight loss, sepsis, lung disease, cellulitis, urinary disorders, or infections.

 azithromycin, clarithromycin, erythromycin, some antivirals, sumatriptan, rizatriptan, zolmitriptan, alcohol, sedating drugs.

Metipranolol Minims

(Chauvin Pharmaceuticals)

Eye drops used as a BETA-BLOCKER to treat high pressure in the eye, and glaucoma in patients who are allergic to preservatives or who wear soft contact lenses. Some of the preparation may be absorbed into the body (*see* side effects, cautions, etc. for propranolol tablets).

Strengths available: 0.1% or 0.3% single-use eye drops.
Dose: for glaucoma, adults 1 drop twice a day. (For other conditions, as advised by doctor.)
Availability: NHS and private prescription.
Contains: metipranolol.

 temporary discomfort or redness in the eye, dry eyes, headache, inflammation of the eye. Rarely, disorders of the cornea.

 in pregnant women, mothers who are breastfeeding, and in patients with a history of breathing disorders, diabetes, overactive thyroid, or those being given a general anaesthetic.

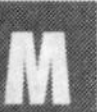

 verapamil, diltiazem, nifedipine, amiodarone, other BETA-BLOCKERS.

 children or for patients suffering from some heart diseases or blocked airways.

---

metoclopramide tablets/modified-release tablets/modified-release capsules/liquid

A tablet, M-R TABLET/capsule, or liquid used as an anti-sickness, anti-spasm drug to treat nausea, vomiting, and migraine.

Strengths available: 5 mg and 10 mg tablets; 15 mg m-r capsules or tablets; 5 mg/5ml liquid.
Dose: adults over 20 years, using m-r products 15 mg twice a day, or using standard tablets/liquid 5-10 mg (according to body weight) three times a day; for migraine, one single dose at onset of symptoms; children and young adults use only for special circumstances such as in sickness caused by cancer

 occasionally, parkinsonian-type symptoms, abnormal movements, drowsiness, diarrhoea, restlessness, depression, high levels of prolactin in the blood, NEUROLEPTIC MALIGNANT SYNDROME.

 in children, the elderly, young adults, pregnant women, and in patients suffering from epilepsy, liver and kidney problems, some forms of breast cancer, PORPHYRIA.

treatment (reduced doses).
Availability: NHS and private prescription.
Contains: metoclopramide hydrochloride.
Brand names: Gastrobid, Gastroflux, Maxolon.
Compound preparations: Migramax, Paramax.

 patients under 20 years (except as above), mothers who are breastfeeding, or for those suffering from PHAEOCHROMOCYTOMA, blocked intestines, or where recent stomach or bowel surgery has taken place.

 alcohol, sedatives.

metolazone tablets

A tablet used as a DIURETIC to treat high blood pressure, fluid retention, swollen abdomen, or toxaemia of pregnancy.

Strengths available: 5 mg tablets.
Dose: for high blood pressure, adults 5 mg a day at first then reduce to 5 mg every other day; for fluid retention, adults 5-10 mg in the morning (or up to 80 mg a day if necessary).
Availability: NHS and private prescription.
Contains: metolazone.
Brand names: Metenix.

low blood pressure on standing, mild stomach upset, reversible impotence, inflamed pancreas, gout, liver disorders, low potassium levels and other blood changes, allergy, rash, sensitivity to light or tiredness.

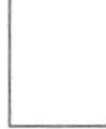 in pregnant women, mothers who are breast-feeding, the elderly, and in patients suffering from liver or kidney disorders, diabetes, gout, LUPUS.

 NON-STEROIDAL ANTI-INFLAMMATORY DRUGS, drugs that alter heart rhythm, carbamazepine, halofantrine, antidiabetics, pimozide, digoxin, lithium, ANTIHYPERTENSIVES.

 children or for patients suffering from severe kidney or liver disorders, Addison's disease, raised blood calcium/uric acid levels, low blood potassium/sodium levels, or PORPHYRIA.

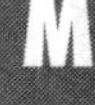

Metopirone *see* metyrapone capsules (Alliance Pharmaceuticals)

metoprolol tablets/modified-release tablets

A tablet or M-R TABLET used as a BETA-BLOCKER to treat angina, high blood pressure, and heart rhythm defects. Also used to prevent migraine and as an additional treatment for overactive thyroid.

Strengths available: 50 mg and 100 mg tablets; 200 mg m-r tablets.
Dose: for angina and heart rhythm defects, adults 50-100 mg 2-3 times a day; for high blood pressure, adults 100 mg a day at first increasing to 200 mg a day if necessary (in a single dose or two divided doses); for overactive thyroid, adults 50 mg four times a day; to prevent migraine, adults 100-200 mg a day in divided doses.
Availability: NHS and private prescription.

cold hands and feet, sleep disturbance, slow heart rate, tiredness, wheezing, heart failure, low blood pressure, stomach upset. Rarely, dry eyes, rash, worsening of psoriasis.

cont.

Contains: metoprolol tartrate.
Brand names: Betaloc, Lopresor.
Compound preparations: Co-Betaloc.

 in pregnant women, mothers who are breast-feeding, the elderly, and in patients suffering from diabetes, kidney or liver disorders, MYASTHENIA GRAVIS, or with a history of allergies. May need to be withdrawn before surgery. Withdraw gradually.

 children or for patients suffering from heart block or failure, asthma, PHAEOCHROMOCYTOMA, or a history of breathing disorders.

 general anaesthetics, CALCIUM-CHANNEL BLOCKERS, ALPHA-BLOCKERS, clonidine, ANTIHYPERTENSIVES, amiodarone, antidiabetics, thymoxamine, theophylline, aminophylline.

Metosyn/Metosyn FAPG *see* topical corticosteroid cream/ointment
(Bioglan Laboratories)

Metrodin *see* urofollitrophin injection
(Serono Laboratories (UK))

Metrogel *see* metronidazole gel
(Novartis Pharmaceuticals UK)

Metrolyl *see* metronidazole suppositories
(Lagap Pharmaceuticals)

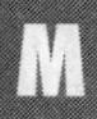

metronidazole dental gel

A gel used, in addition to other treatments, as an ANTIBIOTIC to treat gum disease.

Strengths available: 25% gel.
Dose: used by dentists to fill pocket around tooth. Treatment repeated after 1 week but then not for at least another 6 months.
Availability: NHS and private prescription.
Contains: metronidazole.
Brand names: Elyzol.
Other preparations: metronidazole gel/cream, metronidazole tablets/suspension/suppositories, metronidazole vaginal gel.

 headache, irritation.

 in pregnant women.

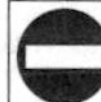 children.

 ANTICOAGULANTS, phenytoin, phenobarbital, disulfiram, lithium, alcohol.

---

metronidazole gel/cream

An ANTIBIOTIC gel or cream used to treat rosacea (a skin disorder of the face) and some other inflammatory or ulcerating skin conditions.

Strengths available: 0.75% and 0.8% gel; 1% cream.
Dose: applied once or twice a day (according to brand).
Availability: NHS and private prescription.
Contains: metronidazole.
Brand names: Anabact, Metrogel, Metrotop, Neutratop, Noritate, Rozex, Zyomet.
Other preparations: metronidazole dental gel, metronidazole tablets/suspension/suppositories, metronidazole vaginal gel.

 irritation.

 in pregnant women. Avoid contact with the eyes. Do not use sunbeds or sunlamps, and avoid strong sunlight after use.

— children or mothers who are breastfeeding.

metronidazole tablets/suspension/suppositories

A tablet, suspension or suppository used as an ANTIBIOTIC to treat infections, including some vaginal infections, leg ulcers, gum disease and dental infections.

Strengths available: 200 mg and 400 mg tablets; 200 mg/5ml suspension; 500 mg suppositories.
Dose: adults, usually 200-400 mg by mouth (or 1000 mg by suppository) every 8 hours (some infections require higher doses in short courses); children use reduced doses according to age and condition.
Availability: NHS and private prescription.
Contains: metronidazole.
Brand names: Flagyl, Metrolyl.
Compound preparations: Flagyl Compak (with Nystatin pessaries).
Other preparations: metronidazole dental gel, metronidazole gel/cream, metronidazole vaginal gel.

 stomach upset, furred tongue, unpleasant taste, skin disorders, severe allergic reaction, liver disorders, muscle or joint pain, lack of co-ordination, dark-coloured urine, numbness in hands and feet, fits, blood changes, dizziness, drowsiness, headache.

 in pregnant women, mothers who are breastfeeding, and in patients with liver disease. Your doctor may advise regular check-ups if treatment exceeds 10 days. Alcohol causes extreme reaction with this medication and should not be taken during treatments or for 48 hours afterwards.

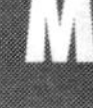

 high doses not recommended for pregnant women or mothers who are breastfeeding.

 ANTICOAGULANTS, phenytoin, phenobarbital, disulfiram, lithium, alcohol, sedating drugs.

metronidazole vaginal gel

A gel used as an ANTIBIOTIC and applied internally to treat vaginal infection.

Strengths available: 0.75% vaginal gel.
Dose: one 5 g dose (1 applicatorful) applied into the vagina at bedtime for 5 nights.
Availability: NHS and private prescription.
Contains: metronidazole.

 abnormal discharge, irritation, additional fungal infection, stomach upset, pressure in pelvis. Occasionally, absorbed and gives systemic effects *see* metronidazole tablets.

 in pregnant women.

cont.

Brand names: Zidoval.
Other preparations: metronidazole dental gel, metronidazole gel/cream, metronidazole tablets/suppositories/suspension.

children, mothers who are breastfeeding, or for women during menstrual periods.

ANTICOAGULANTS, phenytoin, phenobarbital, disulfiram, lithium, alcohol.

Metrotop *see* metronidazole gel
(SSL International)

---

metyrapone capsules

A capsule used as a hormone blocker to treat ADRENAL gland disorders such as Cushing's syndrome and (with other medication) to treat resistant fluid retention caused by increased aldosterone (hormone) production in liver and kidney disease, or heart failure.

Strengths available: 250 mg capsules.
Dose: as advised by doctor.
Availability: NHS and private prescription (hospital supervision only).
Contains: metyrapone.
Brand names: Metopirone.

nausea, vomiting, low blood pressure, dizziness, headache, drowsiness, allergic skin reaction, hair growth, low level of adrenal activity.

in patients suffering from underactive pituitary gland, high blood pressure, underactive thyroid gland, or liver disorders.

pregnant women, mothers who are breastfeeding, or for patients suffering from low adrenal function.

alcohol, sedating drugs.

---

mexiletine capsules/modified-release capsules

A capsule or M-R CAPSULE used as an anti-arrhythmic treatment for abnormal heart rhythm.

Strengths available: 50 mg and 200 mg capsules; 360 mg m-r capsules.
Dose: adults, using standard capsules, 400-600 mg as a single dose to start, then 200-250 mg three times a day; using m-r capsules, 1 capsule twice a day.
Availability: NHS and private prescription.
Contains: mexiletine hydrochloride.
Brand names: Mexitil.

stomach upset, altered heart rhythm, heart conduction disorders, drowsiness, confusion, mental disturbances, fits, lack of articulation or co-ordination, pins and needles, abnormal eye movements, shaking hands, liver and blood disorders.

in pregnant women, mothers who are breastfeeding, and in patients suffering from nerve conduction defects in the heart, slow heart rate, Parkinson's disease, low blood pressure, or heart, liver, or kidney disorders.

other anti-arrhythmic drugs, ritonavir, alcohol, sedating drugs.

children or for patients with heart block or within 3 months of heart attack.

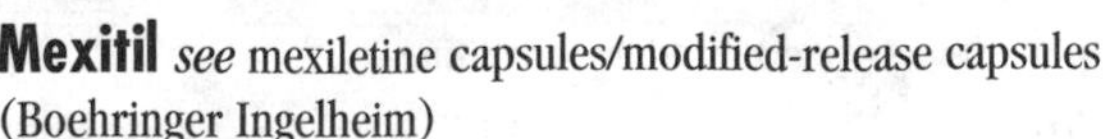

Mexitil *see* mexiletine capsules/modified-release capsules
(Boehringer Ingelheim)

mianserin tablets

A tablet used as an ANTIDEPRESSANT to treat depression.

Strengths available: 10 mg, 20 mg, and 30 mg tablets.
Dose: adults 30-40 mg (elderly patients 30 mg) a day at first increasing gradually if needed to 90 mg a day. May be taken in one dose at bedtime or in divided doses through the day.
Availability: NHS and private prescription.
Contains: mianserin hydrochloride.

Caution: in the elderly, pregnant women, mothers who are breastfeeding, and in patients suffering from heart disease, liver and kidney disorders, thyroid disease, PHAEOCHROMOCYTOMA, epilepsy, diabetes, PORPHYRIA, glaucoma, urine retention, constipation, some other psychiatric conditions. Your doctor may advise regular blood tests. Report any sore throat, fever, or mouth ulcers to your doctor.

Side effects: dry mouth, noises in the ears, tiredness, constipation, difficulty passing urine, blurred vision, stomach upset, palpitations, drowsiness, sleeplessness, dizziness, shaking hands, low blood pressure, weight change, sweating, fever, excitement, confusion in the elderly, skin reactions, jaundice or blood changes, interference with sexual function, changes in heart rhythm, rash, hormone disturbances, fits, movement disorders, blood changes, breast changes in women, menstrual disorders, arthritis, joint pain.

Not to be used for: children or for patients suffering from recent heart attacks, heart rhythm abnormalities, severe liver disease or elevated mood.

Caution needed with: alcohol, sedatives, MAOIS, BARBITURATES, other antidepressants, anti-epileptic drugs.

Micanol *see* dithranol cream
(Medeva Pharma)

Micardis *see* telmisartan tablets
(Boehringer Ingelheim)

Micolette *see* sodium citrate enema
(Dexcel Pharma)

miconazole cream/powder/spray

A cream, powder, or spray used as an antifungal treatment for fungal infections of the skin and nails.

Strengths available: 2% cream and powder; 0.16% spray.
Dose: for skin infections, apply twice a day until 10 days after symptoms disappear; for nail infections, apply once a day under an occlusive dressing.

cont.

Availability: NHS and private prescription, over the counter. Cream also available on nurse prescription.

Side effects: occasionally irritation.

Contains: miconazole nitrate.
Brand names: Daktarin (powder form not available on NHS).
Compound preparations: Daktacort *see* topical CORTICOSTEROID.
Other preparations: miconazole oral gel, miconazole pessaries/vaginal cream.

miconazole oral gel

A gel used as an antifungal to treat or prevent fungal mouth infections.

Caution: in pregnant women and mothers who are breastfeeding.

Not to be used for: children or for patients suffering from PORPHYRIA.

Caution needed with: ANTICOAGULANTS, reboxetine, some antidiabetics, phenytoin, pimozide, cyclosporin, STATINS, tacrolimus.

Strengths available: 24 mg/ml gel.
Dose: adults, 5-10 ml four times a day; children under 2 years, 2.5 ml (aged 2-6 years 5 ml) twice a day; children over 6 years, 5 ml four times a day. Continue for 48 hours after symptoms clear. Place the dose in the mouth and hold as near to infection as possible. Use after meals.
Availability: NHS and private prescription, nurse prescription. (Small quantities available over the counter.)
Contains: miconazole.
Brands: Daktarin Oral Gel.
Other preparations: Dumicoat, miconazole cream/powder/spray, miconazole pessaries/vaginal cream.

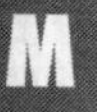

miconazole pessaries/vaginal cream

A pessary and vaginal cream used as an antifungal treatment for thrush of the vulva or vagina.

Side effects: occasionally irritation.

Not to be used for: children.

Strengths available: 100 mg or 1200 mg pessaries; 2% vaginal cream.
Dose: 1 x 100 mg pessary inserted into the vagina once a day for 14 days, or twice a day for 7 days, or 1 x 1200 mg pessary inserted as a single dose at night; vaginal cream used internally once a day for 10-14 days or twice a day for 7 days (1 applicatorful), or for surface infections, applied around the anus and genital area twice a day.
Availability: NHS and private prescription, over the counter.
Contains: miconazole nitrate.
Brand names: Gyno-Daktarin.
Compound preparations: Daktacort *see* topical corticosteroid, Gyno-Daktarin Combi-pack (with miconazole cream).
Other preparations: miconazole cream/powder/spray, miconazole oral gel.

Micralax *see* sodium citrate enema
(Medeva Pharma)

Microfine+ *see* B-D Microfine+

Microgynon 30/ED *see* oral contraceptive (combined)
(Schering Health Care)

Microlet Finger Pricking Device *see* Baylet Lancets, B-D Micro-Fine+ Lancets, Cleanlet Fine Lancets, Milward Steri-Let/Steri-Let Ultra-Fine Lancets, Monolet Lancets, Unilet Universal ComforTouch Lancets, Vitrex Soft Lancets
(Bayer Diagnostics)

Availability: private prescription, over the counter.

Micronor *see* oral contraceptive (progestogen-only)
(Janssen-Cilag)

Micronor HRT

A tablet used, in addition to an oestrogen, as a progestogen for HORMONE REPLACEMENT THERAPY.

Strengths available: 1 mg tablets.
Dose: 1 mg a day from days 15 to 26 of menstrual cycle.
Availability: NHS and private prescription.
Contains: norethisterone.
Compound preparations: hormone replacement therapy (combined), ORAL CONTRACEPTIVES (COMBINED), ORAL CONTRACEPTIVES (PROGESTOGEN-ONLY).
Other preparations: norethisterone tablets (5 mg), norethisterone injection.

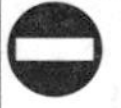 children, pregnant women, mothers who are breastfeeding, or for patients suffering from some cancers, undiagnosed vaginal bleeding, or with a history of liver disease or some skin disorders.

 stomach upset, disorders of the skin and mucous membranes, depression, sleeplessness, drowsiness, hair loss or growth, liver disturbance, severe allergic reaction, breast pain, milk production, abnormal menstrual bleeding, headache, weight gain, fluid retention, changes in sexual desire, worsening of epilepsy or migraine.

 in patients suffering from diabetes, high blood pressure, epilepsy, migraine, asthma, liver or breast disorders, fibroids, gallstones, multiple sclerosis, some skin cancers, LUPUS, POPHYRIA, heart or kidney disease, or who have a history of depression.

 cyclosporin, alcohol, sedating drugs.

Microval *see* oral contraceptive (progestogen-only)
(Wyeth Laboratories)

Mictral *see* nalidixic acid tablets/suspension
(Sanofi Winthrop)

Dose: adults 1 sachet three times a day for 3 days.

Midrid

(Manx Pharma)
A capsule used as an analgesic to treat migraine.

Strengths available: 65 mg + 325 mg capsules.
Dose: adults, 2 capsules at the beginning of the migraine attack, then 1 capsule every hour if needed, to a maximum of 5 capsules in 12 hours.
Availability: NHS and private prescription, over the counter.
Contains: isometheptene mucate and paracetamol.

 dizziness, blood or circulation disorders, rash.

 in patients with heart or circulation disorders, liver or kidney disease, diabetes or overactive thyroid.

 children, pregnant women, mothers who are breastfeeding, or for patients suffering from glaucoma, PORPHYRIA, or severe heart, liver, or kidney disorders, or very high blood pressure.

 MAOIS, bromocriptine, other medicines containing paracetamol.

Migraleve

(Pfizer Consumer Healthcare)
A pink tablet used as an analgesic, ANTIHISTAMINE treatment for migraine. Yellow tablets (containing co-codamol 8/500) also available.

Strengths available: 6.25 mg + 500 mg + 8 mg pink tablets.
Dose: adults, 2 pink tablets at the beginning of the attack, then 2 yellow tablets every 4 hours if needed to a maximum of 2 pink and 6 yellow tablets in 24 hours; children 10-14 years half adult dose.
Availability: NHS and private prescription, over the counter.
Contains: buclizine hydrochloride, paracetamol, and codeine phosphate – pink tablets; paracetamol and

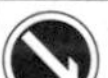 drowsiness, upset stomach (particularly constipation). *See also* co-codamol.

 in pregnant women, women in labour, mothers who are breastfeeding, elderly or weakened patients, and in those suffering from breathing, kidney, or liver problems, low blood pressure, underactive thyroid, enlarged prostate or epilepsy.

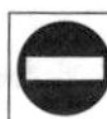 children under 10 years, alcoholics, or patients with head injury, reduced breathing ability, or who are at risk of non-functioning intestines.

codeine phosphate (co-codamol) – yellow tablets.

MAOIS, alcohol, sedating drugs, ritonavir, other drugs containing paracetamol.

Migramax *see* metoclopramide tablets and aspirin 300 mg tablets
(Elan Pharma)

Strengths available: 10 mg metoclopramide + 1.62 g lysine aspirin (equivalent to 900 mg aspirin) in each sachet.
Dose: adults over 20 years, the contents of 1 sachet in water at start of attack, then repeat after 2 hours if needed (maximum of 3 in 24 hours).

Migranal *see* dihydroergotamine nasal spray
(Novartis Pharmaceuticals UK)

Migril *see* ergotamine tablets and cyclizine tablets
(C.P. Pharmaceuticals)

Strengths available: 2 mg + 50 mg tablets (+ 100 mg caffeine).
Dose: adults 1 tablet at start of attack, then half to 1 tablet every 30 minutes if needed, to a maximum of 4 tablets per attack. Do not repeat within 4 days. Maximum of 6 tablets a week.
Contains: ergotamine tartrate, cyclizine hydrochloride, caffeine hydrate.

Mildison Lipocream *see* topical corticosteroid cream
(Yamanouchi Pharma)

M

Milward Steri-Let/Steri-let Ultrafine Lancets
(Entaco)
Diabetics who need to test their blood regularly can use lancets to pierce the skin, either with or without the use of a finger-pricking device.

Lancet width and length: 23G/0.66 mm (Steri-Let) and 28G/0.36 mm (Steri-Let Ultra-Fine) – (Both type A).
Availability: NHS and private prescription, over the counter.
Compatible finger-pricking devices: Autoclix, Autolet Mini, Glucolet, Hypolance, Microlet, Penlet II Plus, Soft Touch. (Autolet II, Autolet Lite, and Autolet Lite Clinisafe also compatible but not recommended by manufacturers.)

---

mineral oil *see* emollient preparations

Min-i-jet Adrenaline *see* adrenaline injection
(Medeva Pharma)

Mini-Wright Peak Flow Meter *see* peak flow meter
(Clement Clarke International)

Minims *see* artificial tears, atropine eye drops, chloramphenicol eye drops, cyclopentolate eye drops, dexamethasone eye drops, gentamicin eye drops, homatropine eye drops, Metipranolol Minims, neomycin eye drops, pilocarpine eye drops, prednisolone eye drops, sodium chloride drops

---

Minims Homatropine *see* homatropine eye drops
(Chauvin Pharmaceuticals)

Minitran *see* glyceryl trinitrate patch
(3M Health Care)

Minocin/Minocin MR *see* minocycline tablets/capsules/modified-release capsules
(Wyeth Laboratories)

---

minocycline tablets/capsules/modified-release capsules

A tablet, capsule, or M-R CAPSULE used as a tetracycline ANTIBIOTIC treatment for chronic bronchitis and other infections, including acne.

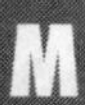

Strengths available: 50 mg or 100 mg tablets; 50 mg or 100 mg capsules; 100 mg m-r capsules.
Dose: adults, usually 100 mg twice a day as standard tablets or capsules, (100 mg once a day or 50 mg twice a day for acne). The m-r capsule used only to treat acne.
Availability: NHS and private prescription.
Contains: minocycline hydrochloride.
Brand names: Aknemin, Blemix, Minocin.

 milk, ANTACIDS, iron supplements, ANTICOAGULANTS, ORAL CONTRACEPTIVES.

 stomach upset, irritation of the oesophagus, skin disorders and pigmentation, headache, disturbed vision, sensitivity to light, additional infections, pressure on the brain, reversible diabetes insipidus, liver disorders, LUPUS, inflamed pancreas or bowel, dizziness, vertigo, discoloration of tears, saliva, and sweat.

 in patients suffering from liver or kidney disorders. Discontinue if reddening of skin occurs. Your doctor may advise regular check-ups with long-term treatment.

 children under 12 years, pregnant women, mothers who are breastfeeding, or for patients suffering from lupus.

Minodiab *see* glipizide tablets
(Pharmacia and Upjohn)

minoxidil tablets

A tablet used in addition to BETA-BLOCKERS and DIURETICS to treat high blood pressure.

Strengths available: 2.5 mg, 5 mg, and 10 mg tablets.
Dose: adults, 5 mg a day at first increasing gradually to a maximum of 50 mg a day (in one single dose or divided into two doses); children use reduced doses according to body weight.
Availability: NHS and private prescription.
Contains: minoxidil.
Brand names: Loniten.
Other preparations: minoxidil topical solution.

 hair growth, fluid retention, weight gain, rapid heart rate, blood changes. Rarely, stomach upset, rash, tender breasts.

 in pregnant women and in patients suffering from angina, recent heart attack, PORPHYRIA, or undergoing dialysis.

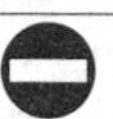 patients suffering from PHAEOCHROMOCYTOMA.

 anaesthetics.

minoxidil topical solution

A liquid used as a hair restorer to treat baldness in men and women.

Strengths available: 2% and 5% solution.
Dose: 1 ml applied to the scalp twice a day. Effect may not be seen for 4 months. Treatment must be continued indefinitely for continued benefit.
Availability: private prescription, over the counter.
Contains: minoxidil.
Brand names: Regaine.
Other preparations: minoxidil tablets.

 dermatitis. Systemic side effects are a possibility *see* minoxidil tablets.

 in patients with high blood pressure and angina. Avoid contact with the eyes, mouth, mucous membranes, or areas of broken, inflamed, or infected skin. Do not inhale the spray.

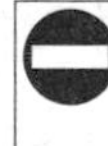 children under 18 years, patients over 65 years, pregnant women, and mothers who are breastfeeding. The 5% solution is not suitable for women.

 some other medications applied to the skin (CORTICOSTEROIDS, isotretinoin, tretinoin, adapalene, petroleum jelly).

Mintec *see* peppermint oil enteric-coated capsules
(Shire Pharmaceuticals)

Mintezol *see* thiabendazole tablets
(Merck Sharp and Dohme)

Minulet *see* oral contraceptive (combined)
(Wyeth Laboratories)

Mirapexin *see* pramipexole tablets
(Pharmacia and Upjohn)

Mirena

(Schering Health Care)

A progestogen form of intra-uterine device used to provide contraception.

Dose: insertion within 7 days of onset of menstrual period (or 6 weeks after birth of a baby), then left in place for 5 years.
Availability: NHS and private prescription.
Contains: levonorgestrel.

 nausea, breast pain, headache, back pain, abdominal pain, abnormal menstrual bleeding, delayed ovulation, skin problems, ovarian cysts, mood changes, vaginal or pelvic inflammation, fluid retention, pelvic infection, perforation of the uterus or cervix. On insertion, pain, epileptic attack, asthma attack, persistent low heart rate.

 in mothers who are breastfeeding, women who have not had children, and in patients suffering from heart disease, high blood pressure, anaemia, endometriosis, HIV infection, diabetes, migraine, some cancers, epilepsy, liver abnormalities, ovarian cysts, or who have had a previous ectopic pregnancy, blood clot, fertility problems, or joint replacement. Your doctor may advise regular examinations.

 pregnant women or for patients suffering from severe heart or blood vessel disease, inflamed pelvis, abnormal or inflamed uterus or cervix, genital infection, severe liver disorders, reduced resistance to infection, PORPHYRIA, undiagnosed vaginal bleeding, some womb or blood disorders, or those who have a history of heart or pelvic infection.

M

↔ BARBITURATES, phenytoin, primidone, carbamazepine, chloral hydrate, ethosuximide, rifampicin, chlorpromazine, meprobamate, griseofulvin, topiramate, modafinil, cyclosporin, nevirapine, celecoxib, ANTICOAGULANTS, CORTICOSTEROIDS.

---

mirtazapine tablets

A tablet used as an ANTIDEPRESSANT to treat depression.

Strengths available: 30 mg tablets.
Dose: 15 mg at night at first then increased to a maximum of 45 mg if needed (either as a single bedtime dose or in two doses during the day).
Availability: NHS and private prescription.
Contains: mirtazapine.
Brand names: Zispin.

 weight gain, increased appetite, drowsiness, liver disorders, fluid retention, low blood pressure on standing, skin disorders, muscle spasm, excitement, shaking hands, blood changes.

 in patients with kidney or liver disorders, epilepsy, heart disorders, low blood pressure, glaucoma, diabetes, mental disorders, difficulty passing urine, or those who have recently had a heart attack. Report any sore throat, mouth ulcers, or fever to your doctor.

 children, pregnant women, or for mothers who are breastfeeding.

 alcohol, sedatives, other antidepressants, MAOIS.

misoprostol tablets

A tablet used to treat stomach ulcers and to prevent those caused by NON-STEROIDAL ANTI-INFLAMMATORY DRUGS.

Strengths available: 200 mcg tablets.
Dose: for treatment, 800 mcg a day (in 2-4 divided doses) with meals and at bedtime for 4-8 weeks; for prevention, 200 mcg 2-4 times a day (at same time as the non-steroidal anti-inflammatory drug).
Availability: NHS and private prescription.
Contains: misoprostol.
Brand names: Cytotec.
Compound preparations: Arthrotec, Napratec.

 upset stomach, menstrual disturbance, vaginal bleeding, rash, dizziness.

 in patients suffering from circulatory disorders. Women of child-bearing age must use adequate contraception.

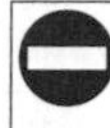 children, pregnant women, mothers who are breastfeeding, or for women planning a pregnancy.

Mistamine *see* mizolastine tablets
(Galderma (UK))

Mixtard *see* insulin

mizolastine modified-release tablets

An M-R TABLET used as an ANTIHISTAMINE to treat allergies such as hayfever and itchy skin rashes.

Strengths available: 10 mg m-r tablets.
Dose: adults and children over 12 years, 10 mg once a day.
Availability: NHS and private prescription.
Contains: mizolastine.
Brand names: Mistamine, Mizollen.

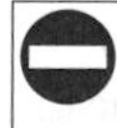 children under 12 years, pregnant women, mothers who are breastfeeding, or for patients with severe liver disorders, slow heart beat, heart disease, or low potassium levels.

 drowsiness, dizziness, weakness, headache, agitation, stomach upset, dry mouth, weight gain.

 in patients suffering from kidney disease.

 drugs affecting heart rhythm, erythromycin, azithromycin, clarithromycin, ANTIDEPRESSANTS, some antifungals, ritonavir, sotalol, cyclosporin, nifedipine, cimetidine, alcohol, sedating drugs.

Mizollen *see* mizolastine tablets
(Schwartz Pharma)

MMR vaccine

A live vaccine used to provide immunization against measles, mumps, and rubella (German measles).

Dose: two doses (usually given at 12-15 months and 3-5 years). Also given to control outbreaks of measles (but not mumps or rubella) with one single dose (within 3 days of exposure to infection).
Availability: NHS and private prescription.
Contains: measles vaccine, mumps vaccine, rubella vaccine.
Brand names: MMR II, Priorix.

 fever, rash, general feeling of being unwell, swollen glands.

 in patients with epilepsy. Women must avoid pregnancy for at least one month after immunization.

 pregnant women or for children with impaired immunity or untreated cancer, feverish illness, or who are allergic to neomycin.

 other live vaccines (within 3 weeks), immunoglobulin (within 3 months), drugs affecting the immune system, high doses of CORTICOSTEROIDS.

MMR II *see* MMR vaccine
(Aventis Pasteur MSD)

Mobic *see* meloxicam tablets
(Boehringer Ingelheim)

Mobiflex *see* tenoxicam tablets
(Roche Products)

M

---

moclobemide tablets

A tablet used as an ANTIDEPRESSANT (similar to MAOIS) to treat serious depression and social phobia.

Strengths available: 150 mg and 300 mg tablets.
Dose: 300 mg a day after food at first increasing gradually to a maximum of 600 mg a day if needed.
Availability: NHS and private prescription.
Contains: moclobemide.
Brand names: Manerix.

 OPIOID ANALGESICS, NON-STEROIDAL ANTI-INFLAMMATORY DRUGS, appetite suppressants, SYMPATHOMIMETICS, other antidepressants, levodopa, sumatriptan, rizatriptan, naratriptan, zolmitriptan.

 sleep disturbance, headache, stomach upset, dizziness, confusion, fluid retention, skin reaction, restlessness, agitation, pins and needles, dry mouth, visual disturbances, liver changes, low blood sodium levels.

 in pregnant women, mothers who are breast-feeding, and in patients suffering from severe liver damage, overactive thyroid, some mental disorders, excitement or agitation. Avoid excessive intake of foods such as cheese, pickled herrings, broad bean pods, fermented soya bean products, and meat/yeast extracts.

 children or for patients who are confused or who suffer from PHAEOCHROMOCYTOMA.

modafinil tablets

A tablet used as a stimulant to treat narcolepsy (a condition that causes the patient to sleep at irregular times).

Strengths available: 100 mg tablets.
Dose: adults, 200-400 mg a day (as a single dose in the morning, or divided into two doses at breakfast and noon). Elderly patients start with 100 mg dose.
Availability: NHS and private prescription.
Contains: modafinil.
Brand names: Provigil.

 children, pregnant women, mothers who are breastfeeding, or for patients with moderate to severe high blood pressure, or a history of heart disorders (including angina) with stimulants.

 loss of appetite, stomach upset, headache, stimulation, excitement, nervousness, dry mouth, palpitations, personality disorders, fast heart beat, high blood pressure, shaking hands, rash, itching, blood changes, abnormal face movements.

 in patients with kidney or liver disorders, high blood pressure, or who may become addicted to the drug. Women of child-bearing age must use adequate contraception.

 ORAL CONTRACEPTIVES, anti-epileptic treatments.

Modalim *see* ciprofibrate tablets
(Sanofi Winthrop)

Modisal LA *see* isosorbide mononitrate modified-release capsules
(Lagap Pharmaceuticals)

Moditen *see* fluphenazine tablets
(Sanofi Winthrop)

Modrasone *see* topical corticosteroid cream/ointment
(Dominion Pharma)

Modrenal *see* trilostane capsules
(Wanskerne)

Moducren *see* timolol tablets, amiloride tablets, and hydrochlorothiazide tablets
(Merck Sharp and Dohme)

Strengths available: 10 mg + 2.5 mg + 25 mg tablets.
Dose: 1-2 tablets a day.

Moduret-25 *see* co-amilozide tablets
(DuPont Pharmaceuticals)

M

Moduretic *see* co-amilozide tablets
(DuPont Pharmaceuticals)

---

moexepril tablets

A tablet used as an ACE-INHIBITOR to treat high blood pressure.

Strengths available: 7.5 mg or 15 mg tablets.
Dose: adults, usually 7.5 mg once a day to start (elderly patients or those also taking DIURETICS or nifedipine, 3.75 mg) increasing if necessary to 15-30 mg a day.
Availability: NHS and private prescription.
Contains: moexepril hydrochloride.
Brand names: Perdix.

Not to be used for: children, pregnant women, or for patients with some heart abnormalities, disorders of the blood supply to the kidney. Not to be taken on the same day as dialysis.

Caution needed with: DIURETICS, anaesthetics, NON-STEROIDAL ANTI-INFLAMMATORY DRUGS, potassium supplements, cyclosporin, lithium, antidiabetics, alcohol, sedating drugs.

Side effects: rash, itching, sore throat, runny nose, stomach upset, cough, blood and liver changes, kidney disorders, low blood pressure, severe allergic reaction, inflamed pancreas. Occasionally, headache, dizziness, tiredness, taste disturbance, fever, pins and needles, muscle or joint pain, sensitivity to sunlight, inflamed membranes or blood vessels, heart rhythm disturbance, angina, chest pain, fainting, stroke, heart attack, appetite and weight changes, dry mouth, flushing, mood change, nervousness, drowsiness, sleep disturbance, influenza-like symptoms, sweating, noises in the ears, difficulty breathing.

Caution: in the elderly, mothers who are breast-feeding, and in patients suffering from kidney disease, auto-immune diseases (such as LUPUS), severe heart failure, or with a history of severe allergies, or in patients undergoing anaesthesia or dialysis. Your doctor may advise regular blood tests.

Mogadon *see* nitrazepam tablets
(ICN Pharmaceuticals)

Moisture-eyes *see* hypromellose eye drops
(Co-Pharma)

Molcer *see* docusate ear drops
(Wallace Manufacturing Chemists)

Molipaxin/Molipaxin CR *see* trazodone tablets/modified-release tablets/capsules/liquid
(Hoechst Marion Roussel)

---

mometasone *see* corticosteroid nasal spray, topical corticosteroid

---

Monit/LS/SR/XL *see* isosorbide mononitrate tablets/modified-release tablets
(Sanofi Synthelabo)

---

mono-amine oxidase inhibitor *see* MAOI

Mono-Cedocard *see* isosorbide mononitrate tablets
(Pharmacia and Upjohn)

Monocor *see* bisoprolol tablets
(Wyeth Laboratories)

Monodur *see* isosorbide mononitrate modified-release tablets
(Waymade)

Monoject *see* insulin injection devices
(Sherwood-Davis and Geck)

Monolet Extra Lancets

(Sherwood-Davis and Geck)
Diabetics who need to test their blood regularly can use lancets to pierce the skin, either with or without the use of a finger-pricking device.

Lancet width and length: 21G/0.8 mm (Type A).
Availability: NHS and private prescription, over the counter.
Compatible finger-pricking devices: Glucolet, Hypolance, Penlet II Plus, Soft Touch.

Monolet Lancets

(Sherwood-Davis and Geck)
Diabetics who need to test their blood regularly can use lancets to pierce the skin, either with or without the use of a finger-pricking device.

Lancet width and length: 21G/0.8 mm (Type A).
Availability: NHS and private prescription, over the counter.
Compatible finger-pricking devices: Autoclix, Autolet Mini, Glucolet, Hypolance, Microlet, Penlet II Plus, Soft Touch.

Monomax/Monomax XL *see* isosorbide mononitrate modified-release capsules/tablets
(Trinity Pharmaceuticals)

Monosorb XL *see* isosorbide mononitrate modified-release tablets
(Approved Prescriptions Services)

Monotard *see* insulin

Monotrim *see* trimethoprim tablets/suspension
(Solvay Healthcare)

Monovent *see* terbutaline syrup
(Lagap Pharmaceuticals)

Monozide *see* bisoprolol tablets and hydrochlorothiazide tablets
(Wyeth Laboratories)

Strengths available: 10 mg + 62.5 mg tablets.
Dose: adults 1 tablet a day.

Monphytol

(LAB)

A paint used as an anti-fungal treatment for fungal infections such as athlete's foot and nail infections.

Dose: adults paint on to the affected area twice a day until 2 weeks after symptoms subside, then once a week.

 children or pregnant women.

Availability: NHS and private prescription, over the counter.
Contains: methyl undecenoate, propyl undecenoate, salicylic acid, methyl salicylate, propyl salicylate, chlorbutanol.

---

montelukast tablets

A tablet or chewable tablet used as an additional treatment to prevent asthma which is not controlled by CORTICOSTEROIDS and bronchodilators.

Strengths available: 5 mg chewable tablets; 10 mg standard tablets.
Dose: adults 10 mg (children aged 6-14 years 5 mg) at night.
Availability: NHS and private prescription.

 stomach upset, dry mouth, weakness, dizziness, severe allergic reaction, headache, sleeplessness, muscle or joint pain, fever, respiratory infection. Report any deterioration in breathing, nasal symptoms, or blood vessel disorders to your doctor.

Contains: montelukast sodium.
Brand names: Singulair.

 phenytoin, phenobarbital, rifampicin.

children under 6 years or for patients with Churg-Strauss syndrome (a condition involving breathing or nasal symptoms and blood vessel disorders). Chewable tablets should not be used by patients with PHENYLKETONURIA.

 in pregnant women and mothers who are breastfeeding.

Moraxen *see* morphine sulphate suppositories (Schwartz Pharma)

Morcap SR *see* morphine modified-release capsules (Sanofi Winthrop)

morphine oral solution/tablets/modified-release tablets/modified-release capsules/modified-release suspension/suppositories

An oral solution, tablet, M-R TABLET/CAPSULE/SUSPENSION, suppository, hydrogel suppository used as an OPIOID ANALGESIC to control chronic severe pain.

Strengths available: 10 mg/5 ml, 30 mg/5 ml, or 100 mg/5 ml solution; 10 mg, 20 mg, and 50 mg standard tablets; 5 mg, 10 mg, 15 mg, 30 mg, 60 mg, 100 mg and 200 mg m-r tablets; 10 mg, 30 mg, 50 mg, 60 mg, 90 mg, 100 mg, 120 mg, 150 mg, and 200 mg m-r capsules; 10 mg, 15 mg, 20 mg, and 30 mg standard suppositories; 35 mg, 50 mg, 75 mg, 100 mg hydrogel suppositories; 20 mg, 30 mg, 60 mg, 100 mg and 200 mg sachets of m-r suspension.
Dose: as advised by doctor according to condition; standard-release preparations given every 4 hours; m-r preparations given once or twice a day (depending on brand); suppositories given every 4 hours; hydrogel suppositories given once a day.
Availability: controlled drug; NHS and private prescription.
Contains: morphine sulphate.

 drowsiness, upset stomach, sweating, dizziness, breathing difficulty, low blood pressure, difficulty passing urine, dry mouth, headache, vertigo, flushing, change in heart rhythm, mood changes, rash, itching, addiction, reduced sexual desire.

 in children, pregnant women, women in labour, mothers who are breastfeeding, elderly or weakened patients, and in those suffering from breathing, kidney, or liver problems, low blood pressure, underactive thyroid, enlarged prostate, or epilepsy. (Higher doses not suitable for some of these categories.) Patients using m-r preparations should continue with the same brand of product when dose is stabilized.

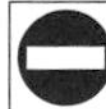 alcoholics or for patients with head injury, reduced breathing ability, PORPHYRIA, or those who have a history of drug addiction or who are suicidal or at risk of non-functioning intestines.

 MAOIS, alcohol, sedating drugs, ritonavir.

cont.

Brand names: Moraxen, Morcap SR, MST Continus, MXL, Oramorph, Sevredol, Zomorph.
Compound preparations: kaolin and morphine mixture (*see* kaolin mixture).

Motens *see* lacidipine tablets
(Boehringer Ingelheim)

Mothers' and Children's Vitamin Drops

(Cupal)
Drops used to supplement the diet of pregnant women and young children.

Strengths available: 700 unit + 20 mg + 300 unit per 5 drops solution.
Dose: mothers and children 5 drops a day.
Availability: NHS and private prescription, over the counter. Also available through maternity and child health clinics.
Contains: vitamins A, C, D.

Motifene *see* diclofenac dual-release capsules
(Sankyo Pharma UK)

Motilium *see* domperidone tablets/suppositories/suspension
(Sanofi Winthrop)

Motipress *see* fluphenazine tablets and nortriptyline tablets
(Sanofi Winthrop)
Used to treat a mixture of anxiety and depression.

Strengths available: 1.5 mg + 30 mg tablets.
Dose: adults 1 at night for up to 3 months.

Motival *see* fluphenazine tablets and nortriptyline tablets
(Sanofi Winthrop)
Used to treat a mixture of anxiety and depression.

Strengths available: 0.5 mg + 10 mg tablets.
Dose: adults 1 tablet three times a day for up to 3 months.

Motrin *see* ibuprofen tablets
(Pharmacia and Upjohn)

---

mouthwash solution tablets NPF

A soluble antimicrobial tablet used to make a mouthwash for dental purposes.

Dose: 1 tablet dissolved in a tumblerful of warm water and used to rinse the mouth as required.
Availability: NHS and private prescription, nurse prescription.

Movelat *see* non-steroidal anti-inflammatory drug (topical)
(Sankyo Pharma UK)

Movicol

(Norgine)
A powder in sachets used as a laxative to treat chronic constipation and impacted faeces.

Dose: adults 1 sachet 2-3 times a day for constipation (or up to 8 a day for impacted faeces); elderly patients start with 1 sachet a day. Treatment continued for 2 weeks for constipation (and repeated if needed) or for 3 days for impacted faeces. Each sachet dissolved in 125 ml water.

bloating, abdominal pain, nausea.

in pregnant women and mothers who are breastfeeding.

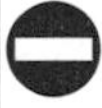
children or for patients with perforated or obstructed intestines, non-functioning bowel, or inflammatory bowel conditions.

Availability: NHS and private prescription, over the counter. Also available on nurse prescription if prescribed generically.
Contains: macrogol '3350', sodium bicarbonate, sodium chloride, potassium chloride.

---

moxisylyte *see* thymoxamine (alternative name)

---

moxonidine tablets

A tablet used to treat high blood pressure.

Strengths available: 200 mcg and 400 mcg tablets.
Dose: 200 mcg each morning increasing if necessary to 400-600 mcg a day (in one single dose or divided into two doses).
Availability: NHS and private prescription.
Contains: moxonidine.
Brand names: Physiotens.

dry mouth, headache, tiredness, weakness, nausea, sleep disturbance, dizziness, widening of blood vessels, skin reactions.

children under 16 years, pregnant women, mothers who are breastfeeding, or for patients with some heart disorders, severe liver or kidney disease, Raynaud's syndrome, epilepsy, depression, Parkinson's disease, glaucoma, lameness/pain when walking, or a history of severe allergic reactions.

in patients suffering from kidney disorders.

sedatives, alcohol.

M

MST Continus *see* morphine modified-release tablets/modified-release suspension
(Napp Pharmaceuticals)

Mucaine *see* aluminium hydroxide mixture and magnesium hydroxide mixture
(Wyeth Laboratories)

Dose: adults 5-10 ml 3-4 times a day before meals and at bedtime, or when required.
Contains: aluminium hydroxide mixture, magnesium hydroxide, oxetacaine (a local anaesthetic also known as oxethazaine).

---

mucin *see* saliva (artificial)

Mucodyne *see* carbocisteine capsules/syrup
(Rhône-Poulenc Rorer)

Mucogel *see* aluminium hydroxide mixture and magnesium hydroxide mixture
(Pharmax)

Dose: adults 10-20 ml three times a day after meals and at bedtime, or when required.

---

mucopolysaccharide polysulphate *see* heparinoid (alternative name)

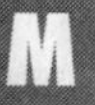

Multiload CU 275/350
(Organon Laboratories)
A copper-bearing coil used as an intra-uterine device to prevent conception.

Dose: insertion usually between the end of the menstrual period and the mid-point of the cycle, then left in place for 3 years.
Availability: NHS and private prescription.
Contains: copper wire.
Other preparations: Nova-T.

 pelvic infection, pain, abnormal bleeding, perforation of the uterus or cervix. On insertion, pain, epileptic attack, asthma attack, persistent low heart rate.

 in women who have not had children and in patients suffering from heart disease, anaemia, endometriosis, HIV infection, diabetes, epilepsy, or who have had a previous ectopic pregnancy, fertility problems, or joint replacement. Your doctor may advise regular examinations.

 ANTICOAGULANTS.

 pregnant women or for patients suffering from inflamed pelvis, abnormal or inflamed uterus or cervix, genital infection, reduced resistance to infection, PORPHYRIA, undiagnosed vaginal bleeding, some cancers, allergy to copper, Wilson's disease, some womb or blood disorders, or who have a history of heart or pelvic infection.

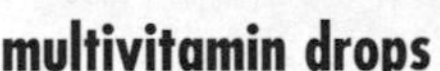

multivitamin drops

Drops used as a multivitamin preparation to prevent vitamin deficiencies.

Dose: children aged 1-12 years 0.6 ml a day: infants under 1 year 0.3 ml a day.
Availability: NHS and private prescription, over the counter.
Contains: vitamins A, D, B_1, B_2, B_3, B_6, C.
Brand names: Abidec, Dalivit.

 in pregnant women. Not recommended for use in adults.

 levodopa, somc DIURETICS.

---

mumps vaccine *see* MMR vaccine

---

mupirocin cream/ointment/nasal ointment

A cream, ointment, or nasal ointment used as an ANTIBIOTIC to treat infections of the nose or skin. (The ointment is used for skin infections such as impetigo, the cream used only to treat skin trauma that later becomes infected.)

Strengths available: 2% cream, ointment, or nasal ointment.
Dose: apply the nasal ointment to the openings of the nose 2-3 times a day for 5-7 days; the cream or ointment applied to the skin up to three times a day for up to 10 days.
Availability: NHS and private prescription.
Contains: mupirocin.
Brand names: Bactroban.

Side effects: stinging.

Caution: in patients with kidney disorders. Avoid the eyes.

Muscinil *see* procyclidine tablets

(Opus Pharmaceuticals)

Muse *see* alprostadil urethral stick

(Abbott Laboratories)

MXL *see* morphine modified-release capsules

(Napp Pharmaceuticals)

---

myasthenia gravis

A progressive form of muscle weakness commonly affecting the muscles used for speaking, eating, and moving the eyes, making these actions difficult.

M

Mycobutin *see* rifabutin capsules
(Pharmacia and Upjohn)

mycophenolate capsules/tablets

A tablet or capsule used (in addition to CORTICOSTEROIDS or cyclosporin) to suppress the immune system and prevent rejection of transplanted organs.

Strengths available: 250 mg capsules; 500 mg tablets.
Dose: for kidney transplantation, adults 100 mg twice a day; for heart and liver transplantation, adults 1500 mg twice a day. The dose taken without food.
Availability: NHS and private prescription (specialist supervision).
Contains: mycophenolate mofetil.
Brand names: CellCept.

upset stomach, abdominal pain, blood disorders, high or low blood pressure, fluid retention, chest pain, cough or breathing difficulty, inflamed nasal passages, dizziness, sleeplessness, shaking hands, headache, infections, chemical disturbances, weakness, kidney disorders, skin disorders, liver disorders, mouth ulcers, inflamed gums, lymph gland disorders, influenza-like symptoms, heart rhythm abnormalities, weight gain, low blood glucose levels, high blood cholesterol levels.

in the elderly and in patients with stomach or intestinal disorders or who are at risk of skin cancer. Your doctor will advise regular blood tests. Report any sore throat, fever, or abnormal bleeding/bruising to your doctor immediately. Women should use adequate contraception and avoid pregnancy for 6 weeks after treatment ends.

children, pregnant women, or mothers who are breastfeeding.

tacrolimus, drugs that affect circulation to the liver or intestines.

Mydrilate *see* cyclopentolate eye drops
(Boehringer Ingelheim)

Myocrisin *see* sodium aurothiomalate injection
(Distriphar)

Myotonine *see* bethanechol tablets
(Glenwood Laboratories)

Mysoline *see* primidone tablets
(Zeneca Pharma)

nabumetone tablets/suspension

A tablet or suspension used as a NON-STEROIDAL ANTI-INFLAMMATORY DRUG to treat the symptoms of osteoarthritis and rheumatoid arthritis.

Strengths available: 500 mg tablets; 500 mg/5 ml suspension.
Dose: adults, 1000 mg at night with an additional 500-1000 mg in the morning if needed; elderly patients, maximum of 1000 mg a day.
Availability: NHS and private prescription.
Contains: nabumetone.
Brand names: Relifex.

 stomach upset and bleeding or ulceration, drowsiness, rash, severe allergy, difficulty breathing, blood or kidney disorders, headache, dizziness, noises in the ears, sensitivity to light, vertigo. Rarely, fluid retention, liver disorders, inflamed pancreas, inflamed bowel, meningitis.

 in the elderly and in patients with heart, liver, or kidney disorders, high blood pressure, asthma, or LUPUS.

ACE-INHIBITORS, aspirin or other non-steroidal anti-inflammatory drugs, some ANTIBIOTICS, ANTICOAGULANTS, some antidiabetic drugs, some antivirals, methotrexate, digoxin, DIURETICS, lithium, tacrolimus, cyclosporin, aluminium hydroxide, alcohol, sedatives.

 children, pregnant women, mothers who are breastfeeding, or for patients with a history of allergy to aspirin or other NSAID, severe kidney disorders, blood clotting disorders, currently active stomach ulcer or intestinal bleeding, inflamed intestines, or severe heart failure.

nadolol tablets

A tablet used as a BETA-BLOCKER to treat heart rhythm disturbances, angina, high blood pressure, as an additional treatment in thyroid disease, and to prevent migraine.

Strengths available: 40 mg and 80 mg tablets.
Dose: adults, usually 40 mg once a day at first increasing to maximum of 160 mg a day; for high blood pressure, start with 80 mg a day increasing to a maximum of 240 mg a day.
Availability: NHS and private prescription.
Contains: nadolol.
Brand names: Corgard.
Compound preparations: Corgaretic.

 children or for patients suffering from heart block or failure, asthma, PHAEOCHROMOCYTOMA, or a history of breathing disorders.

 cold hands and feet, sleep disturbance, slow heart rate, tiredness, wheezing, heart failure, low blood pressure, stomach upset. Rarely, dry eyes, rash, worsening of psoriasis.

 in pregnant women, mothers who are breast-feeding, the elderly, and in patients suffering from diabetes, kidney or liver disorders, MYASTHENIA GRAVIS, or with a history of allergies. May need to be withdrawn before surgery. Withdraw gradually.

 general anaesthetics, CALCIUM-CHANNEL BLOCKERS, ALPHA-BLOCKERS, clonidine, ANTIHYPERTENSIVES, amiodarone, antidiabetics, thymoxamine, theophylline, aminophylline.

nafarelin nasal spray

A nasal spray used as a hormone treatment for endometriosis, and for desensitizing the pituitary gland in *in-vitro* fertilization (IVF) programmes.

Strengths available: 200 mcg per dose nasal spray.
Dose: adults for endometriosis, 1 spray into 1 nostril in the morning and 1 spray into the other nostril in the evening for up to 6 months starting between the 2nd and 4th days of cycle; for IVF programmes, 1 spray into each nostril morning and evening until ovarian down-regulation achieved.
Availability: NHS and private prescription.
Contains: nafarelin acetate.
Brand names: Synarel.

hot flushes, emotional upsets, changes in size of breasts, loss of sexual desire, sweating, rash, reduced bone density, headache, dry vagina, skin reactions, asthma, severe allergy, joint or muscle pain, irritation of nasal passages, vision disturbances, pins and needles, ovarian cysts, temporary changes in blood pressure, changes in head and body hair, acne, palpitations, fluid retention, weight change, bleeding on withdrawal of treatment.

in patients at risk of OSTEOPOROSIS or who have ovarian cysts. Your doctor will advise you to use non-hormonal methods of contraception.

children, pregnant women, mothers who are breastfeeding, or for patients with undiagnosed vaginal bleeding. Not used for more than 6 months (for endometriosis) or 12 weeks (for IVF).

naftidrofuryl capsules

A capsule used to widen blood vessels and treat blood vessel disorders.

Strengths available: 100 mg capsules.
Dose: usually 100-200 mg three times a day; for brain circulation disorders, 100 mg 2-3 times a day.
Availability: NHS and private prescription.
Contains: naftidrofuryl oxalate.
Brand names: Praxilene, Stimlor.

upset stomach, rash, rarely, liver disorders.

children.

Nalcrom *see* sodium cromoglycate capsules
(Pantheon Healthcare)

nalidixic acid tablets/suspension

A tablet/suspension used as an ANTIBIOTIC to treat urinary or intestinal infections.

Strengths available: 500 mg tablets, 300 mg/5 ml suspension.
Dose: adults, 1000 mg four times a day for 7 days reducing to 500 mg four times a day for long-term infections; children use reduced doses according to body weight.
Availability: NHS and private prescription.

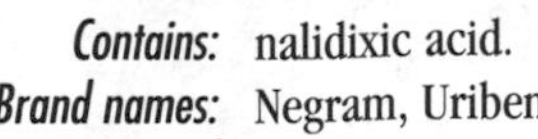

Contains: nalidixic acid.
Brand names: Negram, Uriben.
Compound preparations: Mictral sachets (with sodium citrate, citric acid, sodium bicarbonate)

children under 3 months, mothers who are breastfeeding, or for patients suffering from severe kidney disease, PORPHYRIA, or with a history of epilepsy.

ANTICOAGULANTS, theophylline, aminophylline, cyclosporin, NON-STEROIDAL ANTI-INFLAMMATORY DRUGS, alcohol, sedating drugs.

stomach upset, headache, dizziness, sleep disorders, skin disorders. Rarely, loss of appetite, blood changes, drowsiness, fits, confusion, depression, hallucinations, pins and needles, sensitivity to light, muscle and joint pain, disturbance of the senses, liver and kidney disorders, mental disturbance, face paralysis, chemical disturbances, altered bile flow.

in pregnant women and in patients suffering from kidney disease or with a history of epilepsy or liver disorders. Avoid excessive exposure to sunlight. Your doctor may advise regular blood tests if treatment is long term.

Nalorex *see* naltrexone tablets
(DuPont Pharmaceuticals)

---

naltrexone tablets

A tablet used as an opioid antagonist to treat patients who have been detoxified from opioid addiction.

Strengths available: 50 mg tablets.
Dose: 25 mg a day at first, then 50 mg a day for at least 3 months. (For convenience, weekly dose may be split into three and given on three days of the week.)
Availability: NHS and private prescription (specialist use only).
Contains: naltrexone hydrochloride.
Brand names: Nalorex.

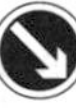

stomach upset, abdominal pain, dizziness, joint or muscle pain, nervousness, difficulty sleeping, headache, reduced energy, loss of appetite, thirst, chest pain, increase in sweating or tear production, chills, rash, delayed ejaculation, liver or blood disorders.

in pregnant women, mothers who are breastfeeding, and in patients suffering from kidney or liver disease.

children or for patients currently addicted to opioids or with active liver disease.

not to be used within 7-10 days of opioids.

N

Napratec *see* naproxen tablets and misoprostol tablets
(Searle)
A combination pack of both tablets.

Dose: adults 1 of each tablet twice a day with food.

Naprosyn *see* naproxen tablets/enteric-coated tablets/modified-release tablets/suppositories/suspension
(Roche Products)

---

naproxen tablets/enteric-coated tablets/modified-release tablets/suppositories/suspension

A tablet, E-C or M-R TABLET, suspension, or suppository used as a NON-STEROIDAL ANTI-INFLAMMATORY DRUG to treat rheumatoid arthritis and other muscle, joint, and bone disorders, period pain, and acute gout.

Strengths available: 250 mg, 275 mg, and 500 mg standard tablets; 250 mg, 375 mg, and 500 mg e-c tablets; 500 mg m-r tablets; 125 mg/ 5 ml suspension; 500 mg suppositories.

Dose: adults, usually 500 mg-1000 mg by mouth each day (as a single dose or divided into 2-4 doses); for gout, 750 mg at first, then 250 mg every 8 hours; for acute muscle or joint disorders and period pain, up to 1250 mg a day. Using suppositories, adults 500 mg once or twice a day; children (for juvenile arthritis only), reduced doses according to body weight.

Availability: NHS and private prescription.

Contains: naproxen.

Brand names: Arthrosin, Naprosyn, Nycopren, Synflex, Timpron.

Compound preparations: Napratec.

stomach upset and bleeding or ulceration, rash, severe allergy, difficulty breathing, blood or kidney disorders, headache, dizziness, noises in the ears, sensitivity to light, vertigo. Rarely, fluid retention, liver disorders, inflamed pancreas, inflamed bowel, meningitis. Suppositories may cause irritation around rectum.

in the elderly, pregnant women, mothers who are breastfeeding, and in patients with heart, liver, or kidney disorders, high blood pressure, asthma or LUPUS.

children under 16 years (except for juvenile arthritis) or for patients with a history of allergy to aspirin or other NSAID, severe kidney disorders, blood clotting disorders, currently active stomach ulcer or intestinal bleeding, inflamed intestines or severe heart failure. Suppositories not to be used for patients with inflammation of the anus or rectum.

ACE-INHIBITORS, aspirin or other non-steroidal anti-inflammatory drugs, some ANTIBIOTICS, ANTICOAGULANTS, some antidiabetic drugs, some antivirals, methotrexate, DIURETICS, lithium, tacrolimus, cyclosporin, aluminium hydroxide, digoxin, ANTACIDS (with e-c tablets).

Naramig *see* naratriptan tablets
(GlaxoWellcome UK)

naratriptan tablets

A tablet used to treat migraine attacks.

Strengths available: 2.5 mg tablets.

Dose: adults, 2.5 mg at start of attack. If migraine then clears, but later recurs, another dose may be taken after 4 hours. (Do not take a second dose if the first

sensations of warmth, tingling, pressure, tightness or heaviness, dizziness, flushing, tiredness, weakness, stomach upset, visual disturbance, heart rhythm disturbance.

in pregnant women, mothers who are breastfeeding, and in patients at risk of heart disease or who suffer from liver or kidney disorders.

fails to work.) Maximum 5 mg in 24 hours.

Availability: NHS and private prescription.
Contains: naratriptan hydrochloride.
Brand names: Naramig.

children under 18 years, adults over 65 years, or for patients with heart disease, severe kidney or liver disease, uncontrolled high blood pressure, or blood vessel disease.

other migraine treatments.

Nardil *see* phenelzine tablets
(Hansam Healthcare)

Narphen *see* phenazocine tablets
(Napp Pharmaceuticals)

Nasacort *see* corticosteroid nasal spray
(Rhône-Poulenc Rorer)

Naseptin cream
(Alliance Pharmaceuticals)
A cream used as an ANTIBIOTIC treatment for infections of the nose.

Dose: apply into each nostril four times a day (for 10 days) to treat infection, or twice a day to prevent infection.
Availability: NHS and private prescription.
Contains: chlorhexidine hydrochloride, neomycin sulphate, peanut oil.

sensitive skin.

avoid prolonged use.

Nasobec *see* corticosteroid nasal spray
(Baker Norton Pharmaceuticals)

Nasonex *see* corticosteroid nasal spray
(Schering-Plough)

Natrilix/Natrilix SR *see* indapamide tablets/modified-release tablets
(Servier Laboratories)

Navidrex *see* cyclopenthiazide tablets
(Goldshield Healthcare)

Navispare *see* amiloride tablets and cyclopenthiazide tablets
(Goldshield Healthcare)

Strengths available: 2.5 mg + 250 mcg tablets.
Dose: adults 1-2 tablets in the morning.

Navoban *see* tropisetron capsules
(Novartis Pharmaceuticals UK)

Nebilet *see* nebivolol tablets
(A. Menarini Pharmaceuticals)

---

nebivolol tablets

A tablet used as a BETA-BLOCKER to treat high blood pressure.

Strengths available: 5 mg tablets.
Dose: adults 5 mg once a day; elderly patients 2.5 mg once a day at first increasing to 5 mg if necessary.
Availability: NHS and private prescription.
Contains: nebivolol hydrochloride.
Brand names: Nebilet.

cold hands and feet, sleep disturbance, slow heart rate, tiredness, wheezing, heart failure, low blood pressure, stomach upset, fluid retention, headache, depression, visual disturbance, pins and needles, impotence. Rarely, dry eyes, rash, worsening of psoriasis.

in pregnant women, mothers who are breast-feeding, the elderly, and in patients suffering from diabetes, kidney disorders, MYASTHENIA GRAVIS, or with a history of allergies. May need to be withdrawn before surgery. Withdraw gradually.

children or for patients suffering from heart block or failure, liver disorders, asthma, PHAEOCHROMOCYTOMA, or with a history of breathing disorders.

general anaesthetics, CALCIUM-CHANNEL BLOCKERS, ALPHA-BLOCKERS, clonidine, ANTIHYPERTENSIVES, amiodarone, antidiabetics, thymoxamine, theophylline, aminophylline.

Nebuhaler
(AstraZeneca UK)
A one-piece spacer device used with Bricanyl and Pulmicort inhalers. Mask available for children and infants.

Availability: NHS and private prescription, over the counter.

---

nedocromil eye drops

An eye drop used as an anti-inflammatory treatment for allergic and other types of conjunctivitis.

Strengths available: 2% eye drops.

Dose: adults and children over 6 years, apply 2-4 times a day. Maximum treatment period 12 weeks for hayfever.
Availability: NHS and private prescription.
Contains: nedocromil sodium.
Brand names: Rapitil.

 temporary irritation, taste in the mouth.

 in pregnant women and in patients who wear hard or gas-permeable contact lenses.

 children under 6 years or for patients wearing soft contact lenses. Long-term treatment for children not recommended.

nedocromil inhaler

An aerosol used as an anti-inflammatory drug to prevent asthma.

Strengths available: 2 mg per dose inhaler.
Dose: adults and children over 6 years, 4 mg (2 puffs) four times a day reducing to twice a day when controlled. Use regularly.
Availability: NHS and private prescription.
Contains: nedocromil sodium.
Brand names: Tilade.

 headache, stomach upset, cough, bitter taste, rarely, wheezing.

 in pregnant women.

 children under 6 years.

nefazodone tablets

A tablet used as an ANTIDEPRESSANT to treat depression.

Strengths available: 50 mg, 100 mg, and 200 mg tablets.
Dose: adults 50-100 mg twice a day at first increasing to a maximum of 300 mg twice a day; elderly patients maximum of 200 mg twice a day.
Availability: NHS and private prescription.
Contains: nefazodone hydrochloride.
Brand names: Dutonin.

 weakness, dry mouth, drowsiness, nausea, dizziness, chills, fever, low blood pressure on standing, constipation, confusion, shaking and unsteadiness, impaired eyesight, pins and needles, fainting, liver disorders, withdrawal reactions.

 in pregnant women, the elderly, and in patients suffering from epilepsy, unstable heart disease, recent heart attack, excitement, liver or kidney disorders, or who are undergoing electric shock treatment.

 alcohol, sedatives, lithium, other antidepressants, digoxin.

 children under 18 years or mothers who are breastfeeding.

nefopam tablets

A tablet used as an ANALGESIC to relieve pain.

Strengths available: 30 mg tablets.

cont.

N

Dose: adults 30-90 mg three times a day.
Availability: NHS and private prescription.
Contains: nefopam hydrochloride.
Brand names: Acupan.

 children or for patients with a history of fits or suffering from heart attack.

 some ANTIDEPRESSANTS, alcohol, sedating drugs.

 stomach upset, nervousness, dry mouth, dizziness, difficulty passing urine, light-headedness, blurred vision, drowsiness or sleeplessness, headache, confusion, hallucinations, sweating, pink colour in urine, fast heart beat.

 in pregnant women, mothers who are breastfeeding, the elderly, and in patients suffering from kidney or liver disease, or difficulty passing urine.

Negram *see* nalidixic acid tablets/suspension
(Sanofi Winthrop)

Neisvac-C *see* meningitis vaccine (C)
(Baxter Healthcare)

---

nelfinavir tablets/powder

A tablet or powder used, in combination with other drugs, as an antiviral to treat HIV infection.

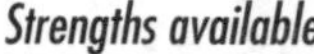

Strengths available: 250 mg tablets; 50 mg/g powder (with 1 g measure).
Dose: adults, 750 mg three times a day or 1250 mg twice a day; children use reduced doses according to body weight.
Availability: NHS and private prescription.
Contains: nelfinavir mesylate.
Brand names: Viracept.

 upset stomach, rash, liver and blood disorders, redistribution of body fat, high blood glucose or lipids.

 in pregnant women and in patients suffering from diabetes, bleeding disorders, liver or kidney disorders.

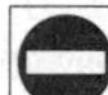 children under 2 years or mothers who are breastfeeding.

 amiodarone, quinidine, rifampicin, rifabutin, carbamazepine, phenytoin, pimozide, midazolam, phenobarbital, ergotamine, simvastatin, ORAL CONTRACEPTIVES, sildenafil, some antifungals and ANTIBIOTICS, some drugs used to reduce blood pressure.

Neo-Bendramax *see* bendrofluazide tablets
(Ashbourne Pharmaceuticals)

Neo-Cortef

(Dominion Pharma)
Drops or an eye ointment used as an ANTIBIOTIC, CORTICOSTEROID treatment for inflammation of the outer ear or infected inflammation of the eye.

Strengths available: 1.5% + 0.5% drops and ointment.
Dose: 1-2 drops into the affected eye(s), or 2-3 drops into the affected ear(s) 3-4 times a day. Ointment may be applied into the eyes 2-3 times a day (or at night if drops used during the day), or once or twice a day into the ears.
Availability: NHS and private prescription.
Contains: hydrocortisone acetate, neomycin sulphate.

 additional infection; thinning of cornea, cataract, or rise in eye pressure when used in the eye.

 in pregnant women and infants.

 patients suffering from non-bacterial infections, glaucoma (if used in the eye), perforated ear drum (if used in the ear).

Neo-Cytamen *see* hydroxocobalamin injection
(Medeva Pharma)

Neo-Mercazole *see* carbimazole tablets
(Roche Products)

Neogest *see* oral contraceptive (progestogen-only)
(Schering Health Care)

---

neomycin cream BPC

A cream used as an ANTIBIOTIC to treat skin infections.

Dose: apply up to three times day for short periods only.
Availability: NHS and private prescription.
Contains: neomycin sulphate.
Compound preparations: Cicatrin, Graneodin, Naseptin. (For skin preparations containing neomycin and a steroid *see* topical corticosteroid.)
Other preparations: Cicatrin dusting powder.

Side effects: allergy may be induced. Ear disorders possible with large doses.

Caution: with large open wounds, and in children, the elderly, patients allergic to other similar antibiotics, and those with kidney disorders.

---

neomycin eye drops/ointment

Eye drops or ointment used as an ANTIBIOTIC to treat bacterial infections of the eye.

Strengths available: 0.5% drops and ointment.
Dose: the drops applied every 2 hours at first, then frequency reduced as infection controlled. The ointment applied at night or 3-4 times a day. Treatment should continue until 48 hours after the infection clears.
Availability: NHS and private prescription.

cont.

Contains: neomycin sulphate.
Brand names: Minims Neomycin Sulphate (single-use drops).
Compound preparations: Maxitrol, Neo-Cortef, Neosporin, Predsol-N (with prednisolone); Betnesol-N and Vista-Methasone N (with betamethasone).
Other preparations: ear products containing neomycin include Audicort, Otomize, Otosporin.

---

neomycin tablets

A tablet used as an ANTIBIOTIC to sterilize the bowel before operations, and in liver failure.

Strengths available: 500 mg tablets.
Dose: adults, to sterilize the bowel 1000 mg every hour for 4 hours, then every 4 hours for 2-3 days; in liver failure up to 4000 mg a day (in divided doses) for up to 14 days. Children over 6 years treated only to sterilize bowel, 250-500 mg every 4 hours for 2-3 days.
Availability: NHS and private prescription.
Contains: neomycin sulphate.
Brand names: Nivemycin.

 ear and kidney damage, low magnesium levels (on prolonged treatment), rash, inflamed intestine, stomach upset, liver changes.

 in elderly patients, pregnant women.

 children under 6 years, mothers who are breastfeeding, or for patients with blocked intestines or MYASTHENIA GRAVIS.

 ANTICOAGULANTS, cyclosporin, DIURETICS, neostigmine, pyridostigmine.

Neo-Naclex *see* bendrofluazide tablets
(Goldshield Healthcare)

Neo-Naclex-K *see* bendrofluazide tablets and potassium chloride tablets
(Goldshield Healthcare)

Strengths available: 2.5 mg + 630 mg tablets.
Dose: adults for high blood pressure, 1-4 tablets once a day; for fluid retention, 2-4 tablets once a day with 1-2 tablets used intermittently for maintenance.

Neoral *see* cyclosporin capsules/liquid
(Novartis Pharmaceuticals UK)

NeoRecormon *see* epoetin beta injection
(Roche Products)

Neosporin *see also* neomycin eye drops
(Dominion Pharma)
A combination of ANTIBIOTICS in eye drops used to treat eye infections.

Dose: apply 2-4 times a day to the affected eye(s), or more frequently if required.
Contains: neomycin, gramicidin, polymixin.

---

neostigmine tablets

A tablet used as an ANTICHOLINESTERASE to treat MYASTHENIA GRAVIS.

Strengths available: 15 mg tablets.
Dose: 15-30 mg as required up to a maximum of 75-300 mg a day. Children given reduced doses (infants 1-5 mg, aged up to 6 years 7.5 mg, aged 6-12 years 15 mg) with a maximum of 15-90 mg according to age.
Availability: NHS and private prescription.
Contains: neostigmine bromide.

 stomach upset. With high doses, increased secretions, low blood pressure, slow heart beat, agitation, weakness, involuntary opening of bowels or passing of urine, shrunken pupils of the eyes, rapid eye movement.

 in pregnant women, mothers who are breast-feeding, and in patients suffering from asthma, heart or kidney disease, epilepsy, Parkinson's disease, disorders of the vagus nerve, low blood pressure, stomach ulcer.

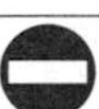 patients with obstructed intestines or urinary system.

 neomycin, clindamycin, colistin.

Neotigason *see* acitretin capsules
(Roche Products)

Nephril *see* polythiazide tablets
(Pfizer)

Nerisone/Nerisone Forte *see* topical corticosteroid cream/oily cream/ointment
(Schering Health Care)

Neulactil *see* pericyazine tablets/syrup
(Distriphar)

---

neuroleptic malignant syndrome

A rare but serious side effect of some drugs (e.g. haloperidol). Symptoms include high body temperature, varying level of consciousness, unstable blood pressure, incontinence, and rigid muscles.

N

Neurontin *see* gabapentin capsules/tablets
(Parke Davis and Co.)

Neutratop *see* metronidazole gel
(Smith and Nephew Healthcare)

Neutrogena dermatological cream *see* emollient cream
(Neutrogena (UK))

nevirapine suspension/tablets

A suspension or tablet used, in combination with other drugs, as an antiviral to treat HIV infection.

Strengths available: 200 mg tablets; 50 mg/5 ml suspension.
Dose: adults, 200 mg once a day at first, increasing to twice a day after 2 weeks; children over 2 months use reduced doses according to body weight.
Availability: NHS and private prescription.
Contains: nevirapine.
Brand names: Viramune.

 skin reactions, liver disorders, stomach upset, headache, drowsiness, tiredness, muscle pain, blood or kidney disorders, fever.

 in pregnant women and in patients with liver or kidney disorders. Your doctor will advise regular blood tests. Report any rash to your doctor.

 children under 2 months or mothers who are breastfeeding.

 ketoconazole, saquinavir, indinavir, ORAL CONTRACEPTIVES, alcohol, sedating drugs.

Nexium *see* esomeprazole tablets
(AstraZeneca UK)

nicardipine capsules/modified-release capsules

A capsule or M-R CAPSULE used as a CALCIUM-CHANNEL BLOCKER to treat high blood pressure and to prevent angina.

Strengths available: 20 mg and 30 mg capsules; 30 mg and 45 mg m-r capsules.
Dose: using standard capsules, adults usually 20-30 mg three times a day (maximum 120 mg a day); using m-r capsules (for high blood pressure only), adults 30-60 mg twice a day.
Availability: NHS and private prescription.
Contains: nicardipine hydrochloride.
Brand names: Cardene.

 chest pain, dizziness, headache, swelling of lower limbs, flushing, feeling warm, palpitations, stomach upset, sleeplessness, low blood pressure, rash, depression, blood disorders, pins and needles, breathing difficulty, impotence, increased need to pass urine.

 in the elderly and in patients suffering from a weak heart, heart failure, liver or kidney disease, or after a stroke.

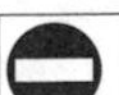

children under 18 years, pregnant women, mothers who are breastfeeding, or for patients with some heart valve disorders, heart shock, unstable or immediate angina, or recent heart attack.

grapefruit juice, amiodarone, rifampicin, anti-epileptic treatments, itraconazole, ALPHA-BLOCKERS, ritonavir, BETA-BLOCKERS, digoxin, cyclosporin, theophylline, aminophylline.

Nicef *see* cephradine capsules
(Galen)

---

nicorandil tablets

A tablet used to treat and prevent angina.

Strengths available: 10 mg and 20 mg tablets.
Dose: adults, 5-10 mg twice a day at first increasing if necessary to a maximum of 30 mg twice a day.
Availability: NHS and private prescription.
Contains: nicorandil.
Brand names: Ikorel.

sildenafil.

headache, widening of blood vessels, flushing, stomach upset, dizziness, low blood pressure and/or rapid heart rate at high doses, weakness, muscle pain, mouth ulcers.

in pregnant women.

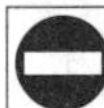
children, mothers who are breastfeeding, or for patients suffering from heart shock or failure, low blood pressure, fluid retention in the lungs, heart attack and other heart abnormalities.

Nicorette *see* nicotine replacement therapy
(Pharmacia and Upjohn)

---

nicotinamide gel

A gel used to treat acne.

dry skin, itching, redness, irritation.

in pregnant women (first 3 months). Avoid contact with eyes and mucous membranes.

Strengths available: 4% gel.
Dose: applied twice a day and reduced to once a day (or alternate days) if irritation occurs.
Availability: NHS and private prescription, over the counter.
Contains: nicotinamide.
Brand names: Papulex.

---

nicotinamide tablets

A tablet used to treat vitamin B_3 deficiency.

Strengths available: 50 mg tablets.
Dose: as advised by doctor.

cont.

Availability: NHS and private prescription, over the counter.
Contains: vitamin B_3.
Compound preparations: vitamin B compound tablets, vitamin B compound strong tablets.

---

nicotine replacement therapy patch/sublingual tablet/nasal spray/inhalation cartridge/lozenge/chewing gum

A patch, sublingual tablet, nasal spray, inhalator, lozenge, or chewing gum used as a source of nicotine to treat nicotine addiction and function as an aid to giving up smoking.

Strengths available: patches releasing 5 mg, 10 mg, or 15 mg in 16 hours; patches releasing 7 mg, 14 mg, or 21 mg in 24 hours; 2 mg and 4 mg chewing gum; 2 mg sublingual tablet; 10 mg inhalation cartridge; 0.5 mg per dose nasal spray; 1 mg lozenges

Dose: for adults, one patch applied to a clean, non-hairy, dry area of skin on upper arm or trunk and changed daily (16-hour patches removed overnight); 1 lozenge sucked slowly every 1-2 hours (maximum of 25 in 24 hours); the chewing gum chewed slowly for 30 minutes (maximum of 15 pieces in 24 hours); 1 spray of nasal spray into each nostril up to twice every hour (maximum 64 sprays a day) at first, reducing after 8 weeks; the inhalation cartridge used for inhalation when needed (maximum of 12 cartridges in 24 hours); 1 sublingual tablet dissolved under the tongue once or twice an hour (maximum 80 mg a day). Initial dose depends on number of cigarettes smoked. Maximum treatment period usually 3-6 months.

addiction, hiccups, stomach upset, irritated throat, increased saliva, headache, dizziness, palpitations, influenza-like symptoms, sleeplessness, muscle pain, chest pain, alteration to blood pressure, anxiety, sleepiness, poor concentration, period pain; skin reaction and inflamed blood vessels (with patches); nose bleeds or irritation, watering eyes, ear disorders (with nasal spray); mouth ulcers, swollen tongue, altered taste (with gum or sublingual tablet); dry mouth (with inhalation cartridge).

in patients with a history of stomach ulcers or inflammation, angina, recent heart attack, or suffering from heart disease, stroke, severe abnormal heart rhythm, high blood pressure, circulation disorders, diabetes, PHAEOCHROMOCYTOMA, kidney or liver disorders, angina, overactive thyroid, skin disorders (with patches). Do not smoke while using this treatment. Exercising while wearing a patch may increase side-effects. Do not drive while using the nasal spray.

children under 18 years, pregnant women, mothers who are breastfeeding, or for patients with severe heart or circulation disorders, recent stroke or other brain blood vessel disorder. Patches not to be used on broken skin.

theophylline, aminophylline, ANTICOAGULANTS, insulin.

Availability: private prescription, over the counter. Some brands also available on NHS.
Contains: nicotine.
Brand names: Nicorette, Nicotinell, NiQuitin CQ.

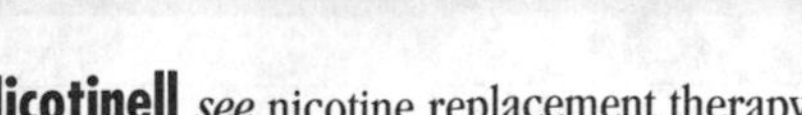

Nicotinell *see* nicotine replacement therapy
(Novartis Pharmaceuticals UK)

nicotinic acid tablets

A tablet used as a lipid-lowering agent to treat high blood lipids.

Strengths available: 50 mg tablets.
Dose: adults, 100-200 mg three times a day increased if necessary to 1000-2000 mg three times a day.
Availability: NHS and private prescription. (Available over the counter in small doses as vitamin supplement only – not for treating high lipid levels.)
Contains: nicotinic acid.

 flushing, dizziness, headache, irregular heartbeat, itching, stomach upset, liver disorders, rash.

 in patients suffering from diabetes, gout, liver disease, stomach ulcers.

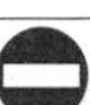 pregnant women or mothers who are breastfeeding.

 STATINS.

nicoumalone tablets

A tablet used as an ANTICOAGULANT to treat and prevent blood clots.

Strengths available: 1 mg tablets.
Dose: as advised by doctor.
Availability: NHS and private prescription.
Contains: nicoumalone (acenocoumarol).
Brand names: Sinthrome.

 bleeding, liver damage, reversible hair loss, stomach upset, headache, skin disorders, inflamed pancreas, purple toes.

 in mothers who are breastfeeding, the elderly, and in patients suffering from high blood pressure, reduced ability of protein in blood to bind drugs, severe heart failure, liver or kidney disease, stomach disorders, vitamin K deficiency. Your doctor will advise regular blood tests to determine correct dose.

 children, pregnant women, or for patients suffering from stomach ulcers, severe high blood pressure, some heart disorders, poor liver or kidney function, some blood disorders.

 alcohol, allopurinol, stanozolol, aspirin, NON-STEROIDAL ANTI-INFLAMMATORY DRUGS, cholestyramine, amiodarone, propafenone, quinidine, ANTIBIOTICS, some ANTIDEPRESSANTS, some antidiabetics, anti-epileptic treatments, antifungals, proguanil, clopidogrel, ticlopidine, ritonavir, chloral, primidone, CORTICOSTEROIDS, disulfiram, danazol, tamoxifen, thyroxine, lipid-lowering drugs, ORAL CONTRACEPTIVES, raloxifene, acitretin, testosterone, sucralfate, cimetidine, omeprazole, sulphinpyrazone, influenza vaccine, vitamin K.

nifedipine capsules and modified-release tablets/capsules

A capsule, M-R TABLET, or M-R CAPSULE used as a CALCIUM-CHANNEL BLOCKER to treat high blood pressure and prevent angina, and to treat Raynaud's phenomenon.

Strengths available: 5 mg and 10 mg capsules; 10 mg, 20 mg, 30 mg, 40 mg, and 60 mg M-R TABLETS;

cont.

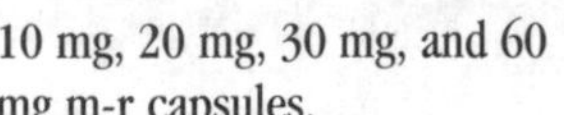

10 mg, 20 mg, 30 mg, and 60 mg m-r capsules.

Dose: adults, for Raynaud's phenomenon, 5-20 mg three times a day (using standard capsules) or 20-40 mg twice a day (using M-R TABLETS); for high blood pressure and angina, up to 90 mg a day (using m-r capsules or tablets) in one single dose or divided into two depending on brand used.

Availability: NHS and private prescription.

Contains: nifedipine.

Brand names: Adalat, Adipine, Angiopine, Calanif, Cardilate, Coracten, Fortipine, Hypolar Retard, Nifedipress, Nifopress, Nimodrel, Nivaten Retard, Slofedipine, Tensipine.

Compound preparations: Beta-Adalat, Tenif.

 headache, flushing, fluid retention, dizziness, chest pain, swollen gums, skin disorders, eye pain, depression, tiredness, abnormal heart rate, upset stomach, increased need to pass urine, pins and needles, muscle pain, shaking hands, impotence, swollen breasts, liver disorders, widened blood vessels.

 in patients with weak hearts, liver or kidney disease, low blood pressure, bowel disorders, or diabetes. Patients using m-r products should use the same brand of preparation once treatment is stabilized.

 children, pregnant women, mothers who are breastfeeding, or for patients suffering from PORPHYRIA, heart shock, narrowed heart valve, unstable or immediate angina attack, or within 1 month of heart attack.

 grapefruit juice, amiodarone, quinidine, rifampicin, antidiabetics, anti-epileptic treatments, itraconazole, ALPHA-BLOCKERS, ritonavir, BETA-BLOCKERS, digoxin, cyclosporin, theophylline, aminophylline.

Nifedipress *see* nifedipine modified-release tablets
(Berk Pharmaceuticals)

Niferex *see* polysaccharide-iron complex liquid/drops
(Tillomed Laboratories)

Nifopress Retard *see* nifedipine modified-release tablets
(Goldshield Healthcare)

---

nimodipine tablets

A tablet used as a CALCIUM-CHANNEL BLOCKER to treat symptoms following stroke.

Strengths available: 30 mg tablets.

Dose: 60 mg every 4 hours (360 mg per day) for 21 days.

Availability: NHS and private prescription.

Contains: nimodipine.

Brand names: Nimotop.

children, within 1 month of heart attack, or for patients with unstable angina.

some drugs used to treat high blood pressure or angina, BETA-BLOCKERS, drugs that may cause kidney disorders, grapefruit juice, amiodarone, ALPHA-BLOCKERS, ritonavir, theophylline, aminophylline, rifampicin, anti-epileptic treatments.

low blood pressure, flushing, headache, changes in heart rate, stomach upset, swollen ankles, dizziness, weakness, pins and needles, muscle pain, shaking hands, skin reactions, increased need to pass urine, liver disturbance, worsening of angina, swollen gums or breasts, visual disturbances.

in pregnant women and in patients suffering from fluid retention in the brain or high pressure in the brain, kidney or liver disorders.

Nimodrel Retard *see* nifedipine modified-release tablets
(Opus Pharmaceuticals)

Nimotop *see* nimodipine tablets
(Bayer Pharma Business Group)

Nindaxa *see* indapamide tablets
(Ashbourne Pharmaceuticals)

Niquitin CQ *see* nicotine replacement therapy
(SmithKline Beecham Consumer Healthcare UK)

---

nisoldipine modified-release tablets

An M-R TABLET used as a CALCIUM-CHANNEL BLOCKER to treat high blood pressure and prevent angina.

Strengths available: 10 mg, 20 mg, and 30 mg m-r tablets.
Dose: adults, 10 mg each morning before food increasing if necessary to a maximum of 40 mg a day.
Availability: NHS and private prescription.
Contains: nisoldipine.
Brand names: Syscor MR.

ALPHA-BLOCKERS, BETA-BLOCKERS, drugs that cause kidney disorders, grapefruit juice, amiodarone, prazosin, ritonavir, theophylline, aminophylline, rifampicin, anti-epileptic treatments, itraconazole.

swollen ankles, headache, flushing, altered heart rhythm, weakness, dizziness, stomach upset, pins and needles, muscle pain, shaking hands, low blood pressure, difficulty breathing, skin disorders, increased need to pass urine, liver disorders, worsening of angina, swollen gums and breasts, visual disturbances.

in the elderly and in patients with low blood pressure.

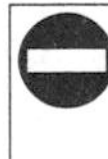
children, pregnant women, mothers who are breastfeeding, or for patients with heart shock, abnormally high blood pressure, narrowed heart valves, unstable or immediate angina attacks, liver disorders, or within 1 week of heart attack.

N

nitrate

A drug used to treat poor blood supply to the heart muscle (angina). Nitrates reduce the work that the heart has to do. Example, glyceryl trinitrate tablets.

---

nitrazepam suspension/tablets

A tablet or suspension used for the short-term treatment of sleeplessness.

Strengths available: 5 mg tablets; 2.5 mg/5 ml suspension.
Dose: adults 5-10 mg (elderly or weak patients 2.5-5 mg) at bedtime.
Availability: NHS (if written generically) and private prescription.
Contains: nitrazepam.
Brand names: Mogadon, Somnite (neither available on NHS).

Side effects: drowsiness, light-headedness, confusion, vertigo, stomach disturbances, loss of memory, aggression, headache, joint immobility, salivation changes, shaking, unsteadiness, low blood pressure, rash, changes in vision, changes in sexual desire, retention of urine, incontinence, blood changes, jaundice. Risk of addiction increases with dose and length of treatment. May impair judgement.

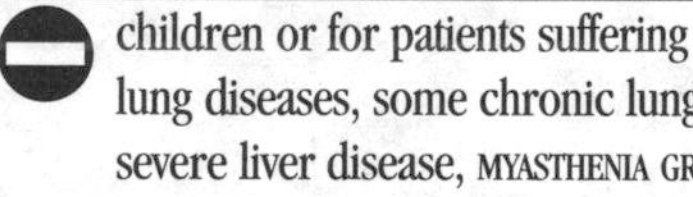

Not to be used for: children or for patients suffering from acute lung diseases, some chronic lung diseases, severe liver disease, MYASTHENIA GRAVIS, some obsessional and psychotic disorders, or who have stopped breathing while asleep.

Caution: in elderly or weak patients, pregnant women, mothers who are breastfeeding, and in patients suffering from lung disorders, kidney or liver disorders, muscle weakness, PORPHYRIA, or with a history of drug or alcohol abuse, or personality disorder. Avoid long-term use, and withdraw gradually.

Caution needed with: alcohol, other sedating drugs, ritonavir, phenytoin.

Nitro-Dur *see* glyceryl trinitrate patches
(Schering-Plough)

N

nitrofurantoin tablets/capsules/modified-release capsules

A tablet, capsule, or M-R CAPSULE used as an antiseptic to treat and prevent infection of the urinary tract.

Strengths available: 50 mg or 100 mg tablets and capsules; 100 mg m-r capsules.
Dose: adults, 50-100 mg four times a day (using standard tablets or capsules) with food or milk for 7 days to treat infection, 50-100 mg at night to prevent infection; children use reduced doses according to body weight; using m-r capsules, adults 100 mg twice a day.
Availability: NHS and private prescription.
Contains: nitrofurantoin.

Side effects: stomach upset, loss of appetite, numbness in hands and feet, severe allergic reaction, symptoms similar to LUPUS, blood changes, liver disorders, temporary hair loss, lung disorders, skin disorders, inflamed pancreas, itching, brown-coloured urine, joint disorders, high pressure in the brain.

Caution: in the elderly and in patients suffering from anaemia, diabetes, chemical disturbance, vitamin B deficiency, lung or liver disorders, and in those prone to nerve disorders in hands and feet.

Brand names: Furadantin, Macrobid, Macrodantin, Urantoin.

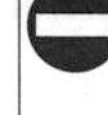 infants under 3 months, pregnant women, mothers who are breastfeeding, or for patients suffering from poor kidney function, PORPHYRIA, or who are prone to anaemia and jaundice caused by drugs.

 magnesium trisilicate.

Nitrolingual *see* glyceryl trinitrate spray
(Lipha Pharmaceuticals)

Nitromin *see* glyceryl trinitrate spray
(Servier Laboratories)

Nivaquine *see* chloroquine tablets/syrup
(Rhône-Poulenc Rorer)

Nivaten Retard *see* nifedipine modified-release tablets
(Cox Pharmaceuticals)

Nivemycin *see* neomycin tablets
(Sovereign Medical)

---

nizatidine capsules

A capsule used as a HISTAMINE H_2-ANTAGONIST to treat and prevent stomach ulcers (including those caused by NON-STEROIDAL ANTI-INFLAMMATORY DRUGS) and to treat acid reflux from the stomach.

Strengths available: 150 mg and 300 mg capsules.
Dose: adult dose to treat ulcers, 300 mg at night or 150 mg twice a day for 4-8 weeks; to prevent ulcers, 150 mg at night; for acid reflux, 150-300 mg twice a day for up to 12 weeks.
Availability: NHS and private prescription.
Contains: nizatidine.
Brand names: Axid, Zinga.

 headache, dizziness, upset stomach, bowel discomfort, liver disorders, tiredness, sweating. Rarely, breast swelling, skin disorders, inflamed pancreas, heart rhythm or conduction disorders, confusion, depression, blood disorders, severe allergic reaction, inflamed blood vessels, high uric acid levels in the blood, fever, muscle or joint pain.

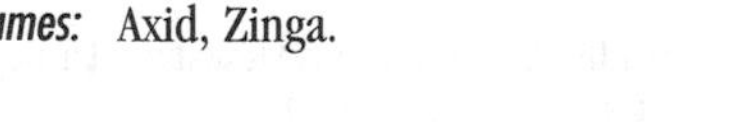

 in pregnant women, mothers who are breastfeeding, in patients who are middle-aged or older, and in those suffering from kidney or liver disorders. Treatment may mask symptoms of stomach cancer.

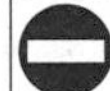 children.

Nizoral *see* ketoconazole tablets and ketoconazole cream/shampoo
(Janssen-Cilag)

Nocutil *see* desmopressin nasal spray
(Norgine)

Nolvadex/D/Forte *see* tamoxifen tablets
(Zeneca Pharma)

---

non-steroidal anti-inflammatory drug (NSAID)

An antirheumatic preparation that has pain-killing properties and reduces inflammation. An NSAID may cause stomach upsets. Example, ibuprofen.

---

non-steroidal anti-inflammatory drug (topical)

A cream, gel, ointment, mousse, or spray applied to the skin and used as a NON-STEROIDAL ANTI-INFLAMMATORY DRUG to relieve symptoms of rheumatic and muscular pain, sprains and strains.

Dose: *see* table below.
Availability: NHS and private prescription. Many are also available over the counter (*marked * in table below*).
Contains: *see* table below.

reddening of skin or rash, sensitivity to sunlight. Rarely (or with excessive use), asthma, kidney disorders, upset stomach or aggravation of stomach ulcer.

in pregnant women and mothers who are breastfeeding (most brands are not recommended), and in patients with kidney disorders, asthma, or stomach ulcers. Avoid broken skin, lips, mucous membranes, and eyes. Do not cover with a dressing. Avoid excessive exposure of treated skin to sunlight.

other non-steroidal anti-inflammatory drugs (whether taken internally, or applied to the skin).

children or for patients suffering from allergy to aspirin or non-steroidal anti-inflammatory drugs.

Product	*Brand names*	*Frequency of application*
benzydamine cream*	Difflam	3-6 times a day for up to 10 days
diclofenac gel	Voltarol Emulgel	3-4 times a day and review after 14 days (or 28 days for osteoarthritis)
felbinac gel/foam	Traxam	2-4 times a day and review after 14 days
heparinoid + salicylic acid cream/gel*	Movelat	up to 4 times a day

ibuprofen 10% gel (some brands*)	Fenbid Forte, Ibugel Forte, Ibuleve Maximum Strength	up to 4 times a day and review after 14 days
ibuprofen 5% cream/ gel/mousse/spray*	Fenbid, Ibugel, Ibuleve, Ibumousse, Ibuspray, Proflex	3-4 times a day
ketoprofen gel	Ketil, Oruvail, Powergel	2-4 times a day for up to 7 days or 2-3 times a day for up to 10 days
piroxicam gel	Feldene	3-4 times a day, and review after 4 weeks

**available over the counter.*

nonoxynol cream/gel/foam/pessaries

A cream, gel, foam, or pessary used in addition to barrier contraceptives (condoms or diaphragms) to prevent pregnancy.

Strengths available: 2% cream or gel; 12.5% foam; 5% pessaries.
Dose: 1 pessary or 1 dose of gel/cream/foam applied into the vagina before intercourse. Cream or gel also applied to the inner surface and rim of the diaphragm before intercourse
Availability: NHS and private prescription, over the counter,
Contains: nonoxynol-9.
Brand names: Delfen, Double Check, Duragel, Gynol II, Ortho-Creme, Orthoforms, Prelude.

Caution: not very effective as contraceptive unless used in conjunction with barriers.

Not to be used for: children.

Nootropil *see* piracetam solution/tablets

(UCB Pharma)

Norditropin *see* somatropin injection

(Novo Nordisk Pharmaceuticals)

norethisterone tablets

A tablet used as a progestogen treatment for postponing menstruation, and for other menstrual and womb disorders (such as endometriosis, painful or heavy periods).

Strengths available: 5 mg tablets.
Dose: usually 5 mg 2-3 times a day.
Availability: NHS and private prescription.
Contains: norethisterone.

Side effects: stomach upset, disorders of the skin and mucous membranes, depression, sleeplessness, drowsiness, hair loss or growth, liver disturbance, severe allergic reaction, breast pain, milk production, abnormal menstrual bleeding, headache, weight gain, fluid retention, changes in sexual desire, worsening of epilepsy or migraine.

cont.

N

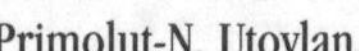

Brand names: Primolut-N, Utovlan.
Compound preparations: HORMONE REPLACEMENT THERAPY (COMBINED), ORAL CONTRACEPTIVE (COMBINED).
Other preparations: norethisterone injection, ORAL CONTRACEPTIVE (PROGESTOGEN-ONLY), Micronor HRT.

 cyclosporin, alcohol, sedating drugs.

 in patients suffering from diabetes, high blood pressure, epilepsy, migraine, asthma, breast disorders, fibroids, gallstones, multiple sclerosis, some skin cancers, LUPUS, heart or kidney disease, or who have a history of depression.

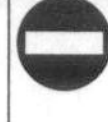 children, pregnant women, or for patients suffering from some cancers, undiagnosed vaginal bleeding, PORPHYRIA, or with a history of liver disease or some skin disorders.

norethisterone injection

An injection used as a progestogen contraceptive (for short-term use).

Strengths available: 200 mg injection.
Dose: 200 mg injected and repeated once if required (after 8 weeks).
Availability: NHS and private prescription.
Contains: norethisterone enantate.
Brand names: Noristerat.
Compound preparations: ORAL CONTRACEPTIVES (COMBINED).
Other preparations: etonogestrel implant, medroxyprogesterone injection, norethisterone tablets, ORAL CONTRACEPTIVE (PROGESTOGEN-ONLY).

 pregnant women or for patients suffering from severe heart or blood vessel disease, benign liver tumours, PORPHYRIA, undiagnosed vaginal bleeding, some womb disorders.

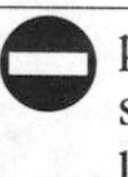

 irregular bleeding, upset stomach, dizziness, depression, skin disorders, change in appetite, weight gain, change in sexual desire, breast discomfort, headache, ovarian cyst, rarely blood clots. There appears to be a small increase in risk of breast cancer but this may be the result of earlier diagnosis through regular examinations.

 in patients suffering from heart disease, high blood pressure, disordered absorption of nutrients from the gut, diabetes, migraine, some cancers, blood lipid disorders, liver abnormalities, ovarian cysts, or those who have had a previous ectopic pregnancy or blood clot, or itching/ear disorders during pregnancy. Your doctor may advise regular examinations. Mothers who are breast-feeding should not feed newborn infants who have severe or persistent jaundice.

 BARBITURATES, phenytoin, primidone, carbamazepine, chloral hydrate, ethosuximide, rifampicin, chlorpromazine, meprobamate, griseofulvin, topiramate, modafinil, cyclosporin, nevirapine, celecoxib.

norfloxacin tablets

A tablet used as an ANTIBIOTIC to treat urinary infections.

Strengths available: 400 mg tablets.
Dose: adults, usually 400 mg twice a day for 3 days (simple urine infections), for 7-10 days (complicated infections), or up to 12 weeks in persistent infections (reducing to 400 mg once a day after 4 weeks if symptoms subside).
Availability: NHS and private prescription.

Contains: norfloxacin.
Brand names: Utinor.

children, pregnant women, or mothers who are breastfeeding.

ANTICOAGULANTS, theophylline, aminophylline, cyclosporin, NON-STEROIDAL ANTI-INFLAMMATORY DRUGS, didanosine, alcohol, sedating drugs.

severe allergy, stomach upset, headache, dizziness, sleep disorders, skin disorders. Rarely, loss of appetite, blood changes, drowsiness, fits, confusion, depression, difficulty breathing, shaking hands, hallucinations, pins and needles, sensitivity to light, muscle and joint pain, disturbance of the senses, liver and kidney disorders, anxiety, inflamed blood vessels, excitement, inflamed pancreas.

in patients suffering from kidney disease, MYASTHENIA GRAVIS, or with a history of epilepsy or liver disorders. Avoid excessive exposure to sunlight.

Norgalax *see* docusate enema
(Norgine)

---

norgestimate *see* oral contraceptive (combined)

Norgeston *see* oral contraceptive (progestogen only)
(Schering Health Care)

---

norgestrel *see* hormone replacement therapy (combined), oral contraceptive (progestogen-only), Schering PC4

Noriday *see* oral contraceptive (progestogen only)
(Searle)

Norimin *see* oral contraceptive (combined)
(Searle)

Norimode *see* loperamide capsules
(Tillomed Laboratories)

Norinyl-1 *see* oral contraceptive (combined)
(Searle)

Noristerat *see* norethisterone injection
(Schering Health Care)

Noritate *see* metronidazole cream
(Kestrel Healthcare)

Normacol/Normacol Plus *see* sterculia granules
(Norgine)

Normasol/Normasol Twist *see* saline solution (sterile)
(SSL International)

Normax *see* co-danthrusate capsules/suspension
(Medeva Pharma)

Norphyllin *see* aminophylline modified-release tablets
(Norton Healthcare)

Norprolac *see* quinagolide tablets
(Novartis Pharmaceuticals UK)

nortriptyline tablets

A tablet used as a TRICYCLIC ANTIDEPRESSANT to treat depression, and bedwetting in children.

Strengths available: 10 mg and 25 mg tablets.
Dose: adults, 25 mg 3-4 times a day (or 75-100 mg once a day) at first increasing to 150 mg a day if needed; elderly and adolescent patients 30-50 mg a day; children aged 7 years and over (for bedwetting only), 10-35 mg at night according to age for up to 3 months.
Availability: NHS and private prescription.
Contains: nortriptyline hydrochloride.
Brand names: Allegron.
Compound preparations: Motipress, Motival.

dry mouth, noises in the ears, tiredness, constipation, difficulty passing urine, blurred vision, stomach upset, palpitations, drowsiness, sleeplessness, dizziness, shaking hands, low blood pressure, weight change, sweating, fever, behavioural changes in children, confusion in the elderly, skin reactions, jaundice or blood changes, interference with sexual function, changes in heart rhythm, rash, hormone disturbances, fits, movement disorders, blood changes, breast changes in women, menstrual disorders.

in the elderly, pregnant women, mothers who are breastfeeding, and in patients suffering from heart disease, liver and kidney disorders, thyroid disease, PHAEOCHROMOCYTOMA, epilepsy, diabetes, PORPHYRIA, glaucoma, urine retention, constipation, some other psychiatric conditions. Your doctor may advise regular blood tests.

children under 7 years or for patients suffering from recent heart attacks, heart rhythm abnormalities, severe liver disease, or elevated mood.

N

 alcohol, sedatives, MAOIS, BARBITURATES, other ANTIDEPRESSANTS, ANTIHYPERTENSIVES, tranquillizers, anti-epileptic drugs, ritonavir, entacapone, selegiline, sotalol, halofantrine, drugs affecting heart rhythm, methylphenidate.

Norvir *see* ritonavir capsules/liquid
(Abbott Laboratories)

Nova T

(Schering Health Care)
A copper wire with silver core used as an intra-uterine device to prevent conception.

Dose: insertion usually between the end of the menstrual period and the mid-point of the cycle, then left in place for 5 years.
Availability: NHS and private prescription.
Contains: copper wire.
Other preparations: Multiload.

 pelvic infection, pain, abnormal bleeding, perforation of the uterus or cervix. On insertion, pain, epileptic attack, asthma attack, persistent low heart rate.

 in women who have not had children and in patients suffering from heart disease, anaemia, endometriosis, HIV infection, diabetes, epilepsy, or who have had a previous ectopic pregnancy, fertility problems, or joint replacement. Your doctor may advise regular examinations.

 ANTICOAGULANTS.

 pregnant women or for patients suffering from inflamed pelvis, abnormal or inflamed uterus or cervix, genital infection, reduced resistance to infection, PORPHYRIA, undiagnosed vaginal bleeding, some cancers, allergy to copper, Wilson's disease, some womb or blood disorders, or who have a history of heart or pelvic infection.

Novofine *see* insulin injection devices
(Novo Nordisk Pharmaceuticals)

Novonorm *see* repaglinide tablets
(Novo Nordisk Pharmaceuticals)

Novopen *see* insulin injection devices
(Novo Nordisk Pharmaceuticals)

Novorapid *see* insulin
(Novo Nordisk Pharmaceuticals)

Nozinan *see* methotrimeprazine tablets
(Link Pharmaceuticals)

NSAID *see* non-steroidal anti-inflammatory drug

Nuelin/Nuelin SA *see* theophylline liquid/tablets/modified-release tablets
(3M Health Care)

Nupercainal *see* cinchocaine ointment
(Eastern Pharmaceuticals)

Nu-Seals *see* aspirin enteric-coated tablets 75 mg and aspirin enteric-coated tablets 300 mg
(Eli Lilly and Co.)

Nutraplus *see* urea cream
(Galderma (UK))

Nutrizym /Nutrizym GR *see* pancreatin capsules
(E. Merck Pharmaceuticals)

Nuvelle /Nuvelle Continuous/Nuvelle TS *see* hormone replacement therapy (combined)
(Schering Health Care)

Nycopren *see* naproxen tablets
(Ardern Healthcare)

Nystaform *see* nystatin cream
(Typharm)

Nystaform-HC *see* nystatin cream/ointment and topical corticosteroid cream/ointment
(Typharm)

Nystan *see* nystatin cream/ointment, nystatin pastilles/suspension, nystatin tablets, nystatin vaginal cream/pessaries
(Bristol-Myers Squibb Pharmaceuticals)

---

nystatin cream/ointment

A cream or ointment used as an antifungal treatment for thrush of the skin.

Strengths available: 100,000 units/g cream and ointment.

Side effects: irritation and burning.

Dose: apply to the affected area 2-4 times a day.
Availability: NHS and private prescription.
Contains: nystatin.
Brand names: Nystan.
Compound preparations: Nystaform (with chlorhexidine), Tinaderm-M, for preparations containing nystatin and steroids *see* topical corticosteroid.
Other preparations: nystatin pastilles/suspension, nystatin tablets, nystatin vaginal cream/pessaries.

---

nystatin pastilles/suspension

A pastille or oral suspension used as an antifungal treatment for thrush in the mouth or intestines (*see also* nystatin tablets).

Strengths available: 100,000 units/ml suspension; 100,000 units per pastille.

Side effects: upset stomach, mouth irritation, skin disorders.

Dose: 100,000 units four times a day after food, usually for 7 days. (Higher doses may be needed if the immune system is not working.) Continue until 48 hours after symptoms disappear. Pastilles are sucked slowly. For suspension, the dose is held in the mouth for as long as possible then swallowed.
Availability: NHS and private prescription, nurse prescription.
Contains: nystatin.
Brand names: Nystan.
Other preparations: nystatin cream/ointment, nystatin tablets, nystatin vaginal cream/pessaries.

N

nystatin tablets

A tablet used as an antifungal to treat and prevent fungal infections in the intestines.

Strengths available: 500,000 units per tablet.

Side effects: upset stomach, mouth irritation, skin disorders.

Dose: adults, 500,000 units every 6 hours (doubled in severe infections). Children use nystatin oral suspension.
Availability: NHS and private prescription.
Contains: nystatin.
Brand names: Nystan.
Other preparations: nystatin cream/ointment, nystatin pastilles/oral suspension, nystatin vaginal cream/pessaries.

---

nystatin vaginal cream/pessaries

A pessary or vaginal cream used as an antifungal treatment for vaginal thrush.

Strengths available: 100,000 units per dose vaginal cream; 100,000 unit pessaries.
Dose: 100,000-200,000 units applied into the vagina at night for at least 14 nights. (Additionally, nystatin cream/ointment may be applied to external genital area.)
Availability: NHS and private prescription.
Contains: nystatin.
Brand names: Nystan.
Compound preparations: Flagyl Compak (with metronidazole tablets).
Other preparations: nystatin cream/ointment, nystatin pastilles/oral suspension, nystatin tablets.

Side effects: temporary irritation.

Caution: in pregnant women and mothers who are breastfeeding. Avoid contact with barrier contraceptives.

Not to be used for: pessaries not to be used by children.

Occlusal *see* salicylic acid collodion
(DermaPharm)

Ocufen *see* flurbiprofen eye drops
(Allergan)

Oculotect *see* povidone eye drops
(CIBA Vision Ophthalmics)

Ocusert Pilo *see* pilocarpine eye drops
(Dominion Pharma)

Odrik *see* trandolapril capsules
(Hoechst Marion Roussel)

---

oestradiol *see* hormone replacement therapy (combined), hormone replacement therapy (oestrogen-only), hormone replacement therapy (topical)

---

oestriol *see* hormone replacement therapy (oestrogen-only), hormone replacement therapy (topical)

Oestrogel *see* hormone replacement therapy (oestrogen-only)
(Hoechst Marion Roussel)

---

oestrogen *see* hormone replacement therapy (combined), hormone replacement therapy (oestrogen-only), oral contraceptive (combined)

oestrone *see* hormone replacement therapy (oestrogen-only)

ofloxacin eye drops

Drops used as an ANTIBIOTIC to treat bacterial infections of the eye.

Strengths available: 0.3% drops.
Dose: 1-2 drops in the affected eye(s) every 2-4 hours for the first 2 days, then reduced to four times a day. (Maximum of 10 days treatment.)
Availability: NHS and private prescription.
Contains: ofloxacin.
Brand names: Exocin.

irritation, intolerance of light. Occasionally, headache, nausea, numbness, dizziness.

in pregnant women and mothers who are breastfeeding.

patients who wear soft contact lenses.

ofloxacin tablets

A tablet used as an ANTIBIOTIC to treat urine, genital, or chest infections.

Strengths available: 200 mg or 400 mg tablets.
Dose: adults, 200-400 mg once or twice a day depending on condition and severity of infection.
Availability: NHS and private prescription.
Contains: ofloxacin.
Brand names: Tarivid.

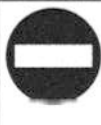
children, pregnant women, mothers who are breastfeeding, or for patients suffering from severe kidney disease.

alcohol, sedatives, ANTICOAGULANTS, cyclosporin, NON-STEROIDAL ANTI-INFLAMMATORY DRUGS, glibenclamide.

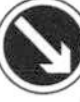
allergy, stomach upset, headache, dizziness, sleep disorders, skin disorders. Rarely, loss of appetite, blood changes, drowsiness, fits, hallucinations, pins and needles, sensitivity to light, muscle and joint pain, disturbance of the senses, liver and kidney disorders, rapid heart beat, temporary low blood pressure, blood vessel disorders, unsteadiness, shaking hands, nerve disorders, mental disorders, change in blood sugar, lung inflammation.

in patients suffering from kidney disease or with a history of epilepsy, liver disorders, or mental disorders. Avoid excessive exposure to sunlight.

Oilatum *see* emollient bath oil/cream/gel/soap
(Stiefel Laboratories (UK))

Oilatum Plus *see* emollient bath oil
(Stiefel Laboratories (UK))

oily cream *see* hydrous ointment (alternative name)

Okacyn *see* lomefloxacin eye drops
(CIBA Vision Ophthalmics)

---

olanzapine tablets

A tablet (standard version or tablet to dissolve on the tongue/disperse in water) used as a sedative to treat schizophrenia.

Strengths available: 2.5 mg, 5 mg, 7.5 mg, and 10 mg standard tablets; 5 mg and 10 mg tablets to dissolve on the tongue/disperse in water.
Dose: adults, up to 10 mg a day at first, adjusted according to response to 5-20 mg a day.
Availability: NHS and private prescription.
Contains: olanzapine.
Brand names: Zyprexa.

Caution needed with: drugs that affect heart rhythm, other sedating drugs, alcohol, ANTIDEPRESSANTS, anti-epileptic treatments, halofantrine, ritonavir.

Side effects: increased appetite, weight gain, dizziness, low blood pressure on standing, drowsiness, ANTIMUSCARINIC effects, rapid heart rate, shaking hands, movement disorders, NEUROLEPTIC MALIGNANT SYNDROME, fluid retention, blood changes, liver disorders. Occasionally, sensitivity to light.

Caution: in the elderly, pregnant women, and in patients with a history of epilepsy or who are suffering from enlarged prostate, glaucoma, heart or circulation disorders, inactive bowel, liver or kidney disorders, diabetes, some blood disorders, or Parkinson's disease.

Not to be used for: children under 18 years, mothers who are breastfeeding, or for patients suffering from some types of glaucoma.

Olbetam *see* acipimox capsules
(Pharmacia and Upjohn)

---

olive oil *see* olive oil ear drops, Rowachol

O

---

olive oil ear drops

An oil used to soften ear wax before syringing the ear.

Dose: for hard wax, use a few drops twice a day for a few days before syringing. Lie with the affected ear uppermost for a few minutes after instilling the drops.
Availability: NHS and private prescription, nurse prescription, over the counter.
Contains: olive oil.

Not to be used for: patients with perforated ear drum.

---

olsalazine capsules/tablets

A tablet or capsule used to treat (and maintain remission of) ulcerative colitis (an inflammatory bowel disorder).

Strengths available: 250 mg capsules; 500 mg tablets.
Dose: adults 1000-3000 mg a day (in divided doses) after food. (500 mg twice a day for maintenance.)
Availability: NHS and private prescription.
Contains: olsalazine sodium.
Brand names: Dipentum.

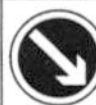

stomach upset, headache, abdominal pain, gallstones, worsening of colitis, rash, LUPUS-like symptoms, kidney disorders, joint pain. Rarely, blood disorders, inflamed pancreas.

in pregnant women. Your doctor may advise regular blood and urine tests. Report any unexplained bruising, bleeding, fever, tiredness, or sore throat to your doctor.

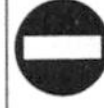

children, mothers who are breastfeeding, or patients with severe kidney damage or who are allergic to aspirin and similar drugs.

---

omega-3 marine triglycerides *see* Maxepa

---

omeprazole capsules/tablets

A capsule or tablet used to treat stomach ulcers (and to treat or prevent those resulting from NON-STEROIDAL ANTI-INFLAMMTORY DRUGS), to treat acid reflux into the oesophagus and other acid-related indigestion symptoms, and for *H. PYLORI* ERADICATION.

Strengths available: 10 mg, 20 mg, and 40 mg tablets and capsules.
Dose: for reflux, usually 20-40 mg once a day for 4-8 weeks to heal the condition, then 10-20 mg a day to prevent relapse; for ulcers, 20-40 mg once a day for 4-8 weeks (then continuing with 10-20 mg once a day for prevention); for acid-related indigestion, 10-20 mg once a day for 2-4 weeks; for other conditions of excess acid (such as Zollinger-Ellison syndrome), up to 120 mg a day (in divided doses) may be required.
Availability: NHS and private prescription.
Contains: omeprazole.
Brand names: Losec.
Compound preparations: *H. pylori* eradication.

headache, upset stomach, skin disorders. Rarely, blood changes, fluid retention, depression, muscle and joint pain, itching, severe allergy, tiredness, dry mouth, skin reactions, hair loss, blurred vision, sensitivity to sunlight, pins and needles, kidney and liver disorders, difficulty breathing, fever, drowsiness, sweating, confusion, agitation, vertigo, hallucinations, sleeplessness, taste disturbance, swollen breasts and impotence.

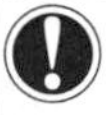

in patients aged over 45 years or with liver disorders. Stomach cancer should be excluded before treatment.

children, pregnant women, or mothers who are breastfeeding.

ANTICOAGULANTS, digoxin, phenytoin, alcohol, sedating drugs.

O

Omnic MR *see* tamsulosin capsules
(Paines and Byrne)

Omnikan *see* insulin injection devices
(B. Braun Medical)

---

ondansetron tablets/syrup/suppository

A tablet (standard version or type to dissolve on the tongue), syrup, or suppository used to treat nausea and vomiting associated with cancer treatment or surgical operation.

Strengths available: 4 mg and 8 mg tablets and mouth-dispersible tablets; 4 mg/5 ml syrup; 16 mg suppositories.
Dose: as advised by doctor.
Availability: NHS and private prescription.
Contains: ondansetron hydrochloride.
Brand names: Zofran.

 constipation, headache, flushing, liver changes, hiccups, abnormal movements, fits, chest pain, low blood pressure, change in heart rhythm. Suppositories may irritate the rectum.

 in pregnant women.

 mothers who are breastfeeding.

One Alpha *see* alfacalcidol capsules/drops
(Leo Pharmaceuticals)

One Touch
(Lifescan)
A plastic reagent strip used in conjunction with One Touch Basic and One Touch Profile meters to detect blood glucose levels. Blood-glucose monitoring enables individual patients suffering from diabetes accurately to control blood glucose and manage their condition.

Availability: NHS and private prescription, nurse prescription, over the counter.

Opilon *see* thymoxamine tablets
(Hansam Healthcare)

---

opioid *see* analgesic

Oprisine *see* azathioprine tablets
(Opus Pharmaceuticals)

Opticrom Aqueous *see* sodium cromoglycate eye drops
(Rhône-Poulenc Rorer)

Optil/Optil XL *see* diltiazem tablets/modified-release tablets
(Opus Pharmaceuticals)

Optilast *see* azelastine eye drops
(ASTA Medica)

Optimax *see* tryptophan tablets
(E. Merck Pharmaceuticals)

Optimine *see* azatadine syrup
(Schering-Plough)

Optipen Pro 1 *see* insulin injection devices
(Aventis Pharma)

Orabase
(Convatec)
An ointment used to protect mucous membranes by forming a layer over mouth ulcers and sore areas of other moist body surfaces.

Dose: apply a thin layer to affected area when needed.
Availability: NHS and private prescription.
Contains: carmellose sodium, pectin, gelatin.
Other preparations: Orahesive.

Orabet *see* metformin tablets
(Lagap Pharmaceuticals)

Orahesive
(Convatec)
A powder used to protect mucous membranes by forming a layer over sore areas of moist body surfaces.

Dose: sprinkle over affected area when needed.
Availability: NHS and private prescription.
Contains: carmellose sodium, pectin, gelatin.
Other preparations: Orabase.

Oraldene *see* hexetidine mouthwash
(Warner Lambert Consumer Healthcare)

oral contraceptive (combined)

A tablet used as an oestrogen and progestogen contraceptive. Low-, normal-, and high-strength preparations are available (*see* table).

Dose: 1 tablet a day (taken in sequence from the pack) for 21 days followed by 7 days without treatment. Some brands (marked * in the table opposite) include 7 inactive tablets to allow one tablet to be taken every day without a break. Usually started on the first day of menstrual bleeding. After child-birth, start the tablets 3 weeks after the birth.

Availability: NHS and private prescription.

Contains: (*see* table opposite).

pregnant women, mothers who are breast-feeding, women over 50 years, patients with a history of heart disease or blood clots, or those suffering from liver disorders, some cancers, severe migraine or migraine associated with visual disturbance, temporary blocking of blood vessels in the brain, PORPHYRIA, undiagnosed vaginal bleeding, or some ear, skin, and kidney disorders.

ACE-INHIBITORS, rifampicin, some other ANTIBIOTICS, ANTICOAGULANTS, ANTIDEPRESSANTS, antidiabetics, some antifungal treatments, ANTIHYPERTENSIVES, modafinil, griseofulvin, BARBITURATES, phenytoin, primidone, carbamazepine, ethosuximide, chloral hydrate, celecoxib, cyclosporin, tretinoin, CORTICOSTEROIDS, tacrolimus, theophylline, aminophylline, lansoprazole, topiramate.

enlarged breasts, bloating and fluid retention, cramps, leg pains, mood change, reduction in sexual desire, headache, upset stomach, vaginal erosion, discharge and bleeding, jaundice, weight gain, skin changes, muscle twitches, raised blood pressure, liver disorder, altered menstrual pattern. Rarely, sensitivity to sunlight. Contact lenses may irritate. There is a slightly increased risk of blood clots (particularly with products containing gestodene or desogestrel) but this is still lower than the risk of blood clots during pregnancy. Also a slightly increased risk of breast cancer but this may be the result of earlier diagnosis through regular examinations. Risk of womb and ovary cancer is decreased.

in women over 35 years, overweight or immobile patients, smokers, or those suffering from high blood pressure, diabetes, varicose veins or other blood vessel disorders, inflammatory bowel disorders, some blood disorders, sickle-cell anaemia, asthma, migraine, depression, kidney disease, multiple sclerosis, womb diseases. Your doctor may advise you not to smoke and to have regular examinations. You should stop treatment at the first sign of serious symptoms such as severe headache or jaundice. Treatment should be stopped 4 weeks before surgery. Depending on when you start the course, you may need additional (barrier) contraceptives for the first 7 days.

Product	*Ingredients*	*Strength*
Binovum	2 different-strength tablets containing norethisterone 0.5-1 mg + ethinyloestradiol 35 mcg at various stages in cycle	normal
Brevinor	norethisterone 0.5 mg + ethinyloestradiol 35 mcg	normal
Cilest	norgestimate 250 mcg + ethinyloestradiol 35 mcg	normal
Eugynon 30	levonorgestrel 250 mcg + ethinyloestradiol 30 mcg	normal
Femodene	gestodene 75 mcg + ethinyloestradiol 30 mcg	normal
Femodene ED*	gestodene 75 mcg + ethinyloestradiol 30 mcg and inactive tablets	normal
Femodette	gestodene 75 mcg , ethinyloestradiol 20 mcg	low
Loestrin 20	norethisterone 1 mg + ethinyloestradiol 20 mcg	low
Loestrin 30	norethisterone 1.5 mg + ethinyloestradiol 30 mcg	normal
Logynon	3 different-strength tablets containing levonorgestrel 50-125 mcg + ethinyloestradiol 30-40 mcg at various stages in cycle	normal
Logynon ED*	3 different-strength tablets containing levonorgestrel 50-125 mcg + ethinyloestradiol 30-40 mcg at various stages in cycle, and inactive tablets	normal
Marvelon	desogestrel 150 mcg + ethinyloestradiol 30 mcg	normal
Mercilon	desogestrel 150 mcg + ethinyloestradiol 20 mcg	low
Microgynon 30	levonorgestrel 150 mcg + ethinyloestradiol 30 mcg	normal
Microgynon 30 ED*	levonorgestrel 150 mcg + ethinyloestradiol 30 mcg and inactive tablets	normal
Minulet	gestodene 75 mcg + ethinyloestradiol 30 mcg	normal
Norimin	norethisterone 1 mg + ethinyloestradiol 35 mcg	normal
Norinyl-1	norethisterone 1 mg + mestranol 50 mcg	high
Ovran	levonorgestrel 250 mcg + ethinyloestradiol 50 mcg	high
Ovran 30	levonorgestrel 250 mcg + ethinyloestradiol 30 mcg	normal
Ovranette	levonorgestrel 150 mcg + ethinyloestradiol 30 mcg	normal
Ovysmen	norethisterone 0.5 mg + ethinyloestradiol 35 mcg	normal
Synphase	3 different-strength tablets containing norethisterone 0.5-1 mg + ethinyloestradiol 35 mcg at various stages in cycle	normal
Triadene	3 different-strength tablets containing gestodene 50-100 mcg + ethinyloestradiol 30-40 mcg at various stages in cycle	normal

cont.

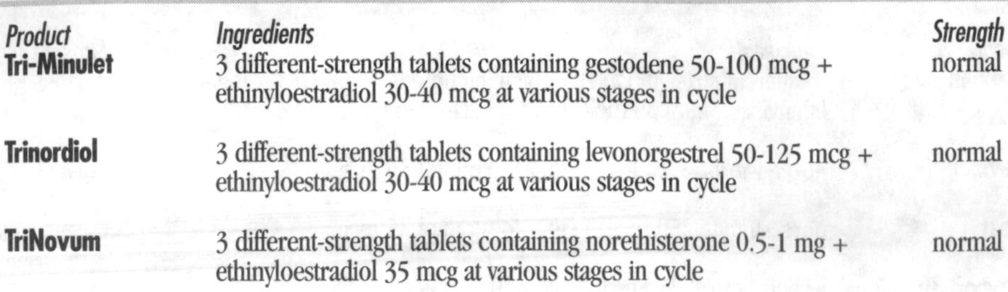

Product	*Ingredients*	*Strength*
Tri-Minulet	3 different-strength tablets containing gestodene 50-100 mcg + ethinyloestradiol 30-40 mcg at various stages in cycle	normal
Trinordiol	3 different-strength tablets containing levonorgestrel 50-125 mcg + ethinyloestradiol 30-40 mcg at various stages in cycle	normal
TriNovum	3 different-strength tablets containing norethisterone 0.5-1 mg + ethinyloestradiol 35 mcg at various stages in cycle	normal

** brands that include 7 inactive tablets in the pack to allow one tablet to be taken every day without a break.*

oral contraceptive (progestogen-only)

A tablet used as a progestogen contraceptive, often suitable for women who are unable to take combined oral contraceptives.

Dose: 1 tablet taken at the same time each day continuously. The course usually started on the first day of menstrual bleeding.
Availability: NHS and private prescription.
Compound preparations: oral contraceptives (combined).
Other preparations: etonogestrel implant, medroxyprogesterone injection, norethisterone injection.
Contains: (*see* table below).

Not to be used for: pregnant women or for patients suffering from severe heart or blood vessel disease, benign liver tumours, PORPHYRIA, undiagnosed vaginal bleeding, some womb disorders.

Side effects: irregular bleeding, upset stomach, dizziness, depression, skin disorders, change in appetite, weight gain, change in sexual desire, breast discomfort, headache, ovarian cyst, rarely blood clots. There appears to be a small increase in risk of breast cancer but this may be the result of earlier diagnosis through regular examinations.

Caution: in patients suffering from heart disease, high blood pressure, disordered absorption of nutrients from the gut, diabetes, migraine, some cancers, liver abnormalities, ovarian cysts, and those who have had a previous ectopic pregnancy or blood clot. Your doctor may advise regular examinations.

Caution needed with: BARBITURATES, phenytoin, primidone, carbamazepine, chloral hydrate, ethosuximide, rifampicin, chlorpromazine, meprobamate, griseofulvin, topiramate, modafinil, cyclosporin, nevirapine, celecoxib.

Brand	*Ingredients*
Femulen	ethynodiol (etynodiol) diacetate 500 mcg
Micronor	norethisterone 350 mcg
Microval	levonorgestrel 30 mcg
Neogest	norgestrel 75 mcg
Norgeston	levonorgestrel 30 mcg
Noriday	norethisterone 350 mcg

oral rehydration solution

A powder that is reconstituted with water and used as a solution to replace fluids and salts lost from the body during diarrhoea.

Strengths available: (individual brands vary slightly in strength).

Dose: reconstitute and use as directed on the packet.

Availability: NHS and private prescription, over the counter.

Contains: sodium chloride, potassium chloride, glucose. Some brands also contain citric acid, sodium citrate, sodium bicarbonate, fructose, or sucrose.

Brand names: Dioralyte, Electrolade, Rehidrat. (Various other brands also available over the counter.)

Compound preparations: Diarrest, Dioralyte Relief (with added rice powder).

Not to be used for: patients with severe kidney disorders, obstructed or non-functioning intestines.

Oralbalance *see* saliva (artificial) gel
(Anglian Pharma)

Oramorph *see* morphine oral solution
(Boehringer Ingelheim)

Orap *see* pimozide tablets
(Janssen-Cilag)

---

orciprenaline tablets/syrup/inhaler

A tablet, syrup, or inhaler used as a BRONCHODILATOR to treat bronchial spasm caused by bronchitis, asthma, or emphysema.

Strengths available: 20 mg tablets; 10 mg/5 ml syrup; 0.75 mg per dose inhaler.

Dose: adults, 20 mg four times a day by mouth or 0.75-1.5 mg (1-2 puffs) of inhaler repeated at intervals of not less than 30 minutes (maximum 12 puffs per day); children, 5-15 mg four times a day by mouth or 1-2 puffs of inhaler up to four times a day (according to age).

Availability: NHS and private prescription.

Contains: orciprenaline sulphate.

Brand names: Alupent.

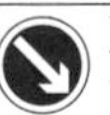
low potassium levels, shaking hands, headache, widening of blood vessels, cramps, altered heart rhythm, nervousness, severe allergic reaction.

in pregnant women, mothers who are breast-feeding, and in patients suffering from weak heart, irregular heart rhythm, high blood pressure, overactive thyroid, diabetes. In severe asthmatics. Blood potassium levels should be checked regularly.

patients suffering from cardiac asthma, overactive thyroid disease, or narrowed blood supply to the heart.

theophylline, aminophylline.

O

Orelox/Orelox Paediatric *see* cefpodoxime tablets/suspension
(Hoechst Marion Roussel)

OrLAAM *see* levacetylmethadol solution
(Britannia Pharmaceuticals)

Orlept *see* sodium valproate tablets/liquid
(C.P. Pharmaceuticals)

---

orlistat capsules

A capsule used as an addition to dietary measures to control obesity.

Strengths available: 120 mg capsules.
Dose: adults, 120 mg taken with each main meal (up to three times a day) for up to 2 years.
Availability: NHS and private prescription.
Contains: orlistat.
Brand names: Xenical.

 oily bowel motions, urgent need to pass motions, wind, pain in abdomen or rectum, headache, tiredness, anxiety, irregular periods, urine or chest infections, influenza, reduced absorption of some vitamins.

 in patients with diabetes. Diet should be rich in fruit and vegetables, and fat intake should be carefully controlled. Do not take a dose if the meal contains no fat.

 children, pregnant women, mothers who are breastfeeding, or for patients with inadequate bile flow or abnormal absorption of nutrients from the intestines.

 cyclosporin, anti-diabetic medications, phentermine, some lipid-lowering drugs.

---

orphenadrine tablets/liquid

A tablet or liquid used as an ANTIMUSCARINIC treatment for Parkinson's disease and similar symptoms caused by medication.

Strengths available: 50 mg tablets; 25 mg/5 ml or 50 mg/5 ml liquid.
Dose: initially 50 mg three times a day increasing gradually to maximum of 400 mg a day.
Availability: NHS and private prescription.
Contains: orphenadrine hydrochloride.
Brand names: Biorphen, Disipal.

 antimuscarinic effects, confusion, euphoria, insomnia, agitation, rash with high doses.

 in children, the elderly, pregnant women, mothers who are breastfeeding, and in patients suffering from heart or blood vessel disease, liver or kidney disorders.

 children or for patients suffering from untreated urine retention, glaucoma, PORPHYRIA, enlarged prostate, some movement disorders, or intestinal blockage.

 other antimuscarinic or sedating drugs.

Ortho Creme *see* nonoxynol cream
(Janssen-Cilag)

Ortho-Dienoestrol *see* hormone replacement therapy (topical)
(Janssen-Cilag)

Ortho-Gynest *see* hormone replacement therapy (oestrogen-only)
(Janssen-Cilag)

Orthoforms *see* nonoxynol pessaries
(Janssen-Cilag)

Orudis *see* ketoprofen capsules/suppositories
(Distriphar)

Oruvail capsules *see* ketoprofen modified-release capsules
(Distriphar)

Oruvail Gel *see* non-steroidal anti-inflammatory drug (topical)
(Rhône-Poulenc Rorer)

Ossopan *see* hydroxyapatite tablets
(Sanofi Winthrop)

---

osteoporosis

A thinning of the bones that occurs in women after the menopause and in elderly men making the bone more likely to fracture. It may also be caused by certain drugs (e.g. CORTICOSTEROIDS).

Ostram *see* calcium phosphate sachets
(E. Merck Pharmaceuticals)

Otomize

(Stafford-Miller)

A suspension supplied in a spray and used as an ANTIBIOTIC and CORTICOSTEROID to treat inflammation of the outer ear.

Dose: 1 spray three times a day until 2 days after the symptoms disappear.

cont.

Availability: NHS and private prescription.
Contains: neomycin sulphate, dexamethasone, glacial acetic acid.

 temporary stinging or burning.

 in pregnant women.

 patients suffering from perforated ear drum.

Otosporin

(GlaxoWellcome UK)

Drops used as an ANTIBIOTIC, CORTICOSTEROID treatment for bacterial infections and inflammation of the outer ear.

Dose: 3 drops into the ear 3-4 times a day, or insert a wick into the ear for 24-48 hours and keep soaked in the drops.
Availability: NHS and private prescription.
Contains: polymixin B sulphate, neomycin sulphate, hydrocortisone.

 stinging or burning.

 in patients receiving ear surgery. Avoid long-term use in infants.

 patients suffering from perforated ear drum or with ear infections not caused by bacteria.

Otrivine-Antistin

(CIBA Vision Ophthalmics)

Eye drops used as a SYMPATHOMIMETIC, ANTIHISTAMINE treatment for allergic conjunctivitis.

Dose: adults 1-2 drops into the eye(s) 2-3 times a day; elderly patients and children over 5 years 1 drop 2-3 times a day.
Availability: NHS and private prescription, over the counter.
Contains: xylometazoline hydrochloride, antazoline sulphate.

 temporary smarting, headache, drowsiness, blurred vision, additional congestion.

 in patients suffering from high blood pressure, overactive thyroid, dry eyes, heart disease, diabetes.

 children under 5 years or for patients suffering from glaucoma or who wear contact lenses.

 alcohol, sedatives, MAOIS, some drugs used to lower blood pressure.

Ovestin *see* hormone replacement therapy (oestrogen-only)
(Organon Laboratories)

Ovran/Ovran 30 *see* oral contraceptive (combined)
(Wyeth Laboratories)

Ovranette *see* oral contraceptive (combined)
(Wyeth Laboratories)

Ovysmen *see* oral contraceptive (combined)
(Janssen-Cilag)

oxazepam tablets

A tablet used as a sedative for the short-term treatment of anxiety.

Strengths available: 10 mg, 15 mg, and 30 mg tablets.
Dose: adults, 15-30 mg (elderly or weak patients 10-20 mg) 3-4 times a day. To control sleeplessness associated with anxiety, 15-50 mg taken at bedtime.
Availability: NHS and private prescription.
Contains: oxazepam.

drowsiness, light-headedness, confusion, vertigo, stomach disturbances, loss of memory, aggression, headache, joint immobility, salivation changes, shaking, unsteadiness, low blood pressure, rash, changes in vision, changes in sexual desire, retention of urine, incontinence, blood changes, jaundice. Risk of addiction increases with dose and length of treatment. May impair judgement.

children or for patients suffering from acute lung diseases, some chronic lung diseases, severe liver disease, MYASTHENIA GRAVIS, some obsessional and psychotic disorders, or who have stopped breathing while asleep.

in the elderly, pregnant women, mothers who are breastfeeding, in women during labour, and in patients suffering from lung disorders, glaucoma, kidney or liver disorders, muscle weakness, PORPHYRIA, or with a history of drug or alcohol abuse. Avoid long-term use and withdraw gradually.

alcohol, other sedating drugs, some anti-epileptic medications, rifampicin, ritonavir.

oxcarbazepine tablets

A tablet used as an anti-epileptic drug to treat epilepsy.

Strengths available: 150 mg, 300 mg, and 600 mg tablets.
Dose: adults, 300 mg twice a day at first, increased to a maximum of 2400 mg a day if needed; children over 6 years use reduced doses according to body weight.
Availability: NHS and private prescription.
Contains: oxcarbazepine.
Brand names: Trileptal.

upset stomach, dizziness, drowsiness, headache, loss of memory, agitation, weakness, unsteadiness, confusion, lack of concentration, shaking, depression, skin disorders, hair loss, blood changes, vertigo, eye disorders, liver disorders, abnormal heart rhythm, LUPUS, severe allergic reaction.

children under 6 years or for mothers who are breastfeeding.

in pregnant women, the elderly, and in patients suffering from liver or kidney disorders, heart failure, heart conduction disorders, low blood sodium levels, or who are allergic to carbamazepine. Women must use non-hormonal methods of contraception or ORAL CONTRACEPTIVES with high oestrogen content. Report any unusual symptoms to your doctor immediately. Treatment should be withdrawn slowly.

other anti-epileptic treatments, MAOIS, oral contraceptives, lithium, alcohol, sedating drugs.

oxerutins capsules

A capsule used as a vein constrictor to treat ankle swelling caused by vein disorders.

Strengths available: 250 mg capsules.
Dose: adults, 500 mg twice a day.
Availability: NHS and private prescription, over the counter.
Contains: oxerutins.
Brand names: Paroven.

 stomach upset, flushes, headache.

 any underlying cause of the fluid retention should be treated.

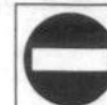 children.

---

oxetacaine *see* oxethazaine (alternative name)

---

oxethazaine *see* Mucaine

Oxis *see* eformoterol powder inhaler
(AstraZeneca UK)

---

oxitropium inhaler

An inhaler used as an ANTIMUSCARINIC treatment for obstructed airways, particularly in bronchitis.

Strengths available: 100 mcg per dose inhaler.
Dose: adults, 200 mcg (2 puffs) 2-3 times a day. Follow instruction supplied with inhaler.
Availability: NHS and private prescription.
Contains: oxitropium bromide.
Brand names: Oxivent.
Other devices: Oxivent Autohaler (breath-activated inhaler).

 dry mouth, constipation, difficulty passing urine, blurred vision, irritation, antimuscarinic effects.

 in patients suffering from enlarged prostate or glaucoma. Avoid getting spray near the eyes.

 children, pregnant women, mothers who are breastfeeding, or for patients who are allergic to ipratropium or atropine.

 other antimuscarinic drugs.

O

Oxivent *see* oxitropium inhaler
(Boehringer Ingelheim)

---

oxpentifylline modified-release tablets

An M-R TABLET used as a blood-cell-altering drug to treat blood vessel disorders such as spasm or blockage (e.g. when causing pain on walking).

Strengths available: 400 mg m-r tablets.

Dose: 400 mg 2-3 times a day.
Availability: NHS and private prescription.
Contains: oxpentifylline (pentoxifylline).
Brand names: Trental.

 children, pregnant women, or for patients with bleeding in the brain, severe bleeding in the eye or heart attack.

 NON-STEROIDAL ANTI-INFLAMMATORY DRUGS, theophylline, aminophylline, antidiabetics, drugs used to lower blood pressure.

 upset stomach, vertigo, flushing, dizziness, sleep disturbance, agitation, headache, rapid heart rate, angina, low blood pressure, blood changes, lack of bile flow, itching, difficulty breathing.

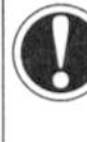 in mothers who are breastfeeding and in patients suffering from low blood pressure, disorder of heart blood vessels, kidney disease, severe liver disease, or PORPHYRIA.

oxprenolol tablets/modified-release tablets

A tablet or M-R TABLET used as a BETA-BLOCKER to treat angina, abnormal heart rhythm, high blood pressure, and anxiety.

Strengths available: 20 mg, 40 mg, 80 mg, and 160 mg tablets; 160 mg m-r tablets.
Dose: adults: for abnormal heart rhythm 40-240 mg a day; for angina 80-320 mg a day; for high blood pressure, 80-320 mg a day; for anxiety 40-80 mg a day. (All in divided doses through the day.)
Availability: NHS and private prescription.
Contains: oxprenolol hydrochloride.
Brand names: Slow Trasicor, Trasicor.
Compound preparations: co-prenozide.

 cold hands and feet, sleep disturbance, slow heart rate, tiredness, wheezing, heart failure, low blood pressure, stomach upset. Rarely, dry eyes, rash, worsening of psoriasis.

 in pregnant women, mothers who are breastfeeding, the elderly, and in patients suffering from diabetes, kidney or liver disorders, MYASTHENIA GRAVIS, or with a history of allergies. May need to be withdrawn before surgery. Withdraw gradually.

 children or for patients suffering from heart block or failure, asthma, PHAEOCHROMOCYTOMA, or with a history of breathing disorders.

 general anaesthetics, CALCIUM-CHANNEL BLOCKERS, ALPHA-BLOCKERS, clonidine, ANTIHYPERTENSIVES, amiodarone, antidiabetics, thymoxamine, theophylline, aminophylline.

oxybutynin tablets/modified-release tablets/elixir

A tablet, M-R TABLET, or elixir used as an anti-spasm and ANTIMUSCARINIC treatment for incontinence, urgency or frequency of urination, or unstable bladder and night-time bedwetting in children.

Strengths available: 2.5 mg, 3 mg, or 5 mg tablets; 5 mg and 10 mg m-r tablets; 2.5 mg/5 ml elixir.
Dose: adults, 5 mg 2-4 times a day; elderly patients, 2.5-5 mg twice a day; children over 5 years (unsta-

 antimuscarinic effects, dry mouth, upset stomach, blurred vision, flushed face, headache, dizziness, drowsiness, dry skin, rash, severe allergic reaction, abnormal heart rhythm, restlessness, disorientation, hallucinations, fits, sensitivity to sunlight.

cont.

ble bladder), 2.5-5 mg 2-3 times a day; children over 7 years (bed-wetting), 2.5-5 mg 2-3 times a day.

Availability: NHS and private prescription.

Contains: oxybutynin hydrochloride.

Brand names: Contimin, Cystrin, Ditropan, Promictuline.

 other antimuscarinic drugs, alcohol, sedatives.

 in pregnant women, the elderly, and in patients suffering from kidney or liver disorders, heart disease, overactive thyroid, nerve disorders, enlarged prostate, hiatus hernia, or PORPHYRIA.

 children under 5 years, mothers who are breastfeeding, or for patients with blocked bowel or bladder, severe bowel disorders, glaucoma or MYASTHENIA GRAVIS.

oxycodone capsules/modified-release tablets/liquid

A capsule, M-R TABLET, or liquid, used as an OPIOID ANALGESIC to treat moderate to severe pain.

Strengths available: 5 mg, 10 mg, and 20 mg capsules; 10 mg, 20 mg, 40 mg, and 80 mg m-r tablets; 5 mg/5 ml and 50 mg/5 ml liquids.

Dose: adults, using capsules or liquid, 5 mg every 4-6 hours increasing to a maximum of 400 mg a day if needed; using m-r tablets, 10 mg twice a day, increased to a maximum of 200 mg twice a day if needed.

Availability: controlled drug; NHS and private prescription.

Contains: oxycodone hydrochloride.

Brand names: Oxycontin, Oxynorm.

 drowsiness, upset stomach, sweating, dizziness, breathing difficulty, low blood pressure, difficulty passing urine, dry mouth, headache, vertigo, flushing, change in heart rhythm, mood changes, rash, itching, addiction, reduced sexual desire.

 in children, women in labour, alcoholics, elderly or weakened patients, and in those suffering from breathing, kidney, or liver problems, inflamed pancreas or bowel, reduced ADRENAL function, disorders of the bile duct and gall bladder, low blood pressure, underactive thyroid, enlarged prostate, or epilepsy. (Higher doses not suitable for some of these categories.)

 MAOIS, alcohol, sedating drugs, ritonavir.

O

 children under 18 years, pregnant women, mothers who are breastfeeding, or for patients with head injury, raised carbon dioxide levels, reduced breathing ability, PORPHYRIA, severe kidney or liver disorders, or those who have a history of drug addiction or who are suicidal or at risk of non-functioning intestines. Not suitable for use within 24 hours of surgery.

Oxycontin *see* oxycodone modified-release tablets (Napp Pharmaceuticals)

Oxymycin *see* oxytetracycline tablets (DDSA Pharmaceuticals)

Oxynorm *see* oxycodone capsules/liquid
(Napp Pharmaceuticals)

---

oxypertine capsules/tablets

A capsule or tablet used as a sedative to treat schizophrenia and other psychological disorders.

Strengths available: 10 mg capsules; 40 mg tablets.
Dose: adults, usually 80-120 mg a day (in divided doses) at first increasing to a maximum of 300 mg a day; for short-term treatment of anxiety, 30-60 mg a day.
Availability: NHS and private prescription.
Contains: oxypertine.

movement disorders, muscle spasms, restlessness, shaking, dry mouth, heart rhythm disturbance, low blood pressure, weight gain, blurred vision, impotence, low body temperature, breast swelling, menstrual changes, blood, liver, eye, and skin changes, drowsiness, apathy, nightmares, sleeplessness, depression, agitation, hyperactivity, blocked nose, difficulty passing water. Rarely, fits, intolerance to light.

unconscious patients or for those suffering from severe kidney or liver impairment, bone marrow depression, or PHAEOCHROMOCYTOMA.

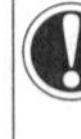
in pregnant women, mothers who are breastfeeding, the elderly, and in patients suffering from heart, lung, or circulation disorders, epilepsy, Parkinson's disease, thyroid disorders, infections, MYASTHENIA GRAVIS, kidney or liver disease, glaucoma, enlarged prostate, or some blood disorders. Should be withdrawn gradually.

alcohol, sedatives, ANTIDEPRESSANTS, some antidiabetic drugs, anaesthetics, anti-epileptic drugs, drugs affecting heart rhythm, ritonavir, halofantrine, sotalol, propranolol, lithium.

---

oxytetracycline tablets/capsules

A tablet used as a tetracycline ANTIBIOTIC to treat infections, including bronchitis and acne.

Strengths available: 250 mg tablets and capsules.
Dose: adults, usually 250-500 mg every 6 hours; for acne, 500 mg twice a day for up to 2 years (or longer in resistant cases).
Availability: NHS and private prescription.
Contains: oxytetracycline dihydrate.
Brand names: Oxymycin, Oxytetramix, Terramycin.
Compound preparations: Terra-Cortril, Terra-Cortril Nystatin and Trimovate *see* topical corticosteroids.

stomach upset, irritation of the oesophagus, reddening of skin, headache, disturbed vision, sensitivity to light, additional infections, pressure on the brain, reversible diabetes insipidus, liver disorders, inflamed pancreas or bowel.

in patients suffering from liver or kidney disorders. Discontinue if reddening of skin occurs.

children under 12 years, pregnant women, mothers who are breastfeeding, or for patients suffering from LUPUS or PORPHYRIA.

milk, ANTACIDS, iron supplements, ANTICOAGULANTS, ORAL CONTRACEPTIVES.

Oxytetramix *see* oxytetracycline tablets
(Ashbourne Pharmaceuticals)

Palfium *see* dextromoramide tablets
(Roche Products)

Palladone/Palladone CR *see* hydromorphone capsules/modified-release capsules
(Napp Pharmaceuticals)

Paludrine *see* proguanil tablets
(Zeneca Pharma)

Paludrine/Avloclor travel pack *see* proguanil tablets and chloroquine tablets
(Zeneca Pharma)

Pancrease/Pancrease HL *see* pancreatin capsules
(Janssen-Cilag)

---

pancreatin capsules/powder/sachets/enteric-coated tablets

A capsule (containing powder or E-C GRANULES), powder, sachet, or E-C TABLET used as a source of pancreatic enzymes to treat deficiency (as in cystic fibrosis and chronic inflammation of the pancreas).

Dose: taken with meals and snacks. Quantity per dose will vary according to brand used (*see* manufacturer's instructions and follow doctor's advice).
Availability: NHS and private prescription, over the counter.
Contains: pancreatin (comprising protease, lipase, amylase).
Brand names: Creon, Nutrizym, Pancrease, Pancrex.

 irritation of the mouth and anus, stomach upset, high levels of uric acid in the blood and urine. Narrowed bowel with high doses in children.

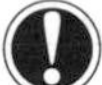 in children (high doses *see* above). Products are degraded by heat – do not mix with hot food or liquids. E-c products must not be chewed. Drink plenty of fluids with high doses.

 patients allergic to pork. Pancrease HL and Nutrizym 22 brands not suitable for children under 15 years with cystic fibrosis.

laxatives, ANTACIDS (for e-c preparations), acarbose.

Pancrex/Pancrex V *see* pancreatin capsules/powder/enteric-coated tablets
(Paines and Byrne)

Panoxyl *see* benzoyl peroxide gel/cream/wash
(Stiefel Laboratories (UK))

pantoprazole enteric-coated tablets

An E-C TABLET used to treat stomach ulcers, acid reflux into the oesophagus, and for *H. PYLORI* ERADICATION.

Strengths available: 20 mg and 40 mg e-c tablets.
Dose: for reflux, usually 40 mg each morning for 4-8 weeks to heal the condition, then 20-40 mg a day to prevent relapse; for ulcers, 40 mg once a day for 2-8 weeks.
Availability: NHS and private prescription.
Contains: pantoprazole sodium sesquihydrate.
Brand names: Protium.
Compound preparations: *H. pylori* eradication.

 headache, upset stomach, skin irritation. Rarely, blood changes, swollen hands and feet, depression, joint pain, itching, severe allergy, dry mouth, skin reactions, blurred vision, liver changes, sleeplessness, fever, liver changes.

 in mothers who are breastfeeding and in patients aged over 45 years or with liver or kidney disorders. Stomach cancer should be excluded before treatment.

 children or pregnant women.

 digoxin, ANTACIDS.

papaveretum *see* Aspav

Papulex *see* nicotinamide gel
(Stevenden Healthcare)

paracetamol tablets/soluble tablets/paediatric soluble tablets/paediatric oral solution/suspension/suppositories

A tablet, soluble tablet, paediatric soluble tablet, paediatric oral solution, suspension, or suppository used as an ANALGESIC to relieve pain and fever.

Strengths available: 500 mg tablets; 120 mg and 500 mg soluble tablets; 120 mg/5 ml paediatric oral solution; 120 mg/5 ml and 250 mg/5 ml suspension; 60 mg, 125 mg, 240 mg, 250 mg, or 500 mg suppositories.
Dose: the following doses taken by mouth or suppository up to 4 times a day: adults, 500-1000 mg; children aged 1-5 years, 120-250 mg; children

 rarely, rash, blood changes, inflamed pancreas, liver or kidney damage with overdose.

 in alcoholics and in patients with liver or kidney disorders.

 children under 3 months (except as above).

 other medicines containing paracetamol, ANTICOAGULANTS (with regular use).

P

cont.

aged 6-12 years, 250-500 mg. Children aged 2 months may be given a single dose or 60 mg after vaccination (or as advised by doctor); children aged 3-12 months, 60-120 mg up to four times a day by mouth. Leave at least 4 hours between doses.

Availability: NHS and private prescription, over the counter (quantity of tablets restricted). Suspension and tablets/soluble tablets available on nurse prescription (quantity of tablets restricted).

Contains: paracetamol.

Brand names: Alvedon, Calpol Paediatric, Calpol Six Plus (available on NHS only if prescribed generically), Disprol Paediatric. Other brands available over the counter (but not all available on NHS).

Compound preparations: co-codamol, co-dydramol, co-methiamol, co-proxamol, Domperamol, Fortagesic (not available on NHS), Midrid, Migraleve, Paramax.

---

paradichlorobenzene *see* Cerumol

Paradote *see* co-methiamol tablets
(Penn Pharmaceuticals)

---

paraffin gauze dressing

A sterile gauze dressing impregnated with paraffin and used to cover burns, wounds, and delicate areas of skin.

Availability: NHS and private prescription, nurse prescription, over the counter.

Contains: white or yellow soft paraffin.

Brand names: Jelonet, Paranet, Paratulle, Unitulle.

Paramax *see* paracetamol tablets and metoclopramide tablets
(Sanofi Synthelabo)
Tablet or sachets of effervescent powder used to treat migraine attacks.

Strengths available: 500 mg + 5 mg tablets; 500 mg + 5 mg sachets.

Dose: adults over 19 years, 2 tablets or sachets at start of attack then every 4 hours if needed (maximum of 6 in 24 hours); young adults aged 12-19, years half adult dose. Not recommended under 12 years.

P

Paranet *see* paraffin gauze dressing
(Vernon-Carus)

Paratulle *see* paraffin gauze dressing
(SSL International)

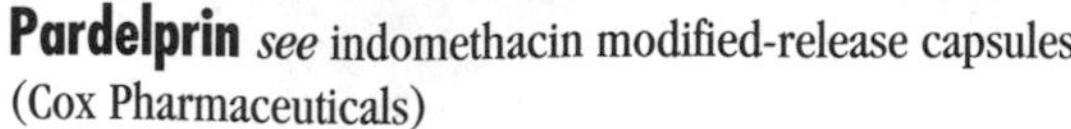

Pardelprin *see* indomethacin modified-release capsules
(Cox Pharmaceuticals)

Pariet *see* rabeprazole tablets
(Eisai)

Parlodel *see* bromocriptine capsules/tablets
(Novartis Pharmaceuticals UK)

Parnate *see* tranylcypromine tablets
(Goldshield Healthcare)

Paroven *see* oxerutins capsules
(Novartis Consumer Health)

---

paroxetine tablets/liquid

A tablet or liquid used as an antidepressant to treat depression, panic disorders, phobias, and obsessive-compulsive disorders.

Strengths available: 20 mg or 30 mg tablets; 10 mg/5 ml liquid.
Dose: adults, usually 10-30 mg each morning up to 50-60 mg a day in severe disorders; elderly patients, 10 mg a day at first, maximum 40 mg a day.
Availability: NHS and private prescription.
Contains: paroxetine hydrochloride.
Brand names: Seroxat.

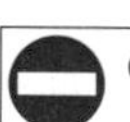 children or for patients with elevated mood.

 ANTICOAGULANTS, other antidepressants, anti-epileptic treatments, ritonavir, sumatriptan, lithium, alcohol, sedatives, selegiline.

 stomach upset, change in appetite and weight, dry mouth, nervousness, drowsiness, sweating, shaking, headache, sleeplessness, dizziness, weakness, fits, change in sexual function, movement disorders, low blood sodium levels, psychiatric disorders, heart rhythm disturbances, low blood pressure on standing, liver disorders.

 in pregnant women, mothers who are breastfeeding, and in patients with epilepsy, liver or kidney disorders, or a history of heart disease, blood clotting disorders, or some psychiatric conditions. Treatment should be withdrawn slowly. Symptoms of panic disorder may get worse in early stages of treatment.

Pavacol-D *see* pholcodine linctus
(Boehringer Ingelheim)

PC4 *see* Schering PC4

peak flow meter

A device used to measure lung function in asthmatics. Available in standard or low-range form (low range used for patients with severely restricted air flow). Usually replaced after 3 years.

Brand names: Asmaplan, Ferraris, Medic-Aid Personal Best, Mini-Wright, Vitalograph, Wright.

peanut oil *see* emollient preparations, Naseptin cream

pectin *see* Orabase, Orahesive

Penbritin *see* ampicillin capsules
(Beecham Research Laboratories)

penciclovir cream

A cream used as an antiviral treatment for cold sores.

Strengths available: 1%.
Dose: adults, apply every 2 hours (during waking hours) for 4 days, starting at the first sign of the attack.
Availability: NHS and private prescription. (Also available over the counter to treat cold sores only.)
Contains: penciclovir.
Brand names: Vectavir.

 temporary stinging or burning, numbness.

 in pregnant women and in patients with poorly functioning immune system. Avoid contact with eyes or mucous membranes.

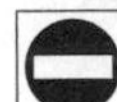 children under 16 years.

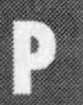

Penfine *see* insulin injection devices
(Disetronic)

penicillamine tablets

A tablet used as an anti-arthritic drug and binding agent to treat severe active rheumatoid arthritis, Wilson's disease (an inherited disorder), inflamed liver, heavy metal poisoning, liver disease, cysteinuria (a rare kidney disease).

Strengths available: 125 mg and 250 mg tablets.
Dose: varies between 125 mg and 3000 mg a day for adults according to condition. (Lower doses used for elderly patients and children.) Usually given only on expert advice.

Availability: NHS and private prescription.
Contains: penicillamine.
Brand names: Distamine.

 in pregnant women, mothers who are breastfeeding, and in patients suffering from kidney disease or who are allergic to penicillin. Your doctor may advise that blood and urine should be checked regularly. Tell your doctor if sore throat, rash, mouth ulcers, bruising, or other unidentified illness develops.

 nausea, loss of appetite, fever, rash, loss of taste, blood changes, blood or protein in the urine, kidney changes, symptoms similar to MYASTHENIA GRAVIS, muscle disease, LUPUS-like symptoms, mouth ulcers, hair loss, lung disorders, enlarged breasts, arthritis symptoms.

 very allergic patients or for patients suffering from LUPUS or blood disorders.

 gold treatments, chloroquine, hydroxychloroquine, drugs that suppress the immune system, iron supplements.

penicillin V tablets/oral solution

A tablet or oral solution used as a penicillin ANTIBIOTIC to treat infection of the ear and throat, some skin infections, and to prevent rheumatic fever or pneumonia.

Strengths available: 250 mg tablets; 125 mg/5 ml or 250 mg/5 ml oral solution.
Dose: adults, 500-750 mg four times a day; children up to 1 year, 62.5 mg (aged 1-5 years 125 mg, aged 6-12 years 250 mg) four times a day.
Availability: NHS and private prescription.
Contains: penicillin V (phenoxymethylpenicillin potassium).
Brand names: Tenkicin.

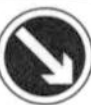 severe allergic reaction, skin rash, itching, fever, joint pain, anaemia, kidney disorders, blood changes, fits, pins and needles, diarrhoea.

 in patients with a history of allergy or kidney disorders.

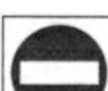 patients allergic to penicillin products.

 ANTICOAGULANTS, methotrexate, oral contraceptives.

Penlet II Plus Finger Pricking Device *see* Baylet Lancets, Cleanlet Fine Lancets, FinePoint Lancets, B-D Micro-Fine+ Lancets, Milward Steri-Let/Steri-Let Ultra-Fine Lancets, Monolet Lancets, Monolet Extra Lancets, Unilet G SuperLite Lancets, Unilet GP Lancets, Unilet Universal ComforTouch Lancets, Vitrex Soft Lancets
(Lifescan)

Availability: private prescription, over the counter.

Pentasa *see* mesalazine enema/modified-release granules/suppositories/tablets
(Ferring Pharmaceuticals)

pentazocine tablets/capsules/suppositories

A tablet, capsule, or suppository used as an OPIOID ANALGESIC to relieve pain.

Strengths available: 25 mg tablets; 50 mg capsules; 50 mg suppositories.
Dose: adults, 25-100 mg (children aged 6-12 years, 25 mg) every 3-4 hours by mouth (after food) or 50 mg up to four times a day by suppository.
Availability: controlled drug; NHS and private prescription.
Contains: pentazocine hydrochloride.
Compound preparations: Fortagesic (not allowed on NHS).

drowsiness, upset stomach, sweating, dizziness, breathing difficulty, low blood pressure, difficulty passing urine, dry mouth, headache, vertigo, flushing, change in heart rhythm, mood changes, rash, itching, addiction, reduced sexual desire, hallucinations.

in children, pregnant women, women in labour, mothers who are breastfeeding, elderly or weakened patients, and in those suffering from breathing, kidney, or liver problems, low blood pressure, underactive thyroid, enlarged prostate, or epilepsy. (Higher doses not suitable for some of these categories.)

MAOIS, alcohol, sedating drugs, ritonavir.

alcoholics or for patients with head injury, reduced breathing ability, heart failure, high blood pressure in arteries or lungs, PORPHYRIA, or those who have a history of drug addiction or who are suicidal or at risk of non-functioning intestines.

pentoxifylline *see* oxpentifylline (alternative name)

Pentrax *see* coal tar shampoo
(DermaPharm)

Pepcid *see* famotidine tablets
(Merck Sharp and Dohme)

peppermint oil enteric-coated capsules

P

An E-C CAPSULE used as an anti-spasm treatment for colic and bloating, as in irritable bowel syndrome. (Some brands are M-R CAPSULES in addition to e-c.)

Strengths available: 0.2 ml e-c capsules.
Dose: adults, 1-2 capsules three times a day for up to 2-3 months.

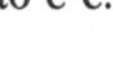

Availability: NHS and private prescription, over the counter.
Contains: peppermint oil.
Brand names: Colpermin, Mintec.

heartburn, irritation around anus, rash, headache, slow heart beat, tremor, loss of co-ordination.

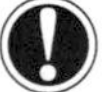
in patients allergic to menthol. Capsules must not be broken or chewed.

children.

ANTACIDS.

Peptac *see* alginate liquid
(Baker Norton Pharmaceuticals)

Peptimax *see* cimetidine tablets
(Ashbourne Pharmaceuticals)

Percutol *see* glyceryl trinitrate 2% ointment
(Dominion Pharma)

Perdix *see* moexepril tablets
(Schwartz Pharma)

---

pergolide tablets

A tablet used to treat Parkinson's disease.

Strengths available: 50 mcg, 250 mcg, or 1000 mcg tablets.
Dose: adults, 50 mcg a day for 2 days, increased gradually to a maximum of 5000 mcg a day but usually no more than 3000 mcg. (levodopa dose reduced gradually as pergolide dose increased).
Availability: NHS and private prescription.
Contains: pergolide mesylate.
Brand names: Celance.

 hallucinations, confusion, movement disorders, drowsiness, low blood pressure, heartbeat abnormalities, stomach upset, inflammation of the nose, breathing difficulty, double vision, dizziness, abdominal disorders, lung or heart disorders, rash, fever, NEUROLEPTIC MALIGNANT SYNDROME.

 in pregnant women, mothers who are breast-feeding, and in patients suffering from heart disease, abnormal heart rhythm, PORPHRIA, or with a history of hallucinations, movement disorders, or confusion. Treatment should be withdrawn gradually.

 some drugs used to treat psychiatric disorders, alcohol, sedating drugs, metoclopramide, domperidone, ANTICOAGULANTS.

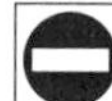 children.

Pergonal *see* human menopausal gonadotrophin injection
(Serono Laboratories (UK))

Periactin *see* cyproheptadine tablets
(Merck Sharp and Dohme)

---

pericyazine tablets/syrup

A tablet or syrup used as a sedative to treat behavioural and character problems, schizophrenia, anxiety, tension, and agitation.

Strengths available: 2.5 mg and 10 mg tablets; 10 mg/5 ml syrup.
Dose: adults, 15-75 mg a day at first increasing to a maximum of 300 mg a day (in divided doses) if needed; elderly patients, 5-30 mg a day at first; children use reduced doses according to body weight.
Availability: NHS and private prescription.
Contains: pericyazine.
Brand names: Neulactil.

 movement disorders, muscle spasms, restlessness, shaking, dry mouth, heart rhythm disturbance, low blood pressure, weight gain, blurred vision, impotence, low body temperature, breast swelling, menstrual changes, blood, liver, eye, and skin changes, drowsiness, apathy, nightmares, sleeplessness, depression, blocked nose, difficulty passing water. Rarely, fits.

 in pregnant women, mothers who are breast-feeding, the elderly, and in patients suffering from heart, lung, or circulation disorders, infections, MYASTHENIA GRAVIS, or some blood disorders. Should be withdrawn gradually.

 alcohol, sedatives, antidepressants, some antidiabetic drugs, anaesthetics, anti-epileptic medications, drugs affecting heart rhythm, ritonavir, halofantrine, sotalol, propranolol, lithium.

 unconscious patients or for patients suffering from bone marrow depression, kidney or liver impairment, epilepsy, Parkinson's disease, thyroid disorders, glaucoma, enlarged prostate, heart failure, or PHAEOCHROMOCYTOMA.

Perinal *see* rectal corticosteroid spray
(Dermal Laboratories)

perindopril tablets

A tablet used as an ACE-INHIBITOR to treat high blood pressure, or as an additional treatment for heart failure.

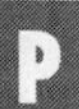

Strengths available: 2 mg and 4 mg tablets.
Dose: adults, 2 mg a day at first increasing to 4-8 mg a day.
Availability: NHS and private prescription.
Contains: perindopril erbumine.
Brand names: Coversyl.

 rash, itching, sore throat, runny nose, stomach upset, cough, blood and liver changes, kidney disorders, low blood pressure, severe allergic reaction, inflamed pancreas. Occasionally, headache, dizziness, tiredness, taste disturbance, fever, pins and needles, muscle or joint pain, sensitivity to sunlight, inflamed membranes or blood vessels, weakness, flushing, sleep disturbance, change in mood.

 in the elderly and in patients suffering from kidney disease, auto-immune diseases (such as LUPUS), severe heart failure, or with a history of severe allergies, or in patients undergoing anaesthesia or dialysis. Your doctor may advise regular blood tests.

 children, pregnant women, mothers who are breastfeeding, or for patients with some heart abnormalities, disorders of the blood supply to the kidney. Not to be taken on the same day as dialysis.

 DIURETICS, anaesthetics, NON-STEROIDAL ANTI-INFLAMMATORY DRUGS, potassium supplements, cyclosporin, lithium, antidiabetics.

Periostat *see* doxycycline capsules
(CollaGenex International)

---

permethrin cream/cream rinse

A cream or cream rinse used a treat scabies (with cream) or head lice (with cream rinse).

Strengths available: 5% skin cream; 1% cream rinse.
Dose: for scabies, apply the cream over whole body and wash off after 8-12 hours (head and neck not treated in adults but included for children under 1 year, elderly patients, and those with inadequate immune system); for head lice, apply the cream rinse to clean, damp hair and rinse off after 10 minutes.
Availability: NHS and private prescription, nurse prescription, over the counter.
Contains: permethrin.
Brand names: Lyclear.

Side effects: itching, redness, stinging. Occasionally fluid retention and rash.

Caution: in pregnant women and mothers who are breastfeeding. Children under 6 months using cream rinse (or 2-24 months using skin cream) must be treated only on the advice of a doctor.

Not to be used for: children under 2 months (cream).

Permitabs *see* potassium permanganate solution
(Bioglan Laboratories)

Peroxyl *see* hydrogen peroxide mouthwash
(Colgate-Palmolive)

P

perphenazine tablets

A tablet used as a sedative to treat vomiting, nausea, anxiety, schizophrenia, and other psychiatric disorders.

Strengths available: 2 mg and 4 mg tablets.
Dose: adults, usually 12 mg a day (in divided doses) up to a maximum of 24 mg a day; elderly patients use a quarter to half the adult dose.
Availability: NHS and private prescription.
Contains: perphenazine.
Brand names: Fentazin.

cont.

Compound preparations: Triptafen/Triptafen-M.

 in pregnant women, mothers who are breast-feeding, the elderly, and in patients suffering from heart, lung, or circulation disorders, epilepsy, Parkinson's disease, thyroid disorders, infections, MYASTHENIA GRAVIS, kidney or liver disease, glaucoma, enlarged prostate, or some blood disorders. Should be withdrawn gradually.

 alcohol, sedatives, antidepressants, some antidiabetic drugs, anaesthetics, anti-epileptic medications, drugs affecting heart rhythm, ritonavir, halofantrine, sotalol, propranolol, lithium.

 movement disorders, muscle spasms, restlessness, shaking, dry mouth, heart rhythm disturbance, low blood pressure, weight gain, blurred vision, impotence, low body temperature, breast swelling, menstrual changes, blood, liver, eye, and skin changes, drowsiness, apathy, nightmares, sleeplessness, depression, blocked nose, difficulty passing water. Rarely, fits.

 unconscious patients or for those suffering from severe kidney or liver impairment, bone marrow depression, or PHAEOCHROMOCYTOMA. Not suitable for treating elderly patients for agitation or restlessness.

Persantin *see* dipyridamole tablets
(Boehringer Ingelheim)

---

pertussis vaccine

A vaccine used to protect against whooping cough, usually given in combination with diphtheria and tetanus vaccines. A single vaccine available for children for whom it was not given or completed as part of this multiple vaccination.

Dose: 3 doses of injection at 1-monthly intervals.
Availability: NHS and private prescription.
Contains: pertussis antigen.
Compound preparations: diphtheria, tetanus, and pertussis vaccine; diphtheria, tetanus, pertussis, and *Haemophilus influenzae* type B vaccine.

 reddening, swelling and hardening of the skin around the injection site, mild fever. Rarely, shock, breathing difficulty, swelling of the throat, collapse, unresponsiveness, screaming, fits.

 in patients with a history (or family history) of feverish fits or in children with developing epilepsy or other brain disorders (delay vaccine until stable).

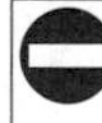 patients suffering from feverish illness or for those who have had severe reaction to previous pertussis vaccine dose.

Peru balsam *see* Anusol, rectal steroid preparations

---

pethidine tablets

A tablet used as an OPIOID ANALGESIC to treat moderate to severe pain.

Strengths available: 50 mg tablets.
Dose: adults, 50-150 mg every 4 hours; children use reduced doses according to body weight.

Availability: controlled drug; NHS and private prescription.
Contains: pethidine hydrochloride.

 in children, pregnant women, women in labour, mothers who are breastfeeding, elderly or weakened patients, and in those suffering from breathing, kidney, or liver problems, low blood pressure, underactive thyroid, enlarged prostate, or epilepsy. (Higher doses not suitable for some of these categories.)

 MAOIS, alcohol, sedating drugs, ritonavir, selegiline.

 drowsiness, upset stomach, sweating, dizziness, breathing difficulty, low blood pressure, difficulty passing urine, dry mouth, headache, vertigo, flushing, change in heart rhythm, mood changes, rash, itching, addiction, reduced sexual desire.

 alcoholics or for patients with head injury, reduced breathing ability, PORPHYRIA, severe kidney disorders, or those who have a history of drug addiction or who are suicidal or at risk of non-functioning intestines. Not suitable for long-term use.

Pevaryl *see* econazole cream/lotion
(Janssen-Cilag)

Pevaryl T.C. *see* econazole cream and topical corticosteroid cream
(Janssen-Cilag)

---

phaeochromocytoma

A tumour of the ADRENAL GLAND which produces excess ADRENALINE-like hormones.

---

phenazocine tablets

A tablet used as an OPIOID ANALGESIC to control severe pain.

Strengths available: 5 mg tablets.
Dose: adults, 5 mg every 4-6 hours (either swallowed or allowed to dissolve under the tongue). Single doses of up to 20 mg may be used.
Availability: controlled drug; NHS and private prescription.
Contains: phenazocine hydrobromide.
Brand names: Narphen.

 drowsiness, upset stomach, sweating, dizziness, breathing difficulty, low blood pressure, difficulty passing urine, dry mouth, headache, vertigo, flushing, change in heart rhythm, mood changes, rash, itching, addiction, reduced sexual desire.

 in women in labour, mothers who are breastfeeding, elderly or weakened patients, and in those suffering from breathing, kidney, or liver problems, low blood pressure, underactive thyroid, or enlarged prostate. (Higher doses not suitable for some of these categories.)

 MAOIS, alcohol, sedating drugs, ritonavir.

 children, pregnant women, alcoholics, or for patients with head injury, reduced breathing ability, PORPHYRIA, epilepsy, or those who have a history of drug addiction or who are suicidal or at risk of non-functioning intestines.

P

phenelzine tablets

A tablet used as an MAOI to treat depression.

Strengths available: 15 mg tablets.
Dose: adults, 15 mg three times a day at first increasing to four times a day if needed (higher doses used in hospital), then reduced to minimum effective dose.
Availability: NHS and private prescription.
Contains: phenelzine sulphate.
Brand names: Nardil.

 severe high blood pressure reactions with certain foods and medicines, sleeplessness, low blood pressure on standing, dizziness, drowsiness, weakness, dry mouth, constipation, stomach upset, blurred vision, difficulty passing urine, fluid retention, rash, weight gain, confusion, agitation, shaking, excitement, abnormal heart rhythm, sweating, fits, blood changes, psychiatric disorders, pins and needles, nerve inflammation, sexual disturbances, headache, abnormal muscle or eye movements, liver disorders.

 alcohol, apraclonidine, brimonidine, pethidine and other opioids, SYMPATHOMIMETIC drugs, other antidepressants, antidiabetics, anti-epileptic treatments, drugs used to lower blood pressure, oxypertine, clozapine, buspirone, levodopa, selegiline, entacapone, some drugs used to treat migraine, tetrabenazine, sedatives. The following foods should be avoided (until 14 days after treatment ends): cheese, meat extracts, broad beans, banana, Marmite, yeast extracts, wine, beer, other alcohol, pickled herrings, egetable proteins.

 in pregnant women, mothers who are breast-feeding, the elderly, and in patients suffering from diabetes, epilepsy, heart or circulatory disorders, blood disorders, agitation, PORPHYRIA, or those currently undergoing electroconvulsive therapy or surgery. Treatment should be withdrawn gradually.

 children or for patients suffering from liver disease, PHAEOCHROMOCYTOMA, or those who are currently excitable or who have disorders of the blood supply to the brain.

Phenergan *see* promethazine hydrochloride tablets/elixir (Rhône-Poulenc Rorer)

---

phenindione tablets

A tablet used as an ANTICOAGULANT to treat and prevent blood clots.

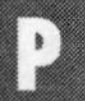

Strengths available: 10 mg, 25 mg, and 50 mg tablets.
Dose: as advised by doctor.
Availability: NHS and private prescription.
Contains: phenindione.

 bleeding, liver or kidney damage, reversible hair loss, stomach upset, headache, skin disorders, inflamed pancreas, purple toes, fever, blood disorders, pink-coloured urine.

 in the elderly and in patients suffering from high blood pressure, reduced ability of protein in blood to bind drugs, severe heart failure, liver or kidney disease, stomach disorders, vitamin K deficiency. Your doctor will advise regular blood tests to determine correct dose.

 children, pregnant women, mothers who are breastfeeding, or for patients suffering from stomach ulcers, severe high blood pressure, some heart disorders, poor liver or kidney function, some blood disorders.

 alcohol, allopurinol, stanozolol, aspirin, NON-STEROIDAL ANTI-INFLAMMATORY DRUGS, cholestyramine, amiodarone, propafenone, quinidine, ANTIBIOTICS, some antidepressants, some antidiabetics, anti-epileptic treatments, antifungals, proguanil, clopidogrel, ticlopidine, ritonavir, chloral, primidone, CORTICOSTEROIDS, disulfiram, danazol, tamoxifen, thyroxine, lipid-lowering drugs, oral contraceptives, raloxifene, acitretin, testosterone, sucralfate, cimetidine, omeprazole, sulphinpyrazone, influenza vaccine, vitamin K.

---

phenobarbital *see* phenobarbitone (alternative name)

---

phenobarbitone tablets/elixir

A tablet or elixir used as a BARBITURATE to treat epilepsy.

Strengths available: 15 mg, 30 mg, and 60 mg tablets; 15 mg/5 ml elixir.
Dose: adults, 60-180 mg at night; children use reduced doses according to body weight.
Availability: controlled drug; NHS and private prescription.
Contains: phenobarbitone (phenobarbital) sodium.

 tolerance, addiction, drowsiness, skin reactions, hangover, dizziness, allergies, headache, confusion, excitement, lack of co-ordination, breathing difficulties, blood disorder.

 in children, elderly or weak patients, pregnant women, mothers who are breastfeeding, and in patients with kidney, liver, or lung disease. Treatment should be withdrawn gradually.

 patients with a history of alcohol or drug abuse or suffering from PORPHYRIA.

 ANTICOAGULANTS, antidepressants, other anti-epileptic medications, griseofulvin, alcohol, sedatives, haloperidol, some antivirals, CALCIUM-CHANNEL BLOCKERS, cyclosporin, CORTICOSTEROIDS, thyroxine, oral contraceptives, tibolone, theophylline, aminophylline, celecoxib.

---

phenol *see* magnesium sulphate paste BP

---

phenothrin lotion/liquid/mousse

An alcoholic lotion, water-based liquid, or mousse used to treat head and pubic lice.

Strengths available: 0.2% lotion; 0.5% liquid; 0.5% mousse.
Dose: lotion used to treat head or pubic lice – rub into dry hair saturating scalp and leave to dry naturally, then shampoo off after 2 hours; alternatively use liquid or mousse to treat head lice only – saturate dry scalp and hair, allow to dry naturally, and shampoo off after 30 minutes (mousse) or 12 hours (liquid).
Availability: NHS and private prescription, nurse prescription.
Contains: phenothrin.

irritation.

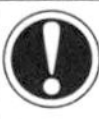 in patients suffering from asthma and eczema. Avoid contact with the eyes. Children under 6 months should be seen by a doctor before using this product.

P

 *cont.*

Brand names: Full Marks.

areas of broken or infected skin. Not to be used more than once a week for 3 weeks. Alcoholic solutions not suitable for asthmatics or patients with eczema.

---

phenoxybenzamine capsules

A capsule used as an ALPHA-BLOCKER to treat high blood pressure associated with PHAEOCHROMOCYTOMA.

Strengths available: 10 mg capsules.
Dose: adults, 10 mg once a day increased as needed; children use reduced doses according to body weight.
Availability: NHS and private prescription.
Contains: phenoxybenzamine hydrochloride.
Brand names: Dibenyline.

low blood pressure on standing, dizziness, tiredness, congested nose, rapid heart rate, failure of ejaculation, vision changes, stomach upset.

in elderly patients and in those suffering from heart failure, severe heart disease, brain blood vessel disorders, or kidney disorders.

patients suffering from heart attack, PORPHYRIA, or with a history of stroke.

---

phenoxymethylpenicillin *see* penicillin V

---

phentermine capsules

A capsule used as a SYMPATHOMIMETIC appetite suppressant to treat obesity.

Strengths available: 15 mg and 30 mg capsules.
Dose: 15-30 mg each morning for 4-6 weeks (maximum 3 months).
Availability: controlled drug; NHS and private prescription.
Contains: phentermine resin complex.
Brand names: Ionamin.

tolerance, addiction, mental disturbances, restlessness, nervousness, agitation, dry mouth, headache, rash, sleeplessness, nausea, vomiting, dizziness, depression, hallucinations, heart rhythm abnormality, constipation, need to pass urine more often, raised blood pressure, fluid retention, hallucinations.

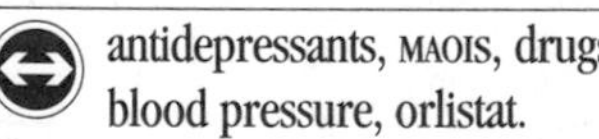
antidepressants, MAOIS, drugs used to lower blood pressure, orlistat.

in patients suffering from high blood pressure, diabetes, or with a history of anxiety or depression.

children, the elderly, pregnant women, mothers who are breastfeeding, or for patients with severe high blood pressure, overactive thyroid gland, epilepsy, heart or circulation disorders, or with a history of mental disorders, alcoholism, or drug addiction.

---

phenylbutazone enteric-coated tablets

An E-C TABLET used as a NON-STEROIDAL ANTI-INFLAMMATORY DRUG to treat ankylosing spondylitis if other treatments are not suitable.

Strengths available: 100 mg e-c tablets.
Dose: adults, 200 mg 2-3 times a day for 2 days then reduced usually to 100 mg three times a day.
Availability: NHS and private prescription (hospitals only).
Contains: phenylbutazone .
Brand names: Butacote.

stomach upset and bleeding or ulceration, skin reactions, severe allergy, difficulty breathing, blood or kidney disorders, headache, dizziness, noises in the ears, sensitivity to light, vertigo, inflamed parotid gland, enlarged thyroid gland, mouth ulcers. Rarely, fluid retention, liver disorders, inflamed pancreas, inflamed bowel, meningitis, lung disorders.

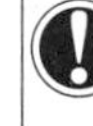
in mothers who are breastfeeding, the elderly, and in patients with fever and breathing difficulties or who are prone to allergies. Your doctor will advise regular blood tests before and during treatment. Report any fever, sore throat, bruising, mouth ulcers, or rash to your doctor immediately.

ACE-INHIBITORS, aspirin or other non-steroidal anti-inflammatory drugs, some ANTIBIOTICS, ANTICOAGULANTS, some antidiabetic drugs, some antivirals, methotrexate, DIURETICS, lithium, tacrolimus, cyclosporin, digoxin, ANTACIDS, thyroxine, misoprostol.

children under 14 years, pregnant women, or for patients with heart or circulation disorders, kidney or liver disorders, thyroid disease, Sjorgen's syndrome (dry eyes or mouth associated with arthritis or LUPUS), PORPHYRIA, lung disorders, or with a history of stomach ulcers or bleeding, inflamed bowel, or blood disorders, or who are allergic to aspirin or other NSAIDs.

---

phenylethyl alcohol *see* Ceanel

---

phenylephrine *see* Isopto frin

---

phenylketonuria (PKU)

A hereditary disease where phenylalanine (an amino acid present in protein) cannot be properly digested in the body. It is treated by using a low-protein diet and avoidance of phenylalanine.

---

phenytoin tablets/chewable tablets/capsules/suspension

A tablet, chewable tablet, capsule, or suspension used as an anticonvulsant to treat epilepsy.

P

Strengths available: 25 mg, 50 mg, and 100 mg capsules; 50 mg and 100 mg tablets; 50 mg chewable tablets; 30 mg/5 ml suspension.
Dose: adults, 150-300 mg a day (as a single dose or in two divided doses) increased to 200-500 mg a day (or more if needed); children use reduced doses according to body weight (maximum 300 mg a day).
Availability: NHS and private prescription.

stomach upset, confusion, dizziness, headache, shaking, sleeplessness, nervousness, movement disorders, numbness in hands or feet, speech and vision disturbances, skin disorders, inflamed arteries, swollen lymph glands, hair growth, LUPUS, blood changes, swollen gums.

cont.

Contains: phenytoin sodium.
Brand names: Epanutin.

patients suffering from PORPHYRIA.

in pregnant women, mothers who are breastfeeding, and in patients suffering from liver disorders. Treatment should be withdrawn slowly. Your doctor may advise regular blood tests. Report any sore throat, rash, fever, mouth ulcers, bruising, or bleeding to your doctor immediately. Doses in tablet, capsule, and liquid forms may not be exactly equivalent – dose should be reassessed if form of medication changed.

aspirin, NON-STEROIDAL ANTI-INFLAMMATORY DRUGS, methadone, ANTACIDS, drugs that affect heart rhythm, some ANTIBIOTICS, ANTICOAGULANTS, antidepressants, tolbutamide, repaglinide, other anti-epileptic treatments, antifungals, pyrimethamine, clozapine, quietapine, sertindole, antivirals, anti-anxiety treatments, CALCIUM-CHANNEL BLOCKERS, cyclosporin, CORTICOSTEROIDS, methotrexate, disulfiram, folic acid, some artificial liquid feeds, lithium, oral contraceptives, tibolone, methylphenidate, theophylline, aminophylline, cimetidine, sucralfate, lansoprazole, omeprazole, sulphinpyrazone, influenza vaccine.

Phiso-Med *see* chlorhexidine solution
(Sanofi Winthrop)

---

pholcodine linctus/paediatric linctus/strong linctus

A linctus used as an OPIOID cough suppressant to treat dry or painful cough.

Strengths available: 2 mg/5 ml, 5 mg/5 ml, or 10 mg/5 ml linctus. (Sugar-free versions available.)
Dose: adults, 5-10 mg 3-4 times a day; children over 1 year, 2-5 mg 3-5 times a day according to age.
Availability: NHS and private prescription, over the counter.
Contains: pholcodine.
Brand names: Galenphol, Pavacol-D. (Other brands available over the counter.)

drowsiness, upset stomach (particularly constipation), sweating, dizziness, breathing difficulty, low blood pressure, difficulty passing urine, dry mouth, headache, vertigo, flushing, change in heart rhythm, mood changes, rash, itching, addiction, reduced sexual desire.

in pregnant women, women in labour, mothers who are breastfeeding, elderly or weakened patients, and in those suffering from breathing, kidney, or liver problems, low blood pressure, underactive thyroid, enlarged prostate, or epilepsy. (Higher doses not suitable for some of these categories.)

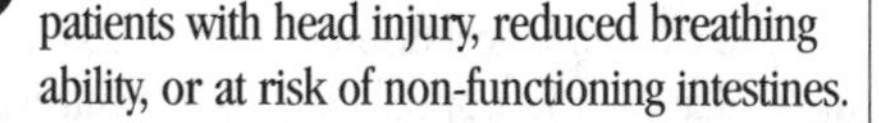
children under 1 year, alcoholics, or for patients with head injury, reduced breathing ability, or at risk of non-functioning intestines.

MAOIS, alcohol, sedating drugs, ritonavir.

Phosex *see* calcium acetate tablets
(Vitaline Pharmaceuticals UK)

Phosphate-Sandoz
(Distriphar)
An effervescent tablet used as a phosphate supplement to treat elevated calcium levels and low phosphate levels.

Dose: adults and children over 5 years up to 6 tablets a day; children under 5 years up to 3 tablets a day.
Availability: NHS and private prescription, over the counter.
Contains: sodium acid phosphate, sodium bicarbonate, potassium bicarbonate.

 diarrhoea, nausea.

 in patients suffering from kidney disease or those on a low-sodium diet.

 ANTACIDS.

Phyllocontin *see* aminophylline modified-release tablets
(Napp Pharmaceuticals)

Physeptone *see* methadone tablets/mixture
(Martindale Pharmaceuticals)

Physiotens *see* moxonidine tablets
(Solvay Healthcare)

---

phytomenadione tablets/oral solution
A tablet or oral solution used as a vitamin K supplement to treat patients with bleeding (or likely to bleed) owing to low levels of clotting factors in the blood (e.g. in newborn babies and as an antidote to ANTICOAGULANT drugs).

Strengths available: 10 mg tablets; 2 mg/0.2 ml oral solution.
Dose: to treat low levels of blood-clotting factors (e.g. after overdose of anticoagulants) adults, 5-20 mg (children 5-10 mg) given once and repeated later if the blood fails to respond; to prevent bleeding in newborn babies, 2 mg given at birth followed by 2 mg 4-7 days later (if baby is breastfed, a third dose given at 1 month).
Availability: NHS and private prescription. (Tablets also available over the counter.)
Contains: phytomenadione (a form of vitamin K).
Brand names: Konakion, Konakion MM.

in pregnant women.

 anticoagulants.

Picolax *see* sodium picosulphate liquid and magnesium sulphate
(Ferring Pharmaceuticals)
A powder in sachets used to evacuate the bowels before surgery or other procedures.

cont.

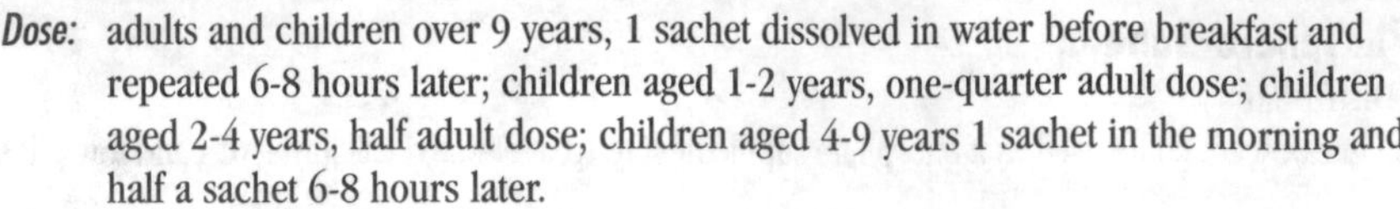

Dose: adults and children over 9 years, 1 sachet dissolved in water before breakfast and repeated 6-8 hours later; children aged 1-2 years, one-quarter adult dose; children aged 2-4 years, half adult dose; children aged 4-9 years 1 sachet in the morning and half a sachet 6-8 hours later.

---

pilocarpine eye drops/eye gel/ocular inserts

An eye drop, eye gel, or eye insert used as a pupil constrictor to treat glaucoma.

Strengths available: 0.5%, 1%, 2%, 3%, and 4% drops; 1%, 2%, and 4% single-use eye drops; 4% eye gel; insert releasing 20 mcg or 40 mcg per hour.

Dose: the drops applied to the affected eye(s) up to four times a day; the gel applied at bedtime only; the insert left in place under eyelid for one week.

Availability: NHS and private prescription.

Contains: pilocarpine hydrochloride or pilocarpine nitrate.

Brand names: Minims Pilocarpine, Ocusert Pilo, Pilogel.

Compound preparations: Isopto Carpine.

 headache, discomfort in the eye, blurred vision, short sight, other changes in the eye. Rarely, low blood pressure, slow heart beat, breathing difficulties, increased saliva or tears, sweating, upset stomach, urgent need to pass urine.

 in patients with dark-coloured eyes and those with damaged eyes, heart disease, high blood pressure, asthma, stomach ulcers, difficulty passing urine, or Parkinson's disease. Patients are advised not to drive because vision may be impaired in poor light (e.g. at night).

 children or for patients with some eye disorders (e.g. iritis, uveitis, some forms of glaucoma) or those wearing soft contact lenses.

 soft contact lenses.

---

pilocarpine hydrochloride tablets

A tablet used to treat the symptoms of underactive salivary glands (dry mouth) after radiation treatment for cancer, and dry mouth or eyes associated with disorders such as rheumatoid arthritis or LUPUS.

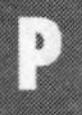

Strengths available: 5 mg tablets.

Dose: adults, 5 mg 3-4 times a day with or after meals increasing to maximum 30 mg a day after 4-8 weeks.

Availability: NHS and private prescription.

Contains: pilocarpine hydrochloride.

Brand names: Salagen.

 sweating, chills, upset stomach, excessive tears, dim or abnormal vision, high or low blood pressure, dizziness, inflamed nasal passages, weakness, increased need to pass urine, widening of blood vessels, headache, breathing disorder, heart rhythm disturbance, low blood pressure, shock, confusion, shaking.

 in patients suffering from asthma, heart or circulation disorders, stomach ulcers, gall bladder disorders, liver or kidney disorders, mental or memory disturbances. Your doctor may advise regular eye examinations. Patients are advised not to drive because vision may be impaired in poor light (e.g. at night).

 children, pregnant women, mothers who are breastfeeding, or for patients with uncontrolled asthma or other severe breathing disorder, eye inflammation, or glaucoma.

⇔ BETA-BLOCKERS, ANTIMUSCARINIC DRUGS.

Pilogel *see* pilocarpine eye gel
(Alcon)

pimozide tablets

A tablet used as a sedative to treat schizophrenia and other mental disorders.

Strengths available: 2 mg and 4 mg tablets.
Dose: adults, 2-4 mg a day at first increasing to a maximum of 20 mg a day; elderly patients half adult dose.
Availability: NHS and private prescription.
Contains: pimozide.
Brand names: Orap.

 movement disorders, muscle spasms, restlessness, shaking, dry mouth, heart rhythm disturbance, low blood pressure, weight gain, blurred vision, impotence, low body temperature, breast swelling, menstrual changes, blood, liver, eye, and skin changes, drowsiness, apathy, nightmares, sleeplessness, depression, blocked nose, difficulty passing water. Rarely, fits. Your doctor will advise brain function tests before treatment starts (and regularly afterwards if dose is above 16 mg a day). Heart check-ups may also be advised.

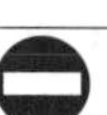 children, mothers who are breastfeeding, unconscious patients, or for those suffering from severe kidney or liver impairment, depression, Parkinson's disease, bone marrow depression, PHAEOCHROMOCYTOMA, or with a history of heart rhythm disturbance.

 in pregnant women, the elderly, and in patients suffering from heart, lung, or circulation disorders, epilepsy, thyroid disorders, infections, MYASTHENIA GRAVIS, chemical imbalance, epilepsy, kidney or liver disease, glaucoma, enlarged prostate, or some blood disorders. Should be withdrawn gradually.

 alcohol, sedatives, antidepressants, some antidiabetic drugs, anaesthetics, anti-epileptic medications, drugs affecting heart rhythm, ritonavir and other antivirals, halofantrine, sotalol, propranolol, lithium, clarithromycin, erythromycin, some antifungals, DIURETICS.

P

Pinadone *see* methadone mixture
(Pinewood Healthcare International)

pindolol tablets

A tablet used as a BETA-BLOCKER to treat high blood pressure and angina.

Strengths available: 5 mg and 15 mg tablets.
Dose: adults, for angina 2.5-5 mg up to three times a day; for high blood pressure,

cont.

10-15 mg a day at first (in divided doses) increasing to a maximum of 45 mg a day.

Availability: NHS and private prescription.
Contains: pindolol.
Brand names: Visken.
Compound preparations: Viskaldix.

 cold hands and feet, sleep disturbance, slow heart rate, tiredness, wheezing, heart failure, low blood pressure, stomach upset. Rarely, dry eyes, rash, worsening of psoriasis.

 in pregnant women, mothers who are breastfeeding, the elderly, and in patients suffering from diabetes, kidney or liver disorders, MYASTHENIA GRAVIS, or with a history of allergies. May need to be withdrawn before surgery. Withdraw gradually.

 children or for patients suffering from heart block or failure, asthma, PHAEOCHROMOCYTOMA, or a history of breathing disorders.

 general anaesthetics CALCIUM-CHANNEL BLOCKERS, ALPHA-BLOCKERS, clonidine, ANTIHYPERTENSIVES, amiodarone, antidiabetics, thymoxamine, theophylline, aminophylline.

---

pinene *see* Rowachol, Rowatinex

---

pioglitazone tablets

A tablet used, in combination with other antidiabetic drugs, to treat diabetes.

Strengths available: 15 mg and 30 mg tablets.
Dose: adults 15-30 mg once a day.
Availability: NHS and private prescription.
Contains: pioglitazone.
Brand names: Actos.

anaemia, low or high blood sugar levels, high cholesterol levels, stomach upset, headache, dizziness, weight gain, fluid retention, heart failure, blood changes, tiredness, weakness, joint pain, impotence, blood in the urine.

 your doctor may advise regular weight checks and blood tests.

 children under 18 years, pregnant women, mothers who are breastfeeding, or for patients with severe kidney disorders, liver disorder, heart failure (or history of heart failure). Not to be used with insulin.

 insulin, cerivastatin, NON-STEROIDAL ANTI-INFLAMMATORY DRUGS.

---

piperazine hydrate *see* Pripsen Elixir

---

piperazine oestrone sulphate *see* estropipate (new name)

---

piperazine phosphate *see* Pripsen Sachets

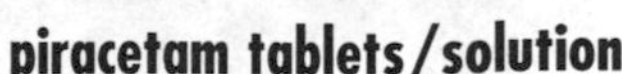

piracetam tablets/solution

A tablet or solution used to treat spasmodic muscle contractions.

Strengths available: 800 mg tablets; 333.3 mg/ml solution.
Dose: adults, 7200 mg a day (in divided doses) at first, increased to a maximum of 20,000 mg a day. (When using oral solution drink water afterwards.)
Availability: NHS and private prescription.
Contains: piracetam.
Brand names: Nootropil.

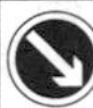 diarrhoea, drowsiness, sleeplessness, nervousness, weight gain, depression, rash, excessive movements.

 in the elderly and in patients with kidney disorders. The treatment should be withdrawn slowly.

 children under 16 years, pregnant women, mothers who are breastfeeding, or for patients with liver disease or severe kidney disorders.

 thyroxine, alcohol, sedating drugs.

Piriton *see* chlorpheniramine tablets/syrup (Stafford-Miller)

---

piroxicam capsules/suppositories/dispersible tablets/or tablet

A capsule, suppository, dispersible tablet, or tablet to melt in the mouth used as a NON-STEROIDAL ANTI-INFLAMMATORY DRUG to treat gout attacks, pain and inflammation in arthritis (including juvenile arthritis), and other muscle or joint problems.

Strengths available: 10 mg or 20 mg capsules; 20 mg melt-in-mouth tablets; 10 mg or 20 mg dispersible tablets; 20 mg suppositories.
Dose: adults, usually 20 mg once a day (10-30 mg for maintenance); 40 mg a day may be used for 2 days (in most disorders or up to 6 days in gout); children use reduced doses according to body weight.
Availability: NHS and private prescription.
Contains: piroxicam.
Brand names: Brexidol, Feldene, Flamatrol, Pirozip.
Other preparations: piroxicam gel *see* non-steroidal anti-inflammatory drug (topical).

 ACE-INHIBITORS, aspirin or other non-steroidal anti-inflammatory drugs, some ANTIBIOTICS, ANTICOAGULANTS, some antidiabetic drugs, some antivirals, methotrexate, DIURETICS, lithium, tacrolimus, cyclosporin, digoxin.

 stomach upset and bleeding or ulceration, rash, severe allergy, difficulty breathing, blood or kidney disorders, headache, dizziness, noises in the ears, sensitivity to light, vertigo. Rarely, fluid retention, liver disorders, inflamed pancreas, inflamed bowel, meningitis. Suppositories may cause irritation around rectum.

 in the elderly, pregnant women, mothers who are breastfeeding, and in patients with heart, liver, or kidney disorders, high blood pressure, asthma or LUPUS.

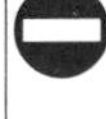 patients with a history of allergy to aspirin or other NSAID, severe kidney disorders, blood-clotting disorders, PORPHYRIA, currently active stomach ulcer or intestinal bleeding, inflamed intestines or severe heart failure. Suppositories not to be used for patients with inflammation of the anus or rectum. Melt-in-the-mouth tablets not to be used by patients with PHENYLKETONURIA.

piroxicam gel *see* non-steroidal anti-inflammatory drug (topical)

Pirozip *see* piroxicam capsules
(Ashbourne Pharmaceuticals)

---

pivmecillinam tablets

A tablet used as an ANTIBIOTIC to treat salmonella infections, cystitis, and other urine infections.

Strengths available: 200 mg tablets
Dose: adults and children over 40 kg, usually 200-400 mg every 6-8 hours (up to 2400 mg a day in salmonella infections); children under 40 kg reduced doses according to body weight.
Availability: NHS and private prescription.
Contains: pivmecillinam hydrochloride.
Brand names: Selexid.

severe allergic reaction, skin rash, itching, fever, joint pain, anaemia, kidney disorders, blood changes, fits, pins and needles, diarrhoea.

in pregnant women and in patients with a history of allergy or kidney disorders. Your doctor may advise liver and kidney tests in long-term treatment. Swallow the tablets with plenty of fluid at meal times in a standing or sitting position.

infants under 3 months, patients allergic to penicillin products, or who suffer from some muscle or liver disorders, narrowed oesophagus, or blocked intestines.

ANTICOAGULANTS, methotrexate, oral contraceptives, sodium valproate, valproic acid.

---

pizotifen tablets/elixir

A tablet or elixir used as a blood-vessel stabilizer to prevent migraine.

Strengths available: 0.5 mg and 1.5 mg tablets; 0.25 mg/5 ml elixir.
Dose: adults, 1.5 mg at night or 500 mcg three times a day at first increasing to maximum of 3 mg per dose and 4.5 mg a day if needed.; children up to 1.5 mg a day in divided doses (maximum of 1 mg in a single dose at night).
Availability: NHS and private prescription.
Contains: pizotifen hydrogen malate.
Brand names: Sanomigran.

drowsiness, weight gain, increased appetite, excitement (in children), ANTIMUSCARINIC effects, Rarely, nausea, dizziness.

in pregnant women and in patients suffering from glaucoma, kidney disorders, or who have difficulty passing urine.

mothers who are breastfeeding.

alcohol, sedatives.

PKU *see* phenylketonuria

Plaquenil *see* hydroxychloroquine tablets
(Sanofi Winthrop)

Plavix *see* clopidogrel tablets
(Sanofi Winthrop)

Plendil *see* felodipine tablets
(AstraZeneca UK)

Plesmet *see* ferrous glycine sulphate syrup
(Link Pharmaceuticals)

pneumococcal vaccine

A vaccination used to provide immunization against pneumonia.

Dose: adults and children over 2 years, one single dose of 0.5 ml. There may be a need to repeat after 5-10 years in patients whose immunity declines more than usual (e.g. if the spleen is removed).

Availability: NHS and private prescription.

Contains: pneumococcal polysaccharide vaccine.

Brand names: Pneumovax II, Pnu-Imune.

drugs that suppress the immune system.

mild fever, discomfort at the site of the injection, relapse in patients suffering from skin rash caused by low blood platelet levels, severe allergic reaction.

in patients with severely weak heart or lungs or who have previously suffered from pneumonia. Revaccination may result in more serious reactions.

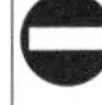
children under 2 years, pregnant women, mothers who are breastfeeding, or for patients who have an infection or who are suffering from feverish breathing illness or active infection, or have been given radio- or chemotherapy to treat Hodgkin's disease, or less than 10 days before or during any treatment that suppresses the immune system.

Pneumovax II *see* pneumococcal vaccine
(Aventis Pasteur MSD)

Pnu-Imune *see* pneumococcal vaccine
(Wyeth Laboratories)

Pocketscan

(Lifescan)

A reagent strip used in conjunction with the Pocketscan meter to detect blood glucose levels. Blood-glucose monitoring enables individual patients suffering from diabetes accurately to control blood glucose and manage their condition.

Availability: NHS and private prescription, nurse prescription, over the counter.

---

podophyllin compound paint

A paint used as a skin softener to treat genital warts.

Strengths available: 15% paint.
Dose: applied by trained nurses or doctors once a week. The solution should be left on the skin for no longer than 6 hours then washed off.
Availability: NHS and private prescription.
Contains: podophyllum resin in compound benzoin tincture.
Other preparations: podophyllotoxin cream/solution.
Compound preparations: Posalfilin ointment.

 irritation, toxicity.

 in patients with large numbers of warts (a few treated at a time to prevent toxicity). Keep well away from the face.

 children, pregnant women, mothers who are breastfeeding, or for application to normal or broken skin.

---

podophyllotoxin cream/solution

A cream or solution used as a skin softener to treat genital warts.

Strengths available: 0.5% solution; 0.15% cream.
Dose: adults, applied twice a day for 3 days and may be repeated at weekly intervals to a maximum of 4-5 periods of treatment (depending on brand).
Availability: NHS and private prescription.
Contains: podophyllotoxin.
Brand names: Condyline, Warticon, Warticon Fem.
Other preparations: podophyllin paint compound BP.

 irritation, toxicity.

 in patients with large numbers of warts (a few treated at a time to prevent toxicity). Keep well away from the face.

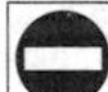 children, pregnant women, mothers who are breastfeeding, or for application to normal or broken skin.

P

---

poliomyelitis vaccine

A live vaccine taken by mouth, or an inactivated vaccine given by injection, used to prevent poliomyelitis.

Dose: 3 doses at 1-month intervals required for course (usually given in infancy) with boosters given when starting and leaving school and every 10 years afterwards if at particular risk (e.g. because of occupation or travel).

Availability: NHS and private prescription.

Contains: poliomyelitis virus.

patients with feverish illness. Live (oral) vaccine not to be used in patients with poorly functioning immune system (or people living with them), HIV infection, some forms of cancer, or those with stomach upset.

discomfort at site of injection (with inactivated vaccine), mild fever.

live (oral) vaccine not given to pregnant women unless benefit outweighs risk to baby.

oral typhoid vaccine (with live vaccine).

---

poloxamer *see* co-danthramer

---

polyacrylic acid *see* carbomer eye drops

---

polyethylene glycol *see* macrogol (alternative name)

Polyfax

(Dominion Pharma)

An ointment or eye ointment used as an ANTIBIOTIC to treat styes, conjunctivitis, other eye inflammations, skin infections, impetigo, burns.

Dose: for eye infections, apply the eye ointment at least twice a day; for skin infections, apply the standard ointment 2-3 times a day.

Availability: NHS and private prescription.

Contains: polymyxin B sulphate, bacitracin zinc.

may induce allergy to the ingredients. Also possible kidney disorders.

for the skin ointment: in children, the elderly, and in patients suffering from large or open wounds, kidney disorders.

---

polymyxin *see* Gregoderm, Maxitrol, Neosporin, Otosporin, Polyfax, Polytrim

---

polysaccharide-iron complex elixir/drops

An elixir (available with or without dropper bottle) used as an iron supplement to treat or prevent iron-deficiency anaemia.

Strengths available: equivalent to 100 mg iron in 5 ml (elixir) or 0.5 mg iron per drop (from dropper bottle).

Dose: adults, 5 ml once or twice a day to treat anaemia or 2.5 ml a day to prevent the condition (once a

stomach upset.

in patients with inflamed bowel, constipation, other intestinal disorders, or who have a history of stomach ulcers.

cont.

day only in mid- to late pregnancy); children aged 6-12 years, 5 ml (aged 2-6 years 2.5 ml) once a day; younger children use drops three times a day (number of drops depends on body weight).

Availability: private prescription, over the counter. Elixir available on NHS. (Drops available on NHS only if given to premature babies.)

Contains: polysaccharide-iron complex.

Brand names: Niferex.

 some ANTIBIOTICS.

---

polystyrene sulphonate resin

A powder used (either rectally or by mouth) as an ion-exchange resin to treat raised potassium levels.

 raised calcium or sodium levels, low potassium levels, hard immovable faeces, stomach upset, ulcerated rectum or bowel disorder after enema.

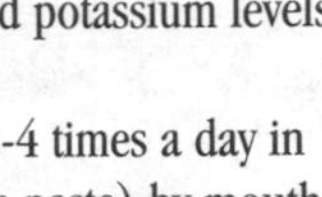

Dose: adults, 15 g 3-4 times a day in water (or as a paste) by mouth, or 30 g a day in methylcellulose solution as an enema used rectally; children use reduced doses according to body weight. (Newborn infants only treated rectally.)

Availability: NHS and private prescription, over the counter.

Contains: calcium polystyrene sulphonate or sodium polystyrene sulphonate.

Brand names: Calcium Resonium, Resonium A.

 in children, pregnant women, mothers who are breastfeeding, or in patients with heart failure, high blood pressure, kidney disorders, or fluid retention. Your doctor will advise regular blood tests.

 patients suffering from overactive parathyroid glands, sarcoidosis (a disease causing raised calcium levels), certain forms of cancer, blocked bowels, low potassium levels, or newborn infants with low gut activity.

Polytar/Polytar AF/Polytar Emollient/Polytar Plus *see* coal tar shampoo/solution (Stiefel Laboratories (UK))

---

polythiazide tablets

A tablet used as a DIURETIC to treat fluid retention and high blood pressure.

Strengths available: 1 mg tablets.

Dose: adults, usually 1-4 mg a day (but 0.5 mg may be sufficient to treat high blood pressure).

Availability: NHS and private prescription.

Contains: polythiazide.

Brand names: Nephril.

 low blood pressure on standing, mild stomach upset, reversible impotence, loss of appetite, dizziness, inflamed pancreas, gout, liver disorders, low potassium levels and other blood changes, allergy, rash, sensitivity to light, or tiredness.

 in pregnant women, mothers who are breastfeeding, the elderly, and in patients suffering from liver or kidney disorders, diabetes, gout, LUPUS. Your doctor may advise regular blood and urine checks.

 patients suffering from severe kidney or liver disorders, lack of urine output, Addison's disease, raised blood calcium/uric acid levels, low blood potassium/sodium levels, PORPHYRIA, or who are allergic to some antibiotics.

 NON-STEROIDAL ANTI-INFLAMMATORY DRUGS, drugs that alter heart rhythm, carbamazepine, halofantrine, antidiabetics, pimozide, digoxin, lithium, ANTIHYPERTENSIVES.

Polytrim

(Dominion Pharma)

Drops or an ointment used as an ANTIBIOTIC combination to treat eye infections.

 in pregnant women and mothers who are breastfeeding.

Dose: 1 drop applied into the affected eye(s) 3-4 times a day (the ointment applied 3-4 times a day) until 2 days after the symptoms have gone.
Availability: NHS and private prescription.
Contains: polymyxin B sulphate, trimethoprim.

---

polyvinyl alcohol eye drops

Drops used to lubricate dry eyes.

 patients who wear soft contact lenses.

Strengths available: 1% or 1.4% eye drops.
Dose: 1-2 drops used in the affected eye(s) as required.
Availability: NHS and private prescription, over the counter.
Contains: polyvinyl alcohol.
Brand names: Liquifilm Tears, Sno-Tears.
Compound preparations: Hypotears (with macrogol, another lubricant), Liquifilm Tears preservative-free (with povidone).

Ponstan *see* mefenamic acid tablets/capsules/suspension
(Elan Pharma)

Pork Actrapid *see* insulin

Pork Insulatard *see* insulin

Pork Mixtard *see* insulin

Posalfilin *see* podophyllin compound paint and salicylic acid collodion
(Norgine)
Used to treat verrucae on the feet.

Strengths available: 20% + 25% ointment.
Dose: apply daily.

Postmi 75 *see* aspirin 75 mg tablets
(Ashbourne Pharmaceuticals)

Potaba *see* potassium aminobenzoate tablets/capsules/powder
(Glenwood Laboratories)

---

potassium acid tartrate *see* potassium effervescent tablets

---

potassium aminobenzoate capsules/tablets/powder
A capsule, tablet, or powder in a sachet used as a fibrous tissue dissolver to treat thickened skin (as in scleroderma or Peyronie's disease).

Strengths available: 0.5 g capsules; 0.5 g tablets; 3 g sachets of powder.
Dose: adults up to 12 g a day in divided doses after food.
Availability: NHS and private prescription, over the counter.
Contains: potassium aminobenzoate.
Brand names: Potaba.

 loss of appetite, nausea.

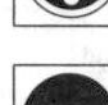 in patients suffering from kidney disease.

children.

 some ANTIBIOTICS.

---

potassium benzoate *see* Kloref

P

potassium bicarbonate *see* alginate liquid/tablets, Effercitrate sachets, Kloref, Phosphate-Sandoz, potassium effervescent tablets, Sando-K

---

potassium chloride *see* Diarrest, Klean-Prep, Kloref, Movicol, oral rehydration solution

---

potassium chloride modified-release tablets/syrup
An M-R TABLET or syrup used as a potassium supplement to treat potassium deficiency.

Strengths available: 600 mg m-r tablets; 75 mg/ml syrup.

Dose: as advised by doctor.
Availability: NHS and private prescription, over the counter.
Contains: potassium chloride.
Brand names: Kay-Cee-L, Slow-K.
Compound preparations: Kloref, Diumide-K, Lasikal, Neo-Naclex, Sando-K effervescent tablets (with potassium bicarbonate).
Other preparations: potassium effervescent tablets.

Caution needed with: some DIURETICS, ACE-INHIBITORS, cyclosporin.

Side effects: nausea and vomiting, obstruction and ulceration of the bowel or oesophagus.

Caution: in the elderly and in patients suffering from kidney disorders, narrowed or ulcerated intestines, or who have a history of stomach ulcers. (Caution also in patients with hiatus hernia for m-r tablets.) With m-r tablets, the dose should be taken with plenty of fluid while standing or sitting.

Not to be used for: patients with severe kidney failure or high chloride or acid levels in the blood.

potassium citrate mixture BP

A solution used as an alkalinizing treatment for the relief of discomfort in mild urine infections.

Dose: 10 ml diluted in water three times a day.
Availability: NHS and private prescription, over the counter.
Contains: potassium citrate, citric acid monohydrate.
Compound preparations: Effercitrate tablets (with potassium bicarbonate).

Side effects: raised potassium levels on high doses, mild DIURETIC effects.

Caution: in the elderly and in patients suffering from kidney problems or heart disease.

Caution needed with: some diuretics, ACE-INHIBITORS, cyclosporin.

potassium clorazepate capsules

A capsule used as a sedative for the short-term treatment of anxiety.

Strengths available: 7.5 mg or 15 mg capsules.
Dose: adults, 7.5-22.5 mg a day (elderly 7.5 mg a day).
Availability: private prescription only.
Contains: potassium clorazepate (dipotassium clorazepate).
Brand names: Tranxene.

Not to be used for: children under 16 years or for patients suffering from acute lung diseases, some chronic lung diseases, severe liver disease, MYASTHENIA GRAVIS, some obsessional and psychotic disorders, or who have stopped breathing while asleep.

Side effects: drowsiness, light-headedness, confusion, ver-tigo, stomach disturbances, loss of memory, aggression, headache, joint immobility, salivation changes, shaking, unsteadiness, low blood pressure, rash, changes in vision, changes in sexual desire, retention of urine, incontinence, blood changes, jaundice. Risk of addiction increases with dose and length of treatment. May impair judgement.

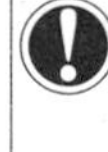
Caution: in children, the elderly, pregnant women, mothers who are breastfeeding, women during labour, and in patients suffering from lung disorders, glaucoma, kidney or liver disorders, muscle weakness, PORPHYRIA, or with a history of drug or alcohol abuse. Avoid long-term use and withdraw gradually.

cont.

 alcohol, other sedating drugs, some antivirals and anti-epileptic medications.

---

potassium effervescent tablets

An effervescent tablet used to correct potassium deficiency in patients with high chloride and acid levels in the blood.

Strengths available: 500 mg + 300 mg tablets.
Dose: as advised by doctor.
Availability: NHS and private prescription, over the counter.
Contains: potassium bicarbonate and potassium acid tartrate.
Other preparations: potassium chloride modified-release tablets/syrup, Sando-K effervescent tablets (potassium chloride with potassium bicarbonate).

 nausea and vomiting.

 in patients with kidney failure or heart disease.

 patients with low levels of chloride or high levels of potassium in the blood.

 some DIURETICS, ACE-INHIBITORS, cyclosporin.

---

potassium hydroxyquinoline sulphate *see* Quinocort, Quinoderm, Quinoped

---

potassium iodide *see* Vitamin Tablets for Nursing Mothers

---

potassium permanganate solution/tablets

A solution or tablet to dissolve in water used to cleanse and deodorize weeping eczema and wounds.

Strengths available: 0.1% solution; 400 mg tablets.
Dose: apply as a wet dressing, or soak the affected part using the solution (diluted 1 part in 10 with water) or the tablet (1 dissolved in 4 litres of water).
Availability: NHS and private prescription, over the counter.
Contains: potassium permanganate.
Other preparations: Permitabs (tablets dissolved to make solution).

irritation of mucous membranes.

 stains skin and clothing. The tablets must not be swallowed (for external use only).

P

---

potassium sorbate *see* sodium citrate enema

Poviderm *see* povidone iodine dressing

(SSL International)

---

povidone eye drops

An eye drop available as single-dose containers and used to treat dry eyes.

Strengths available: 5% drops.
Dose: 1 drop to be applied to the affected eye(s) four times a day.
Availability: NHS and private prescription, over the counter.
Contains: povidone.
Brand names: Oculotect.
Compound preparations: Liquifilm Tears preservative-free (with polyvinyl alcohol).

povidone iodine dressing/paint/solution/cream/ointment/spray/shampoo/skin cleanser

A range of products used as an antiseptic to treat skin or scalp infections (including scaly scalp disorders). Dressings are used on leg ulcers, pressure sores, and minor wounds.

Dose: most skin products used once or twice a day (once or twice a week for scalp preparations).
Availability: NHS and private prescription, over the counter. Solution and dressing also available on nurse prescription.
Contains: povidone-iodine.
Brand names: Betadine, Inadine, Poviderm, Videne.
Other preparations: povidone iodine gargle/mouthwash, povidone iodine pessaries/vaginal gel/vaginal cleansing kit.

may induce allergy.

in pregnant women, mothers who are breast-feeding, and in patients with kidney disorders or broken skin conditions.

patients with thyroid disorders. Many products not recommended for children under 2 years,

lithium.

povidone-iodine gargle/mouthwash

A solution used as an antiseptic to treat mouth infections.

Strengths available: 1% solution.
Dose: wash the mouth or gargle (using neat or diluted solution) for 30 seconds up to four times a day for up to 14 days.
Availability: NHS and private prescription, over the counter.
Contains: povidone-iodine.
Brand names: Betadine.
Other preparations: povidone iodine dressing/paint/solution/cream/ointment/spray/shampoo/skin cleanser, povidone iodine pessaries/vaginal gel/vaginal cleansing kit.

irritation, may induce allergy.

in pregnant women, mothers who are breast-feeding, and in patients with kidney disorders or broken skin conditions.

children under 6 years or for patients with thyroid disorders.

lithium.

povidone-iodine pessaries/vaginal gel/vaginal cleansing kit

A pessary, vaginal gel, or vaginal cleansing kit used as an antiseptic to treat some vaginal infections.

Strengths available: 200 mg pessaries; 10% vaginal gel; 10% solution in vaginal cleansing kit.
Dose: 1 pessary inserted into the vagina twice a day or 5 g vaginal gel inserted at night; or the vaginal cleansing kit used each morning. Products may be used in combination with each other (using one product in the morning and another at night). Maximum treatment period 14 days.
Availability: NHS and private prescription, over the counter.
Contains: povidone-iodine.
Brand names: Betadine.
Other preparations: povidone iodine dressing/paint/solution/cream/ointment/spray/shampoo/skin cleanser, povidone iodine gargle/mouthwash.

Side effects: irritation, may induce allergy.

Caution: in patients with kidney disorders. The solution in the cleansing kit must be diluted before use. These products may not be suitable for use with barrier contraceptives.

Not to be used for: children, pregnant women, mothers who are breastfeeding, or for patients with thyroid disorders.

Caution needed with: lithium, barrier contraceptives.

Powergel *see* non-steroidal anti-inflammatory drug (topical)
(Searle)

Pragmatar *see* coal tar cream
(Alliance Pharmaceuticals)

Pralenal *see* enalapril tablets
(Opus Pharmaceuticals)

P

pramipexole tablets

A tablet used in combination with levodopa to treat Parkinson's disease.

Strengths available: 88 mcg, 180 mcg, and 700 mcg tablets.
Dose: 88 mcg three times a day at first increasing gradually to a maximum of 3.3 mg a day (in three divided doses).
Availability: NHS and private prescription.
Contains: pramipexole dihydrochloride monohydrate.

stomach upset, drowsiness, sudden onset of sleep, movement disorders, hallucinations, low blood pressure.

in pregnant women and in patients with severe heart or circulation disorders, mental disorders, or kidney disease. Your doctor may advise regular eye tests. Do not drive or undertake other hazardous activities.

Brand names: Mirapexin.

 children or mothers who are breastfeeding.

 digoxin, sedatives, alcohol.

---

pramocaine *see* pramoxine (alternative name)

---

pramoxine *see* rectal corticosteroid

---

pravastatin tablets

A tablet used as a STATIN to reduce cholesterol levels in patients who have not responded to dietary changes, to slow down the narrowing of heart blood vessels, and to reduce the possibility of heart attack or stroke in some patients who are particularly vulnerable. Also used to reduce the number of days in hospital after a heart attack.

Strengths available: 10 mg, 20 mg, and 40 mg tablets.
Dose: adults, usually 10-40 mg at night.
Availability: NHS and private prescription.
Contains: pravastatin sodium.
Brand names: Lipostat.

 children under 18 years, pregnant women, mothers who are breastfeeding, or for patients with current liver disease or some inherited cholesterol disorders.

 tiredness, rash, chest pain, muscle pain and inflammation, headache, stomach upset, liver changes. Report any unexplained muscle pain to your doctor.

 in patients with liver disorders. Your doctor may advise regular blood tests. Women of child-bearing age should use adequate contraception during treatment and for 1 month afterwards.

 cyclosporin, other lipid-lowering drugs.

Praxilene *see* naftidrofuryl capsules (Lipha Pharmaceuticals)

prazosin tablets

A tablet used as an ALPHA-BLOCKER to treat heart failure, high blood pressure, Raynaud's phenomenon, and enlarged prostate gland.

Strengths available: 0.5 mg, 1 mg, and 2 mg tablets.
Dose: for heart failure, 0.5 mg 2-4 times a day increasing to a maximum of 20 mg a day if needed; for high blood pressure, 0.5 mg 2-3 times a day up to a maxi-

 low blood pressure on standing, dizziness, stomach upset, weakness, depression, dry mouth, headache, palpitations, fluid retention, blocked nose, lack of energy, increased need to pass urine, drowsiness.

cont.

mum of 20 mg a day if needed; for Raynaud's phenomenon 0.5 mg twice a day up to a maximum of 2 mg twice a day; for enlarged prostate 0.5 mg twice a day up to a maximum of 2 mg twice a day.

Availability: NHS and private prescription.
Contains: prazosin hydrochloride.
Brand names: Alphavase, Hypovase.

in the elderly, pregnant women, mothers who are breastfeeding, and in patients suffering from heart conditions, kidney or liver disorders. Take the first dose at bedtime.

children or for patients who have low blood pressure on standing or those suffering from fainting when they urinate.

sedatives, alcohol, anaesthetics, anti-depressants, BETA-BLOCKERS, some other drugs used to treat high blood pressure or angina, DIURETICS, thymoxamine.

Preconceive *see* folic acid tablets
(Lane Health Products)

Precortisyl Forte *see* prednisolone tablets
(Hoechst Marion Roussel)

Predenema *see* corticosteroid enema
(Pharmax)

Predfoam *see* corticosteroid internal foam
(Pharmax)

Pred-Forte *see* prednisolone eye drops
(Allergan)

---

prednisolone *see* corticosteroid enema/internal foam, prednisolone enteric-coated tablets/soluble tablets/tablets, prednisolone eye drops, rectal corticosteroid

P

---

prednisolone tablets/soluble tablets/enteric-coated tablets

A tablet, soluble tablet, or E-C TABLET used as a CORTICOSTEROID to suppress inflammation and allergies. It is useful in conditions such as asthma, rheumatoid arthritis, and inflammatory bowel disease, and to suppress the immune system.

Strengths available: 1 mg, 5 mg, and 25 mg tablets; 2.5 mg and 5 mg e-c tablets; 5 mg soluble tablets.
Dose: adults, usually up to 60 mg a day (maintenance usually 2.5-15 mg). Children use reduced doses.
Availability: NHS and private prescription.

Contains: prednisolone (or prednisolone sodium phosphate in soluble tablets).
Brand names: Deltacortril, Precortisyl Forte.

 high blood sugar, thin bones, mood changes, stomach ulcers, fluid retention, potassium loss, high blood pressure, menstrual irregularity, hairiness, increased likelihood of infection, euphoria, depression, sleeplessness, aggravation of schizophrenia and epilepsy, eye disorders, thinning of skin, acne, bruising, blood changes, stomach upset, inflamed pancreas, muscle abnormality, suppression of the ADRENAL GLANDS, ulcerated or infected oesophagus, general feeling of being unwell, hiccups, reduced growth in children.

 in pregnant women, mothers who are breast-feeding, and in patients who have had recent bowel surgery or who are suffering from inflamed veins, psychiatric disorders, thinning of the bones, stomach ulcers, tuberculosis or other infections, high blood pressure, glau-coma, epilepsy, diabetes, underactive thyroid, liver disease, stress. Withdraw gradually. Avoid contact with chicken pox for 3 months after treatment ends and seek medical attention if exposed.

 infants under 1 year or for patients who have untreated infections.

 live vaccines, some ANTIBIOTICS and anti-epileptics, ANTICOAGULANTS, antidiabetics, some anti-fungals, digoxin, cyclosporin. ANTACIDS should not be taken at the same time as e-c tablets.

prednisolone eye drops

Eye drops used as a CORTICOSTEROID for the short-term treatment of eye inflammation when no infection is present.

Strengths available: 0.5% or 1% eye drops. Also 0.5% single-use drops.
Dose: usually 1-2 drops into the affected eye(s) every 1-2 hours, reducing when symptoms sub-side.
Availability: NHS and private prescription.
Contains: prednisolone sodium phosphate.
Brand names: Pred Forte, Prednisolone Minims, Predsol.
Compound preparations: Predsol-N (with neomycin).

 rise in eye pressure, thinning of cornea, cataract, eye infection.

 avoid prolonged use in pregnant women or infants.

 patients suffering from eye infections, glaucoma, corneal ulcer, or who wear contact lenses.

 contact lenses.

Prednisolone Minims *see* prednisolone eye drops
(Chauvin Pharmaceuticals)

Predsol *see* prednisolone eye drops, corticosteroid enema, rectal corticosteroid
(Medeva Pharma)

Predsol-N *see* prednisolone eye drops and neomycin eye drops
(Medeva Pharma)

Pregaday *see* ferrous fumarate tablets and folic acid tablets
(Medeva Pharma)
A tablet used to treat anaemia in mid- to late pregnancy.

Strengths available: equivalent to 100 mg iron + 350 mcg folic acid.
Dose: 1 a day.

Pregnyl *see* chorionic gonadotrophin injection
(Organon Laboratories)

Prelude *see* nonoxynol pessaries
(W. J. Rendell)

Premarin *see* hormone replacement therapy (oestrogen-only), hormone replacement therapy (topical)
(Wyeth Laboratories)

Premique/Premique cycle *see* hormone replacement therapy (combined)
(Wyeth Laboratories)

Prempak-C *see* hormone replacement therapy (combined)
(Wyeth Laboratories)

Prepadine *see* dothiepin tablets
(Berk Pharmaceuticals)

Prescal *see* isradipine tablets
(Novartis Pharmaceuticals UK)

Preservex *see* aceclofenac tablets
(UCB Pharma)

Prestim *see* timolol tablets and bendrofluazide tablets
(Leo Pharmaceuticals)

Strengths available: 10 mg + 2.5 mg tablets.
Dose: adults, usually 1-2 tablets a day (maximum 4 a day).

Priadel *see* lithium liquid/modified-release tablets
(Sanofi Synthelabo)

---

prilocaine *see* EMLA

---

primidone tablets

A tablet used as an anticonvulsant to treat epilepsy and involuntary shaking (tremor).

Strengths available: 250 mg tablets.
Dose: to treat epilepsy, adults 125 mg a day at first increasing to a maximum of 1500 mg a day (in divided doses); children 250-1000 mg a day in divided doses depending on age. To treat tremor, adults 50 mg a day increasing to a maximum of 750 mg a day.
Availability: NHS and private prescription.
Contains: primidone.
Brand names: Mysoline.

 drowsiness, hangover, dizziness, breathing difficulty, headache, confusion, excitement, anaemia, skin reactions, tolerance, addiction, lack of co-ordination, blood disorders, visual disturbances.

 in children, elderly or weak patients, pregnant women, mothers who are breastfeeding, and in patients with kidney, liver, or lung disease. Treatment should be withdrawn gradually.

 patients with a history of alcohol or drug abuse or suffering from PORPHYRIA.

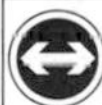 alcohol, sedatives, ANTICOAGULANTS, antidepressants, other anti-epileptic treatments, antivirals, CALCIUM-CHANNEL BLOCKERS, cyclosporin, oral contraceptives, tibolone, theophylline, aminophylline.

Primolut-N *see* norethisterone tablets
(Schering Health Care)

Primoteston Depot *see* testosterone injection
(Cambridge Laboratories)

Prioderm *see* malathion lotion/shampoo
(SSL International)

Priorix *see* MMR vaccine
(SmithKline Beecham Pharmaceuticals)

Pripsen sachets/elixir

(SSL International)
A sachet or liquid used to treat worm infestations in the intestines.

Dose: for sachets, to treat threadworm, adults and children over 6 years 1 sachet (infants 3-12 months 2.5 ml powder, children aged 1-6 years 5 ml powder) dissolved in water or milk, repeated after 14 days; for elixir, adults 15 ml once a day for 7 days (to treat threadworm) or 30 ml as a single dose (repeated after 14 days) to treat roundworm (children given reduced doses according to age and body weight).
Availability: NHS and private prescription, nurse prescription (if prescribed generically), over the counter.
Contains: piperazine hydrate (elixir) or piperazine phosphate and senna (sachets).

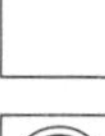 stomach upset, itchy rash, breathing difficulty, severe allergic reaction, skin disorders, dizziness, lack of co-ordination, drowsiness, confusion, muscle spasm.

 in pregnant women, mothers who are breast-feeding, and in patients suffering from kidney or liver disorders, epilepsy or other brain disorders. Very young children should be treated only on advice of a doctor.

 children under 3 months or for patients with severe kidney disorders.

 alcohol, sedating drugs.

Pripsen tablets *see* mebendazole tablets
(SSL International)

Pro-Banthine *see* propantheline tablets
(Hansam Healthcare)

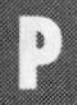

Pro-Viron *see* mesterolone tablets
(Schering Health Care)

procainamide tablets

A tablet used to treat abnormal heart rhythm.

Strengths available: 250 mg tablets.
Dose: adults, as advised by doctor (according to body weight).
Availability: NHS and private prescription.

 stomach upset, LUPUS-like symptoms, blood changes, rash, mental disorders, fever, heart disorders.

Contains: procainamide hydrochloride.
Brand names: Pronestyl.

 other drugs affecting heart rhythm, TRICYCLIC ANTIDEPRESSANTS, reboxetine, mizolastine, halofantrine, sedatives, alcohol, sotalol, muscle relaxants, cimetidine.

 in the elderly, pregnant women, and in patients suffering from liver or kidney disorders, asthma, or MYASTHENIA GRAVIS. Your doctor may advise regular blood tests.

 children, mothers who are breastfeeding, or for patients suffering from lupus or some heart disorders.

---

prochlorperazine tablets/buccal tablets/syrup/suppositories/sachets

A tablet, buccal tablet, syrup, suppository, or sachet of effervescent powder used to treat severe nausea, vomiting, vertigo, inner ear disturbances, severe anxiety, schizophrenia, and other mental disturbances.

Strengths available: 5 mg and 25 mg tablets; 3 mg buccal tablets (left between upper lip and gum to dissolve); 5 mg/5 ml syrup; 5 mg sachets; 5 mg and 25 mg suppositories.
Dose: to treat nausea and vomiting, adults 20 mg at first then 10 mg after 2 hours; to prevent nausea and vomiting, adults 5-10 mg 2-3 times a day (children reduced doses according to body weight). For ear disturbances, adults 5 mg three times a day increasing to a maximum of 30 mg a day then reducing for maintenance. For anxiety, adults 15-40 mg a day in divided doses. For mental disturbances, adults 12.5 mg twice a day at first increasing usually to 75-100 mg a day.
Availability: NHS and private prescription.
Contains: prochlorperazine maleate (tablets and suppositories) or prochlorperazine mesylate (syrup and sachets).
Brand names: Buccastem, Prozière 5, Stemetil.

 movement disorders, muscle spasms, restlessness, shaking, dry mouth, heart rhythm disturbance, low blood pressure, weight gain, blurred vision, impotence, low body temperature, breast swelling, menstrual changes, blood, liver, eye, and skin changes, drowsiness, apathy, nightmares, sleeplessness, depression, blocked nose, difficulty passing water. Rarely, fits.

 in pregnant women, mothers who are breastfeeding, the elderly, and in patients suffering from heart, lung, or circulation disorders, infections, MYASTHENIA GRAVIS. Should be withdrawn gradually.

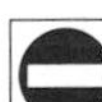 children (except for treatment of nausea and vomiting), unconscious patients, or for patients suffering from severe kidney or liver impairment, bone marrow depression, Parkinson's disease, glaucoma, epilepsy, thyroid disorders, enlarged prostate, kidney or liver disease, some blood disorders, or PHAEOCHROMOCYTOMA. The sachets are not suitable for patients with PHENYLKETONURIA.

 alcohol, sedatives, antidepressants, some antidiabetic drugs, anaesthetics, anti-epileptic medications, drugs affecting heart rhythm, ritonavir, halofantrine, sotalol, lithium.

Proctofoam-HC *see* rectal corticosteroid
(Stafford-Miller)

P

Proctosedyl *see* rectal corticosteroid
(Hoechst Marion Roussel)

---

procyclidine tablets/syrup

A tablet or syrup used as an ANTIMUSCARINIC treatment for Parkinson's disease and similar symptoms caused by medication.

Strengths available: 5 mg tablets; 2.5 mg/5 ml or 5 mg/5 ml syrup.
Dose: initially 2.5 mg (½ tablet) three times a day increasing gradually to a usual maximum of 30 mg a day. Elderly patients use lower doses.
Availability: NHS and private prescription.
Contains: procyclidine hydrochloride.
Brand names: Arpicolin, Kemadrin, Muscinil.

antimuscarinic effects, confusion, agitation, rash with high doses.

in the elderly, pregnant women, mothers who are breastfeeding, and in patients suffering from heart or blood vessel disease, enlarged prostate, liver or kidney disorders.

children or for patients suffering from untreated urine retention, glaucoma, some movement disorders, or intestinal blockage.

other antimuscarinic or sedating drugs.

Profasi *see* chorionic gonadotrophin injection
(Serono Laboratories (UK))

---

proflavine cream BPC

A cream used to treat minor burns and abrasions.

Dose: apply as necessary.
Availability: NHS and private prescription, over the counter.
Contains: proflavine hemisulphate, liquid paraffin.

stains clothing.

Proflex *see* non-steroidal anti-inflammatory drug (topical)
(Novartis Consumer Health)

P

---

progesterone injection

An injection used as a hormone treatment for abnormal menstrual bleeding, to maintain pregnancy in women who habitually abort, and as part of *in-vitro* fertilization (IVF) methods.

Strengths available: 25 mg, 50 mg, or 100 mg injections.
Dose: as advised by doctor.
Availability: NHS and private prescription.

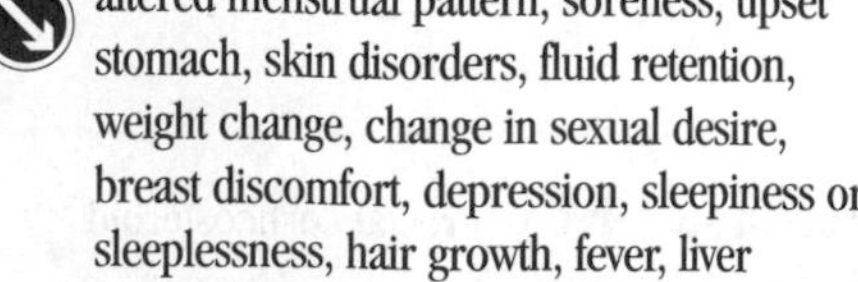
altered menstrual pattern, soreness, upset stomach, skin disorders, fluid retention, weight change, change in sexual desire, breast discomfort, depression, sleepiness or sleeplessness, hair growth, fever, liver disorders, reaction at injection site.

Contains: progesterone.
Brand names: Gestone.
Other preparations: progesterone suppositories/pessaries, progesterone vaginal gel.

 in mothers who are breastfeeding and in patients with diabetes, epilepsy, heart disease, liver or kidney disorders, high blood pressure, migraine, or with a history of depression.

 children or for patients suffering from abnormal vaginal bleeding, breast cancer, PORPHYRIA, severe blood vessel disorders, failed or incomplete abortion, or severe liver disorders.

cyclosporin.

progesterone suppositories/pessaries

A suppository/pessary used as a hormone treatment for post-natal depression and premenstrual syndrome.

Strengths available: 200 mg and 400 mg suppositories/pessaries.
Dose: adults 200-400 mg twice a day given either by vagina or rectum. (For pre-menstrual syndrome start on day 12-14 of cycle and continue until period starts.)
Availability: NHS and private prescription.
Contains: progesterone.
Brand names: Cyclogest.
Other preparations: progesterone injection, progesterone vaginal gel.

 altered menstrual pattern, soreness, upset stomach, skin disorders, fluid retention, weight change, change in sexual desire, breast discomfort, depression, sleepiness or sleeplessness, hair growth, fever, liver disorders. Pain with rectal use.

 in mothers who are breastfeeding and in patients with diabetes, epilepsy, heart disease, liver or kidney disorders, high blood pressure, migraine, or with a history of depression. Use rectally if barrier contraceptives are used.

 barrier contraceptives, cyclosporin.

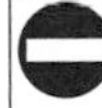 children or for patients suffering from abnormal vaginal bleeding, breast cancer, PORPHYRIA, severe blood vessel disorders, failed or incomplete abortion, or severe liver disorders. Not intended for use in pregnant women.

progesterone vaginal gel

A vaginal gel used as a hormone treatment for progesterone deficiency, infertility, or (in conjunction with oestrogen) to treat menopausal symptoms. Also used in *in-vitro* fertilization (IVF) methods.

Strengths available: 4% or 8% gel.
Dose: adults, usually 1 application of 4% gel on alternate days from days 15 to 25 of cycle for progesterone deficiency, or with the last 12 days of hormone

 altered menstrual pattern, soreness, upset stomach, skin disorders, fluid retention, weight change, change in sexual desire, breast discomfort, depression, sleepiness or sleeplessness, hair growth, fever, liver disorders.

 in mothers who are breastfeeding and in patients with diabetes, epilepsy, heart disease, liver or kidney disorders, high blood pressure, migraine, or with a history of depression.

cont.

replacement therapy (oestrogen only). For infertility or IVF use, 1 application of 8% gel on the days specified by doctor.

Availability: NHS and private prescription.

Contains: progesterone.

Brand names: Crinone.

Other preparations: progesterone injection, progesterone suppositories/pessaries.

 children or for patients suffering from abnormal vaginal bleeding, breast cancer, PORPHYRIA, severe blood vessel disorders, failed or incomplete abortion, or severe liver disorders.

barrier contraceptives, cyclosporin.

Prograf *see* tacrolimus capsules
(Healthcare Logistics)

---

proguanil tablets

A tablet used as an anti-malarial drug to treat and (in combination with other drugs) to prevent malaria.

Strengths available: 100 mg tablets.

Dose: to prevent malaria, adults and children over 12 years, 200 mg once a day; children under 14 years use reduced doses according to age. Begin taking the tablets at least 24 hours before entering infected area and continue for at least 4 weeks after leaving. (Doses for treating malaria as advised by doctor.)

Availability: NHS and private prescription, over the counter (if for prevention of malaria). Not generally prescribed on NHS for prevention of malaria.

Contains: proguanil hydrochloride.

Brand names: Paludrine.

Compound preparations: Malarone, Paludrine/Avloclor travel pack (combined with chloroquine tablets in one pack).

 mild stomach upset, skin reactions, hair loss, mouth ulcers, inflammation of the mouth.

 in pregnant women and in patients suffering from kidney disorders.

 warfarin.

Progynova/Progynova TS *see* hormone replacement therapy (oestrogen-only)
(Schering Health Care)

P

Proluton Depot *see* hydroxyprogesterone injection
(Schering Health Care)

---

promazine tablets/solution/suspension

A tablet, solution, or suspension used as a sedative to treat agitation or restlessness in the elderly, or as additional short-term treatment for other types of agitation.

Strengths available: 25 mg and 50 mg tablets; 25 mg/5 ml and 50 mg/5 ml solution; 50 mg/5 ml suspension.

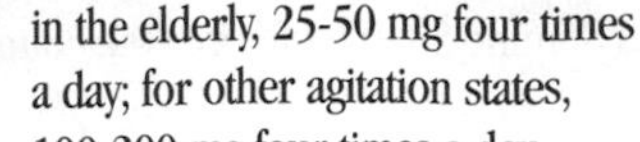

Dose: in the elderly, 25-50 mg four times a day; for other agitation states, 100-200 mg four times a day.
Availability: NHS and private prescription.
Contains: promazine hydrochloride (tablets or solution), promazine hydrochloride embonate (suspension).

 children, unconscious patients, or for patients suffering from severe kidney or liver impairment, bone marrow depression, or PHAEOCHROMOCYTOMA.

 alcohol, sedatives, antidepressants, some anti-diabetic drugs, anaesthetics, anti-epileptic medications, drugs affecting heart rhythm, ritonavir, halofantrine, sotalol, propranolol, lithium.

 movement disorders, muscle spasms, restlessness, shaking, dry mouth, heart rhythm disturbance, low blood pressure, weight gain, blurred vision, impotence, low body temperature, breast swelling, menstrual changes, blood, liver, eye, and skin changes, drowsiness, apathy, nightmares, sleeplessness, depression, blocked nose, difficulty passing water. Rarely, fits.

 in pregnant women, mothers who are breastfeeding, the elderly, and in patients suffering from heart, lung, or circulation disorders, epilepsy, Parkinson's disease, thyroid disorders, infections, MYASTHENIA GRAVIS, kidney or liver disease, glaucoma, enlarged prostate, or some blood disorders. Should be withdrawn gradually.

---

promethazine hydrochloride tablets/elixir

A tablet or elixir used as an ANTIHISTAMINE treatment for allergies, travel sickness, and as a sedative for the short-term treatment of insomnia.

Strengths available: 5 mg and 25 mg tablets; 5 mg/5 ml elixir.
Dose: for allergies, adults 25 mg at night (or twice a day if needed), or 10 mg 2-3 times a day; children aged 2-5 years 5-15 mg a day (aged 5-10 years 10-25 mg a day) in divided doses. For travel sickness, adults 20-25 mg the night before the journey, repeated the next morning if needed; children aged 2-5 years 5 mg (aged 5-10 years 10 mg) the night before and the following morning if needed. For sedation, adults 25-50 mg at bedtime; children 2-5 years 15-20 mg (5-10 years 20-25 mg) at bedtime.
Availability: NHS and private prescription, over the counter (except for sedation in children).
Contains: promethazine hydrochloride.

 drowsiness, reduced reactions. Rarely, dizziness, excitation, movement disorders, headache, ANTIMUSCARINIC effects. Rarely heart rhythm disturbances, severe allergic reaction, skin disorders, noises in the ears, sensitivity to sunlight, Parkinson-like symptoms, confusion, depression, fits, shaking, sweating, muscle pain, pins and needles, liver disorders, hair loss, sleep disturbances.

 in the elderly, pregnant women, mothers who are breastfeeding, and in patients with enlarged prostate, severe heart failure, low blood pressure, difficulty passing urine, Parkinson's disease, glaucoma, epilepsy, or liver disease.

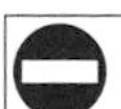 children under 2 years.

 MAOIS, TRICYCLIC ANTIDEPRESSANTS, some ANALGESICS, ritonavir, alcohol, other sedating drugs.

P

cont.

Brand names: Phenergan. Other brands, such as Sominex, available over the counter to treat insomnia in adults.
Other preparations: promethazine teoclate tablets.

promethazine teoclate tablets

A tablet used as an ANTIHISTAMINE treatment for nausea, vertigo, ear disorders, travel sickness, and to treat severe vomiting in pregnancy.

Strengths available: 25 mg tablets.
Dose: for travel sickness, adults 25 mg the night before the journey (or 1-2 hours before the journey); for other conditions, 25-75 mg (rarely 100 mg) a day; children aged 5-10 years half adult dose (maximum 37.5 mg a day); for vomiting in pregnancy, 25-100 mg at night.
Availability: NHS and private prescription, over the counter (for travel sickness only).
Contains: promethazine hydrochloride.
Brand names: Avomine.
Other preparations: promethazine hydrochloride tablets.

 drowsiness, reduced reactions. Rarely, dizziness, excitation, movement disorders, headache, ANTIMUSCARINIC effects. Rarely heart rhythm disturbances, severe allergic reaction, skin disorders, noises in the ears, sensitivity to sunlight, Parkinson-like symptoms, confusion, depression, fits, shaking, sweating, muscle pain, pins and needles, liver disorders, hair loss, sleep disturbances.

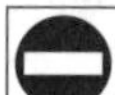 in the elderly, pregnant women, mothers who are breastfeeding, and in patients with enlarged prostate, severe heart failure, low blood pressure, difficulty passing urine, Parkinson's disease, glaucoma, epilepsy, or liver disease.

 children under 5 years.

MAOIS, TRICYCLIC ANTIDEPRESSANTS, some ANALGESICS, ritonavir, alcohol, other sedating drugs.

Promictuline *see* oxybutynin tablets
(Ashbourne Pharmaceuticals)

Prominal *see* methylphenobarbitone tablets
(Sanofi Winthrop)

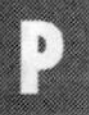

Pronestyl tablets *see* procainamide tablets
(Bristol-Myers Squibb Pharmaceuticals)

Propaderm *see* topical corticosteroid cream/ointment
(GlaxoWellcome UK)

propafenone tablets

A tablet used as an anti-arrhythmic drug to treat heart rhythm disturbances.

Strengths available: 150 mg and 300 mg tablets.

Dose: adults, 150 mg three times a day at first (in hospital) then up to 300 mg three times a day; patients under 70 kg and the elderly may use lower doses.
Availability: NHS and private prescription.
Contains: propafenone hydrochloride.
Brand names: Arythmol.

upset stomach, dizziness, headache, tiredness, rash, bitter taste in mouth, slow heart rate, low blood pressure on standing, heart conduction defects, lack of bile flow, blood disorders, LUPUS, fits, muscle spasm.

in the elderly, mothers who are breastfeeding, patients with pacemakers, and in patients suffering from heart failure, breathing disorders, liver or kidney disorders.

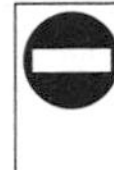
children, pregnant women, or for patients suffering from uncontrolled heart failure, heart shock, severe breathing disorders, chemical imbalance, some heart rhythm or conduction disturbances, very low blood pressure, MYASTHENIA GRAVIS.

rifampicin, ANTICOAGULANTS, TRICYCLIC ANTI-DEPRESSANTS, reboxetine, ritonavir, digoxin, cimetidine, theophylline, aminophylline.

---

propantheline tablets

A tablet used as an anti-spasm, ANTIMUSCARINIC treatment for intestinal spasm, bed wetting, or sweating.

Strengths available: 15 mg tablets.
Dose: adults, usually 15-20 mg 2-3 times a day (maximum of 120 mg a day).
Availability: NHS and private prescription.
Contains: propantheline bromide.
Brand names: Pro-Banthine.

antimuscarinic effects, skin reactions, stomach upset, altered heart rhythm, difficulty passing urine, disturbed vision, dry mouth, intolerance of light, flushing, dry skin, confusion, dizziness.

in children, pregnant women, mothers who are breastfeeding, elderly patients, and those with diarrhoea or inflamed bowel, high blood pressure, abnormal heart rhythm, fever, reflux oesophagitis, or heart attack.

patients with glaucoma, MYASTHENIA GRAVIS, enlarged prostate, or non-functioning intestines.

other antimuscarinic drugs.

Propecia *see* finasteride 1 mg tablets
(Merck Sharp and Dohme)

Propine *see* dipivefrine eye drops
(Allergan)

---

propiverine tablets

A tablet used as an ANTIMUSCARINIC treatment for unstable bladder, increased need or urgency of passing urine, or incontinence.

Strengths available: 15 mg tablets.
Dose: adults, 15 mg 2-4 times a day; elderly patients, 15 mg 2-3 times a day.
Availability: NHS and private prescription.
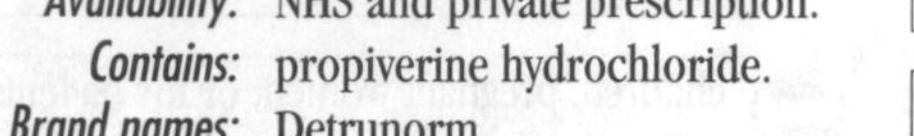
Contains: propiverine hydrochloride.
Brand names: Detrunorm.

 other antimuscarinic drugs, alcohol, sedating drugs.

 dry mouth, blurred vision, drowsiness, difficulty passing urine, low blood pressure, stomach upset, tiredness, irritability, restlessness, hot flushes, abnormal heart rhythm, rash.

 in the elderly and in patients suffering from overactive thyroid gland, heart disease, enlarged prostate, reflux oesophagitis, hiatus hernia, or numb nerves.

 children, pregnant women, mothers who are breastfeeding, or for patients suffering from severe kidney disorders, blocked intestines, some bowel disorders, glaucoma, MYASTHENIA GRAVIS, or liver disorders.

---

propranolol tablets/modified-release capsules

A tablet or M-R CAPSULE used as a BETA-BLOCKER to treat high blood pressure, PHAEOCHROMOCYTOMA (with ALPHA-BLOCKERS only), angina, heart rhythm disturbances, anxiety, and to prevent migraine and further heart attacks after a first one.

Strengths available: 10 mg, 40 mg, 80 mg, and 160 mg tablets; 80 mg and 160 mg m-r capsules.
Dose: 40-320 mg a day depending on condition. Standard tablet doses taken divided through the day. M-r capsules taken either as a single daily dose or twice a day.
Availability: NHS and private prescription.
Contains: propranolol hydrochloride.
Brand names: Bedranol SR, Beta-Prograne, Half Beta-Prograne, Half-Inderal LA, Inderal, Inderal LA.
Compound preparations: Inderetic, Inderex.

 cold hands and feet, sleep disturbance, slow heart rate, tiredness, wheezing, heart failure, low blood pressure, stomach upset. Rarely, dry eyes, rash, worsening of psoriasis.

 in pregnant women, mothers who are breast-feeding, the elderly, and in patients suffering from diabetes, kidney or liver disorders, MYASTHENIA GRAVIS, or with a history of allergies. May need to be withdrawn before surgery. Withdraw gradually.

 children or for patients suffering from heart block or failure, asthma, PHAEOCHROMOCYTOMA (apart from specific use with alpha-blockers), or a history of breathing disorders.

 general anaesthetics, CALCIUM-CHANNEL BLOCKERS, alpha-blockers, clonidine, ANTIHYPERTENSIVES, amiodarone, antidiabetics, thymoxamine, theophylline, aminophylline, fluvoxamine, chlorpromazine, propafenone.

---

propyl salicylate *see* Monphytol

---

propyl undecenoate *see* Monphytol

propylene glycol *see* Aserbine

propylthiouracil tablets

A tablet used to treat overactive thyroid.

Strengths available: 50 mg tablets.
Dose: adults, 300-600 mg a day until symptoms controlled then 50-150 mg a day for maintenance.
Availability: NHS and private prescription.
Contains: propylthiouracil.

rash, headache, nausea, mild stomach upset, joint pain, bone marrow depression, blood or liver disorders, inflamed blood vessels, rash, itching, LUPUS-like symptoms. Tell the doctor immediately if you develop sore throat, mouth ulcers, tiredness, unexplained bruising, or fever.

in pregnant women, mothers who are breastfeeding, and in patients with liver or kidney disorders.

Proscar *see* finasteride 5 mg tablets
(Merck Sharp and Dohme)

Prostap SR *see* leuprorelin injection
(Wyeth Laboratories)

protease *see* pancreatin capsules

Prothiaden *see* dothiepin capsules/tablets
(Knoll)

Protium *see* pantoprazole enteric-coated tablets
(Knoll)

Provera *see* medroxyprogesterone tablets
(Pharmacia and Upjohn)

Provigil *see* modafinil tablets
(Cephalon UK)

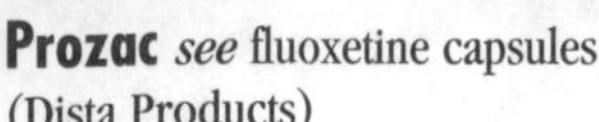

Prozac *see* fluoxetine capsules
(Dista Products)

Prozière 5 *see* prochlorperazine tablets
(Ashbourne Pharmaceuticals)

---

pseudoephedrine tablets/elixir/linctus

A tablet, elixir, or linctus used as a SYMPATHOMIMETIC decongestant to relieve congestion of the nose, sinuses, and upper respiratory tract.

Strengths available: 60 mg tablets; 30 mg/5 ml linctus or elixir.
Dose: adults, 60 mg four times a day; children aged 2-5 years 15 mg (aged 6-12 years 30 mg) 3-4 times a day.
Availability: NHS and private prescription, over the counter.
Contains: pseudoephedrine hydrochloride.
Brand names: Galpseud, Sudafed. (Other brands available over the counter.)
Compound preparations: Galpseud Plus, Sudafed Plus.

Side effects: rapid heart beat, sleeplessness, restlessness, anxiety. More rarely, irregular heart beat, shaking, dry mouth, cold hands and feet.

in the elderly and in patients with high blood pressure, narrowed blood supply to the heart, overactive thyroid, diabetes, kidney disease, or enlarged prostate.

children under 2 years.

MAOIS, drugs used to lower blood pressure, other sympathomimetics.

Psoriderm *see* coal tar preparations
(Dermal Laboratories)

Psorin *see* coal tar ointment/solution, dithranol ointment, and salicylic acid ointment
(Ayrton Saunders)

Strengths available: 1% + 0.11% + 1.6% ointment; scalp gel contains dithranol 0.25% + salicylic acid 1.6%, and methyl salicylate.
Dose: ointment applied up to twice a day; scalp gel applied on alternate days and washed off after 10-20 minutes, increasing to daily use (left on for 1 hour) if necessary.

Pulmicort/Pulmicort LS *see* budesonide inhaler
(AstraZeneca UK)

Pulmozyme *see* dornase alfa nebulizer solution
(Roche Products)

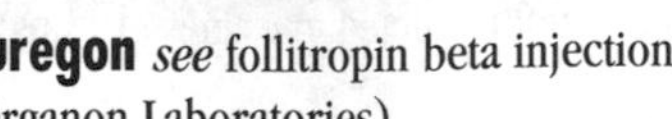

Puregon *see* follitropin beta injection
(Organon Laboratories)

Pylorid *see* ranitidine bismuth citrate tablets
(GlaxoWellcome UK)

Pyralvex

(Norgine)
A liquid used as an anti-inflammatory treatment for mouth ulcers and soreness caused by dentures.

Strengths available: 5% + 1% liquid.
Dose: adults, apply 3-4 times a day.
Availability: NHS and private prescription, over the counter.
Contains: anthraquinone glycosides and salicylic acid.

 irritation.

 children.

---

pyrazinamide tablets

A tablet used, in combination with other drugs, as an anti-tubercular drug to treat tuberculosis.

Strengths available: 500 mg tablets.
Dose: as advised by doctor.
Availability: NHS and private prescription.
Contains: pyrazinamide.
Brand names: Zinamide.
Compound preparations: Rifater.

 liver disorders, fever, loss of appetite, stomach upset, joint pain, blood disorders, itchy rash.

 in patients with diabetes, gout, liver or kidney disorders. Your doctor may advise that liver function and blood should be checked regularly.

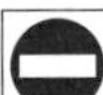 children or for patients with liver damage or PORPHYRIA.

---

pyridostigmine tablets

A tablet used as a nerve conduction enhancer to treat non-functioning bowel, MYASTHENIA GRAVIS, and to relieve urine retention after operations.

Strengths available: 60 mg tablets.
Dose: for myasthenia gravis, adults 30-120 mg up to 10 times a day; children use reduced doses (usually 30-360 mg a day). For non-functioning bowel or urine retention, adults 60-240 mg (children 15-60 mg) as required.
Availability: NHS and private prescription.
Contains: pyridostigmine bromide.

 stomach upset. With high doses, increased secretions, low blood pressure, slow heart beat, agitation, weakness, involuntary opening of bowels or passing of urine, shrunken pupils of the eyes, rapid eye movement.

 in pregnant women, mothers who are breast-feeding, patients suffering from asthma, heart or kidney disease, epilepsy, Parkinson's disease, disorders of the vagus nerve, low blood pressure, stomach ulcer.

cont.

Brand names: Mestinon.

patients with obstructed intestines or urinary system.

neomycin, clindamycin, colistin.

pyridoxine tablets

A tablet used to treat vitamin B_6 deficiency, nerve disorders caused by isoniazid treatment, some forms of anaemia, and premenstrual syndrome.

Strengths available: 20 mg and 50 mg tablets.
Dose: to treat deficiency, 20-50 mg up to three times a day; for nerve disorders 50 mg three times a day (treatment) or 10 mg a day (prevention); for anaemia 100-400 mg a day in divided doses; for premenstrual syndrome 50-100 mg a day.
Availability: NHS and private prescription, over the counter.
Contains: vitamin B_6.
Brand names: various brands available over the counter.

high dose may give toxic effects.

levodopa.

pyrimethamine tablets

A tablet used, in combination with other similar drugs, as an anti-malarial drug to prevent malaria for residents in malarial areas. Not recommended for travellers.

Strengths available: 25 mg tablets.
Dose: adults, 25 mg (children aged 5-10 years 12.5 mg) once a week. Continue until 4 weeks after leaving the malarious area.
Availability: NHS and private prescription.
Contains: pyrimethamine.
Brand names: Daraprim.
Compound preparations: Fansidar, Maloprim.

rash, anaemia, sleeplessness.

in pregnant women, mothers who are breast-feeding, and in patients with liver or kidney disorders.

children under 5 years.

co-trimoxazole, trimethoprim, phenytoin, methotrexate.

P

Pyrogastrone

(Sanofi Winthrop)

A tablet or liquid used as an ANTACID and stomach-lining protection to treat inflammation and ulceration of the oesophagus and acid reflux from the stomach.

Strengths available: 20 mg + 600 mg + 240 mg + 60 mg + 210 mg tablets; 10 mg + 150 mg in 5 ml liquid.

sodium and water retention, low blood potassium levels, low blood pressure, heart failure, muscle and kidney damage.

Dose: adults 1 tablet (chewed) or 10 ml liquid three times a day, with double dose at night, for 6-12 weeks.
Availability: NHS and private prescription.
Contains: carbenoxolone sodium, alginic acid, aluminium hydroxide, magnesium trisilicate, sodium bicarbonate (tablets); carbenoxolone sodium and aluminium hydroxide (liquid).

 in the elderly and in patients suffering from heart disease, high blood pressure, liver or kidney disorders, sodium or water retention.

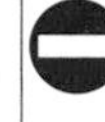 children, pregnant women, adults over 75 years, or for patients with liver or kidney failure, heart failure, or low blood potassium levels.

 preparations coated to protect the stomach (E-C products), digoxin, spironolactone, amiloride.

Other preparations: carbenoxolone gel, carbenoxolone granules.

Quellada M *see* malathion liquid/shampoo
(Stafford-Miller)

Questran/Questran Light *see* cholestyramine sachets
(Bristol-Myers Squibb Pharmaceuticals)

---

quietapine tablets

A tablet used as a sedative to treat schizophrenia.

Strengths available: 25 mg, 100 mg, 150 mg, and 200 mg tablets.
Dose: adults, 25 mg twice a day at first increasing each day and finally adjusted to 300-450 mg a day in two divided doses; elderly patients 25 mg once a day at first.
Availability: NHS and private prescription.
Contains: quietapine.
Brand names: Seroquel.

 weight gain, dizziness, low blood pressure on standing, rapid heart rate, shaking hands, movement disorders, NEUROLEPTIC MALIGNANT SYNDROME, drowsiness, stomach upset, weakness, inflamed nasal passages, fever, anxiety, muscle pain, rash, heart rhythm abnormality, blood changes, liver disorders.

 in the elderly, pregnant women, and in patients with a history of epilepsy or suffering from heart or circulation disorders (including brain circulation), liver or kidney disorders, or Parkinson's disease.

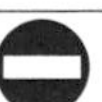 children or mothers who are breastfeeding.

 drugs that affect heart rhythm, other sedating drugs, alcohol, antidepressants, anti-epileptic treatments, halofantrine, ritonavir.

Quinaband *see* zinc paste, clioquinol, and calamine bandage
(SSL International)

---

quinagolide tablets

A tablet used as a treatment for high prolactin levels in the blood (which may cause menstrual disorders and infertility in women, impotence in men, and other effects such as headache, vision disorders, and other brain disturbances).

Strengths available: 25 mcg, 50 mcg, 75 mcg, and 150 mcg tablets.
Dose: adults 25 mcg at bedtime for 3 nights, then increased gradually to 75-150 mcg a day (or more if needed).
Availability: NHS and private prescription.
Contains: quinagolide hydrochloride.
Brand names: Norprolac.

low blood pressure on standing, dizziness, upset stomach, headache, drowsiness, poor circulation, fainting, loss of appetite, abdominal pain, sleeplessness, flushing, fluid retention, congested nose. With high doses, confusion, hallucinations, movement disorders, dry mouth, leg cramps, lung changes.

in patients with a history of mental disorder, or suffering from severe heart or circulation disorder, Raynaud's syndrome, or PORPHYRIA. Your doctor may advise regular check-ups. Women not intending to become pregnant should use barrier contraceptives. Those being treated for infertility should discontinue the treatment as soon as pregnancy is confirmed.

children, mothers who are breastfeeding, women who have experienced complications of pregnancy, or for patients with kidney or liver disorders. Should not be given to women who have recently given birth if they also have high blood pressure.

alcohol, other sedating drugs.

quinalbarbitone capsules

A capsule used as a BARBITURATE for the short-term treatment of severe sleeplessness in patients already taking these drugs.

Strengths available: 50 mg and 100 mg capsules.
Dose: adults 100 mg at night.
Availability: controlled drug; NHS and private prescription.
Contains: quinalbarbitone (secobarbital) sodium.
Brand names: Seconal Sodium.
Compound preparations: Tuinal.

drowsiness, hangover, dizziness, allergies, headache, shaky movements, breathing difficulties, confusion, excitement, withdrawal reactions.

in patients suffering from liver, kidney, or lung disease. Addiction may develop. Must be withdrawn slowly.

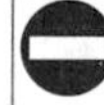
children, young adults, pregnant women, mothers who are breastfeeding, elderly or weak patients, or those with a history of drug or alcohol abuse, or suffering from PORPHYRIA, or in the management of pain.

ANTICOAGULANTS, alcohol, antiviral drugs, CALCIUM-CHANNEL BLOCKERS, cyclosporin, thyroxine, tibolone, theophylline, aminophylline, gestrinone, antidepressants, other sedatives, CORTICOSTEROIDS, oral contraceptives, rifampicin, phenytoin.

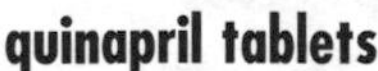

quinapril tablets

A tablet used as an ACE-INHIBITOR to treat high blood pressure and heart failure.

Strengths available: 5 mg, 10 mg, 20 mg, and 40 mg tablets.
Dose: to treat high blood pressure, 10 mg once a day at first (or 2.5 mg in elderly patients and those with kidney disorders or who are taking diuretics) then adjusted according to response to a maximum of 80 mg a day; to treat heart failure, 2.5 mg once a day at first then adjusted to maximum of 40 mg a day.
Availability: NHS and private prescription.
Contains: quinapril.
Brand names: Accupro.
Compound preparations: Accuretic.

 headache, dizziness, fluid retention, wind, nervousness, depression, sleeplessness, blurred vision, impotence, high potassium levels, runny nose, blood changes, liver or kidney disorder, inflamed pancreas, rash, low blood pressure, severe allergy, inflammation of the nose, cough, upper respiratory tract infection, tiredness, nausea, and pain in stomach, back, abdomen, chest, or muscles.

 in patients with kidney disease, severe heart failure, some diseases of the blood vessels, and in those undergoing anaesthesia. Your doctor may advise regular blood and urine checks.

 children, pregnant women, mothers who are breastfeeding, or for patients with some heart valve disorders.

 some diuretics, potassium supplements, NON-STEROIDAL ANTI-INFLAMMATORY DRUGS, some ANTIBIOTICS, lithium, anaesthetics, cyclosporin, alcohol, antidiabetics.

quinidine tablets/modified-release tablets

A tablet or M-R TABLET used as an anti-arrhythmic drug to treat abnormal heart rhythm.

Strengths available: 200 mg tablets; 250 mg m-r tablets.
Dose: adults, 200-400 mg 3-4 times a day using standard tablets; 500 mg twice a day (then adjusted according to response) using m-r tablets.
Availability: NHS and private prescription.
Contains: quinidine sulphate (tablets) or quinidine bisulphate (m-r tablets).
Brand names: Kinidin.

 stomach upset, LUPUS-like symptoms, blood changes, rash, mental disorders, fever, heart rhythm disorders, low blood pressure, liver disorders.

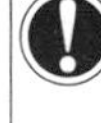 in the elderly and in patients with liver or kidney disorders, low blood pressure, slow heart rate, low potassium levels, blocked oesophagus, asthma, and MYASTHENIA GRAVIS. Your doctor may advise regular blood tests.

 children, pregnant women, mothers who are breastfeeding, or for patients suffering from LUPUS, digoxin overdose, or some heart disorders.

 other drugs affecting heart rhythm, rifampicin, rifabutin, ANTICOAGULANTS, TRICYCLIC ANTIDEPRESSANTS, reboxetine, mizolastine, halofantrine, mefloquine, pimozide, sertindole, thioridazine, nifedipine, verapamil, nelfinavir, ritonavir, digoxin, DIURETICS, sedatives, alcohol, sotalol, muscle relaxants, cimetidine.

quinine sulphate/bisulphate tablets

A tablet used to treat malaria and leg cramps at night.

Strengths available: 200 mg quinine sulphate tablets; 300 mg quinine bisulphate tablets.
Dose: for cramp, adults 200-300 mg at night; for malaria, as advised by doctor.
Availability: NHS and private prescription.
Contains: quinine sulphate or bisulphate.

 noises in the ears, headache, nausea, stomach pain, rash, disturbance of vision, confusion, blood or kidney disorders, low blood sugar, flushing, severe allergic reaction.

 in pregnant women and in patients suffering from some heart conditions and enzyme deficiency that causes anaemia/jaundice with some drugs.

 halofantrine, flecainide, amiodarone, pimozide, sedatives, mefloquine, digoxin.

 patients suffering from some blood disorders or inflammation of the optic nerve.

Quinocort *see* topical corticosteroid cream
(Quinoderm)

Quinoderm *see* benzoyl peroxide cream
(Quinoderm)

Quinoped

(Quinoderm)
A cream used as an antifungal treatment for athlete's foot and other fungal skin infections.

Strengths available: 5% + 0.5% cream.
Dose: apply twice a day.
Availability: NHS and private prescription, over the counter.
Contains: benzoyl peroxide, potassium hydroxyquinoline sulphate.

Caution: may bleach fabrics.

Qvar *see* beclomethasone CFC-free inhaler
(3M Health Care)

---

rabeprazole tablets

R

An E-C TABLET used to treat stomach ulcers and acid reflux into the oesophagus. Also used for *H. PYLORI* ERADICATION.

Strengths available: 10 mg and 20 mg e-c tablets.
Dose: for reflux, usually 20 mg each morning for 4-8 weeks to heal the condition then 10-20 mg a day to prevent relapse; for ulcers, 20 mg once a day for 4-12 weeks.
Availability: NHS and private prescription.

Brand names: Pariet.

 in mothers who are breastfeeding and in patients aged over 45 years or with liver disorders. Stomach cancer should be excluded before treatment.

 children or pregnant women.

 headache, upset stomach, skin irritation. Rarely, blood changes, swollen hands and feet, depression, joint pain, itching, severe allergy, dry mouth, skin reactions, blurred vision, liver changes, sleeplessness, mouth inflammation, chest pain, weakness, drowsiness, nervousness, loss of appetite, influenza-like symptoms, sweating, weight gain.

 digoxin, ANTACIDS, alcohol, sedating drugs.

---

rabies vaccine

A vaccination used to prevent and treat rabies.

Dose: as advised by doctor (depends on level of exposure and previous vaccination record).
Availability: NHS and private prescription.
Contains: inactivated rabies vaccines.
Brand names: Rabipur.

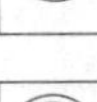 skin reaction at injection site, fever, general illness.

 chloroquine.

Rabipur *see* rabies vaccine
(Masta)

Raciran *see* ranitidine tablets
(Opus Pharmaceuticals)

---

raloxifene tablets

A tablet used to treat and prevent osteoporosis in women who have passed the menopause.

Strengths available: 60 mg tablets.
Dose: adults, 60 mg once a day.
Availability: NHS and private prescription.
Contains: raloxifene hydrochloride.
Brand names: Evista.

 ANTICOAGULANTS, other medications that might cause blood clots.

 blood clots, hot flushes, leg cramp, swollen hands and feet, influenza-like symptoms, rash, stomach upset.

 in women who are already at risk of blood clots.

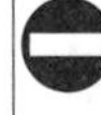 children, pregnant women, mothers who are breastfeeding, men, women who are not mobile, or for patients with a history of blood clots, undiagnosed vaginal bleeding, liver or severe kidney disorders, breast or womb cancer, lack of bile flow.

ramipril capsules

A capsule used as an ACE-INHIBITOR to treat high blood pressure and as an additional treatment in heart failure. Also used to reduce risk of heart attack or stroke (or reduce need for surgery on heart blood vessels) in susceptible patients.

Strengths available: 1.25 mg, 2.5 mg, 5 mg, and 10 mg capsules.
Dose: usually 1.25 mg a day at first increasing to a maximum of 10 mg a day; dose starts at 1.25-2.5 mg twice a day for patients who have just had a heart attack; to reduce risk of heart attack or stroke in susceptible patients, start at 2.5 mg once a day.
Availability: NHS and private prescription.
Contains: ramipril.
Brand names: Tritace.
Compound preparations: Triapin, Triapin Mite.

rash, itching, sore throat, runny nose, stomach upset, cough, blood and liver changes, kidney disorders, low blood pressure, severe allergic reaction, inflamed pancreas. Occasionally, headache, dizziness, tiredness, taste disturbance, fever, pins and needles, muscle or joint pain, sensitivity to sunlight, inflamed membranes or blood vessels, sleep disturbance, change in mood, abnormal heart rhythm, chest pain or infection, fainting, stroke, heart attack, inflamed or dry mouth, skin reactions, loss of appetite, Raynaud's phenomenon, confusion, impotence, reduced sexual desire, hair loss, eye inflammation, loose nails.

children, pregnant women, mothers who are breastfeeding, or for patients with some heart abnormalities, disorders of the blood supply to the kidneys. Not to be taken on the same day as dialysis.

in the elderly and in patients suffering from kidney or liver disease, blood disorders, autoimmune diseases (such as LUPUS), severe heart failure, or with a history of severe allergies, or in patients undergoing anaesthesia or dialysis. Your doctor may advise regular blood tests.

DIURETICS, anaesthetics, NON-STEROIDAL ANTI-INFLAMMATORY DRUGS, potassium supplements, cyclosporin, lithium, antidiabetics.

Ranbaxy Cefaclor M-R *see* cefaclor modified-release tablets
(Ranbaxy UK)

Ranitic *see* ranitidine tablets
(Tillomed Laboratories)

R

ranitidine tablets/effervescent tablets/syrup

A tablet, effervescent tablet, or syrup used as a HISTAMINE H_2-ANTAGONIST to treat stomach ulcers, acid reflux that irritates the oesophagus, conditions involving excess stomach acid (e.g. Zollinger-Ellison syndrome), indigestion, and *H. PYLORI* ERADICATION. Also used to treat and prevent stomach ulcers caused by NON-STEROIDAL ANTI-INFLAMMATORY DRUGS.

Strengths available: 150 mg and 300 mg tablets; 150 mg and 300 mg effervescent tablets; 75 mg/5 ml syrup.

Dose: adults, usually 150 mg twice a day or 300 mg at night, reducing to 150 mg at night for long-term maintenance if appropriate. Up to 6000 mg a day may be needed in Zollinger-Ellison syndrome. Children treated only for stomach ulcer (reduced dose according to body weight).

Availability: NHS and private prescription. (Lower-strength preparations available over the counter to treat indigestion, heartburn, and excess acid related to food and drink.)

Contains: ranitidine hydrochloride.

Brand names: Raciran, Ranitic, Rantec, Zaedoc, Zantac.

 headache, dizziness, upset stomach, dry mouth, skin disorders, bowel discomfort, liver disorders, loss of appetite, tiredness. Rarely, breast swelling, severe skin disorders, inflamed pancreas, heart rhythm or conduction disorders, confusion, depression, blood disorders, severe allergic reaction, fever, muscle or joint pain, agitation, vision disturbance, hair loss.

 in pregnant women, patients who are middle-aged or older, and in patients suffering from kidney or liver disorders. Treatment may mask symptoms of stomach cancer.

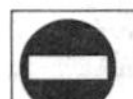 children or mothers who are breastfeeding.

---

ranitidine bismuth citrate tablets

A tablet used as a HISTAMINE H_2-ANTAGONIST to treat stomach ulcers and for *H. PYLORI* ERADICATION.

Strengths available: 400 mg tablets.

Dose: adults to treat ulcers, 400 mg twice a day for 4-8 weeks. (Maximum of 16 weeks treatment in 1 year.)

Availability: NHS and private prescription.

Contains: ranitidine bismuth citrate.

Brand names: Pylorid.

 headache, dizziness, upset stomach, dry mouth, skin disorders, bowel discomfort, liver disorders, loss of appetite, tiredness. Rarely, breast swelling, severe skin disorders, inflamed pancreas, heart rhythm or conduction disorders, confusion, depression, blood disorders, severe allergic reaction, fever, muscle or joint pain, dark colour of tongue, black bowel motions, agitation, vision disturbance, hair loss, stomach upset.

children, pregnant women, mothers who are breastfeeding, or for patients suffering from PORPHYRIA or moderate to severe kidney disorders.

 in patients who are middle-aged or older and in patients suffering from kidney or liver disorders. Treatment may mask symptoms of stomach cancer.

Rantec *see* ranitidine tablets
(Berk Pharmaceuticals)

Rapitil *see* nedocromil eye drops
(Rhône-Poulenc Rorer)

R

reboxetine tablets

A tablet used as an antidepressant to treat depression.

Strengths available: 4 mg tablets.
Dose: adults, 4 mg twice a day increased to 12 mg a day if needed.
Availability: NHS and private prescription.
Contains: reboxetine mesylate.
Brand names: Edronax.

low blood pressure on standing, sweating, dizziness, vertigo, impotence, pins and needles, difficulty or pain passing urine, dry mouth, rapid heart rate, constipation, low potassium levels.

in patients with liver or severe kidney disorders, some mental disorders, difficulty passing urine, enlarged prostate, glaucoma, or who have a history of heart or circulation disorders, or epilepsy.

erythromycin, azithromycin, clarithromycin, other antidepressants, MAOIS, antifungals.

children, pregnant women, or mothers who are breastfeeding,

rectal corticosteroid

A preparation used as a CORTICOSTEROID to treat haemorrhoids (piles) or other disorders of the anus or rectum. Most products have additional soothing or anaesthetic ingredients.

Dose: (*see* table below). Limited to a maximum of 7 days' treatment.
Availability: NHS and private prescription.
Contains: (*see* table below).

continuous use, especially in pregnant women and children, or for patients suffering from infected conditions. Many preparations not suitable for children (*marked * in table below*).

thinning of the anal skin, worsening of untreated infections, dermatitis. Few side effects from mild to moderate preparations used short term. With longer-term treatment – fluid retention, suppression of ADRENAL GLANDS, and general corticosteroid effects *see* prednisolone tablets.

in children and pregnant women.

Product	*Forms available*	*Corticosteroid ingredient*	*Other ingredients*	*Dose*
Anugesic-HC*	cream	hydrocortisone	benzyl benzoate, bismuth oxide, Peru balsam, pramoxine, zinc oxide	apply twice a day and after bowel movements.
	suppositories	hydrocortisone	benzyl benzoate, bismuth oxide, bismuth subgallate, Peru balsam, pramoxine, zinc oxide	1 inserted into the rectum twice a day and after bowel movements.

Product	*Forms available*	*Corticosteroid ingredient*	*Other ingredients*	*Dose*
Anusol-HC*	ointment and suppositories	hydrocortisone	benzyl benzoate, bismuth oxide, bismuth subgallate, Peru balsam, zinc oxide	apply ointment or insert 1 suppository into rectum twice a day and after bowel movements.
Betnovate Rectal	ointment	betamethasone	lignocaine, phenylephrine	apply 2-3 times a day. (Used with caution in children over 1 year.)
Perinal*	spray	hydrocortisone	lignocaine	apply 2-3 times a day.
Proctofoam HC*	foam in aerosol	hydrocortisone	pramoxine (pramocaine)	1 applicatorful applied into the rectum 2-3 times a day and after bowel movements.
Proctosedyl	ointment and suppositories	hydrocortisone	cinchocaine	apply ointment or insert 1 suppository into rectum twice a day and after bowel movements.
Scheriproct	ointment and suppositories	prednisolone	cinchocaine	apply ointment 2-4 times a day or insert 1 suppository 1-3 times a day after bowel movements.
Ultraproct*	ointment and suppositories	fluocortolone	cinchocaine	apply ointment 2-4 times a day or insert 1 suppository 1-3 times a day.
Uniroid-HC*	ointment and suppositories	hydrocortisone	cinchocaine	apply ointment or insert 1 suppository into rectum twice a day and after bowel movements.
Xyloproct	ointment	hydrocortisone	lignocaine, zinc oxide	apply several times a day.

* indicates not suitable for children.

Rectubes *see* diazepam rectal solution
(C.P. Pharmaceuticals)

Refolinon *see* calcium folinate tablets
(Pharmacia and Upjohn)

Regaine *see* minoxidil topical solution
(Pharmacia and Upjohn)

Regranex *see* becaplermin gel
(Janssen-Cilag)

Regulan *see* ispaghula husk
(Proctor and Gamble Pharmaceuticals UK)

Regulose *see* lactulose solution
(Novartis Consumer Health)

Regurin *see* trospium tablets
(Galen)

Rehidrat *see* oral rehydration solution
(Searle)

Relaxit *see* sodium citrate enema
(Crawford Pharmaceuticals)

Relenza *see* zanamavir disks/suspension
(GlaxoWellcome UK)

Relifex *see* nabumetone tablets/suspension
(SmithKline Beecham Pharmaceuticals)

Remedeine/Remedeine Forte *see* co-dydramol tablets
(Napp Pharmaceuticals)

Reminyl *see* galantamine tablets
(Shire Pharmaceuticals)

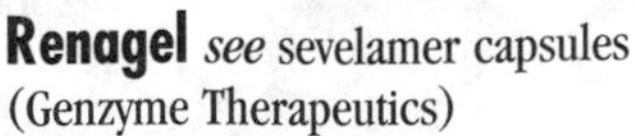

Renagel *see* sevelamer capsules
(Genzyme Therapeutics)

---

repaglinide tablets

A tablet used as an antidiabetic treatment for diabetes (either alone or in combination with metformin).

Strengths available: 0.5 mg, 1 mg, and 2 mg tablets.
Dose: adults, 0.5 mg immediately before each main meal adjusted to a maximum of 16 mg a day. (1 mg starting dose needed if transferring from another anti-diabetic.)
Availability: NHS and private prescription.
Contains: repaglinide.
Brand names: Novonorm.

 stomach upset, rash, liver disorders, abdominal pain, vision disturbance.

 in patients with kidney disorders. Insulin may be needed instead at times of illness or surgery.

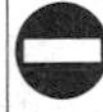 children under 18 years, elderly patients over 75 years, pregnant women, mothers who are breastfeeding, or for patients with liver or severe kidney disorders, increased acid content of the blood due to uncontrolled diabetes.

 erythromycin, rifampicin, phenytoin, fluconazole, itraconazole, ketoconazole, MAOIS, BETA-BLOCKERS, ACE-INHIBITORS, alcohol, diuretics, thyroxine, SYMPATHOMIMETICS.

---

reproterol inhaler

An inhaler used as a BRONCHODILATOR to treat asthma, bronchitis, and emphysema (a breathing disorder).

Strengths available: 0.5 mg per dose.
Dose: adults, 0.5-1.0 mg (1-2 puffs) up to three times a day for persistent symptoms or every 3-6 hours for immediate attacks; children aged 6-12 years use 0.5 mg (1 puff) only (at same frequency as for adults).
Availability: NHS and private prescription.
Contains: reproterol hydrochloride.
Brand names: Bronchodil.

 low potassium levels, shaking hands, headache, widening of blood vessels, cramps, altered heart rhythm, nervousness, severe allergic reaction.

 in pregnant women, mothers who are breast-feeding, and in patients suffering from weak heart, irregular heart rhythm, high blood pressure, overactive thyroid, diabetes, angina. In severe asthmatics, blood potassium levels should be checked regularly.

 children.

 BETA-BLOCKERS, theophylline, aminophylline, SYMPATHOMIMETICS.

Requip *see* ropinorole tablets
(SmithKline Beecham Pharmaceuticals)

Resonium A *see* polystyrene sulphonate resin
(Sanofi Winthrop)

R

Respillin *see* amoxycillin capsules/suspension
(OPD Pharmaceuticals)

Respontin *see* ipratropium bromide nebulizer solution
(GlaxoWellcome UK)

Restandol *see* testosterone capsules
(Organon Laboratories)

Retcin *see* erythromycin tablets
(DDSA Pharmaceuticals)

Retin-A *see* tretinoin cream/gel/lotion
(Janssen-Cilag)

Retinova *see* tretinoin cream
(Johnson and Johnson Medical)

Retrovir *see* zidovudine capsules/syrup
(GlaxoWellcome UK)

Rheumacin LA *see* indomethacin modified-release capsules
(Hillcross Pharmaceuticals)

Rheumatac Retard *see* diclofenac modified-release tablets
(Sovereign Medical)

Rheumox/Rheumox 600 *see* azapropazone capsules/tablets
(Goldshield Healthcare)

Rhinocort Aqua *see* corticosteroid nasal spray
(AstraZeneca UK)

Rhinolast *see* azelastine nasal spray
(ASTA Medica)

Rhumalgan CR *see* diclofenac modified-release tablets
(Lagap Pharmaceuticals)

---

riboflavin/riboflavine *see* vitamin B_2

Ridaura *see* auranofin tablets
(Yamanouchi Pharma)

---

rifabutin capsules

A capsule used as an anti-tubercular drug to treat some mycobacterial infections and tuberculosis of the lungs, and to prevent mycobacterial infections in patients with low immunity.

Strengths available: 150 mg capsules.
Dose: adults, 150-600 mg a day depending on condition.
Availability: NHS and private prescription.
Contains: rifabutin.
Brand names: Mycobutin.

 upset stomach, anaemia, orange discoloration of skin, urine, and other secretions, blood changes, joint or muscle pain, eye disorders, liver disorders, influenza-like symptoms, difficulty breathing, fever, rash, shock.

 in patients with liver or kidney disorders or PORPHYRIA. Soft contact lenses may be stained. Report any persistent nausea, vomiting, tiredness, or jaundice to your doctor. Your doctor may advise regular blood tests and eye checks. Women on oral contraceptives may need to take additional contraceptive precautions.

 children, pregnant women, or mothers who are breastfeeding.

 drugs affecting heart rhythm, clarithromycin, azithromycin, erythromycin, ANTICOAGULANTS, some antidiabetics, phenytoin, carbamazepine, antifungals, antivirals, cyclosporin, CORTICOSTEROIDS, azathioprine, oral contraceptives, digitoxin.

Rifadin *see* rifampicin capsules/syrup
(Hoechst Marion Roussel)

---

rifampicin capsules/syrup

A capsule or syrup used, in combination with other drugs, as an ANTIBIOTIC to treat tuberculosis and other similar infections. Also used to prevent meningitis in patients at risk of contracting the disease.

Strengths available: 150 mg and 300 mg capsules; 100 mg/5 ml syrup.

 upset stomach, inflamed bowel, kidney failure, fluid retention, anaemia, orange discoloration of skin, urine, and other secretions, blood changes, joint pain, muscle pain or weakness, disturbed menstrual cycle, liver disorders, influenza-like symptoms, difficulty breathing, fever, rash, shock, blood clots, and vein inflammation.

R

cont.

Dose: as advised by doctor (depends on condition).
Availability: NHS and private prescription.
Contains: rifampicin.
Brand names: Rifadin, Rimactane.
Compound preparations: Rifater, Rifinah, Rimactazid.

 in pregnant women, mothers who are breast-feeding, elderly or very young patients, undernourished patients, or those with liver or kidney disorders or PORPHYRIA. Soft contact lenses may be stained. Report any persistent nausea, vomiting, tiredness, or jaundice to your doctor. Your doctor may advise regular blood tests. Women on oral contraceptives may need to take additional contraceptive precautions.

 drugs affecting heart rhythm, chloramphenicol, ANTICOAGULANTS, some antidiabetics, phenytoin, antifungals, antivirals, cyclosporin, CORTICOSTEROIDS, azathioprine, oral contraceptives, digitoxin, atovaquone, some drugs used to treat high blood pressure or angina, tacrolimus, theophylline, aminophylline, celecoxib.

Rifater *see* rifampicin capsules, isoniazid tablets, and pyrazinamide tablets
(Hoechst Marion Roussel)

Strengths available: 120 mg + 50 mg + 300 mg capsules.
Dose: as advised by doctor.

Rifinah *see* rifampicin capsules and isoniazid tablets
(Hoechst Marion Roussel)

Strengths available: 150 mg + 100 mg or 300 mg + 150 mg tablets.
Dose: as advised by doctor.

Rilutek *see* riluzole tablets
(Rhône-Poulenc Rorer)

---

riluzole tablets

A tablet used to delay progression of motor neurone disease.

Strengths available: 50 mg tablets.
Dose: adults, 50 mg twice a day.
Availability: NHS and private prescription. (Specialist use only.)
Contains: riluzole.
Brand names: Rilutek.

 stomach upset, weakness, drowsiness, dizziness, vertigo, rapid heart rate, abdominal pain, pins and needles around the mouth, liver disorders.

 report any fever to your doctor. Your doctor may advise regular blood tests.

 children, pregnant women, mothers who are breastfeeding, or for patients suffering from kidney or liver disorders.

 alcohol, sedating drugs. (Other interactions not yet determined.)

R

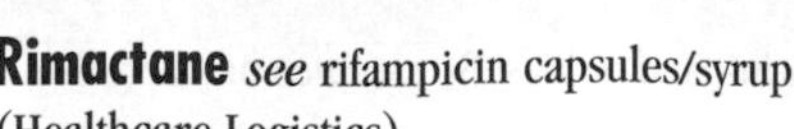

Rimactane *see* rifampicin capsules/syrup
(Healthcare Logistics)

Rimactazid *see* isoniazid tablets and rifampicin capsules
(Healthcare Logistics)

Strengths available: 150 mg + 100 mg or 300 mg + 150 mg tablets.
Dose: as advised by doctor.

---

rimexolone eye drops

An eye drop used as a CORTICOSTEROID for the short-term treatment of eye inflammation.

Strengths available: 1% eye drops.
Dose: adults, usually 1 drop into the eye(s) four times a day but more often for severe conditions. Maximum treatment period 4 weeks. In uveitis dose reducing to once a day.
Availability: NHS and private prescription.
Contains: rimexolone.
Brand names: Vexol.

 rise in eye pressure, thinning of cornea, cataract, eye infection.

 in pregnant women, mothers who are breast-feeding, and in patients suffering from glaucoma or corneal ulcers.

 children or for patients suffering from eye infections.

Rinatec *see* ipratropium nasal spray
(Boehringer Ingelheim)

---

risedronic acid tablets

A tablet used to treat OSTEOPOROSIS and reduce the risk of bone fractures, or to treat Paget's disease (another bone disorder). Also used to prevent osteoporosis and to maintain bone mass in women taking CORTICOSTEROIDS after the menopause.

Strengths available: 5 mg and 30 mg tablets.
Dose: to treat and prevent osteoporosis, adults one 5 mg tablet once a day. Dose for Paget's disease is 30 mg once a day for 2 months with re-treatment beginning 2 months after the first course if necessary. Tablet should be taken either 20 minutes before the first food/drink of the day or

 upset stomach, abdominal pain, wind, muscle or bone pain, headache, rash, and possibly disorders of the oesophagus.

 in patients with problems swallowing or disorders of the oesophagus, or in those unable to stay upright. Do not lie down for 30 minutes after taking the tablet.

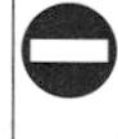 children, adolescents, pregnant women, mothers who are breastfeeding, patients with low blood levels of calcium, or who have severe kidney disorders.

 food and drink (*see* above).

cont.

at least 2 hours before/after any food or drink and at least 30 minutes before going to bed.

Availability: NHS and private prescription.
Contains: risedronic acid.
Brand names: Actonel.

Risperdal *see* risperidone liquid/tablets
(Janssen-Cilag)

---

risperidone liquid/tablets

A tablet and liquid used as a sedative to treat schizophrenia and other mental disorders.

Strengths available: 0.5 mg, 1 mg, 2 mg, 3 mg, 4 mg, and 6 mg tablets; 1 mg/ml liquid.
Dose: adults, 2 mg a day at first, then increase to a maximum of 16 mg a day (but not usually more than 10 mg). Dose may be taken as a single daily dose or divided into two; elderly patients start with 0.5 mg twice a day.
Availability: NHS and private prescription.
Contains: risperidone.
Brand names: Risperdal.

 drugs that affect heart rhythm, other sedating drugs, alcohol, antidepressants, anti-epileptic treatments, halofantrine, ritonavir.

 weight gain, dizziness, low blood pressure on standing, drowsiness, rapid heart rate, shaking hands, movement disorders, NEUROLEPTIC MALIGNANT SYNDROME, sleeplessness, agitation, anxiety, headache, blurred vision, stomach upset, rash, blood changes, liver disorders, disorders of sexual function, incontinence, chemical disturbance, fits, abnormal temperature regulation.

 in the elderly, pregnant women, mothers who are breastfeeding, and in patients with a history of epilepsy or suffering from heart or circulation disorders, liver or kidney disorders, or Parkinson's disease.

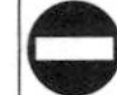 children.

Ritalin *see* methylphenidate tablets
(Novartis Pharmaceuticals UK)

---

ritonavir capsules/liquid

A capsule or liquid used, in combination with other antivirals, as an antiviral treatment for HIV infections.

Strengths available: 100 mg capsules; 400 mg/5 ml liquid.
Dose: adults 600 mg twice a day; children use reduced doses according to size.
Availability: NHS and private prescription.
Contains: ritonavir.
Brand names: Norvir.

 upset stomach, taste disturbance, abdominal pain, loss of appetite, irritated throat, headache, pins and needles; widening of blood vessels, dizziness, enhanced feeling, weakness, skin disorders, sleep disturbance, blood or liver disorders, dry or ulcerated mouth, cough, fever, pain, muscle pain, anxiety, weight loss, sweating, itching, chemical imbalance, low thyroxine levels, inflamed pancreas, defective fat metabolism, diabetes.

 in pregnant women and in patients suffering from diabetes, diarrhoea, bleeding disorders, liver disorders.

 children under 2 years, mothers who are breastfeeding, or for patients with severe liver disease.

 bupropion, pain killers (ANALGESICS), NON-STEROIDAL ANTI-INFLAMMATORY DRUGS, drugs affecting heart rhythm, rifabutin, erythromycin, clarithromycin, azithromycin, ANTICOAGULANTS, antidepressants, St John's Wort (*Hypericum*), tolbutamide, carbamazepine, antifungals, sedatives, pimozide, clozapine, other antivirals, drugs used to treat anxiety or sleeplessness, some drugs used to treat high blood pressure or angina, cyclosporin, ergotamine, simvastatin, oral contraceptives, oestrogens, progestogens, sildenafil, tacrolimus, theophylline, aminophylline.

rivastigmine capsules

A capsule used to treat Alzheimer's disease.

Strengths available: 1.5 mg, 3 mg, 4.5 mg, and 6 mg capsules.
Dose: adults, 1.5 mg twice a day at first increasing to a maximum of 6 mg twice a day.
Availability: NHS and private prescription.
Contains: rivastigmine hydrogen tartrate.
Brand names: Exelon.

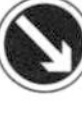 weakness, loss of appetite, weight loss, depression, confusion, agitation, stomach upset or bleeding, abdominal pain, headache, sleeplessness, shaking, sweating, tiredness, angina, fainting, difficulty passing urine.

 in pregnant women and in patients suffering from kidney or liver disorders, some heart disorders, stomach ulcers (or at risk of stomach ulcers), or those with a history of asthma or other breathing obstruction.

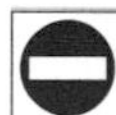 children or mothers who are breastfeeding.

Rivotril *see* clonazepam tablets
(Roche Products)

rizatriptan tablets/wafers

A tablet or wafer (to be dissolved on the tongue) used to treat migraine attacks.

Strengths available: 1 mg and 10 mg tablets; 10 mg wafers.
Dose: 10 mg at start of attack repeated after 2 hours if migraine is relieved but then recurs (do not take a second dose if the first fails to take effect). Maximum of 20 mg in 24 hours.

cont.

Availability: NHS and private prescription.
Contains: rizatriptan benzoate.
Brand names: Maxalt.

 children under 18 years, adults over 65 years, or for patients with heart disease, severe kidney or liver disease, uncontrolled high blood pressure, blood vessel disease, or who have had a stroke or other disorder of brain blood vessels.

 other migraine treatments, ergotamine, propranolol, MAOIS, moclobemide, alcohol, sedating drugs.

 sensations of warmth, tingling, pressure, tightness or heaviness, dizziness, flushing, tiredness, weakness, stomach upset, drowsiness, palpitations, rapid heart rate, stomach upset, dry mouth and thirst, sore mouth and throat, difficulty breathing, pins and needles, headache, reduced alertness, sleeplessness, shaking, nervousness, vertigo, abnormal movements, muscle pain and weakness, sweating, itching, rash, blurred vision, high blood pressure, fainting.

 in pregnant women, mothers who are breast-feeding, and in patients at risk of heart disease or who suffer from liver or kidney disorders.

Roaccutane *see* isotretinoin capsules
(Roche Products)

Robaxin *see* methocarbamol tablets
(Shire Pharmaceuticals)

Rocaltrol *see* calcitriol capsules
(Roche Products)

---

rofecoxib suspension/tablets

A tablet or suspension used as a NON-STEROIDAL ANTI-INFLAMMATORY DRUG to treat pain and inflammation in osteoarthritis.

Strengths available: 12.5 mg and 25 mg tablets; 12.5 mg/5 ml suspension.
Dose: 12.5-25 mg once a day.
Availability: NHS and private prescription.
Contains: rofecoxib.
Brand names: Vioxx.

R

 children, mothers who are breastfeeding, women in late pregnancy, or for patients with a history of allergy to aspirin or other NSAID, blood clotting disorders, currently active stomach ulcer or intestinal bleeding, kidney disorders, inflamed intestines, or heart failure.

 stomach upset and bleeding or ulceration, rash, severe allergy, difficulty breathing, blood or kidney disorders, headache, dizziness, noises in the ears, sensitivity to light, vertigo, mouth ulcers, chest pain, weight gain, sleep disturbance, eczema, muscle cramps. Rarely, fluid retention, liver disorders, inflamed pancreas, inflamed bowel, meningitis.

 in the elderly, pregnant women, mothers who are breastfeeding, and in patients with heart or liver disorders, high blood pressure, asthma, or LUPUS.

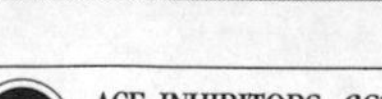

 ACE-INHIBITORS, aspirin or other non-steroidal anti-inflammatory drugs, some ANTIBIOTICS, ANTICOAGULANTS, some antidiabetic drugs, some antivirals, methotrexate, DIURETICS, lithium, digoxin, tacrolimus, cyclosporin, aluminium hydroxide.

Rohypnol *see* flunitrazepam tablets
(Roche Products)

Ronmix *see* erythromycin suspension/tablets
(Ashbourne Pharmaceuticals)

---

ropinorole tablets

A tablet used alone or in combination with levodopa to treat Parkinson's disease.

Strengths available: 0.25 mg, 1 mg, 2 mg, and 5 mg tablets.
Dose: adults 0.25 mg three times a day at first increasing gradually to a maximum of 24 mg a day (in three divided doses).
Availability: NHS and private prescription.
Contains: ropinorole hydrochloride.
Brand names: Requip.

 sulpiride, metoclopramide, theophylline, aminophylline, HORMONE REPLACEMENT THERAPY, sedatives, alcohol.

 stomach upset, drowsiness, sudden onset of sleep, movement disorders, hallucinations, low blood pressure, swollen legs, fainting, confusion, slow heart rate.

 in patients with severe heart, circulation, or mental disorders. Do not drive or undertake other hazardous activities. Treatment should be withdrawn slowly.

 children, pregnant women, mothers who are breastfeeding, or for patients with liver or severe kidney disorders.

---

rosiglitazone tablets

A tablet used, in combination with other antidiabetic drugs, to treat diabetes.

Strengths available: 4 mg and 8 mg tablets.
Dose: initially 4 mg a day increasing if necessary to 8 mg once a day (or 4 mg twice a day) if used with metformin.
Availability: NHS and private prescription.
Contains: rosiglitazone.
Brand names: Avandia.

insulin, cerivastatin, NON-STEROIDAL ANTI-INFLAMMATORY DRUGS.

 anaemia, low or high blood sugar levels, high cholesterol levels, stomach upset, headache, dizziness, weight gain, fluid retention, heart failure, blood changes, tiredness, weakness.

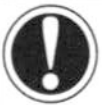 your doctor may advise regular weight checks and blood tests.

 children under 18 years old, pregnant women, mothers who are breastfeeding, or patients with severe kidney disorders, liver disorder, heart failure (or history of heart failure). Not to be used with insulin.

Rowachol

(Meadow Laboratories)

A capsule of essential oils used as an additional treatment for gallstones.

Dose: adults, 1 capsule three times a day at first, increasing to 1-2 capsules three times a day before meals.
Availability: NHS and private prescription.
Contains: menthol, menthone, pinene, camphene, cineole, borneol, olive oil.

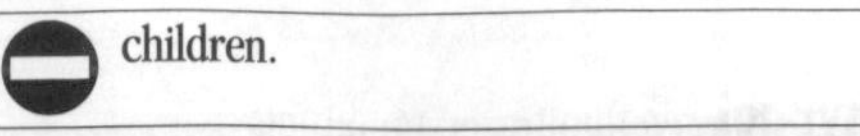
children.

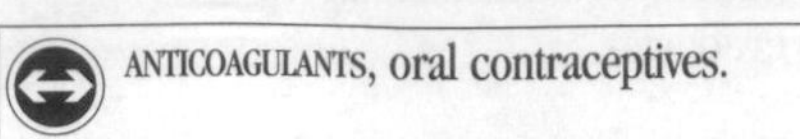
ANTICOAGULANTS, oral contraceptives.

Rowatinex

(Meadow Laboratories)

A capsule of essential oils used to treat stones in the kidney or urinary tract.

Dose: adults, 1-2 capsules 3-4 times a day before meals.
Availability: NHS and private prescription.
Contains: anethol, fenchone, pinene, camphene, cineole, borneol.

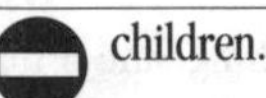
children.

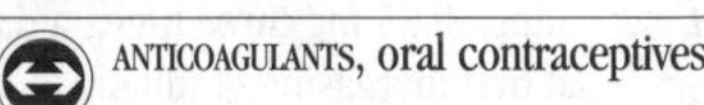
ANTICOAGULANTS, oral contraceptives.

Rozex *see* metronidazole cream/gel
(Galderma (UK))

rubella vaccine

Rubella, or German measles, is an active virus that in childhood is usually quite mild but, if contracted by pregnant women, can lead to defects in the baby. An attack of rubella usually gives the sufferer immunity for life. Formerly, this vaccine was used only to immunize females of child-bearing age but this has now been extended to both sexes to eliminate rubella.

Dose: 1 dose only needed.
Availability: NHS and private prescription.
Contains: live rubella vaccine.
Brand names: Ervevax.
Compound preparations: MMR vaccine.

Side effects: fever, rash, joint pain, swelling of lymph glands.

Caution: women should not become pregnant within 1 month of receiving the vaccine.

Caution needed with: CORTICOSTEROIDS, other live vaccines, some cancer treatments, radiation, transfusions, immunoglobulin.

Not to be used for: women in early pregnancy or for patients suffering from changes to immunity systems, acute feverish illness, cancer.

Rynacrom *see* sodium cromoglycate nasal spray
(Pantheon Healthcare)

R

Rynacrom Compound *see* sodium cromoglycate nasal spray and xylometazoline nasal spray
(Pantheon Healthcare)

Strengths available: 2% + 0.025% nasal spray.
Dose: adults and children, 1 spray into each nostril four times a day.

Rythmodan *see* disopyramide capsules/modified-release tablets
(Borg Medicare)

Sabril *see* vigabatrin tablets/sachets
(Hoechst Marion Roussel)

Safe Clip *see* B-D Safe Clip

Saizen *see* somatropin injection
(Serono Laboratories (UK))

Salactol *see* salicylic acid collodion
(Dermal Laboratories)

Salagen *see* pilocarpine hydrochloride tablets
(Chiron UK)

Salamol inhaler/Easibreathe *see* salbutamol inhaler
(Baker Norton Pharmaceuticals/Norton Healthcare)

Salamol Steri-Neb *see* salbutamol nebulizer solution
(Baker Norton Pharmaceuticals)

Salatac *see* salicylic acid collodion
(Dermal Laboratories)

Salazopyrin/Salazopyrin-EN *see* sulphasalazine tablets/enteric-coated tablets/enema/suspension/suppositories
(Pharmacia and Upjohn)

Salbulin *see* salbutamol CFC-free inhaler
(3M Health Care)

salbutamol inhaler/nebulizer solution/syrup/tablets/modified-release tablets/modified-release capsules

An inhaler, nebulizer solution, syrup, tablet or M-R CAPSULE/TABLET used as a BRONCHODILATOR to treat asthma and other breathing disorders caused by obstructed airways. Dry powder inhalation devices are also available (*see* 'other devices' below).

low potassium levels, shaking hands, headache, widening of blood vessels cramps, altered heart rhythm, nervousness, severe allergic reaction.

in pregnant women, mothers who are breast-feeding, and in patients suffering from kidney damage, weak heart, irregular heart rhythm, high blood pressure, overactive thyroid, diabetes. In severe asthmatics, blood potassium levels should be checked regularly.

BETA-BLOCKERS, theophylline, aminophylline, SYMPATHOMIMETICS.

Strengths available: 100 mcg per dose inhaler; 2.5 mg or 5 mg nebulizer solution; 2 mg/5 ml syrup; 2 mg and 4 mg tablets; 4 mg and 8 mg m-r tablets/capsules.

Dose: using tablets/syrup, adults 4 mg 3-4 times a day (2 mg used for elderly or sensitive patients) with 8 mg maximum single dose; children aged 2-6 years 1-2 mg (aged 6-12 years 2 mg) 3-4 times a day. Using m-r preparations, adults 8 mg (children aged 3-12 years 4 mg) twice a day. Using inhaler, adults and children 100-200 mcg (1-2 puffs) up to 3-4 times a day. Using dry powder devices (*see* below), adults 200-400 mcg (children 200 mcg) 3-4 times a day. Using nebulizer solution, adults and children over 18 months 2.5- 5.0 mg up to four times a day via nebulizer. To prevent exercise-induced attack, a single dose of 400 mcg inhaled dry powder in adults (200 mcg in children).

Availability: NHS and private prescription.

Contains: salbutamol sulphate.

Brand names: Aerolin, Airomir, Asmasal, Maxivent, Salamol, Salbulin, Steripoules, Ventmax, Ventolin, Volmax.

Compound preparations: Aerocrom, Combivent, Ventide.

Other devices: Asmasal Clickhaler, Ventodisks, Ventolin Accuhaler (all breath-activated dry powder devices); Aerolin Autohaler, Airomir Autohaler, Salamol Easi-Breathe (all breath-activated inhalers); Ventolin Rotacaps (dry powder capsules for inhalation); Asmasal Spacehaler (lower-velocity device).

salicylamide *see* analgesic (topical)

salicylic acid *see* Monphytol, Movelat, Pyralvex, salicylic acid collodion, salicylic acid ointment/lotion

salicylic acid collodion

A liquid used as a skin softener to treat warts and calluses.

irritation of the treated area.

protect surrounding skin and avoid broken skin.

patients suffering from diabetes, poor circulation, or for treating the face, anal, or genital areas.

Strengths available: 12% solution.
Dose: apply once a day or every other day. Rub down the surface of the wart or callus once a week. Treatment may last for up to 3 months.
Availability: NHS and private prescription, over the counter.
Contains: salicylic acid, flexible collodion.
Compound preparations: Cuplex (with lactic acid and copper acetate), Duofilm, Occlusal (with polyacrylic solution), Posalfilin, Salatac and Salactol (with lactic acid).
Other preparations: salicylic acid lotion/ointment/shampoo, Verrugon (salicylic acid 50% in ointment base).

---

salicylic acid lotion/ointment/shampoo

A lotion, ointment, or shampoo used to treat acne and scaly skin or scalp disorders (e.g. psoriasis).

irritation, dryness. Excessive use may lead to absorption and aspirin-like effects.

avoid contact with mouth, eyes, and mucous membranes.

areas of broken or inflamed skin.

Strengths available: 2% solution; 2% ointment; 3% shampoo available only in combination with sulphur (Meted).
Dose: the lotion applied up to three times a day; the ointment applied twice a day; the shampoo used twice a week.
Availability: NHS and private prescription, over the counter.
Contains: salicylic acid.
Brand names: Acnisal.
Compound preparations: Aserbine, benzoic acid compound ointment BP, Capasal, coal tar and salicylic acid ointment BP, Diprosalic (*see* topical corticosteroids), Ionil T, Meted shampoo (with sulphur), Psorin, salicylic acid and sulphur cream/ointment (with sulphur), zinc and salicylic acid paste.
Other preparations: salicylic acid collodion.

---

saline solution (sterile)

A sterile solution (available in sachets, tubes, or sprays) used to cleanse wounds, burns, or eyes. Also used to dilute some nebulizer solutions before use.

Strengths available: 0.9% solution.
Dose: used as needed for cleansing. Dilute nebulizer solutions according to manufacturer's directions.
Availability: NHS and private prescription, nurse prescription, over the counter.

cont.

Contains: sodium chloride.
Brand names: Amidose Saline, Askina, Irriclens, Normasol, Saline Steripoules, Sterac, Steripod Wound Cleanser.
Other preparations: sodium chloride eye drops BP.

saliva (artificial) pastilles/spray/lozenges/gel

A pastille, spray, gel, or lozenge used to provide artificial saliva for dry mouth and throat.

Dose: usually 1 pastille or 2-3 sprays used as required but *see* individual product labels for detail.
Availability: NHS and private prescription, over the counter. (Some brands available on NHS only if used to treat dry mouth caused by radiotherapy or Sjorgen's Syndrome.)
Contains: (*see* table below).

Product	*Main ingredients*
Glandosane spray	carmellose sodium
Luborant spray	carmellose sodium
Oralbalance gel	xylitol
Salivace spray	xylitol, carmellose sodium
Saliveze spray	carmellose sodium, xylitol.
Salivix pastilles	malic acid
Saliva Orthana lozenges	xylitol
Saliva Orthana Spray	xylitol, mucin

Salivace *see* saliva (artificial) spray
(Penn Pharmaceuticals)

Saliveze *see* saliva (artificial) spray
(Wyvern Medical)

Salivix *see* saliva (artificial) pastilles
(Provalis Healthcare)

Saliva Orthana *see* saliva (artificial) spray/lozenges
(Nycomed Amersham)

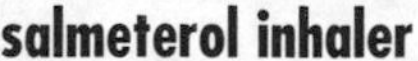

salmeterol inhaler

An inhaler used as a long-acting BRONCHODILATOR to treat asthma and other breathing disorders in those patients who require long-term regular treatment and who are already taking CORTICOSTEROIDS or sodium cromoglycate. Dry powder inhalation devices are also available (*see* 'other devices' below).

Strengths available: 25 mcg per dose inhaler; 50 mcg per dose dry powder devices.
Dose: adults and children over 4 years 50 mcg (2 puffs of inhaler or 1 dose of dry powder) inhaled twice a day (doubled for adults with severe asthma conditions).
Availability: NHS and private prescription.
Contains: salmeterol xinafoate.
Brand names: Serevent.
Compound preparations: Seretide.
Other devices: Serevent Accuhaler, Serevent Diskhaler (dry powder devices).

 children under 4 years or for patients with severe or unstable asthma or for relief of immediate asthma attack.

 low potassium levels, shaking hands, headache, widening of blood vessels, cramps, altered heart rhythm, nervousness, severe allergic reaction, breathing difficulty, skin reactions, muscle cramp, chest pain, joint pain, irritation.

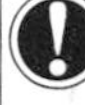 in pregnant women, mothers who are breast-feeding, and in patients suffering from kidney damage, weak heart, irregular heart rhythm, high blood pressure, overactive thyroid, diabetes. In severe asthmatics, blood potassium levels should be checked regularly. Anti-inflammatory treatment (corticosteroid or sodium cromoglycate) should be continued with this treatment.

 BETA-BLOCKERS, theophylline, aminophylline, SYMPATHOMIMETICS.

Salofalk *see* mesalazine enteric-coated tablets/enema/suppositories
(Provalis Healthcare)

Sando-K *see* potassium effervescent tablets
(Distriphar)

Sandocal/Calcium-Sandoz

(Novartis Pharmaceuticals UK)

A tablet (Sandocal) or syrup (Calcium-Sandoz) used as a calcium supplement to treat calcium deficiency or OSTEOPOROSIS.

Dose: as advised by doctor.
Availability: NHS and private prescription, over the counter.
Contains: calcium lactate gluconate and calcium carbonate (Sandocal); calcium glubionate and calcium lactobionate (Calcium-Sandoz syrup).

Side effects: mild stomach upset.

Caution: in patients with kidney disorders or sarcoidosis.

Not to be used for: patients with high levels of calcium in the blood or urine, some tumours, overactive parathyroid glands.

Sandrena *see* hormone replacement therapy (oestrogen-only)
(Organon Laboratories)

SangCya *see* cyclosporin oral solution
(Imtix Sangstat UK)

Sanomigran *see* pizotifen tablets/elixir
(Novartis Pharmaceuticals UK)

---

saquinavir capsules

A capsule used, in combination with other antiviral drugs, as an antiviral to treat HIV infection.

Strengths available: 200 mg capsules.
Dose: adults, either 1200 mg every 8 hours (using Fortovase brand) or 600 mg every 8 hours (using Invirase brand).
Availability: NHS and private prescription.
Contains: saquinavir (Fortovase brand), saquinavir mesylate (Invirase brand).
Brand names: Fortovase, Invirase.

 upset stomach, ulcers on mucous membranes, abdominal pain, headache, pins and needles, numbness in hands and feet, dizziness, muscle pain or inflammation, joint pain, fever, skin disorders, weakness, itching, liver or blood disorders, inflamed pancreas, kidney stones, abnormal fat metabolism.

 in the elderly, pregnant women, and in patients with diabetes, diarrhoea, kidney or liver disorders, bleeding disorders, or those who are not able to absorb nutrients normally.

 rifampicin, rifabutin, anti-epileptic treatments, pimozide, other antivirals, midazolam, dexamethasone, ergotamine, simvastatin, sildenafil.

 children under 16 years, mothers who are breastfeeding, or for patients with severe liver disease.

Schering PC4

(Schering Health Care)
A tablet used as an oestrogen, progestogen contraceptive in an emergency within 72 hours of unprotected intercourse.

Strengths available: 500 mcg + 50 mcg tablets.
Dose: 2 tablets as soon as possible after intercourse (within 72 hours) then a further 2 tablets 12 hours later.
Availability: NHS and private prescription.
Contains: norgestrel and ethinyloestradiol.

 upset stomach, disturbed menstrual pattern. Rarely, blood clots, raised blood pressure, jaundice, breast discomfort, headache, dizziness.

in mothers who are breastfeeding, women over 35 years, and in patients with diabetes, high blood pressure, epilepsy, PORPHYRIA, tetanus, liver and kidney disease, gallstones, heart or circulation disorders, overweight or immobile patients, smokers, or those suffering from varicose veins or other blood vessel disorder, inflammatory bowel disorders, some blood disorders, asthma, migraine, depression, multiple sclerosis, womb diseases. Use barrier contraceptives until the next menstrual period.

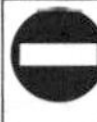
pregnant women or for patients with a history of heart disease or blood clots or those suffering from liver disorders, some cancers, migraine associated with visual disturbance (at the time of taking the tablets), porphyria, sickle-cell anaemia, undiagnosed vaginal bleeding, or some ear, skin, and kidney disorders. Do not use if intercourse took place more than 72 hours ago. Not for regular use.

rifampicin, some other ANTIBIOTICS, ANTICOAGULANTS, antidiabetics, griseofulvin, BARBITURATES, phenytoin, primidone, carbamazepine, ethosuximide.

Scheriproct *see* rectal corticosteroid
(Schering Health Care)

Scopoderm *see* hyoscine patches
(Novartis Pharmaceuticals UK)

Seasorb *see* alginate dressing
(Coloplast)

Secadrex *see* acebutolol tablets and hydrochlorothiazide tablets
(Akita Pharmaceuticals)

Strengths available: 200 mg + 12.5 mg tablets.
Dose: adults 1-2 tablets each day.

---

secobarbital *see* quinalbarbitone (alternative name)

Seconal Sodium *see* quinalbarbitone capsules
(Flynn Pharma)

Sectral *see* acebutolol tablets
(Akita Pharmaceuticals)

Securon/Securon SR *see* verapamil tablets/modified-release tablets
(Knoll)

selegiline tablets/syrup

A tablet, tablet to dissolve on the tongue, or syrup used to treat Parkinson's disease either alone or in combination with levodopa.

Strengths available: 5 mg and 10 mg standard tablets; 1.25 mg tablets to dissolve on the tongue; 10 mg/5 ml syrup.
Dose: using syrup or standard tablets, adults 10 mg each morning, or 5 mg in the morning and 5 mg at midday. (Elderly patients may start with only 2.5 mg in the morning.) Using tablets that dissolve on the tongue (Zelapar), adults 1.25 mg each morning (and do not drink or rinse mouth for 5 minutes afterwards).
Availability: NHS and private prescription.
Contains: selegiline hydrochloride.
Brand names: Eldepryl, Zelapar.

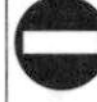
levodopa, pethidine, other OPIOID ANALGESICS, antidepressants, MAOIS, some migraine treatments, alcohol, SYMPATHOMIMETICS.

low blood pressure, upset stomach, confusion, mental disorders, inflamed mouth, sore throat, depression, agitation, headache, ver-tigo, sleep disturbance, dizziness, shaking, back or joint pain, muscle cramp, skin reactions, difficulty passing urine, liver disorders. Side effects of levodopa may be increased if used at the same time.

in patients with uncontrolled high blood pressure, angina, heart rhythm abnormality, liver disorders, mental disorders, or a history of stomach ulcers. The 1.25 mg tablet that dissolves on the tongue (Zelapar) is equivalent to 10 mg as standard tablet or syrup.

children, pregnant women, mothers who are breastfeeding, or for patients with current stomach ulcers. The tablets that dissolve on the tongue are not suitable for patients with PHENYLKETONURIA.

selenium sulphide shampoo

A suspension used as an antidandruff shampoo to treat dandruff and scaly scalp disorders.

Strengths available: 2.5% shampoo.
Dose: use twice a week for 2 weeks, then once a week for 2 weeks, then as needed.
Availability: NHS and private prescription.
Contains: selenium sulphide.
Brand names: Selsun.

keep away from the eyes or broken skin; do not use within 48 hours of hair-waving or colouring substances.

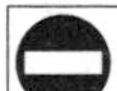
children under 5 years.

S

Selexid *see* pivmecillinam tablets
(Leo Pharmaceuticals)

Selsun *see* selenium sulphide shampoo
(Abbott Laboratories)

Semi-Daonil *see* glibenclamide tablets
(Hoechst Marion Roussel)

Semprex *see* acrivastine capsules
(GlaxoWellcome UK)

---

senna tablets/syrup/granules

A tablet, syrup, or granules used as a stimulant laxative to treat constipation.

Strengths available: 7.5 mg tablets; 7.5 mg/5 ml syrup; 15 mg/5 ml granules.
Dose: adults 15-30 mg at night; children aged 6-12 years half adult dose (taken in the morning); children aged 2-6 years 3.75-7.5 mg taken as syrup (2.5-5 ml) in the morning.
Availability: NHS and private prescription, nurse prescription, over the counter.
Contains: sennosides.
Brand names: Senokot (tablets not available on NHS).
Compound preparations: Manevac, Pripsen sachets.

 stomach cramps, low potassium levels and non-functioning bowels (with prolonged use).

 not generally recommended for prolonged use.

 children under 2 years or for patients suffering from blocked intestine.

Senokot *see* senna tablets/syrup/granules
(Reckitt and Colman Products)

Septrin *see* co-trimoxazole suspension/tablets
(GlaxoWellcome UK)

Serc *see* betahistine tablets
(Solvay Healthcare)

Serenace *see* haloperidol tablets/capsules/solution
(Baker Norton Pharmaceuticals)

S

Seretide *see* fluticasone inhaler and salmeterol inhaler
(Allen and Hanburys)

Strengths available: 100 mcg + 50 mcg, 250 mcg + 50 mcg, or 500 mcg + 50 mcg per dose of Accuhaler (dry powder inhalation device); 50 mcg + 25 mcg, 125 mcg + 25 mcg, and 250 mcg + 25 mcg CFC-free inhalers.
Dose: adults, 1 dose of Accuhaler or 2 puffs of inhaler (of any strength) twice a day; children aged 4-12 years use lowest strength of Accuhaler only.

Serevent *see* salmeterol inhaler
(Allen and Hanburys)

Serophene *see* clomiphene tablets
(Serono Laboratories (UK))

Seroquel *see* quietapine tablets
(Zeneca Pharma)

Serotulle *see* chlorhexidine dressings
(SSL International)

Seroxat *see* paroxetine tablets/liquid
(SmithKline Beecham Pharmaceuticals)

---

sertraline tablets

A tablet used to treat the symptoms of depression and obsessive compulsive disorders.

Strengths available: 50 mg and 100 mg tablets.
Dose: adults, 50 mg a day at first, increasing to a maximum of 200 mg if necessary, then reducing to 50 mg for maintenance.
Availability: NHS and private prescription.
Contains: sertraline hydrochloride.
Brand names: Lustral.

Side effects: stomach upset, change in appetite and weight, dry mouth, nervousness, drowsiness, sweating, shaking, headache, sleeplessness, dizziness, weakness, fits, change in sexual function, movement disorders, low blood sodium levels, skin disorders, rapid heart rate, confusion, loss of memory, mental disturbances, aggression, sensitivity to light, severe allergic reaction, muscle and joint pain, inflamed pancreas, milk production from breasts, menstrual disturbance, pins and needles, blood changes, heart rhythm disturbances, liver disorders.

Caution: in pregnant women, mothers who are breastfeeding, and in patients with epilepsy, liver or kidney disorders, or a history of heart disease, blood clotting disorders, or some psychiatric conditions. Treatment should be withdrawn slowly. Symptoms of panic disorder may get worse in early stages of treatment.

 children or for patients with elevated mood or poor liver function.

 ANTICOAGULANTS, other antidepressants, ritonavir, sumatriptan, lithium, alcohol, sedatives, selegiline.

sevelamer capsules

A capsule used as a phosphate binder to treat high phosphate levels in patients receiving kidney dialysis.

Strengths available: 403 mg capsules.
Dose: adults, 6-12 capsules a day at first, then as advised by doctor (according to response).
Availability: NHS and private prescription.
Contains: sevelamer.
Brand names: Renagel.

 in pregnant women, mothers who are breastfeeding, and in patients with stomach or intestinal disorders. Your doctor may advise regular blood tests.

 patients with blocked bowel.

Sevredol *see* morphine tablets/oral solution
(Napp Pharmaceuticals)

sildenafil tablets

A tablet used to treat impotence in men.

Strengths available: 25 mg, 50 mg, and 100 mg tablets.
Dose: adults, 50 mg at first (25 mg in the elderly) taken one hour before sexual activity. May be increased to 100 mg per dose if needed. Maximum of 1 dose in 24 hours.
Availability: private prescription, and on NHS prescription for men with certain specified causes of impotence (e.g. spinal cord injury).
Contains: sildenafil citrate.
Brand names: Viagra.

 indigestion, headache, flushing, dizziness, congested nose, fainting, rapid heart beat, eye disorders, visual disturbance, persistent painful erection, rash, heart attack, blockage or rupture of blood vessels in brain.

 in patients with heart or circulation disorders, liver or kidney disorders, deformity of penis, bleeding disorders, stomach ulcers, or in patients prone to prolonged erection.

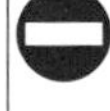 children, women, or for patients with low blood pressure, some eye disorders, or who have recently had a stroke or heart attack, or where sexual activity would be inadvisable.

 grapefruit juice, erythromycin, itraconazole, ketoconazole, antivirals, nicorandil, cimetidine, glyceryl trinitrate, isosorbide dinitrate, ALPHA-BLOCKERS, isosorbide mononitrate.

silver nitrate stick

A caustic pencil used to remove warts and verrucae.

Strengths available: 95% + 5% stick.
Dose: moisten the tip and apply for 1-2 minutes. Repeat after 24 hours, to a maximum of 3 applications for warts or 6 applications for verrucae.
Availability: NHS and private prescription, over the counter.
Contains: silver nitrate and potassium nitrate.
Brand names: Avoca.

 stains skin and fabrics. Protect surrounding skin before use.

 areas of broken skin, the face, around the anus or genital areas, or for application to large areas.

silver sulphadiazine cream

A cream used as an antibacterial treatment for wounds, burns, infected leg ulcers, bed sores, and where skin has been removed for grafting.

Strengths available: 1% cream.
Dose: applied once a day to burns, once a day or on alternate days for leg ulcers and bed sores, three times a week for other conditions.
Availability: NHS and private prescription.
Contains: silver sulphadiazine (sulfadiazine).
Brand names: Flamazine.

 burning, itching, rash, silver poisoning (with prolonged use) resulting in grey colour of skin and eyes.

 in pregnant women, mothers who are breast-feeding, and in patients suffering from kidney or liver disease, or where application is to large areas.

 newborn babies, women in late pregnancy, or patients who are allergic to sulphonamides (such as sulphadiazine or sulphamethoxazole).

 ANTICOAGULANTS, amiodarone, phenytoin, pyrimethamine, cyclosporin, azathioprine, methotrexate, some other wound treatments.

simethicone *see* activated dimethicone, Kolanticon

simple eye ointment

An eye ointment used to lubricate and protect the eye particularly where the cornea has eroded.

Dose: applied to the affected eye(s) as required.
Availability: NHS and private prescription, over the counter.
Contains: liquid paraffin, wool fat, yellow soft paraffin.

 vision may be blurred.

 contact lenses.

simple linctus BP/simple paediatric linctus BP

A linctus used to soothe a dry irritating cough.

Strengths available: adult and children's (paediatric) strengths. Sugar-free versions also available.

Dose: adults, 5 ml of adult-strength linctus 3-4 times a day; children 5-10 ml of paediatric-strength linctus 3-4 times a day.

Availability: NHS and private prescription, over the counter.

Contains: citric acid monohydrate.

ordinary linctus not to be used for patients with diabetes (use sugar-free version).

Simplene *see* adrenaline eye drops
(Chauvin Pharmaceuticals)

---

simvastatin tablets

A tablet used as a STATIN to reduce cholesterol levels in patients who have not responded to dietary changes, to slow down the narrowing of heart blood vessels, and to reduce the possibility of heart attack in some patients who are particularly vulnerable.

Strengths available: 10 mg, 20 mg, 40 mg, and 80 mg tablets.

Dose: adults, usually 10-80 mg a day at night but higher doses divided through the day.

Availability: NHS and private prescription.

Contains: simvastatin.

Brand names: Zocor.

rash, hair loss, anaemia, dizziness, pins and needles, liver disorders, inflamed pancreas, severe allergic reaction, dizziness, muscle pain and inflammation, headache, stomach upset, liver changes. Report any unexplained muscle pain to your doctor.

in patients with liver or severe kidney disorders. Your doctor may advise regular blood tests. Women of child-bearing age should use adequate contraception during treatment and for 1 month afterwards.

children under 18 years, pregnant women, mothers who are breastfeeding, or for patients with current liver disease or PORPHYRIA.

cyclosporin, other lipid-lowering drugs, ANTICOAGULANTS, antifungals, antivirals.

Sinemet-110/Sinemet-275, Sinemet-Plus/Sinemet-CR *see* co-careldopa tablets
(Du Pont Pharmaceuticals)

Sinequan *see* doxepin capsules
(Pfizer)

S

Singulair *see* montelukast tablets
(Merck Sharp and Dohme)

Sinthrome *see* nicoumalone tablets
(Alliance Pharmaceuticals)

Siopel
(Bioglan Laboratories)
A cream used as a barrier to protect against water-based irritants.

Dose: apply as needed.
Availability: NHS and private prescription, nurse prescription, over the counter.
Contains: dimethicone, cetrimide, arachis (peanut) oil.

 contains arachis (peanut) oil.

 patients who are allergic to peanuts.

Skelid *see* tiludronic acid tablets.
(Sanofi Winthrop)

Skinoren *see* azeleic acid cream
(Schering Health Care)

SLE *see* lupus

Slofedipine MR/XL *see* nifedipine modified-release tablets
(Sterwin Medicines)

Slofenac *see* diclofenac modified-release tablets
(Sterwin Medicines)

Slo-Phyllin *see* theophylline modified-release capsules
(Lipha Pharmaceuticals)

Slow Fe *see* ferrous sulphate modified-release tablets
(Novartis Consumer Health)

Slow Fe Folic *see* ferrous sulphate modified-release tablets and folic acid tablets
(Novartis Consumer Health)
Used to prevent iron and folic acid deficiency in pregnant women.

Strengths available: 160 mg + 400 mcg tablets.
Dose: adults 1-2 a day.

Slow K *see* potassium chloride modified-release tablets
(Alliance Pharmaceuticals)

Slow Sodium *see* sodium chloride modified-release tablets
(Distriphar)

Slow Trasicor *see* oxprenolol modified-release tablets
(Sovereign Medical)

Slozem *see* diltiazem modified-release capsules
(Lipha Pharmaceuticals)

Sno-Phenicol *see* chloramphenicol eye drops
(Chauvin Pharmaceuticals)

Sno-Tears *see* polyvinyl alcohol eye drops
(Chauvin Pharmaceuticals)

---

soap spirit BP
A liquid used as a soap to remove crusts from the skin.

Dose: applied as needed.
Availability: NHS and private prescription, over the counter.
Contains: soft soap (in alcohol).

---

sodium acid phosphate *see* Carbalax, Fleet Enema, Fletchers' Phosphate Enema, Phosphate-Sandoz

---

sodium alginate *see* alginate tablets/liquid/sachets, Pyrogastrone

---

sodium alkylsulphoacetate *see* sodium citrate enema

Sodium Amytal *see* amylobarbitone capsules (Flynn Pharma)

---

sodium aurothiomalate injection

A gold salt injection used to treat rheumatoid arthritis.

Strengths available: 10 mg, 20 mg, and 50 mg injections.
Dose: as advised by doctor.
Availability: NHS and private prescription (on specialist advice only).
Contains: sodium aurothiomalate.
Brand names: Myocrisin.

 any other medication that might cause kidney or blood disorders, aspirin, some NON-STEROIDAL ANTI-INFLAMMATORY DRUGS.

 protein in the urine, mouth ulcers, skin reactions, blood disorders. Rarely, inflamed intestines, inflamed nerves, lung or liver disorders, kidney disorders, hair loss.

 in the elderly and in patients with a history of eczema, bowel inflammation, liver or kidney disorders, or allergic skin reactions. Your doctor will advise blood, skin, and urine tests before each dose, and annual chest X-rays. Report any metallic taste in the mouth, bruising, vaginal bleeding, diarrhoea, or disorders of the mouth or throat to your doctor immediately.

pregnant women, mothers who are breastfeeding, or for patients suffering from severe liver or kidney disease, LUPUS, PORPHYRIA, flaky skin disorders, some chest or intestinal conditions, or who have a history of blood disorders or defective bone marrow.

---

sodium bicarbonate *see* alginate tablets/liquid, Carbalax, gentian mixture (alkaline), Klean-Prep, magnesium carbonate aromatic mixture BP, magnesium trisilicate mixture BP/magnesium trisilicate compound oral powder BP, Mictral, Movicol, oral rehydration solution, Phosphate-Sandoz, Pyrogastrone, sodium bicarbonate ear drops BP, sodium bicarbonate tablets/capsules/powder, sodium chloride mouthwash compound BP

---

sodium bicarbonate ear drops

Ear drops used to remove ear wax.

Strengths available: 5% solution.
Dose: use as needed. Lie down with treated ear uppermost for 5-10 minutes after inserting the drops.
Availability: NHS and private prescription, nurse prescription, over the counter.
Contains: sodium bicarbonate.

---

sodium bicarbonate tablets/capsules/powder

A tablet/capsule/powder used as an ANTACID to relieve indigestion, correct chemical imbalance in the kidney, and to relieve discomfort in mild urine infections.

Strengths available: 300 mg and 600 mg tablets; 500 mg capsules; or 100% powder.
Dose: for indigestion, 600-1800 mg (using 300 mg tablets) sucked as needed; for chemical imbal-

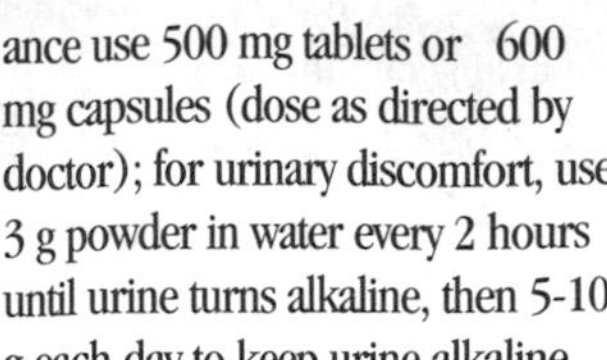

ance use 500 mg tablets or 600 mg capsules (dose as directed by doctor); for urinary discomfort, use 3 g powder in water every 2 hours until urine turns alkaline, then 5-10 g each day to keep urine alkaline.

Availability: NHS and private prescription, over the counter.

Contains: sodium bicarbonate.

Compound preparations: alginate tablets/liquid/sachets, magnesium trisilicate mixture BP/compound powder BP, Mictral, Pyrogastrone, various antacid preparations.

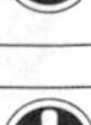

belching, high alkaline levels in the body with prolonged use.

in pregnant women, the elderly, and in patients with liver, kidney, or heart disease, and those on diets that are restricted in sodium. Avoid prolonged use

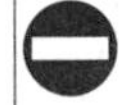

patients with general chemical imbalance in the body.

---

sodium cellulose phosphate sachets

A powder supplied in sachet and used as an ion-exchange compound to treat raised calcium levels in the urine or blood, recurring kidney stones, osteopetrosis (a condition where excess bone is formed).

Strengths available: 5 g sachets.

Dose: adults, 1 sachet three times a day (children, 2 sachets a day divided into 3 doses) dispersed in water or sprinkled on to food.

Availability: NHS and private prescription, over the counter.

Contains: sodium cellulose phosphate.

Brand names: Calcisorb.

diarrhoea, magnesium deficiency.

in growing children (treatment should be monitored) and in patients with kidney disorders. Treatment should be accompanied by a low-calcium diet with foods rich in oxalates restricted.

pregnant women, mothers who are breast-feeding, or for patients suffering from kidney or heart failure or conditions where sodium intake is restricted.

---

sodium chloride *see* Klean-Prep, Movicol, oral rehydration solution, saline solution (sterile), sodium chloride eye drops/solution, sodium chloride modified-release tablets, sodium chloride mouthwash compound BP

---

sodium chloride eye drops/solution

A saline solution or drops used to irrigate the eye (e.g. for first aid).

Strengths available: 0.9% solution.

Dose: used as needed.

Availability: NHS and private prescription, over the counter.

Contains: sodium chloride.

Brand names: Sodium Chloride Minims (preservative-free drops).

Compound preparations: Artificial Tears Minims.

Other preparations: saline solution (sterile).

Sodium Chloride Minims *see* sodium chloride eye drops/solution
(Chauvin Pharmaceuticals)

---

sodium chloride mouthwash compound BP

A solution used to clean and freshen the mouth.

Dose: dilute with an equal amount of water before use.
Availability: NHS and private prescription, over the counter.
Contains: sodium bicarbonate, sodium chloride.

---

sodium chloride modified-release tablets

An M-R TABLET used as a salt supplement to treat and prevent salt deficiency.

Strengths available: 600 mg m-r tablets.
Dose: adults, 4-20 tablets a day to treat low sodium levels, 4-8 tablets a day to prevent the condition; children given reduced doses according to body weight.
Availability: NHS and private prescription, over the counter.
Contains: sodium chloride.
Brand names: Slow Sodium.
Compound preparations: oral rehydration solution.

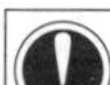 drink plenty of fluids with this treatment.

 patients suffering from fluid retention, heart disease, ADRENAL tumour, or for any patient whose diet is restricted in sodium.

 medicines used to treat high blood pressure, lithium, DIURETICS.

---

sodium citrate *see* Diarrest, Mictral, oral rehydration solution, sodium citrate enema

---

sodium citrate enema

A small-volume enema used as a softener and lubricant to treat constipation, and for evacuation of the bowels.

Strengths available: 450 mg in 5 ml.
Dose: adults and children over 3 years 5-10 ml (depending on brand); children under 3 years may use the Relaxit brand, inserting nozzle only to half the length.
Availability: NHS and private prescription, nurse prescription, over the counter.
Contains: sodium citrate, glycerol, sorbitol. Also: potassium sorbate, sodium laurylsulphoacetate and citric acid (Micolette); sodium alkylsulphoacetate (Micralax); sorbic acid (Micralax and Relaxit); sodium lauryl sulphate (Relaxit).
Brand names: Micolette, Micralax, Relaxit.

Caution: in elderly and weak patients.

Not to be used for: children under 3 years (some brands) or for patients suffering from inflammatory bowel disease or other immediate stomach or intestinal disorder.

S

sodium cromoglicate *see* sodium cromoglycate (alternative name)

sodium cromoglycate capsules

A capsule used as an anti-allergy drug to treat food allergies.

Strengths available: 100 mg capsules.
Dose: adults, 200 mg (children over 2 years, 100 mg) four times a day before meals, swallowed whole or opened and the contents dissolved in hot water then diluted with cold water before drinking. Dose may be increased to a maximum of 40 mg/kg body weight per day.
Availability: NHS and private prescription.
Contains: sodium cromoglycate (sodium cromoglicate).
Brand names: Nalcrom.
Other preparations: sodium cromoglycate eye drops, sodium cromoglycate inhaler/nebulizer solution, sodium cromoglycate nasal spray.

Side effects: rarely, rash, joint pain, nausea.

Not to be used for: children under 2 years.

sodium cromoglycate eye drops

Eye drops used as an anti-inflammatory preparation to treat allergic eye inflammation.

Strengths available: 2% drops.
Dose: 1-2 drops into the eyes four times a day.
Availability: NHS and private prescription, over the counter.
Contains: sodium cromoglycate (sodium cromoglicate).
Brand names: Hay-Crom Aqueous, Opticrom, Vividrin, Viz-On.
Other preparations: sodium cromoglycate capsules, sodium cromoglycate inhaler/nebulizer solution, sodium cromoglycate nasal spray.

Side effects: temporary discomfort.

Not to be used for: patients who wear soft contact lenses.

Caution needed with: soft contact lenses.

sodium cromoglycate inhaler/nebulizer solution

An inhaler or nebulizer solution used as an anti-inflammatory preparation to prevent asthma.

Strengths available: 5 mg per dose inhaler; 20 mg/2ml nebulizer solution.
Dose: adults and children, 10 mg (2 puffs) of inhaler four times a day (or up to 8 times a day if severe), with extra doses before exercise if needed; using nebulizer, 20 mg solution four times a day (or up to 6 times a day if severe). Regular use essential for effect.
Availability: NHS and private prescription.
Contains: sodium cromoglycate (sodium cromoglicate).
Brand names: Cromogen, Intal.
Other devices: Cromogen Easibreathe (breath-activated inhaler), Intal Fisonair (inhaler with spacer *cont.*

Side effects: temporary cough or difficulty breathing, irritated throat.

device), Intal Spincaps and Spinhaler (dry powder capsules and inhalation device used 4-8 times a day, as for inhaler).

Compound preparations: Aerocrom.

Other preparations: sodium cromoglycate capsules, sodium cromoglycate eye drops, sodium cromoglycate nasal spray.

---

sodium cromoglycate nasal spray

A nasal spray used as an anti-inflammatory preparation to prevent allergic rhinitis (hayfever).

Strengths available: 4% or 2% spray.

Dose: adults and children, 1 puff of 4% spray in each nostril 2-4 times a day (or 1 puff of 2% 4-6 times a day).

Availability: NHS and private prescription, over the counter.

Contains: sodium cromoglycate (sodium cromoglicate).

Brand names: Rynacrom, Vividrin.

Compound preparations: Rynacrom Compound.

Other preparations: sodium cromoglycate capsules, sodium cromoglycate eye drops, sodium cromoglycate inhaler/nebulizer solution.

Side effects: irritation of nose. Rarely, difficulty breathing.

---

sodium dihydrogen phosphate dihydrate *see* Fleet phospho-soda solution

---

sodium feredetate *see* sodium ironedetate (alternative name)

---

sodium fluoride *see* fluoride

---

sodium fusidate *see* fusidic acid tablets

---

sodium ironedetate elixir

An elixir used as an iron supplement to treat iron-deficiency anaemia.

Strengths available: 190 mg/5 ml elixir.

Dose: adults, 5-10 ml three times a day; children under 1 year, 2.5 ml twice a day; children 1-5 years, 2.5 ml three times a day; children 6-12 years 5 ml 3 times a day.

Availability: NHS and private prescription, over the counter.

Contains: sodium ironedetate (feredetate).

Brand names: Sytron.

stomach upset.

in patients with inflamed bowel, constipation, other intestinal disorders, or who have a history of stomach ulcers.

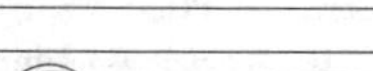

some ANTIBIOTICS.

S

sodium lactate *see* emollient preparations

sodium laurylsulphate *see* sodium citrate enema

sodium laurylsulphoacetate *see* sodium citrate enema

sodium perborate *see* Bocasan

sodium phenylbutyrate tablets/granules

A tablet or granules used to treat patients with enzyme deficiencies that prevent the formation of urea (urea cycle disorders).

Strengths available: 500 mg tablets; 940 mg/g granules.
Dose: as advised by doctor (specialist use only). Granules should be mixed with food before taking.
Availability: NHS and private prescription.
Contains: sodium phenylbutyrate.
Brand names: Ammonaps.

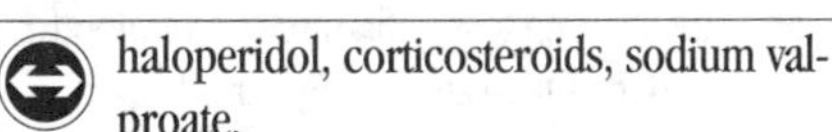
haloperidol, corticosteroids, sodium valproate.

absence or disturbance of menstrual periods, chemical disturbances, body odour, decreased appetite, taste disturbance, upset stomach, abdominal pain, stomach ulcer, fainting, inflamed pancreas, rectal bleeding, heart rhythm abnormality, fluid retention, depression, rash, weight gain, headache, bruising, blood disorders.

in patients with heart failure, liver or kidney disorders. Your doctor will advise regular blood tests.

pregnant women or mothers who are breast-feeding.

sodium phosphate *see* Fleet Enema, Fletchers' Phosphate Enema

sodium picosulfate *see* sodium picosulphate (alternative name)

sodium picosulphate elixir

An elixir used as a stimulant laxative to treat constipation and to clear the bowels before medical procedures.

Strengths available: 5 mg/5 ml elixir.
Dose: adults 5-15 ml (children 2-5 years 2.5 ml, aged 5-10 years 2.5-5 ml) at night.
Availability: NHS and private prescription, nurse prescription, over the counter.

stomach cramps, low potassium levels and non-functioning bowels (with prolonged use).

not generally recommended for prolonged use.

S

cont.

Contains: sodium picosulphate (picosulfate).
Brand names: Dulco-Lax liquid, Laxoberal (not available on NHS).
Compound preparations: Picolax sachets.

 children under 2 years or for patients suffering from blocked intestine.

---

sodium polystyrene sulphonate *see* polystyrene sulphonate resin

---

sodium pyrrolidone carboxylate *see* emollient preparations

---

sodium sulphate *see* Klean-prep

---

sodium valproate/valproic acid enteric-coated tablets/modified-release tablets/crushable tablets/enteric-coated capsules/liquid/syrup

An E-C TABLET, M-R TABLET, crushable tablet, E-C CAPSULE, liquid, or syrup used as an anti-epileptic treatment for all forms of epilepsy.

Strengths available: for sodium valproate: 100 mg crushable tablets; 200 mg and 500 mg e-c tablets; 200 mg and 500 mg m-r tablets; 200 mg/5 ml liquid or syrup. For valproic acid: 150 mg, 300 mg, and 500 mg e-c capsules.
Dose: as advised by doctor.
Availability: NHS and private prescription.
Contains: sodium valproate or valproic acid.
Brand names: Epilim, Orlept (sodium valproate); Convulex (valproic acid).

 stomach upset, drowsiness, skin disorders, weight gain, hair loss, fluid retention, inflamed pancreas, blood changes, liver disorders, disturbance of menstrual periods, breast swelling, unsteadiness, shaking, increased appetite, hearing loss, inflammation of blood vessels, dementia, Fanconi's Syndrome (a disease resulting in kidney disorders and rickets).

 in children, pregnant women, mothers who are breastfeeding, and in patients suffering from kidney disorders, LUPUS, or who are undergoing major surgery or who have a history of liver disorders. Your doctor will advise regular liver checks in the first few months of treatment. Treatment should be withdrawn gradually.

ANTICOAGULANTS, antidepressants, other anti-epileptic treatments, chloroquine, mefloquine, alcohol, sedatives. ANTACIDS should not be taken at the same time as e-c tablets/capsules.

 patients suffering from active liver disease, PORPHYRIA, or who have a family history of severe liver disorders.

S

Sofra-Tulle *see* framycetin dressings
(Hoechst Marion Roussel)

Sofradex

(Distriphar)

Drops or ointment used as an antibiotic, CORTICOSTEROID treatment for inflammation of the outer ear or eye.

Strengths available: 0.05% + 0.5% + 0.005% drops or ointment.

Dose: apply 2-3 drops 3-4 times a day (or ointment once or twice a day) to the affected ear(s); apply 1-2 drops up to six times a day (or ointment 2-3 times a day) to the affected eye(s); or use drops during the day and ointment at night.

Availability: NHS and private prescription.

Contains: dexamethasone sodium metasulphobenzoate, framycetin sulphate, gramicidin.

additional infection; temporary stinging or burning (when used in ear); cataract, thinning cornea, fungal infection, rise in eye pressure (when used in eye).

in pregnant women and infants – do not use for extended periods.

patients suffering from perforated ear drum (if used in the ear); patients suffering from eye infections not responsive to antibiotics, glaucoma, or for patients who wear soft contact lenses (if used in the eye).

ANTIMUSCARINICS.

Soframycin *see* framycetin eye drops/ointment

(Distriphar)

Softclix II Finger Pricking Device *see* Baylet Lancets, Cleanlet Fine Lancets, FinePoint Lancets, B-D Micro-Fine+ Lancets, Milward Steri-Let/Steri-Let Ultra-Fine Lancets, Monolet Lancets, Monolet Extra Lancets, Unilet G SuperLite Lancets, Unilet GP Lancets, Unilet Universal ComforTouch Lancets, Vitrex Soft Lancets

(Roche Diagnostics)

Availability: private prescription, over the counter.

Softclix II Lancets

(Roche Diagnostics)

Diabetics who need to test their blood regularly can use lancets to pierce the skin, either with or without the use of a finger-pricking device.

Lancet width and length: 28G/0.4 mm (Type C).

Availability: NHS and private prescription, over the counter.

Compatible finger-pricking devices: Softclix II.

---

soft soap *see* soap spirit BP

Soft Touch Finger Pricking Device *see* Softclix Lancets
(Roche Diagnostics)

Availability: private prescription, over the counter.

Solian *see* amisulpride tablets
(Sanofi Synthelabo)

Solpadol *see* co-codamol tablets/effervescent tablets 30/500
(Sanofi Winthrop)

Soltamox *see* tamoxifen solution
(Rosemont Pharmaceuticals)

Solvazinc *see* zinc sulphate tablets
(Provalis Healthcare)

---

somatropin injection

An injection used as a growth hormone to treat conditions associated with deficiency (e.g. Turner syndrome, poor kidney function in children).

Strengths available: various strengths between 0.6 units and 45 units per injection.
Dose: as advised by doctor.
Availability: NHS and private prescription.
Contains: somatropin.
Brand names: Genotropin, Humatrope, Norditropin, Saizen, Zomacton.

headache, eye disorders, stomach upset, high fluid pressure in the brain, fluid retention, muscle and joint pain, pins and needles, underactive thyroid, skin reactions at injection site, high glucose levels, weakness, decreased fat.

in patients suffering from diabetes, swollen optic disc, underactive thyroid, hip disorders, high pressure in the brain, or with a history of cancer. Your doctor will advise regular eye checks.

pregnant women, mothers who are breast-feeding, or for children with closed bone ends, patients with tumours, or after kidney transplantation.

CORTICOSTEROIDS.

Somnite *see* nitrazepam suspension
(Norgine)

Sonata *see* zaleplon capsules
(Wyeth Laboratories)

Soneryl *see* butobarbitone tablets
(Hansam Healthcare)

Sorbalgon /Sorbalgon T *see* alginate dressing
(Paul Hartmann)

Sorbid-SA *see* isosorbide dinitrate modified-release capsules
(Zeneca Pharma)

sorbic acid *see* sodium citrate enema

sorbitol *see* sodium citrate enema

Sorbsan/Sorbsan Plus/Sorbsan SA 2000 *see* alginate dressing
(Maersk Medical)

Sotacor *see* sotalol tablets
(Bristol-Myers Squibb Pharmaceuticals)

sotalol tablets

A tablet used as a BETA-BLOCKER to treat abnormal heart rhythm.

Strengths available: 40 mg, 80 mg, and 160 mg tablets.
Dose: 80 mg a day at first increasing gradually to a maximum of 320 mg a day (or 640 mg under specialist supervision) in 2-3 divided doses.
Availability: NHS and private prescription.
Contains: sotalol hydrochloride.
Brand names: Beta-Cardone, Sotacor.

cold hands and feet, sleep disturbance, slow heart rate, tiredness, wheezing, heart failure, low blood pressure, stomach upset. Rarely, dry eyes, rash, worsening of psoriasis, abnormally fast heart rhythm.

in pregnant women, mothers who are breast-feeding, the elderly, and in patients suffering from diabetes, severe or prolonged diarrhoea, kidney or liver disorders, MYATHENIA GRAVIS, or with a history of allergies. Chemical imbalance in the blood may need to be corrected. May need to be withdrawn before surgery. Withdraw gradually.

children or for patients suffering from heart block or failure, kidney failure, asthma, PHAEOCHROMOCYTOMA, a history of breathing disorders, or who have certain types of abnormal heart rhythm.

S

cont.

 general anaesthetics, CALCIUM-CHANNEL BLOCKERS, ALPHA-BLOCKERS, clonidine, ANTIHYPERTENSIVES, amiodarone, antidiabetics, thymoxamine, theophylline, aminophylline, fluvoxamine, chlorpromazine, propafenone, disopyramide, procainamide, quinidine, TRICYCLIC ANTIDEPRESSANTS, mizolastine, halofantrine, mefloquine, sedatives, pimozide.

soya oil *see* emollient preparations

Spasmonal/Spasmonal Forte *see* alverine capsules
(Norgine)

Spasmonal Fibre (formerly Alvercol) *see* alverine capsules and sterculia granules
(Norgine)
Granules used to treat irritable bowel syndrome.

Strengths available: 0.5% + 62% granules.
Dose: adults, 1-2 heaped 5 ml spoonsful swallowed with water (without chewing) once or twice a day after meals (but not immediately before bedtime).

spironolactone tablets

A tablet used as a DIURETIC to treat fluid retention in liver cirrhosis, kidney disorders, heart failure, and excessive ADRENAL hormones.

Strengths available: 25 mg, 50 mg, and 100 mg tablets.
Dose: for fluid retention, 100-200 mg a day increasing to 400 mg if required (children use reduced doses). For heart failure, usually 25 mg once a day.
Availability: NHS and private prescription.
Contains: spironolactone.
Brand names: Aldactone, Spirospare.
Compound preparations: co-flumactone (with hydroflumethiazide), Lasilactone.

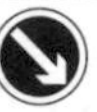 breast enlargement, impotence, tiredness, raised potassium levels, irregular periods, stomach upset, rash, headache, confusion, low sodium levels, liver and blood disorders, soft bones.

 in the elderly and in patients suffering from kidney or liver disease, PORPHYRIA. Your doctor may advise regular blood tests.

 pregnant women, mothers who are breast-feeding, or for patients suffering from severe kidney disorders, raised potassium or low sodium levels, Addison's disease.

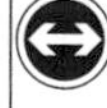 ACE-INHIBITORS, NON-STEROIDAL ANTI-INFLAMMATORY DRUGS, potassium supplements, carbamazepine, ANTIHYPERTENSIVES, halofantrine, digoxin, cyclosporin, lithium.

S

Spirospare *see* spironolactone tablets
(Ashbourne Pharmaceuticals)

Sporonox/Sporonox Pulse *see* itraconazole capsules/liquid
(Janssen-Cilag)

Sprilon

(Smith and Nephew Healthcare)
An aerosol spray used as a barrier to protect the skin from faeces and urine, and to treat eczema, leg ulcers, bedsores, and cracked skin.

Dose: spray for 2-3 seconds from a distance of 20 cm.
Availability: NHS and private prescription, nurse prescription, over the counter.
Contains: dimethicone, zinc oxide.

stanozolol tablets

A tablet used as an anabolic STEROID to treat blood vessel disorders.

Strengths available: 5 mg tablets.
Dose: adults, 2.5 mg-10 mg a day according to condition; children over 1 year used reduced doses according to age.
Availability: NHS and private prescription.
Contains: stanozolol.
Brand names: Stromba.

masculinization, hair growth, fluid and sodium retention, voice changes, disorders of menstrual periods, skin disorders, liver disorders, indigestion, cramp, headache, thyroid effects, change in mood, blood disorders.

in children (avoid long-term use), women before the menopause, and in patients suffering from heart or kidney disease, breast cancer, diabetes, or with a history of jaundice. Your doctor may advise blood tests for liver function.

ANTICOAGULANTS, antidiabetics.

children under 1 year, pregnant women, mothers who are breastfeeding, or for patients suffering from prostate cancer, liver disease, PORPHYRIA, insulin-dependent diabetes. Not to be used to treat weight loss or children who fail to thrive.

Staril *see* fosinopril tablets
(Bristol-Myers Squibb Pharmaceuticals)

statin

A lipid-lowering drug used to reduce high levels of lipids (such as cholesterol or triglycerides) in the blood which are known to increase the risk of developing coronary heart disease where blood vessels in the heart become narrowed and blocked. By reducing these high lipid levels, it may be possible to halt the progression of this disease (where it is established) and to prevent heart attack or stroke which may otherwise result. Example, simvastatin.

stavudine capsules/solution

A capsule or solution used in combination with other antiviral drugs to treat patients infected with HIV.

Strengths available: 15 mg, 20 mg, and 30 mg capsules; for making into a solution 1 mg/ml.
Dose: adults, 30-40 mg, according to weight, every 12 hours (at least 1 hour before food); children over 3 months use reduced doses according to body weight.
Availability: NHS and private prescription.
Contains: stavudine.
Brand names: Zerit.

 numbness in hands and feet, inflamed pancreas, liver and blood disorders, stomach upset, loss of appetite, chest or abdominal pain, headache, dizziness, sleeplessness, difficulty breathing, weakness, mood change, muscle or joint pain, influenza-like symptoms, skin disorders, enlarged lymph glands, abnormal tissue growth.

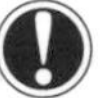 in pregnant women and in patients with kidney or liver disease, or a history of numb hands or feet, or inflamed pancreas.

 zidovudine, trimethoprim.

 mothers who are breastfeeding.

Stelazine *see* trifluoperazine tablets/modified-release capsules/syrup
(Goldshield Healthcare)

Stemetil *see* prochlorperazine tablets/buccal tablets/sachets/suppositories/syrup
(Distriphar)

Sterac *see* saline solution
(Galen)

---

sterculia granules

Granules (available in sachets or in a bulk pack) used as a bulking agent to treat constipation caused by lack of fibre in the diet.

Strengths available: 62% granules.
Dose: adults, 1-2 sachets or 1-2 heaped 5 ml spoonsful once or twice a day after meals; children aged 6-12 years, half adult dose. Children under 6 years treated only as advised by doctor. The dose should be swallowed without chewing but with plenty of liquid.
Availability: NHS and private prescription, nurse prescription, over the counter.
Contains: sterculia.

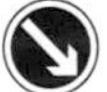 wind, bloating, obstructed intestines.

 in elderly, weak, or, diabetic patients or those with narrowed or poorly functioning intestines. Do not take a dose immediately before going to bed.

 patients with blocked intestines, difficulty swallowing, or relaxed bowel.

Brand names: Normacol.
Compound preparations: Normacol Plus (with added frangula – another laxative. Caution needed in pregnant women), Spasmonal Fibre.

Sterexidine *see* chlorhexidine solution
(Galen)

Steri-Let *see* Milward Steri-Let

Steri-Neb Ipratropium *see* ipratropium bromide nebulizer solution
(Baker Norton Pharmaceuticals)

Steripaste *see* zinc paste bandage
(SSL International)

Steripod antimicrobial cleanser *see* chlorhexidine solution
(SSL International)

Steripod wound and burn cleanser *see* chlorhexidine solution
(SSL International)

Steripod wound cleanser *see* saline solution (sterile)
(SSL International)

Steripoules *see* salbutamol nebulizer solution, saline solution (sterile)
(Galen)

Ster-Zac bath concentrate *see* triclosan liquid
(SSL International)

Ster-Zac powder *see* hexachlorophane powder
(SSL International)

Stesolid *see* diazepam rectal tubes
(Cox Pharmaceuticals)

Stiedex/Stiedex Lp *see* topical corticosteroid lotion/oily cream
(Stiefel Laboratories (UK))

Stiemycin *see* erythromycin topical solution
(Stiefel Laboratories (UK))

stilboestrol *see* diethylstilbestrol (new name)

Stilnoct *see* zolpidem tablets
(Sanofi Synthelabo)

Strefen *see* flurbiprofen throat lozenges
(Crookes Healthcare)

Stromba *see* stanozolol tablets
(Sanofi Winthrop)

Stugeron/Stugeron Forte *see* cinnarizine tablets/capsules
(Janssen-Cilag)

Subutex *see* buprenorphine sublingual tablets
(Schering-Plough)

sucralfate tablets/suspension

A tablet or suspension used as a cell-surface protector in the treatment of stomach inflammation and ulcers, and to prevent bleeding from stomach ulcers in seriously ill patients.

Strengths available: 1 g tablets; 1 g/5 ml suspension.
Dose: adults, for treatment 2 g twice a day or 1 g four times a day 1 hour before meals and at bedtime (usually taken for 4-12 weeks – up to 8 g a day may be needed); to prevent ulcers, 1 g (as suspension) six times a day (maximum eight times a day).
Availability: NHS and private prescription.
Contains: sucralfate.
Brand names: Antepsin.

stomach upset, dry mouth, rash, back pain, dizziness, drowsiness, headache, vertigo, intestinal obstruction.

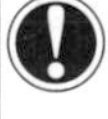
in pregnant women, mothers who are breast-feeding, and in patients who are seriously ill or who have kidney disorders.

children or for patients with severe kidney disorders.

ANTICOAGULANTS, some antidiabetics, alcohol, sedating drugs, phenytoin, theophylline, aminophylline.

sucrose *see* alginate tablets/liquid, oral rehydration solution

Sudafed *see* pseudoephedrine tablets/liquid
(Warner Lambert Consumer Healthcare)

Sudafed Plus

A tablet or syrup used as a SYMPATHOMIMETIC and ANTIHISTAMINE treatment for allergic inflammations of the nose (such as hayfever).

Strengths available: 60 mg + 2.5 mg tablets; 30 mg + 1.25 mg in 5 ml syrup.
Dose: adults, 1 tablet or 10 ml syrup four times a day; children aged 2-5 years, 2.5 ml syrup (aged 6-12 years 5 ml syrup) four times a day.
Availability: NHS and private prescription.
Contains: pseudoephedrine hydrochloride and triprolidine hydrochloride.

 drowsiness, rash, fast heart beat, sleeplessness, restlessness, anxiety. More rarely, irregular heart beat, shaking, dry mouth, cold hands and feet, hallucinations.

 in the elderly and in patients with high blood pressure, narrowed blood supply to the heart, glaucoma, overactive thyroid, diabetes, kidney disease, or enlarged prostate.

 children under 2 years.

 MAOIS, drugs used to lower blood pressure, alcohol, sedatives, other sympathomimetics.

Sudocrem

(Tosara Products (UK))
A cream used as an antiseptic emollient to treat bedsores, eczema, burns, and nappy rash.

Dose: apply a thin layer to the affected area as needed.
Availability: NHS and private prescription, over the counter.
Contains: benzyl alcohol, benzyl benzoate, benzyl cinnamate, hydrous wool fat, zinc oxide.

Sulazine EC *see* sulphasalazine enteric-coated tablets
(Chatfield Laboratories)

sulconazole cream

A cream used as an antifungal treatment for fungal infections of the skin.

Strengths available: 1% cream.
Dose: apply once or twice a day and continue for 2-3 weeks after the symptoms disappear.
Availability: NHS and private prescription.
Contains: sulconazole nitrate.
Brand names: Exelderm.

 irritation.

 keep out of the eyes. Stop treatment if irritation occurs.

Suleo M *see* malathion liquid
(SSL International)

---

sulfacetamide *see* sulphacetamide (alternative name)

---

sulfadiazine *see* sulphadiazine (alternative name)

---

sulfadoxine *see* Fansidar

---

sulfamethoxazole *see* sulphamethoxazole (alternative name)

---

sulfametopyrazine tablets

A tablet used as an ANTIBIOTIC to treat bronchitis and urine infections.

Strengths available: 2 g tablets.
Dose: adults, 2 g once a week.
Availability: NHS and private prescription.
Contains: sulfametopyrazine.
Brand names: Kelfizine W.

Side effects: upset stomach, mouth or tongue inflammation, rash, blood changes, folate (vitamin) deficiency. Rarely, skin changes, liver or pancreas disorders, inflamed bowel, headache, depression, kidney disorders, fits, lack of co-ordination, nerve inflammation or meningitis, vertigo, noises in the ears, muscle or joint pain, breathing disorders.

Not to be used for: children, mothers who are breastfeeding, women in late pregnancy, or for patients suffering from severe kidney or liver disease, PORPHYRIA, or blood disorders.

Caution: in the elderly, pregnant women, and in patients suffering from kidney or liver disease, blood disorders, asthma, or sensitivity to light. Drink plenty of non-alcoholic fluids. Your doctor may advise regular blood tests during prolonged treatment.

Caution needed with: amiodarone, ANTICOAGULANTS, some antidiabetic drugs, phenytoin, pyrimethamine, cyclosporin, azathioprine, methotrexate.

---

sulfasalazine *see* sulphasalazine (alternative name)

---

sulfathiazole *see* sulphathiazole (alternative name)

---

sulfinpyrazone *see* sulphinpyrazone (alternative name)

---

sulindac tablets

A tablet used as a NON-STEROIDAL ANTI-INFLAMMATORY DRUG to treat arthritis, ankylosing spondylitis, acute gout, and other muscle or joint disorders.

Strengths available: 100 mg and 200 mg tablets.
Dose: adults, 200 mg twice a day.
Availability: NHS and private prescription.
Contains: sulindac.
Brand names: Clinoril.

 stomach upset and bleeding or ulceration, rash, severe allergy, difficulty breathing, blood or kidney disorders, headache, dizziness, noises in the ears, sensitivity to light, vertigo. Rarely, fluid retention, liver disorders, inflamed pancreas, inflamed bowel, meningitis, discoloured urine.

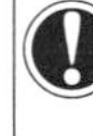 in the elderly, pregnant women, mothers who are breastfeeding, and in patients with heart, liver, or kidney disorders, high blood pressure, asthma, LUPUS or a history of kidney stones. Drink plenty of fluids.

 ACE-INHIBITORS, aspirin or other non-steroidal anti-inflammatory drugs, some ANTIBIOTICS, ANTICOAGULANTS, some antidiabetic drugs, some antivirals, methotrexate, DIURETICS, lithium, tacrolimus, cyclosporin, digoxin.

 children or for patients with a history of allergy to aspirin or other NSAID, severe kidney disorders, blood clotting disorders, currently active stomach ulcer or intestinal bleeding, inflamed intestines, or severe heart failure.

Sulparex *see* sulpiride tablets
(Bristol-Myers Squibb Pharmaceuticals)

---

sulphabenzamide *see* Sultrin

---

sulphacetamide *see* Sultrin

---

sulphadiazine tablets

A tablet used as an ANTIBIOTIC to prevent recurrence of rheumatic fever.

Strengths available: 500 mg tablets.
Dose: for patients weighing more than 30 kg, 1000 mg a day; for patients weighing less than 30 kg, 500 mg a day.
Availability: NHS and private prescription.
Contains: sulphadiazine (sulfadiazine).

 upset stomach, mouth or tongue inflammation, rash, blood changes, folate (vitamin) deficiency. Rarely, skin changes, liver or pancreas disorders, inflamed bowel, headache, depression, kidney disorders, fits, lack of co-ordination, nerve inflammation or meningitis, vertigo, noises in the ears, muscle or joint pain, breathing disorders.

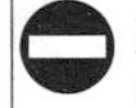 patients suffering from severe kidney or liver disease, PORPHYRIA, or blood disorders.

cont.

 amiodarone, ANTICOAGULANTS, some antidiabetic drugs, phenytoin, pyrimethamine, cyclosporin, azathioprine, methotrexate.

 in the elderly, pregnant women, mothers who are breastfeeding, and in patients suffering from kidney disease, asthma, or sensitivity to light. Drink plenty of non-alcoholic fluids. Your doctor may advise regular blood tests during prolonged treatment.

sulphamethoxazole *see* co-trimoxazole

sulphasalazine tablets/enteric-coated tablets/suspension/suppositories/enema

A tablet, E-C TABLET, suspension, suppository, or enema used to treat ulcerative colitis or Crohn's disease (inflammatory bowel diseases) and rheumatoid arthritis that does not respond to NON-STEROIDAL ANTI-INFLAMMATORY DRUGS.

Strengths available: 500 mg tablets or e-c tablets; 250 mg/5 ml suspension; 500 mg suppositories; 3000 mg enema.

Dose: for bowel disorders, adults 1000-2000 mg four times a day (using tablets or suspension), reducing to 500 mg four times a day when symptoms subside; children use reduced doses, according to body weight. Using suppositories, adults 500-1000 mg twice a day (after bowel movements); children use reduced doses. Using enema, 3000 mg at night, retained for at least an hour. For rheumatoid arthritis, 500 mg a day at first increasing to a maximum of 2000-3000 mg a day in divided doses if needed.

Availability: NHS and private prescription.

Contains: sulphasalazine (sulfasalazine).

Brand names: Salazopyrin, Sulazine.

 ANTACIDS should not be taken at the same time as e-c tablets.

 headache, skin disorders, high temperature, loss of appetite, stomach upset, liver or kidney disorders, worsening of some intestinal disorders, blood changes, diminished sperm production, sensitivity to light, urine disorders, severe allergic reaction, lung and eye disorders, mouth inflammation, inflamed parotid gland or pancreas, unsteadiness, vertigo, noises in the ears, hair loss, meningitis, numbness in hands and feet, sleeplessness, depression, hallucinations, LUPUS-like symptoms. Urine may be coloured orange.

 in pregnant women, mothers who are breast-feeding, and in patients with liver or kidney disease, PORPHYRIA, a history of allergy or anaemia/jaundice caused by drugs, or patients who are at risk of blood or liver disorders, or who are 'slow acetylators' (can clear some drugs only slowly from the body). Contact lenses may be stained. Your doctor may advise regular blood tests. Tell your doctor if sore throat, fever, or unidentified illness occurs.

 children under 2 years or for patients allergic to aspirin or salicylates. Enema not to be used for children.

S

sulphathiazole *see* Sultrin

sulphinpyrazone tablets

A tablet used as a uric acid-lowering drug to treat high uric acid levels and to prevent gout.

Strengths available: 100 mg and 200 mg tablets.
Dose: 100-200 mg a day with food at first, increasing to 600-800 mg a day over 2-3 weeks, then reducing to minimum effective dose.
Availability: NHS and private prescription.
Contains: sulphinpyrazone (sulfinpyrazone).
Brand names: Anturan.

 stomach upset, skin reactions, fluid and salt retention, blood disorders, stomach ulcers or bleeding, kidney and liver disorders.

 in pregnant women, mothers who are breastfeeding, and in patients with kidney or heart disease or who have anaemia and jaundice caused by medication. Drink plenty of fluids.

 children or for patients suffering from some blood disorders, a history of stomach ulcers, severe liver or kidney disorders, PORPHYRIA, or those who are allergic to NON-STEROIDAL ANTI-INFLAMMATORY DRUGS. Not suitable for treating an immediate gout attack.

 ANTICOAGULANTS, some antidiabetics, phenytoin, theophylline, aminophylline, aspirin, non-steroidal anti-inflammatory drugs.

---

sulphur *see* Actinac, Cocois, Meted, Pragmatar

---

sulpiride tablets

A tablet used as a sedative to treat schizophrenia.

Strengths available: 200 mg and 400 mg tablets.
Dose: adults, 200-400 mg twice a day (or up to 2400 mg a day for some types of symptoms); elderly patients start with lower doses and increase gradually.
Availability: NHS and private prescription.
Contains: sulpiride.
Brand names: Dolmatil, Sulparex, Sulpitil.

 movement disorders, muscle spasms, restlessness, shaking, dry mouth, heart rhythm disturbance, low blood pressure, weight gain, blurred vision, impotence, low body temperature, breast swelling, menstrual changes, blood, liver, eye, and skin changes, drowsiness, apathy, nightmares, sleeplessness, depression, blocked nose, difficulty passing water. Rarely, fits.

 in pregnant women, the elderly, and in patients suffering from heart, lung, or circulation disorders, epilepsy, Parkinson's disease, thyroid disorders, infections, MYASTHENIA GRAVIS, kidney or liver disease, glaucoma, enlarged prostate, or some blood disorders. Should be withdrawn gradually.

 children under 14 years, mothers who are breastfeeding, unconscious patients, severe kidney or liver impairment, or for patients suffering from bone marrow depression, PORPHYRIA, or PHAEOCHROMOCYTOMA.

 alcohol, sedatives, antidepressants, some antidiabetic drugs, anaesthetics, anti-epileptic medications, drugs affecting heart rhythm, ritonavir, halofantrine, sotalol, propranolol, lithium.

Sulpitil *see* sulpiride tablets
(Pharmacia and Upjohn)

Sultrin
(Janssen-Cilag)
A cream used as an antibacterial treatment for vaginal infections.

Dose: adults, 1 applicatorful of cream inserted into the vagina twice a day for 10 days, then reducing to once a day if necessary.
Availability: NHS and private prescription.
Contains: sulphathiazole (sulfathiazole), sulphacetamide (sulfacetamide), sulfabenzamide.

allergy. With prolonged treatment, risk of sulphonamide being absorbed (for side-effects *see* co-trimoxazole).

damages condoms and diaphragms.

children, pregnant women, mothers who are breastfeeding, or for patients with kidney disease or who are allergic to peanuts.

barrier contraceptives (*see* above).

sumatriptan tablets/injection/nasal spray
A tablet, injection, or nasal spray used to treat migraine attacks.

Strengths available: 50 mg and 100 mg tablets; 6 mg injections; 20 mg per dose nasal spray.
Dose: adults, 50-100 mg by mouth, 6 mg by injection, or 20 mg (one dose) of nasal spray into one nostril. This dose should be used as soon as possible after start of attack. If migraine responds but then recurs, repeat the dose (but leave at least 1 hour for injection or 2 hours for nasal spray). Second dose should not be used if migraine did not respond initially. Maximum of 2 doses in 24 hours.
Availability: NHS and private prescription.
Contains: sumatriptan (nasal spray), sumatriptan succinate (tablets and injection).
Brand names: Imigran.

tiredness, pain, dizziness, feelings of heaviness and weakness, raised blood pressure, sensation of heat, flushing, stomach upset, altered heart rate, tight throat or chest pain (stop treatment), liver disorders; rarely, fits, low blood pressure, serious heart circulation disorders, severe allergic reaction.

in pregnant women, mothers who are breast-feeding, and in patients suffering from heart disease, high blood pressure, allergy to some ANTIBIOTICS, or a history of epilepsy, liver or kidney disorders.

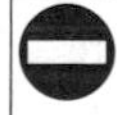
children under 18 years or for patients with heart blood vessel disorders, angina, uncontrolled high blood pressure, or anyone who has suffered a heart attack or stroke. Do not take within 24 hours of ERGOTAMINE.

ergotamine (*see* above), antidepressants, lithium.

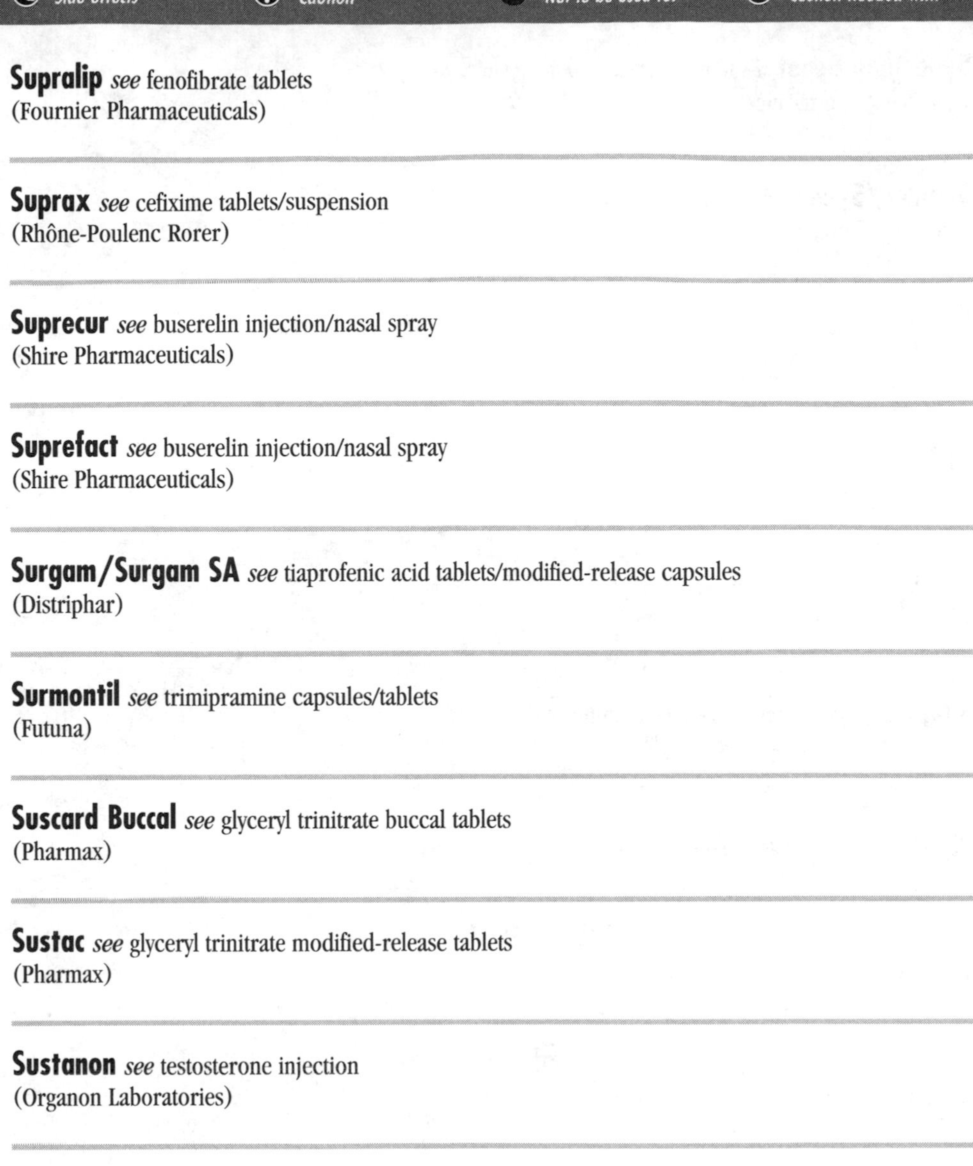

Supralip *see* fenofibrate tablets
(Fournier Pharmaceuticals)

Suprax *see* cefixime tablets/suspension
(Rhône-Poulenc Rorer)

Suprecur *see* buserelin injection/nasal spray
(Shire Pharmaceuticals)

Suprefact *see* buserelin injection/nasal spray
(Shire Pharmaceuticals)

Surgam/Surgam SA *see* tiaprofenic acid tablets/modified-release capsules
(Distriphar)

Surmontil *see* trimipramine capsules/tablets
(Futuna)

Suscard Buccal *see* glyceryl trinitrate buccal tablets
(Pharmax)

Sustac *see* glyceryl trinitrate modified-release tablets
(Pharmax)

Sustanon *see* testosterone injection
(Organon Laboratories)

Sustiva *see* efavirenz capsules
(DuPont Pharmaceuticals)

Symmetrel *see* amantadine capsules
(Alliance Pharmaceuticals)

---

sympathomimetic
A drug that functions like ADRENALINE and causes narrowing of the blood vessels but which may open other organs, such as the bronchial tubes. Example, pseudoephedrine.

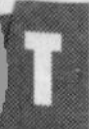

Synacthen Depot *see* tetracosactrin depot injection
(Alliance Pharmaceuticals)

Synalar/Synalar-C *see* topical corticosteroid cream/gel/ointment
(Bioglan Laboratories)

Synalar-N *see* topical corticosteroid cream/ointment and neomycin cream
(Bioglan Laboratories)

Synarel *see* nafarelin nasal spray
(Searle)

Synflex *see* naproxen tablets
(Roche Products)

Synphase *see* oral contraceptive (combined)
(Searle)

Syntaris *see* corticosteroid nasal spray
(Roche Products)

Synuretic *see* co-amilozide tablets
(DDSA Pharmaceuticals)

Syscor *see* nisoldipine modified-release tablets
(Pharmax)

Sytron *see* sodium ironedetate elixir
(Link Pharmaceuticals)

T-Gel *see* coal tar shampoo
(Neutrogena (UK))

---

tacalcitol ointment

An ointment used as a vitamin D product to treat psoriasis (including that on the scalp).

Strengths available: 4 mcg/g ointment.
Dose: apply sparingly at bedtime (maximum of 10 g per day if used all over including the scalp). Maximum period of use 12 months.
Availability: NHS and private prescription.
Contains: tacalcitol monohydrate.
Brand names: Curatoderm.

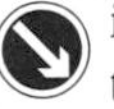 irritation, itching, reddening of skin, burning, tingling or numbness. Rarely, dermatitis, worsening of psoriasis.

 in pregnant women, mothers who are breast-feeding, and in patients with kidney disorders, certain types of psoriasis, or who are at risk of high calcium levels. Avoid contact with the eyes and accidental transfer to other body areas. Avoid exposure to sunlight or sunbeds immediately after application.

 sunlight and sunbeds (*see* above).

 children or for patients with high calcium levels.

tacrolimus capsules

A capsule used to suppress the immune system and prevent rejection following liver or kidney transplants.

Strengths available: 0.5 mg, 1 mg, and 5 mg capsules.
Dose: as advised by doctor.
Availability: NHS and private prescription.
Contains: tacrolimus.
Brand names: Prograf.

 stomach upset or ulcer, angina, rapid or irregular heart beat, high blood pressure, low blood pressure, heart disorders, shaking, sleeplessness, headache, dizziness, hallucinations, depression, anxiety, migraine, decreased reflexes, fits, eye disorders, confusion, deafness or noises in the ears, blood or kidney disorders, thyroid disorder, imbalance of acid and alkali in the body, sweating, hair growth or loss, abnormal processing of glucose in the body, fluid retention, severe allergic reaction, itching, redness, liver disorders, inflamed pancreas, weight and appetite changes, lung disorders.

 pregnant women, mothers who are breastfeeding, or for patients with allergy to erythromycin, azithromycin, or clarithromycin.

 grapefruit juice, NON-STEROIDAL ANTI-INFLAMMATORY DRUGS, clarithromycin, erythromycin, rifampicin, nefazodone, antifungals, ritonavir, nifedipine, diltiazem, cyclosporin, some DIURETICS, oral contraceptives, potassium.

 in patients suffering from chicken pox or shingles, PORPHYRIA, or with high potassium/uric acid levels. Your doctor may advise regular tests during treatment. Avoid excessive exposure to sunlight. Women must use non-hormonal contraception.

Tagamet *see* cimetidine tablets/effervescent tablets/syrup (SmithKline Beecham Pharmaceuticals)

T

Tambocor *see* flecainide tablets
(3M Health Care)

Tamofen *see* tamoxifen tablets
(Pharmacia and Upjohn)

tamoxifen tablets/solution

A tablet or solution used as an anti-oestrogen treatment for infertility in women caused by failure of ovulation, and to treat and prevent breast cancer.

Strengths available: 10 mg, 20 mg, and 40 mg tablets; 10 mg/5 ml solution.
Dose: adults, usually 20 mg a day. For infertility, the dose is given on days 2-5 of menstrual cycle (with dose increased to 40-80 mg a day for subsequent courses if necessary).
Availability: NHS and private prescription.
Contains: tamoxifen citrate.
Brand names: Emblon, Nolvadex, Soltamox, Tamofen.

hot flushes, vaginal bleeding or itching, stomach upset, dizziness, disturbed vision, blood changes, fluid retention, headache, light-headedness, skin disorders, fibroids in the womb, severe allergic reaction, blood clots (if other similar drugs also used), hair loss, liver changes, menstrual periods may stop. Rarely, ovarian cysts, high calcium levels, womb cancer (very small risk).

in women before the menopause and in patients suffering from secondary bone tumours or PORPHYRIA. Report any abnormal vaginal bleeding/discharge or irregularity of menstrual cycle to your doctor. Use non-hormonal methods of contraception.

children, pregnant women, or mothers who are breastfeeding.

other anti-cancer drugs, ANTICOAGULANTS, rifampicin.

Tampovagan *see* hormone replacement therapy (oestrogen-only)
(Co-Pharma)

tamsulosin modified-release capsules

An M-R CAPSULE used to treat enlarged prostate gland in men.

Strengths available: 400 mcg capsules.
Dose: 400 mcg once a day after breakfast.
Availability: NHS and private prescription.
Contains: tamsulosin hydrochloride.
Brand names: Flomax MR, Omnic MR.

dizziness, vertigo, stomach upset, low blood pressure on standing, fainting, dry mouth, changes in urine flow, rapid heart rate, palpitations, fluid retention, chest pain, tiredness, drowsiness, rash, itching, flushing, headache.

in elderly patients, and those suffering from low blood pressure, or heart, liver or kidney disorders. Your doctor may advise regular blood pressure checks. Treatment should be withdrawn if chest pain worsens, or 24 hours before anaesthesia. The first dose should be taken when going to bed.

 children or for patients suffering from severe liver disorder, or with a history of low blood pressure on standing, or fainting while passing urine.

 other ALPHA-BLOCKERS, ANTIHYPERTENSIVES, some drugs used to treat heart or circulation disorders, anaesthetics, NON-STEROIDAL ANTI-INFLAMMATORY DRUGS, alcohol, sedatives.

Tanatril *see* imidapril tablets
(Trinity Pharmaceuticals)

Tarband *see* zinc paste and coal tar bandage
(SSL International)

Tarivid *see* ofloxacin tablets
(Hoechst Marion Roussel)

Tarka *see* trandolapril capsules and verapamil modified-release tablets
(Knoll)

Strengths available: 2 mg + 180 mg M-R CAPSULES.
Dose: adults 1 a day.

Tavanic *see* levofloxacin tablets
(Hoechst Marion Roussel)

Tavegil *see* clemastine tablets/elixir
(Novartis Consumer Health)

tazarotene gel

A gel used to treat psoriasis.

Strengths available: 0.02% and 0.1% gel.
Dose: apply each evening for up to 12 weeks.
Availability: NHS and private prescription.
Contains: tazarotene.
Brand names: Zorac.

 irritation, burning, reddening or descaling of skin, rash, dermatitis, worsening of psoriasis. Rarely, inflammation, dryness, stinging, painful skin.

 avoid contact with eyes, face, scalp, skinfolds, or areas of inflammation or eczema. Avoid strong sunlight and sunbeds. Do not apply other skin preparations within 1 hour of treatment. Women should use adequate contraception.

 children under 18 years, pregnant women, or mothers who are breastfeeding.

 other skin preparations.

T

Tears Naturale *see* hypromellose eye drops
(Alcon)

Tegagen *see* alginate dressing
(3M Health Care)

Tegretol/Tegretol Retard *see* carbamazepine tablets/modified-releasetablets/chewable tablets/syrup/suppositories
(Novartis Pharmaceuticals UK)

Telfast *see* fexofenadine tablets
(Hoechst Marion Roussel)

---

telmisartan tablets

A tablet used as an ACE-II ANTAGONIST to treat high blood pressure.

Strengths available: 40 mg and 80 mg tablets.
Dose: 20-80 mg once a day.
Availability: NHS and private prescription.
Contains: telmisartan.
Brand names: Micardis.

low blood pressure, high potassium levels, severe allergic reaction, blood changes, headache, dizziness, muscle or joint pain, stomach upset or bleeding, back pain, sore throat, urine or respiratory infection, tiredness, cough. Occasionally, anaemia, high uric acid levels.

in patients with heart, liver, stomach, or intestinal disorders. Your doctor may advise regular blood tests.

children, pregnant women, mothers who are breastfeeding, or for patients with blocked bile duct, severe kidney or liver disorders, or who cannot digest fructose.

anaesthetics, NON-STEROIDAL ANTI-INFLAMMATORY DRUGS, cyclosporin, DIURETICS, lithium, potassium, digoxin.

---

temazepam tablets/capsules/solution

A tablet, capsule, or solution used as a short-term treatment for sleeplessness.

Strengths available: 10 mg or 20 mg tablets; 10 mg/5 ml solution; 10 mg, 15 mg, 20 mg, and 30 mg capsules.
Dose: adults, usually 10-20 mg at bedtime (rarely 30-40 mg); elderly patients usually 10 mg (rarely 20 mg).

drowsiness, light-headedness, confusion, vertigo, stomach disturbances, loss of memory, aggression, headache, joint immo-bility, salivation changes, shaking, unsteadiness, low blood pressure, rash, changes in vision, changes in sexual desire, retention of urine, incontinence, blood changes, jaundice. Risk of addiction increases with dose and length of treatment. May impair judgement.

Availability: controlled drug; NHS and private prescription. (Capsules not available on NHS.)

Contains: temazepam.

alcohol, other sedating drugs, ritonavir, phenytoin.

in elderly or weak patients, pregnant women, mothers who are breastfeeding, and in patients suffering from lung disorders, kidney or liver disorders, muscle weakness, PORPHYRIA, or with a history of drug or alcohol abuse, or personality disorder. Avoid long-term use and withdraw gradually.

children or for patients suffering from acute lung diseases, some chronic lung diseases, severe liver disease, MYASTHENIA GRAVIS, some obsessional and psychotic disorders, or who have stopped breathing while asleep.

Temgesic *see* buprenorphine sublingual tablets
(Schering-Plough)

Tenben *see* atenolol tablets and bendrofluazide tablets
(Galen)

Strengths available: 25 mg + 1.25 mg capsules.

Dose: adults 1-2 a day.

Tenchlor *see* co-tenidone tablets
(Berk Pharmaceuticals)

Tenif *see* atenolol tablets and nifedipine modified-release tablets
(Zeneca Pharma)

Strengths available: 50 mg + 20 mg M-R CAPSULES.

Dose: for high blood pressure, adults 1 capsule once or twice a day; elderly patients 1 a day. For angina 1 capsule twice a day.

Tenkicin *see* penicillin V tablets
(OPD Pharmaceuticals)

Tenoretic/Tenoret-50 *see* co-tenidone tablets
(Zeneca Pharma)

Tenormin/Tenormin LS *see* atenolol tablets/syrup
(Zeneca Pharma)

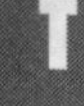

tenoxicam tablets

A tablet used as a NON-STEROIDAL ANTI-INFLAMMATORY DRUG to treat rheumatic disorders, and for the short-term treatment of strains, sprains, and other similar injuries.

Strengths available: 20 mg tablets.
Dose: adults, 20 mg a day. Treatment time for injuries is usually 7 days (maximum of 14 days).
Availability: NHS and private prescription.
Contains: tenoxicam.
Brand names: Mobiflex.

 stomach upset and bleeding or ulceration, rash, severe allergy, difficulty breathing, blood or kidney disorders, headache, dizziness, noises in the ears, sensitivity to light, vertigo. Rarely, fluid retention, liver disorders, inflamed pancreas, inflamed bowel, meningitis.

 in the elderly, pregnant women, mothers who are breastfeeding, and in patients with heart, liver, or kidney disorders, high blood pressure, asthma, or LUPUS.

 ACE-INHIBITORS, aspirin or other non-steroidal anti-inflammatory drugs, some ANTIBIOTICS, ANTICOAGULANTS, some antidiabetic drugs, some antivirals, methotrexate, DIURETICS, lithium, tacrolimus, cyclosporin, digoxin, aluminium hydroxide.

 children or for patients with a history of allergy to aspirin or other NSAID, severe kidney disorders, blood clotting disorders, currently active stomach ulcer or intestinal bleeding, inflamed intestines, or severe heart failure.

Tensipine MR *see* nifedipine modified-release tablets
(Genus Pharmaceuticals)

Tensopril *see* captopril tablets
(Norton Healthcare)

Teoptic *see* carteolol eye drops
(CIBA Vision Ophthalmics)

---

terazosin tablets

A tablet used as an ALPHA-BLOCKER to treat high blood pressure, and enlarged prostate gland in men.

Strengths available: 1 mg, 2 mg, and 5 mg tablets.
Dose: for high blood pressure, adults 1 mg at bedtime at first, increasing gradually to 2-20 mg a day. For enlarged prostate, adults 1 mg at bedtime, increased gradually if necessary to a maximum of 10 mg a day.
Availability: NHS and private prescription.

 fainting with first dose, dizziness, low blood pressure on standing, tiredness, swollen limbs, dizziness, vertigo, stomach upset, dry mouth, changes in urine flow, rapid heart rate, palpitations, chest pain, drowsiness, rash, itching, flushing, headache.

Contains: terazosin hydrochloride.
Brand names: Hytrin (for treating high blood pressure), Hytrin BPH (for treating enlarged prostate).

 in elderly patients and in those suffering from heart, liver, or kidney disorders. Your doctor may advise regular blood pressure checks. Treatment should be withdrawn if chest pain worsens, or 24 hours before anaesthesia. The first dose should be taken when going to bed.

 other alpha-blockers, ANTIHYPERTENSIVES, some drugs used to treat heart or circulation disorders, anaesthetics, NON-STEROIDAL ANTI-INFLAMMATORY DRUGS, alcohol, sedatives.

 children or for patients suffering from severe liver disorder, or with a history of low blood pressure on standing, or fainting while passing urine.

---

terbinafine tablets/cream

A tablet or cream used as an antifungal treatment for fungal skin infections such as ringworm. Tablet treatment also used for nail infections.

Strengths available: 250 mg tablets; 1% cream.
Dose: adults, 250 mg once a day by mouth for 2-12 weeks (depending on infection) or longer for toenail infections; the cream applied thinly once or twice a day, usually for 1-2 weeks.
Availability: NHS and private prescription.
Contains: terbinafine hydrochloride.
Brand names: Lamisil.

 with cream: redness, itching, stinging. With tablets: upset stomach, headache, loss of appetite, skin disorders, muscle or joint pain, taste disturbance, liver disorders, sensitivity to sunlight.

 in pregnant women, mothers who are breast-feeding, and in patients with liver or kidney disorders.

 children.

 oral contraceptives (with tablets).

---

terbutaline inhaler/tablets/modified-release tablets/syrup/nebulizer solution

An inhaler, tablet, M-R TABLET, syrup, or nebulizer solution used as a BRONCHODILATOR to treat asthma and other breathing disorders caused by obstructed airways.

Strengths available: 250 mcg per dose inhaler; 5 mg/2 ml nebulizer solution (single units ready for use) or 10 mg/ml nebulizer solution (bottle for dilution before use); 5 mg tablets; 1.5 mg/5 ml syrup; 7.5 mg m-r tablets.
Dose: using tablets/syrup, adults 2.5 mg three times a day for 1-2 weeks, increased to 5 mg three times a day if needed; children aged 7-15 years, 2.5 mg 2-3 times a day; younger children

 low potassium levels, shaking hands, headache, widening of blood vessels, cramps, altered heart rhythm, nervousness, severe allergic reaction, sleep and behaviour problems in children.

 in pregnant women, mothers who are breast-feeding, and in patients suffering from kidney damage, weak heart, irregular heart rhythm, high blood pressure, overactive thyroid, diabetes. In severe asthmatics, blood potassium levels should be checked regularly.

cont.

use reduced doses according to body weight. Using m-r tablets, adults 7.5 mg twice a day (not suitable for children). Using inhaler, adults and children, 250-500 mcg (1-2 puffs) up to 3-4 times a day. Using nebulizer solution, adults 5-10 mg (children 2-5 mg according to age) 2-4 times a day, using a nebulizer.

m-r tablets not to be used for children.

BETA-BLOCKERS, theophylline, aminophylline, SYMPATHOMIMETICS.

Availability: NHS and private prescription.
Contains: terbutaline sulphate.
Brand names: Bricanyl, Monovent.
Other devices: Bricanyl Turbohaler (dry powder inhaler device – 500 mcg per dose).

Teril Cr *see* carbamazepine modified-release tablets
(Lagap Pharmaceuticals)

Terra-Cortril *see* topical corticosteroid ointment
(Pfizer)

Terra-Cortril Nystatin *see* topical corticosteroid cream and nystatin cream
(Pfizer)

Terramycin *see* oxytetracycline tablets
(Pfizer)

Tertroxin *see* liothyronine tablets
(Goldshield Healthcare)

Testoderm *see* testosterone patches
(Ferring Pharmaceuticals)

---

testosterone capsules/patches/implant/injection

A capsule, patch, implant, or injection used as a male hormone to treat underdeveloped male sexual organs and other disorders caused by low hormone levels. Menopausal women may be treated with implants as an addition to hormone replacement therapy.

Strengths available: 40 mg capsules; patches releasing 2.5 mg, 5 mg, or 6 mg in 24 hours; 100 mg or 200 mg implant; various injection strengths according to type of testosterone.
Dose: adults, by mouth 120-160 mg a day for 2-3 weeks reducing to 40-120 mg a day for maintenance; using patches, 2.5-7.5 mg a day (the patches applied to a clean, dry patch of skin and replaced after 24 hours); the 6 mg patch applied to clean, dry,

shaved, scrotal skin and replaced after 22-24 hours. Menopausal women treated with implants (50-100 mg, replaced every 4-8 months). Injections given every 2-6 weeks (dose as directed by doctor).

Availability: NHS and private prescription.

Contains: testosterone undecanoate (capsules), testosterone (implant and patches), testosterone enantate/propionate/phenylpropionate/isocaproate/decanoate (injection).

Brand names: Andropatch, Primoteston Depot, Restandol, Sustanon, Testoderm, Virormone.

headache, depression, stomach upset or bleeding, jaundice, swollen breasts, anxiety, weakness, changes in sexual desire, prostate abnormalities, pins and needles, chemical imbalance, fluid retention, high blood calcium levels, hair growth, baldness, skin disorders, bone growth, erect penis, early sexual development, suppressed sperm production, early closure of epiphyses (bone ends), liver disorders, masculinization in women. Also skin allergies and irritation with patches.

in boys before puberty and in patients suffering from heart, liver, or kidney disorders, high blood pressure, epilepsy, migraine, or bone tumours.

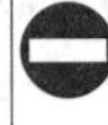
children (except to treat delayed puberty in males), pregnant women, mothers who are breastfeeding, or for patients with prostate or liver cancer, kidney or heart disorders, high calcium levels.

ANTICOAGULANTS, antidiabetics.

tetanus vaccine

A vaccine used to stimulate the body's immune system to provide immunity to tetanus infection.

Dose: in untreated patients, 3 injections at 4-week intervals. Boosters may be given after a further 10 years if necessary. After 5 doses, the patient should have life-long immunity.

Availability: NHS and private prescription.

Contains: tetanus vaccine.

Brand names: Clostet.

Compound preparations: diphtheria and tetanus vaccine; diphtheria, tetanus, and pertussis vaccine; diphtheria, tetanus, pertussis, and *Haemophilus influenzae* type B vaccine.

fever, general feeling of being unwell, skin reaction at injection site.

in patients with a history of allergy to tetanus.

patients suffering from infectious diseases (unless definitely at immediate risk of contracting tetanus).

tetrabenazine tablets

A tablet used as a sedative to treat movement disorders (as in Huntington's chorea, senile chorea).

Strengths available: 25 mg tablets.

Dose: adults, 12.5 mg twice a day (elderly patients once a day)

drowsiness, stomach upset, depression, shaking hands, low blood pressure, Parkinson-like symptoms, NEUROLEPTIC MALIGNANT SYNDROME.

cont.

at first, increasing to a maximum of 200 mg a day if needed.

Availability: NHS and private prescription.

Contains: tetrabenazine.

Brand names: Xenazine 25.

 in pregnant women.

 children or mothers who are breastfeeding.

 MAOIS, sedating drugs, alcohol.

---

tetracaine *see* amethocaine (alternative name)

---

tetracosactide *see* tetracosactrin (alternative name)

---

tetracosactrin depot injection

An injection used as an alternative to CORTICOSTEROIDS in the short-term treatment of rheumatic disorders or inflamed bowel disorders (such as Crohn's disease or ulcerative colitis).

Strengths available: 1 mg injection.

Dose: adults, 1 mg given by injection once or twice a day at first, reducing to 1 mg every 2-3 days (or less) for maintenance; children over 3 years given reduced doses according to body weight.

Availability: NHS and private prescription.

Contains: tetracosactrin (tetracosactide) acetate.

Brand names: Synacthen Depot.

 high blood sugar, thin bones, mood changes, stomach ulcers, fluid retention, potassium loss, high blood pressure, menstrual irregularity, hairiness, increased likelihood of infection, euphoria, depression, sleeplessness, aggravation of schizophrenia and epilepsy, eye disorders, thinning of skin, acne, bruising, blood changes, stomach upset, inflamed pancreas, muscle abnormality, suppression of the ADRENAL GLANDS, ulcerated or infected oesophagus, general feeling of being unwell, hiccups, reduced growth in children, severe allergic reaction.

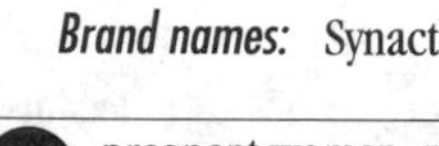 pregnant women, mothers who are breastfeeding, children under 3 years, or for patients who have untreated infections, asthma, mental disorders, stomach ulcers, heart failure, or some adrenal disorders.

 live vaccines, some ANTIBIOTICS and anti-epileptics, ANTICOAGULANTS, antidiabetics, some antifungals, digoxin, cyclosporin.

 in patients who have had recent bowel surgery or who are suffering from inflamed veins, psychiatric disorders, thinning of the bones, stomach ulcers, tuberculosis or other infections, high blood pressure, glaucoma, epilepsy, diabetes, underactive thyroid, liver disease, stress. Withdraw gradually. Avoid contact with chicken pox for 3 months after treatment ends and seek medical attention if exposed.

---

tetracycline tablets/capsules

A tablet or capsule used as an ANTIBIOTIC to treat infections, especially chest infections and acne.

Strengths available: 250 mg tablets and capsules.

Dose: usually 250-500 mg four times a day. For acne, 500 mg tablets twice a day reducing to 250 mg twice a day after 3 months. The dose to be taken with plenty of fluid while sitting or standing.
Availability: NHS and private prescription.
Contains: tetracycline hydrochloride.
Brand names: Achromycin.
Compound preparations: Deteclo (with chlortetracycline and demeclocycline).
Other preparations: tetracycline ointment.

 stomach upset, irritation of the oesophagus, reddening of skin, headache, disturbed vision, sensitivity to light, additional infections, pressure on the brain, reversible diabetes insipidus, liver disorders, inflamed pancreas or bowel.

 in patients suffering from liver or kidney disorders. Discontinue if reddening of skin occurs.

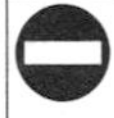 children under 12 years, pregnant women, mothers who are breastfeeding, or for patients suffering from LUPUS.

 milk, ANTACIDS, iron supplements, ANTICOAGULANTS, oral contraceptives.

tetracycline ointment

An ointment used as an ANTIBIOTIC to treat skin infection.

Strengths available: 3% ointment.
Dose: adults, apply on gauze 1-3 times a day.
Availability: NHS and private prescription.
Contains: tetracycline hydrochloride.
Brand names: Achromycin.
Other preparations: tetracycline tablets/capsules.

 additional infection.

 children, pregnant women, or mothers who are breastfeeding.

tetracycline solution

A solution applied to the skin and used as an ANTIBIOTIC treatment for acne.

Strengths available: 0.22% solution.
Dose: apply twice a day with enough lotion to wet the skin.
Availability: NHS and private prescription.
Contains: tetracycline hydrochloride.
Brand names: Topicycline.

 stinging, burning.

 in pregnant women, mothers who are breast-feeding, and in patients with kidney disorders. Avoid the eyes, mouth, and mucous membranes.

 children.

tetrahydrofurfuryl salicylate *see* analgesic (topical)

Tetralysal 300 *see* lymecycline capsules
(Galderma (UK))

Teveten *see* eprosartan tablets
(Solvay Healthcare)

Theo-Dur *see* theophylline modified-release tablets
(AstraZeneca UK)

theophylline tablets/modified-release tablets/modified-release capsules/liquid

A tablet, M-R TABLET/CAPSULE, or liquid used as a BRONCHODILATOR to treat bronchial spasm associated with severe acute asthma, chronic bronchitis, emphysema.

Strengths available: 125 mg tablets; 60 mg/5 ml liquid; 60 mg, 125 mg, or 250 mg m-r capsules; 175 mg, 200 mg, 300 mg, or 400 mg m-r tablets.
Dose: 120-240 mg 3-4 times a day after food using standard tablets/liquid, or 200-400 mg twice a day using m-r preparations. Children use lower doses according to body weight.
Availability: NHS and private prescription, over the counter.
Contains: theophylline.
Brand names: Nuelin, Slo-Phyllin, Theo-Dur, Uniphyllin Continus.
Compound preparations: Franol, Franol plus.

upset stomach, headache, sleeplessness, fits, abnormal heart rhythm, skin reactions.

in pregnant women, mothers who are breast-feeding, the elderly, and in patients suffering from heart disease, high blood pressure, over-active thyroid, liver disease, stomach ulcer, epilepsy, fever. Patients taking m-r forms of theophylline should remain on the same brand once stabilized. Smokers who alter their smoking habits may need dose adjusting.

patients suffering from PORPHYRIA.

cimetidine, some ANTIBIOTICS and anti-fungal treatments, CORTICOSTEROIDS, ritonavir, some ANTIHYPERTENSIVES, disulfiram, zafirlukast, DIURETICS, some other bronchodilators, fluvoxamine, diltiazem, verapamil, lithium, some anti-epileptics, methotrexate, nizatidine, oral contraceptives (combined), SYMPATHOMIMETICS, sulfinpyrazone, influenza vaccine, ticlopidine, alcohol, smoking.

thiabendazole tablets

A chewable tablet used to treat worms and other associated conditions and infections.

Strengths available: 500 mg chewable tablets.
Dose: dose as advised by doctor (according to body weight). Maximum 1500 mg twice a day with food.
Availability: NHS and private prescription.
Contains: thiabendazole (tiabendazole).

stomach upset, liver disorders, changes in eyesight, noises in the ears, low blood pressure, bedwetting, headache, itching, drowsiness, fever, severe allergic reaction, skin disorders.

T

Brand names: Mintezol.

 pregnant women, mothers who are breast-feeding, or for patients suffering from mixed infections with roundworms.

in the elderly and in patients suffering from kidney or liver disorders. Nutritional deficiencies must be corrected before starting treatment.

 alcohol, sedatives, theophylline, aminophylline.

thiamine tablets

A tablet used as a source of vitamin B_1 to treat deficiency.

Strengths available: 50 mg and 100 mg tablets.
Dose: 10-300 mg a day according to condition.
Availability: NHS and private prescription, over the counter.
Contains: thiamine hydrochloride (vitamin B_1).
Brand names: Benerva (not available on NHS).
Compound preparations: Ketovite, multivitamin drops, vitamin B compound tablets, vitamins capsules BPC.

thioridazine tablets/suspension/syrup/solution

A tablet, suspension, syrup, or oral solution used as a treatment for schizophrenia when other treatments have failed.

Strengths available: 25 mg, 50 mg, and 100 mg tablets; 25 mg/5 ml and 100 mg/5 ml suspension; 25 mg/5 ml syrup and solution.
Dose: adults, 75-600 mg a day in divided doses; elderly patients 30-100 mg a day; children over 1 year (treated for severe mental or behavioural problems only) given reduced doses according to body weight.
Availability: NHS and private prescription.
Contains: thioridazine (liquid forms) or thioridazine hydrochloride (tablets).
Brand names: Melleril.

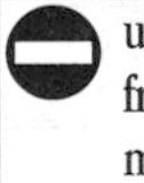 unconscious patients or for patients suffering from severe kidney or liver impairment, bone marrow depression, PORPHYRIA, or PHAEOCHROMOCYTOMA, significant heart disease or who have low potassium/magnesium levels.

 movement disorders, muscle spasms, restlessness, shaking, dry mouth, heart rhythm disturbance, low blood pressure, weight gain, blurred vision, impotence, low body temperature, breast swelling, menstrual changes, blood, liver, eye, and skin changes, drowsiness, apathy, nightmares, sleeplessness, depression, blocked nose, difficulty passing water. Rarely, fits.

 in pregnant women, mothers who are breast-feeding, the elderly, and in patients suffering from heart, lung, or circulation disorders, epilepsy, Parkinson's disease, thyroid disorders, infections, MYASTHENIA GRAVIS, kidney or liver disease, glaucoma, enlarged prostate, or some blood disorders. Should be withdrawn gradually. Your doctor may advise regular eye checks during prolonged treatment.

 alcohol, sedatives, antidepressants, some antidiabetic drugs, anaesthetics, anti-epileptic medications, drugs affecting heart rhythm, ritonavir, halofantrine, sotalol, lithium, OPIOID ANALGESICS.

T

threonine *see* Cicatrin

thymol glycerin compound BP 1988

A solution used to clean and freshen the mouth.

Dose: dilute with an equal amount of water before use.
Availability: NHS and private prescription, nurse prescription, over the counter.
Contains: glycerol, thymol.

thymoxamine tablets

A tablet used to widen blood vessels and treat Raynaud's syndrome (a condition caused by spasms of arteries in the hands).

Strengths available: 40 mg tablets.
Dose: 40 mg four times a day at first increasing if necessary to 80 mg four times a day.
Availability: NHS and private prescription.
Contains: thymoxamine hydrochloride (moxisylyte).
Brand names: Opilon.

 upset stomach, vertigo, headache, liver disorder, flushing, dizziness.

 in patients suffering from diabetes.

 children, pregnant women, mothers who are breastfeeding, or for patients with liver disease.

 BETA-BLOCKERS, some drugs used to treat high blood pressure or enlarged prostate gland.

thyroxine tablets

A tablet used as a thyroid hormone to treat thyroid deficiency.

Strengths available: 25 mcg, 50 mcg, and 100 mcg tablets.
Dose: adults, 50-100 mcg a day at first (50 mcg for patients over 50 years old) adjusted according to doctor's instructions (usually to 100-200 mcg a day); elderly patients, children, and patients with heart disorders take lower doses as advised by doctor.
Availability: NHS and private prescription.
Contains: thyroxine (levothyroxine) sodium.
Brand names: Eltroxin.

 abnormal heart rhythm, chest pain, rapid heart rate, muscle cramp or weakness, headache, shaking, restlessness, flushing, excitability, sweating, upset stomach, fever, intolerance of heat, rapid weight loss.

 in the elderly, pregnant women, mothers who are breastfeeding, and in patients suffering from diabetes, disorders of the pituitary gland, or poor ADRENAL function.

 patients suffering from excessive levels of thyroid hormones, heart or circulation problems, or where effort causes anginal chest pain.

 ANTICOAGULANTS.

tiabendazole *see* thiabendazole (alternative name)

tiagabine tablets

A tablet used as an additional treatment for epilepsy in patients not controlled on other medications.

Strengths available: 5 mg, 10 mg, and 15 mg tablets.
Dose: adults, 5 mg twice a day at first increasing as necessary to a maximum of 45 mg a day (in divided doses).
Availability: NHS and private prescription.
Contains: tiagabine hydrochloride.
Brand names: Gabitril.

upset stomach, dizziness, tiredness, shaking, nervousness, lack of concentration, emotional upset, drowsiness, depression, confusion, speech disorders, blood disorders, mental disturbance.

in pregnant women, mothers who are breast-feeding, and in patients with liver disorders or a history of serious behavioural problems.

children under 12 years or for patients with severe liver disorders.

other anti-epileptic treatments, alcohol, sedating drugs.

tiaprofenic acid tablets/modified-release capsules

A tablet or M-R CAPSULE used as a NON-STEROIDAL ANTI-INFLAMMATORY DRUG to treat pain and inflammation in arthritis and other muscle and joint disorders.

Strengths available: 200 mg and 300 mg tablets; 300 mg m-r capsules.
Dose: adults, 600 mg a day (in divided doses if using standard tablets or as a single daily dose using m-r capsules).
Availability: NHS and private prescription.
Contains: tiaprofenic acid.
Brand names: Surgam.

stomach upset and bleeding or ulceration, rash, severe allergy, difficulty breathing, blood or kidney disorders, headache, dizziness, noises in the ears, sensitivity to light, vertigo, severe cystitis. Rarely, fluid retention, liver disorders, inflamed pancreas, inflamed bowel, meningitis.

in the elderly, pregnant women, mothers who are breastfeeding, and in patients with heart, liver, or kidney disorders, high blood pressure, asthma, or LUPUS. Report any abnormal urinary symptoms to your doctor immediately.

children or for patients with a history of allergy to aspirin or other NSAID, severe kidney disorders, bladder or prostate disorders, blood clotting disorders, currently active stomach ulcer or intestinal bleeding, inflamed intestines, or severe heart failure.

ACE-INHIBITORS, aspirin or other non-steroidal anti-inflammatory drugs, some ANTIBIOTICS, ANTICOAGULANTS, some antidiabetic drugs, some antivirals, methotrexate, DIURETICS, lithium, tacrolimus, cyclosporin, digoxin.

tibolone tablets

A tablet used to treat symptoms of the menopause and to prevent thinning of the bones in women after the menopause.

Strengths available: 2.5 mg tablets.

cont.

Dose: adults, 2.5 mg a day.
Availability: NHS and private prescription.
Contains: tibolone.
Brand names: Livial.

 ANTICOAGULANTS.

 children, pregnant women, mothers who are breastfeeding, or for patients suffering from some tumours, undiagnosed vaginal bleeding, blood vessel disorders of the brain or heart, severe liver disorders.

 changes in body weight, dizziness, headache, depression, muscle or bone pain, scaly skin disorders, vaginal bleeding, stomach upset, liver disorder, facial hair growth, fluid retention, visual disturbance, skin irritation, itching, migraine.

 in patients who have transferred from another form of HORMONE REPLACEMENT THERAPY medication and in those suffering from epilepsy, migraine, diabetes, a history of kidney disorders or high cholesterol levels.

Ticlid *see* ticlopidine tablets
(Sanofi Winthrop)

---

ticlopidine tablets

A tablet used to reduce the risk of stroke or heart attack in patients who already have narrowed blood vessels (e.g. patients who have suffered a stroke or who have difficulty walking because of poor blood supply to the legs).

Strengths available: 250 mg tablets.
Dose: adults, 250 mg twice a day with meals.
Availability: NHS and private prescription.
Contains: ticlopidine hydrochloride.
Brand names: Ticlid.

 children or for patients at risk of abnormal bleeding or suffering from stomach ulcers or blood disorders.

 blood disorders, increased bleeding tendency, upset stomach, liver disorders, severe allergic reaction, inflamed blood vessels, LUPUS-like symptoms, kidney disorders, increased lipid levels in the blood, rash, itching.

 in pregnant women, mothers who are breast-feeding, and in patients who suffer from liver or kidney disorders. Your doctor will advise regular blood tests. Report any symptoms of infection to your doctor.

 NON-STEROIDAL ANTI-INFLAMMATORY DRUGS, aspirin, ANTICOAGULANTS, cyclosporin, theophylline, aminophylline, digoxin, phenytoin.

Tilade *see* nedocromil inhaler
(Pantheon Healthcare)

Tildiem/Tildiem LA/Tildiem Retard *see* diltiazem modified-release tablets/capsules
(Sanofi Synthelabo)

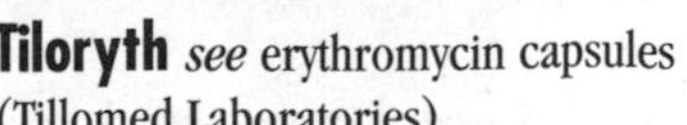

Tiloryth *see* erythromycin capsules
(Tillomed Laboratories)

tiludronic acid tablets

A tablet used to treat Paget's disease (a bone disorder).

Strengths available: 200 mg tablets.
Dose: adults, 400 mg once a day for 12 weeks. Course may be repeated after 6 months if needed.
Availability: NHS and private prescription.
Contains: tiludronic acid.
Brand names: Skelid.

 stomach upset, weakness, dizziness, skin disorders, headache.

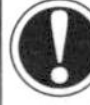 in patients suffering from kidney disorders. Vitamin D deficiency or low calcium levels should be corrected before starting treatment and adequate levels maintained in the diet.

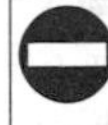 children, pregnant women, mothers who are breastfeeding, or for patients suffering from severe kidney disorders.

 indomethacin. Avoid food, ANTACIDS, and cal-cium (in diet or supplements) for 2 hours before and after the dose.

Timodine *see* topical corticosteroid cream and nystatin cream
(Reckitt and Colman Products)

timolol eye drops

An eye drop (available as standard and long-acting formulations) used as a BETA-BLOCKER to treat high pressure in the eye, and glaucoma. Some of the preparation may be absorbed into the body (*see* side-effects, cautions, etc. as for timolol tablets).

Strengths available: 0.25% and 0.5% standard eye drops; 0.25% and 0.5% long-acting eye drops.
Dose: adults, 1 drop of long-acting solution in the affected eye once a day or 1 drop of standard solution twice a day. Start with 0.25% strength and increase to 0.5% if needed.
Availability: NHS and private prescription.
Contains: timolol maleate.
Brand names: Glau-Opt, Timoptol.
Compound preparations: Cosopt.
Other preparations: timolol tablets.

 temporary discomfort or redness in the eye, dry eyes. Rarely, disorders of the cornea.

 in pregnant women, mothers who are breast-feeding, and in patients suffering from diabetes, overactive thyroid, or those being given a general anaesthetic.

 children or for patients using soft contact lenses, or those with a history of breathing disorders (e.g. asthma) or suffering from some heart diseases.

 verapamil, diltiazem, nifedipine, amiodarone.

T

timolol tablets

A tablet used as a BETA-BLOCKER to treat high blood pressure and angina. Also used after heart attack to prevent further attack, and to prevent migraine.

Strengths available: 10 mg tablets.
Dose: adults for high blood pressure, 5 mg twice a day or 10 mg once a day at first increasing to a maximum of 60 mg a day (in divided doses) if necessary; for angina, 5 mg 2-3 times a day at first increasing to a maximum of 45 mg a day; after heart attack, 5 mg twice a day increasing to 10 mg twice a day after 2 days; to prevent migraine 10-20 mg once a day.
Availability: NHS and private prescription.
contains: timolol maleate.
Brand names: Betim.
Compound preparations: Moducren, Prestim.
Other preparations: timolol eye drops.

cold hands and feet, sleep disturbance, slow heart rate, tiredness, wheezing, heart failure, low blood pressure, stomach upset. Rarely, dry eyes, rash, worsening of psoriasis.

in pregnant women, mothers who are breast-feeding, the elderly, and in patients suffering from diabetes, kidney or liver disorders, MYASTHENIA GRAVIS, or with a history of allergies. May need to be withdrawn before surgery. Withdraw gradually.

children or for patients suffering from heart block or failure, asthma, PHAEOCHROMOCYTOMA, or with a history of breathing disorders.

general anaesthetics, CALCIUM-CHANNEL BLOCKERS, ALPHA-BLOCKERS, clonidine, ANTIHYPERTENSIVES, amiodarone, antidiabetics, thymoxamine, theophylline, aminophylline, propafenone.

Timonil Retard *see* carbamazepine modified-release tablets
(C.P. Pharmaceuticals)

Timoptol/Timoptol LA *see* timolol eye drops
(Merck Sharp and Dohme)

Timpron *see* naproxen tablets/enteric-coated tablets
(Berk Pharmaceuticals)

Tinaderm-M

(Schering-Plough)

A cream used as an antifungal treatment for fungal skin and nail infections.

Dose: apply 2-3 times a day (usually for 2-3 weeks).
Availability: NHS and private prescription.
Contains: tolnaftate, nystatin.

---

tinidazole tablets

A tablet used as an ANTIBIOTIC to treat and prevent infections, and for *H. PYLORI* ERADICATION.

Strengths available: 500 mg tablets.
Dose: adults, usually 500 mg twice a day for 5-6 days, or 2000 mg on first day followed by 1000 mg a day on subsequent days. To treat vaginal and mouth (gum) infections, 2000 mg once (as a single dose). To treat intestinal infections, adults usually 2000 mg once a day for 2-3 days (children given reduced doses according to body weight).
Availability: NHS and private prescription.
Contains: tinidazole.
Brand names: Fasigyn.

stomach upset, furred tongue, unpleasant taste, skin disorders, severe allergic reaction, liver disorders, muscle or joint pain, lack of co-ordination, dark-coloured urine, numbness in hands and feet, fits, blood changes, dizziness, drowsiness, headache.

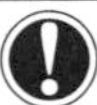

in pregnant women, mothers who are breastfeeding, and in patients with liver disease. Your doctor may advise regular check-ups if treatment exceeds 10 days. Alcohol causes extreme reaction with this medication and should not be taken during treatments or for 48 hours afterwards.

children (except for intestinal infections as above), women in the first 3 months of pregnancy, or for mothers who are breastfeeding.

alcohol, sedating drugs.

---

tioconazole nail solution

A solution used as an antifungal treatment for fungal nail infections.

Strengths available: 28% solution.
Dose: apply the solution to the nails and surrounding skin twice a day for up to 12 months.
Availability: NHS and private prescription.
Contains: tioconazole.
Brand names: Trosyl.

irritation.

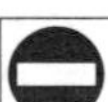

pregnant women.

Tisept *see* chlorhexidine solution
(SSL International)

---

titanium dioxide *see* Metanium

---

titanium peroxide *see* Metanium

---

titanium salicylate *see* Metanium

Titralac *see* calcium carbonate tablets
(3M Health Care)

---

tizanidine tablets

A tablet used to treat muscle spasm associated with multiple sclerosis, injury to the spinal cord, or other disease.

Strengths available: 2 mg tablets.
Dose: adults, 2 mg a day, increased to a maximum of 36 mg a day (in divided doses).
Availability: NHS and private prescription.
Contains: tizanidine hydrochloride.
Brand names: Zanaflex.

drowsiness, dizziness, dry mouth, upset stomach, tiredness, low blood pressure, hallucinations, sleeplessness, slow heart rate, liver disorders.

in pregnant women, mothers who are breast-feeding, and in patients suffering from kidney disorders. Your doctor may advise regular blood tests.

children, the elderly, or for patients suffering from severe liver disorders.

procainamide, quinidine, sedatives, alcohol, digoxin.

Tobi *see* tobramycin nebulizer solution
(PathoGenesis)

---

tobramycin nebulizer solution

A solution for inhalation used as an ANTIBIOTIC to manage infections in patients with cystic fibrosis.

Strengths available: 300 mg/5 ml solution.
Dose: adults and children over 6 years, 300 mg via nebulizer every 12 hours for 28 days, then course repeated after 28-day interval.
Availability: NHS and private prescription.
Contains: tobramycin.
Brand names: Tobi.

change in voice, cough, ear damage, kidney disorders. Rarely, low magnesium levels, inflamed bowel, stomach upset, rash.

in pregnant women, mothers who are breast-feeding, and in patients who are coughing up blood or suffering from muscular weakness, kidney or ear disorders. Your doctor will advise regular checks on your kidney and lung function.

children under 6 years or for patients suffering from MYASTHENIA GRAVIS.

ANTICOAGULANTS, cyclosporin, DIURETICS, neostigmine, pyridostigmine, some drugs used during surgery.

---

tocopheryl acetate *see* vitamin E tablets/suspension

Tofranil *see* imipramine tablets/syrup
(Novartis Pharmaceuticals UK)

tolbutamide tablets

A tablet used as an antidiabetic drug to treat diabetes.

Strengths available: 500 mg tablets.
Dose: adults, 500-2000 mg a day in divided doses.
Availability: NHS and private prescription.
Contains: tolbutamide.

allergy (including skin rash, fever, and jaundice), stomach upset, headache. Rarely, blood disorders.

in the elderly and in patients suffering from kidney or liver disorders.

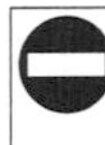
children, pregnant women, mothers who are breastfeeding, during surgery, or for patients suffering from juvenile diabetes, hormone disorders, stress, infections, PORPHYRIA, severe illness, or severe liver or kidney disorders.

ACE-INHIBITORS, alcohol, ANABOLIC STEROIDS, non-STEROIDAL ANTI-INFLAMMATORY DRUGS, some ANTIBIOTICS, ANTICOAGULANTS, MAOIS, fluconazole, miconazole, some tranquillizers, BETA-BLOCKERS, nifedipine, CORTICOSTEROIDS, DIURETICS, some drugs used to lower blood cholesterol or lipids, lithium, oral contraceptives, testosterone, cimetidine, sulfinpyrazone, ritonavir.

tolfenamic acid tablets

A tablet used as a NON-STEROIDAL ANTI-INFLAMMATORY DRUG to treat migraine attacks.

Strengths available: 200 mg tablets.
Dose: adults, 200 mg at start of attack, repeated once after 1-2 hours if needed.
Availability: NHS and private prescription.
Contains: tolfenamic acid.
Brand names: Clotam Rapid.

stomach upset and bleeding or ulceration, rash, severe allergy, difficulty breathing, blood or kidney disorders, discomfort when passing urine, headache, dizziness, noises in the ears, sensitivity to light, vertigo. Rarely, fluid retention, liver disorders, inflamed pancreas, inflamed bowel, meningitis.

ACE-INHIBITORS, aspirin or other non-steroidal anti-inflammatory drugs, some ANTIBIOTICS, ANTICOAGULANTS, some antidiabetic drugs, some antivirals, methotrexate, DIURETICS, lithium, tacrolimus, cyclosporin, digoxin.

in the elderly, pregnant women, mothers who are breastfeeding, and in patients with heart, liver, or kidney impairment, high blood pressure, asthma, LUPUS, or with a history of stomach ulcers.

children, women in the late stages of pregnancy, or for patients with a history of allergy to aspirin or other NSAID, liver or kidney disorders, blood clotting disorders, currently active stomach ulcer or intestinal bleeding, inflamed intestines, or severe heart failure. Suppositories not to be used for patients with inflammation of the anus or rectum.

T

tolnaftate *see* Tinaderm-M

tolterodine tablets

A tablet used as an ANTIMUSCARINIC treatment for unstable bladder and symptoms such as incontinence, urgent need to pass urine, or increased frequency of passing urine.

Strengths available: 1 mg and 2 mg tablets.
Dose: adults, 2 mg twice a day. (If side effects are a problem reduce to 1 mg twice a day.) Treatment reassessed after 6 months.
Availability: NHS and private prescription.
Contains: tolterodine tartrate.
Brand names: Detrusitol.

antimuscarinic effects, dry mouth, upset stomach, headache, dry skin and eyes, nervousness, drowsiness, blurred vision, confusion, difficulty passing urine, chest pain, pins and needles.

in patients suffering from blocked bladder outlet, hiatus hernia, blocked intestine, nerve disorders, liver or kidney disorders.

children, pregnant women, mothers who are breastfeeding, or for patients suffering from glaucoma, MYASTHENIA GRAVIS, difficulty passing urine, some bowel disorders.

other antimuscarinic drugs, sedatives, alcohol.

Topal *see* alginate tablets
(Ceuta Healthcare)

Topamax *see* topiramate tablets/capsules
(Janssen-Cilag)

topical corticosteroid cream/ointment/lotion/scalp application/ear ointment

A preparation used as a CORTICOSTEROID treatment to relieve symptoms of inflammatory conditions of the skin or scalp such as eczema.

Dose: apply thinly, usually once or twice a day (but check prescription label for individual products).
Availability: NHS and private prescription. (Simple hydrocortisone preparations are available over the counter for short-term treatment of allergic contact dermatitis, irritant dermatitis, insect bite reactions, and mild to moderate eczema only. Other restrictions also apply to over the counter sales.)

thinning, spotting, or streaking of the skin, worsening of untreated infections, acne, dermatitis around the mouth, contact dermatitis, and loss of pigment. Few side effects from mild to moderate preparations used short term. With longer-term treatment or potent preparations – fluid retention, suppression of ADRENAL GLANDS and general corticosteroid effects, *see* prednisolone tablets.

T

Contains: (*see* tables below).

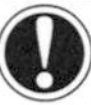 use for short periods of time only especially in children, on vulnerable parts of the body (such as thin areas of skin, raw surfaces, the face or skin folds), and in patients suffering from psoriasis.

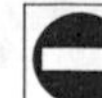 continuous use especially in pregnant women, or for patients suffering from leg ulcers, acne, dermatitis around the mouth, rosacea, scabies or any infected skin condition (unless also being treated). More potent products should not be used on children under 1 year old, on the face, or for patients with widespread psoriasis or acne.

Ingredient	*Brands*
alclometasone	**Modrasone** (Mo)
beclomethasone (beclometasone)	**Propaderm** (S)
betamethasone	**Betacap** (S), **Betnovate** (S), **Betnovate-RD** (Mo), **bettamousse** (S), **Diprosone** (S)
clobetasol	**Dermovate** (VS)
clobetasone butyrate	**Eumovate** (Mo)
desoxymethasone (desoximetasone)	**Stiedex LP** (Mo), **Steidex** (S)
diflucortolone	**Nerison** (S), **Nerisone Forte** (VS)
fluocinolone	**Synalar** (S), **Synalar 1 in 4** (Mo), **Synalar 1 in 10** (Mi)
fluocinonide	**Metosyn** (S)
fluocortolone	**Ultralanum Plain** (Mo)
flurandrenolone (fludroxycortide)	**Haelan*** (Mo)
fluticasone	**Cutivate** (S)
halcinonide	**Halciderm Topical** (S)
hydrocortisonc butyratc	**Locoid** (S), **Locoid Crelo** (S)
hydrocortisone	**Dioderm** (Mi), **Efcortelan** (Mi), **Mildison** (Mi)
mometasone	**Elocon** (S)

* *cream and ointment available on prescription, but tape restricted to use in hospitals.*

Strength indicated in brackets as follows:
Mi = mild Mo = moderate S = strong VS = very strong

Compound preparations: products with added antibiotic or antifungal ingredients are used to treat infected conditions, *see* table.

cont.

Brand	Corticosteroid ingredient	Other ingredients	Uses
Adcortyl with Graneodin (S)	triamcinolone	gramicidin, neomycin	inflamed skin with bacterial infection, infected insect bites
Alphaderm (Mo)	hydrocortisone	urea	eczema, inflamed skin
Alphosyl HC	hydrocortisone	coal tar, allantoin	psoriasis
Aureocort (S)	triamcinolone	chlortetracycline	inflamed and infected skin
Betnovate-C (S)	betamethasone	clioquinol	inflammatory conditions with suspected fungal or bacterial infection
Betnovate-N (S)	betamethasone	neomycin	inflammatory conditions with suspected bacterial infection
Calmurid HC (Mo)	hydrocortisone	urea, lactic acid	Dry eczema or inflammation
Canesten HC (Mi)	hydrocortisone	clotrimazole	inflamed skin with fungal infection
Daktacort (Mi)	hydrocortisone	miconazole	inflamed and infected skin
Dermovate-NN (VS)	clobetasol	neomycin, nystatin	inflammatory conditions with suspected infection
Diprosalic (S)	betamethasone	salicylic acid	Dry and flaky inflamed conditions
Econacort (Mi)	hydrocortisone	econazole	inflammation with fungal or bacterial infection
Eurax-Hydrocortisone (Mi)	hydrocortisone	crotamiton	eczema and itching skin conditions
Fucibet (S)	betamethasone	fusidic acid	eczema with bacterial infection
Fucidin H (Mi)	hydrocortisone	fusidic acid	eczema and dermatitis with bacterial infection
Gregoderm (Mi)	hydrocortisone	neomycin, polymyxin, nystatin	infected inflammatory conditions, psoriasis of scalp
Locoid-C (S)	hydrocortisone butyrate	chlorquinaldol	infected eczema, psoriasis, or inflamed skin
Lotriderm (S)	betamethasone	clotrimazole	fungal infections
Nystaform-HC (Mi)	hydrocortisone	nystatin, chlorhexidine	inflammation with fungal or bacterial infection

Brand	Corticosteroid ingredient	Other ingredients	Uses
Pevaryl TC (S)	triamcinolone	econazole	inflammation with fungal or bacterial infection
Quinocort (Mi)	hydrocortisone	potassium hydroxy-quinolone sulphate	infected inflammatory conditions
Synalar C (S)	fluocinolone	clioquinol	infected inflammatory conditions
Synalar N (S)	fluocinolone	neomycin	infected inflammatory conditions
Terra-Cortril (Mi)	hydrocortisone	oxytetracycline	weeping, infected eczema, infected dermatitis, insect bites.
Terra-Cortril Nystatin (Mi)	hydrocortisone	oxytetracycline, nystatin	infected inflammatory conditions
Timodine (Mi)	hydrocortisone	nystatin, benzalkonium chloride, dimethicone	inflammation or nappy rash with fungal infection
Tri-Adcortyl (S)	triamcinolone	gramicidin, neomycin	inflammation with bacterial or fungal infection
Trimovate (Mo)	clobetasone butyrate	oxytetracycline, nystatin	inflammation in moist skin areas where infection likely
Vioform-hydrocortisone (Mi)	hydrocortisone	clioquinol	Infected inflammation, infected skin in anal or genital areas

Strength indicated in brackets as follows:
Mi = mild Mo = moderate S = strong VS = very strong

Topicycline *see* tetracycline solution
(Shire Pharmaceuticals)

topiramate capsules/tablets

A tablet or capsule (which can be opened and the contents sprinkled on to food) used as an additional anti-epileptic treatment for epilepsy in patients not adequately controlled on other drugs.

Strengths available: 25 mg, 50 mg, 100 mg, and 200 mg tablets; 15 mg and

stomach upset, weight loss, loss of concentration and memory, confusion, mood changes, altered behaviour, speech disorders, unsteadiness, pins and needles, dizziness, tiredness, weakness, drowsiness, eye and taste disorders, aggression, mental disorders, blood disorders.

cont.

T

25 mg sprinkle capsules.

Dose: adults and children over 2 years, 25 mg at night at first, increasing to a maximum of 800 mg a day (in divided doses) for adults (lower maximum doses for children). Usual adult dose 100-200 mg twice a day.

Availability: NHS and private prescription.

Contains: topiramate.

Brand names: Topamax.

 in pregnant women and in patients suffering from liver or kidney disorders. Drink plenty of fluids. Withdraw treatment slowly.

 children under 2 years or mothers who are breastfeeding.

other anti-epileptic treatments, oral contraceptives, alcohol, sedating drugs.

Toradol *see* ketorolac tablets
(Roche Products)

torasemide tablets

A tablet used as a DIURETIC to treat fluid retention in the lungs or kidneys, and high blood pressure.

Strengths available: 2.5 mg, 5 mg, and 10 mg tablets.

Dose: adults for fluid retention, 5 mg each morning increasing to 40 mg if necessary; for high blood pressure, 2.5 mg each morning increasing to 5 mg if necessary.

Availability: NHS and private prescription.

Contains: torasemide.

Brand names: Torem.

 low blood potassium, magnesium, or sodium, stomach upset, rash, cramps, headache, blood changes, breast enlargement, gout, high blood sugar. Rarely, sensitivity to light.

 in patients suffering from kidney or liver damage, low levels of sodium or potassium, diabetes, gout, enlarged prostate, or impaired urination.

children, pregnant women, mothers who are breastfeeding, or for patients suffering from cirrhosis of the liver, low blood pressure, or kidney failure where urine production is absent.

 ANTIHYPERTENSIVES, NON-STEROIDAL ANTI-INFLAMMATORY DRUGS, drugs affecting heart rhythm, some ANTIBIOTICS, antidiabetics, halofantrine, pimozide, digoxin, lithium, theophylline, aminophylline.

Torem *see* torasemide tablets
(Roche Products)

tramadol capsules/modified-release capsules/modified-release tablets/sachets/soluble tablets

A capsule, M-R CAPSULE/TABLET, tablet, or powder (in a sachet) used as an OPIOID ANALGESIC to treat moderate to severe pain.

Strengths available: 50 mg capsules; 50 mg and 100 mg sachets; 50 mg soluble tablets; 50 mg, 100 mg, 150 mg, and 200 mg m-r capsules; 100 mg, 150 mg, and 200 mg twice-daily m-r tablets;

150 mg, 200 mg, 300 mg, and 400 mg once-daily m-r tablets.

Dose: adults using capsules, tablets, soluble tablets, or sachets, 50-100 mg up to four times a day (at least 4 hours between doses); using m-r capsules and twice-daily formulations of m-r tablets, 50-200 mg twice a day; using once-daily formulations of m-r tablets, up to 400 mg once a day.

Availability: NHS and private prescription.

Contains: tramadol hydrochloride.

Brand names: Tramake Insts (sachets), Zamadol, Zydol; Dromadol SR, Zamadol SR and Zydol SR (twice daily m-r products), Zydol XL (once daily m-r tablet).

drowsiness, upset stomach, sweating, dizziness, breathing difficulty, low or high blood pressure, difficulty passing urine, dry mouth, headache, vertigo, flushing, change in heart rhythm, mood changes, rash, itching, addiction, reduced sexual desire, severe allergic reaction, hallucinations, confusion.

in women in labour, elderly or weakened patients, and in those suffering from breathing, kidney, or liver problems, head injury, reduced breathing ability, low blood pressure, underactive thyroid, enlarged prostate or with a history of epilepsy or drug addiction. (Higher doses not suitable for some of these categories.)

MAOIS, antidepressants, alcohol, sedating drugs, ritonavir.

children, pregnant women, mothers who are breastfeeding, alcoholics, or for patients with PORPHYRIA or who are suicidal or at risk of non-functioning intestines.

Tramake *see* tramadol capsules/sachets
(Galen)

---

tramazoline *see* Dexa-Rhinaspray Duo

Trandate *see* labetolol tablets
(Medeva Pharma)

---

trandolapril capsules

A capsule used as an ACE-II ANTAGONIST to treat high blood pressure, and patients who are left with abnormal heart function after heart attack.

Strengths available: 0.5 mg, 1 mg, and 2 mg capsules.

Dose: adults, 0.5 mg once a day at first increasing to a maximum of 4 mg a day.

Availability: NHS and private prescription.

Contains: trandolapril.

rash, itching, sore throat, runny nose, stomach upset, cough, blood and liver changes, kidney disorders, low blood pressure, severe allergic reaction, inflamed pancreas. Occasionally, headache, dizziness, tiredness, taste disturbance, fever, pins and needles, muscle or joint pain, sensitivity to sunlight, inflamed membranes or blood vessels, rapid or abnormal heart rhythm, angina, bleeding in the brain, heart attack, reduced blood supply to the brain, bowel obstruction, skin reactions, dry mouth, weakness, hair loss, breathing disorders.

cont.

Brand names: Gopten, Odrik.
Compound preparations: Tarka.

children, pregnant women, mothers who are breastfeeding, or for patients with some heart abnormalities, disorders of the blood supply to the kidney. Not to be taken on the same day as dialysis.

in the elderly and in patients suffering from kidney disease, auto-immune diseases (such as LUPUS), severe heart failure, or with a history of severe allergies, or in patients undergoing anaesthesia or dialysis. Your doctor may advise regular blood tests.

DIURETICS, anaesthetics, NON-STEROIDAL ANTI-INFLAMMATORY DRUGS, potassium supplements, cyclosporin, lithium, antidiabetics.

---

tranexamic acid tablets

A tablet used as a blood-clotting agent to treat heavy periods and other heavy bleeding disorders.

Strengths available: 500 mg tablets.
Dose: adults, usually 1000-1500 mg 2-4 times a day (depending on condition).Treatment continued for 3-4 days to treat heavy periods. Children treated with reduced doses (according to body weight).
Availability: NHS and private prescription.
Contains: tranexamic acid.
Brand names: Cyklokapron.

stomach upset, disturbance of colour vision (stop taking the treatment if this occurs). Rarely, blood clots.

in pregnant women and in patients with kidney disorders or blood in the urine. Your doctor may advise regular eye and liver checks.

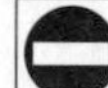
patients with a history of blood clots.

Tranquilyn *see* methylphenidate tablets
(Genus Pharmaceuticals)

Transiderm-Nitro *see* glyceryl trinitrate patches
(Novartis Pharmaceuticals UK)

Transvasin *see* analgesic (topical)
(SSL International)

Tranxene *see* potassium clorazepate capsules
(Boehringer Ingelheim)

---

tranylcypromine tablets

A tablet used as an MAOI to treat depression.

Strengths available: 10 mg tablets.
Dose: adults, 10 mg twice a day at first (the second dose taken no later than 3 p.m. in the afternoon) increasing if necessary to 20 mg for the second dose, then reducing to 10 mg once a day for maintenance.
Availability: NHS and private prescription.
Contains: tranylcypromine sulphate.
Brand names: Parnate.

Side effects: severe high blood pressure reactions with certain foods and medicines, sleeplessness, low blood pressure on standing, dizziness, drowsiness, weakness, dry mouth, constipation, stomach upset, blurred vision, difficulty passing urine, fluid retention, rash, weight gain, confusion, agitation, shaking, excitement, abnormal heart rhythm, sweating, fits, blood changes, psychiatric disorders, pins and needles, nerve inflammation, sexual disturbances, headache, abnormal muscle or eye movements, liver disorders.

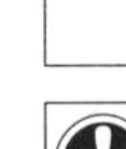

Caution: in pregnant women, mothers who are breast-feeding, the elderly, and in patients suffering from diabetes, epilepsy, heart or circulatory disorders, blood disorders, agitation, POR-PHYRIA, or those currently undergoing electroconvulsive therapy or surgery. Treatment should be withdrawn gradually.

Not to be used for: children or for patients suffering from liver disease, PHAEOCHROMOCYTOMA, or those who are currently excitable or who have disorders of the blood supply to the brain.

Caution needed with: alcohol, apraclonidine, brimonidine, pethidine and other OPIOIDS, SYMPATHOMIMETICS, other anti-depressants, antidiabetics, anti-epileptic treatments, drugs used to lower blood pressure, oxypertine, clozapine, buspirone, levodopa, selegiline, entacapone, some drugs used to treat migraine, tetrabenazine, sedatives. The following foods should be avoided (until 14 days after treatment ends): cheese, meat extracts, broad beans, banana, Marmite, yeast extracts, wine, beer, other alcohol, pickled herrings, vegetable proteins.

Trasicor *see* oxprenolol tablets
(Sovereign Medical)

Trasidrex *see* co-prenozide tablets
(Goldshield Healthcare)

Travasept *see* chlorhexidine solution
(Baxter Healthcare)

Traxam *see* non-steroidal anti-inflammatory drug (topical)
(Wyeth Laboratories)

T

trazodone tablets/modified-release tablets/capsules/liquid

A tablet, M-R TABLET, capsule, or liquid used as an antidepressant to treat depression.

Strengths available: 50 mg and 100 mg capsules; 150 mg tablets; 50 mg/5 ml liquid; 150 mg m-r tablets.
Dose: adults, 150 mg a day (as one dose at night, or divided through the day), increasing if necessary to 300 mg a day (or up to 600 mg in hospital patients); elderly patients start with 100 mg a day.
Availability: NHS and private prescription.
Contains: trazodone hydrochloride.
Brand names: Molipaxin.

children, women in the first 3 months of pregnancy, or for patients suffering from recent heart attacks, heart rhythm abnormalities, severe liver disease or elevated mood.

alcohol, sedatives, MAOIS, other antidepressants, anti-epileptic drugs, digoxin.

dry mouth, noises in the ears, tiredness, constipation, difficulty passing urine, blurred vision, stomach upset, palpitations, drowsiness, sleeplessness, dizziness, shaking hands, low blood pressure, weight change, sweating, fever, behavioural changes in children, confusion in the elderly, skin reactions, jaundice or blood changes, interference with sexual function, changes in heart rhythm, rash, hormone disturbances, fits, movement disorders, blood changes, breast changes in women, menstrual disorders.

in the elderly, pregnant women, mothers who are breastfeeding, and in patients suffering from heart disease, liver and kidney disorders, thyroid disease, PHAEOCHROMOCYTOMA, epilepsy, diabetes, PORPHYRIA, glaucoma, urine retention, constipation, some other psychiatric conditions. Your doctor may advise regular blood tests.

Trental *see* oxpentifylline modified-release tablets (Borg Medicare)

---

tretinoin cream/gel/lotion

A cream, gel, or lotion used as a vitamin A derivative to treat acne and skin disorders caused by excessive exposure to sunlight (pigmentation, roughness, and fine wrinkling).

Strengths available: 0.025% and 0.05% cream; 0.01% and 0.025% gel; 0.025% lotion.
Dose: adults, for acne apply a 0.01% or 0.025% preparation thinly once or twice a day for at least 6-8 weeks (gel recommended for oily or dark skin, cream for dry or fair skin, and lotion for large areas such as the back); for sun damage, apply the

irritation, reddening or dryness of skin, itching, crusting or peeling, increased sensitivity to sunlight, temporary change in skin colour, severe acne, swollen or irritated eyes.

on sensitive areas of skin and the angles of the nose. Women of childbearing age must use adequate contraception.

children, pregnant women, mothers who are breastfeeding, or for patients with a family history of skin cancer. Not for application to mouth, eyes, mucous membranes, damaged or sunburned skin, areas of eczema. Avoid exposure to sunlight and do not use sunlamps/sunbeds.

0.05% cream thinly at night, reducing to 1-3 times a week.

Availability: private prescription. All except the 0.05% cream also available on NHS.

Contains: tretinoin.

Brand names: Acticin, Retin-A, Retinova (0.05% – not available on NHS).

Compound preparations: Aknemycin Plus.

products that cause the skin to peel (e.g. benzoyl peroxide and some cosmetic products) or which might cause irritation.

Tri-Adcortyl *see* topical corticosteroid cream/ointment/ear ointment, neomycin cream and nystatin ointment
(Bristol-Myers Squibb Pharmaceuticals)

Triadene *see* oral contraceptive (combined)
(Schering Health Care)

TriamaxCo *see* co-triamterzide
(Ashbourne Pharmaceuticals)

---

triamcinolone *see* Adcortyl with Graneodin, Audicort, Aureocort, corticosteroid nasal spray, Tri-Adcortyl, triamcinolone dental paste/intra-articular injection

---

triamcinolone dental paste

A paste used as a CORTICOSTEROID treatment for mouth ulcers, inflamed gums, and other mouth inflammation.

Strengths available: 0.1% paste.

Dose: apply a thin layer of paste to the affected area 2-4 times a day. Do not rub in. Treat children for 5 days only. Short courses also recommended in the elderly.

Availability: NHS and private prescription. (Also available over the counter for treatment of mouth ulcers.)

Contains: triamcinolone acetonide.

Brand names: Adcortyl in Orabase.

may make infections worse. Long-term use (or covering the paste with dentures) may result in general corticosteroid effects, *see* prednisolone tablets.

in children and pregnant women.

patients with untreated mouth infection.

---

triamcinolone injection

An injection used as a CORTICOSTEROID to treat joint pain and swelling due to conditions such as arthritis, and to treat allergic states such as hayfever, and other disorders requiring corticosteroid treatment.

Strengths available: 20 mg/1ml injection, in 1ml, 2 ml, or 5 ml quantities; also 25 mg/5 ml injection.
Dose: as advised by doctor.
Availability: NHS and private prescription.
Contains: triamcinolone acetonide or triamcinolone hexacetonide.
Brand names: Adcortyl, Kenalog, Lederspan.

in pregnant women, mothers who are breast-feeding, and in patients who have had recent bowel surgery or who are suffering from inflamed veins, psychiatric disorders, thinning of the bones, stomach ulcers, tuberculosis or other infections, high blood pressure, glaucoma, epilepsy, diabetes, underactive thyroid, liver disease, stress. Withdraw gradually. Avoid contact with chicken pox for 3 months after treatment ends and seek medical attention if exposed.

high blood sugar, thin bones, mood changes, stomach ulcers, fluid retention, potassium loss, high blood pressure, menstrual irregularity, hairiness, increased likelihood of infection, euphoria, depression, sleeplessness, aggravation of schizophrenia and epilepsy, eye disorders, thinning of skin, acne, bruising, blood changes, stomach upset, inflamed pancreas, muscle abnormality, suppression of the ADRENAL GLANDS, ulcerated or infected oesophagus, general feeling of being unwell, hiccups, reduced growth in children.

children under 6 years or for patients who have untreated infections.

live vaccines, some ANTIBIOTICS and anti-epileptics, ANTICOAGULANTS, antidiabetics, some antifungals, digoxin, cyclosporin.

Triam-Co *see* co-triamterzide
(Baker Norton Pharmaceuticals)

---

triamterene capsules

A capsule used as a potassium-sparing DIURETIC to treat fluid retention (especially when due to heart failure, kidney or liver disease) or with other diuretics to prevent potassium depletion.

Strengths available: 50 mg capsules.
Dose: adults, 150-250 mg a day at first reducing to alternate days for maintenance. The daily dose is divided into two and taken at breakfast and lunch. (Lower dose at breakfast if given with other diuretics.)
Availability: NHS and private prescription.
Contains: triamterene.
Brand names: Dytac.

stomach upset, rash, dry mouth, confusion, low blood pressure on standing, high potassium or low sodium levels in the blood, sensitivity to sunlight, blood disorders. May cause blue colour in urine. Rarely, kidney failure.

in pregnant women, mothers who are breast-feeding, elderly patients, diabetics, and in patients with gout, liver or kidney disease. Your doctor may advise blood tests for potassium levels.

children or for patients suffering from high potassium levels, Addison's disease, or kidney failure.

Compound preparations: co-triamterzide tablets, Dytide, Frusene, Kalspare.

potassium supplements, other potassium-sparing diuretics, ACE-INHIBITORS, NON-STEROIDAL ANTI-INFLAMMATORY DRUGS, carbamazepine, ANTI-HYPERTENSIVES, cyclosporin, lithium.

Triapin/Triapin Mite *see* felodipine tablets and ramipril capsules (Hoechst Marion Roussel)

---

triclofos oral solution

A solution used as a sedative for the short-term treatment of sleeplessness.

Strengths available: 500 mg/5 ml solution.
Dose: adults, 1000-2000 mg (10-20 ml) at bedtime; children use up to 1000 mg (10 ml) according to age.
Availability: NHS and private prescription.
Contains: triclofos sodium.

stomach upset, wind, rash, urine changes, headache, excitement, addiction, confusion in the elderly, vertigo, lack of co-ordination, general feeling of being unwell, blood changes.

in the elderly and in patients with general debility or a history of drug/alcohol addiction, or suffering from respiratory disease or some psychiatric disorders. Withdraw slowly and avoid contact with the skin.

pregnant women, mothers who are breast-feeding, or for patients suffering from heart disease, stomach inflammation, liver or kidney disorders, or PORPHYRIA.

alcohol, other sedatives, WARFARIN.

---

triclosan *see* emollient preparations, triclosan liquid

---

triclosan liquid

A liquid used as a disinfectant to cleanse and disinfect the skin.

Strengths available: 2% skin cleanser, 0.5% hand rub, 2% bath concentrate.
Dose: used as needed.
Availability: NHS and private prescription, over the counter.
Contains: triclosan.
Brand names: Aquasept, Ster-Zac Bath Concentrate.
Compound preparations: Manusept (with isopropyl alcohol), Oilatum Plus (see emollient).

keep out of the eyes.

---

tricyclic antidepressant

A drug used to treat depression but which may cause sedation and dry mouth. Example, amitriptyline tablets.

Tridestra *see* hormone replacement therapy (combined)
(Orion Pharma (UK))

trientine capsules

A capsule used as an alternative to penicillamine in Wilson's disease.

Strengths available: 300 mg capsules.
Dose: 1200-2400 mg a day in 2-4 divided doses before food.
Availability: NHS and private prescription.
Contains: trientine dihydrochloride.

nausea.

in pregnant women.

iron preparations.

trifluoperazine tablets, modified-release capsules/solution/syrup

A tablet, M-R CAPSULE, solution, or syrup used as a sedative to treat nausea, vomiting, severe anxiety (and associated symptoms), agitation, schizophrenia, and other mental disorders.

Strengths available: 1 mg and 5 mg tablets; 5 mg/5 ml solution; 1 mg/5 ml syrup; 2 mg, 10 mg, and 15 mg m-r capsules.
Dose: for anxiety, adults usually 2-4 mg a day (maximum 6 mg a day), children over 3 years 1-4 mg a day according to age; for schizophrenia and other mental disorders, adults 10 mg (children up to 5 mg) a day at first then adjusted according to response; for nausea and vomiting, adults 2-6 mg a day, children up to 4 mg a day according to age. Doses are usually divided throughout the day but 10 mg and 15 mg m-r capsules may be used as once-daily doses.
Availability: NHS and private prescription.
Contains: trifluoperazine hydrochloride.
Brand names: Stelazine.

movement disorders, muscle spasms, restlessness, shaking, dry mouth, heart rhythm disturbance, low blood pressure, weight gain, blurred vision, impotence, low body temperature, breast swelling, menstrual changes, blood, liver, eye, and skin changes, drowsiness, apathy, nightmares, sleeplessness, depression, blocked nose, difficulty passing water. Rarely, fits.

in pregnant women, mothers who are breast-feeding, the elderly, and in patients suffering from heart, lung, or circulation disorders, epilepsy, Parkinson's disease, thyroid disorders, infections, MYASTHENIA GRAVIS, kidney or liver disease, glaucoma, or enlarged prostate. Should be withdrawn gradually.

unconscious patients or for patients suffering from bone marrow depression, blood disorders, severe kidney or liver impairment, uncontrolled heart failure, or PHAEOCHROMOCYTOMA.

alcohol, sedatives, antidepressants, some antidiabetic drugs, anaesthetics, anti-epileptic medications, drugs affecting heart rhythm, ritonavir, halofantrine, sotalol, propranolol, lithium.

Trifyba
(Sanofi Winthrop)

A powder used as a bulking agent to treat constipation, diverticular disease, irritable bowel, piles, and fissures.

Strengths available: 80% powder in 3.5 g sachets.
Dose: adults, 1 sachet 2-3 times a day; children half to one sachet once or twice a day according to age and size. Powder should be mixed with food or liquid.
Availability: NHS and private prescription, over the counter.
Contains: wheat fibre (bran).

 wind, bloating, obstructed intestines.

 in elderly, weak, or diabetic patients, and in those with narrowed or poorly functioning intestines. Drink plenty of fluids.

children (except for intestinal conditions) or for patients with blocked intestines, difficulty swallowing, relaxed bowel, or who are unable to tolerate gluten in the diet (e.g. coeliac disease).

---

trihexyphenidyl *see* benzhexol (alternative name)

Trileptal *see* oxcarbazepine tablets
(Novartis Pharmaceuticals UK)

---

trilostane capsules
A capsule used as an ADRENAL inhibitor when the adrenal glands are overactive.

Strengths available: 60 mg and 120 mg capsules.
Dose: adults, 60 mg four times a day for the first 3 days then adjust as needed up to a maximum of 960 mg a day.
Availability: NHS and private prescription.
Contains: trilostane.
Brand names: Modrenal.

 flushing, upset stomach, running nose, tingling and swollen mouth, rash, blood disorders.

 in patients suffering from kidney or liver disorders, stress, or breast cancer. Your doctor may wish to confirm there is no tumour of the adrenal glands before starting treatment. Women should use non-hormonal methods of contraception.

 children, pregnant women, mothers who are breastfeeding, or for patients who have severe kidney or liver disorders.

 some DIURETICS, potassium.

---

trimeprazine tablets/syrup
A tablet or syrup used as an ANTIHISTAMINE treatment for itching and allergies.

Strengths available: 10 mg tablets; 7.5 mg/5 ml and 30 mg/5 ml syrup.
Dose: adults, 10 mg 2-3 times a day (or up to 100 mg a day in severe cases); elderly patients *cont.*

10 mg once or twice a day; children over 2 years 2.5-5 mg 3-4 times a day according to age.
Availability: NHS and private prescription.
Contains: trimeprazine (alimemazine) tartrate.
Brand names: Vallergan.

 children under 2 years, pregnant women, mothers who are breastfeeding, unconscious patients, or for patients suffering from epilepsy, underactive thyroid, glaucoma, Parkinson's disease, MYASTHENIA GRAVIS, kidney or liver disease, enlarged prostate, bone marrow depression, or PHAEOCHROMOCYTOMA.

 alcohol, sedatives, antidepressants, some antidiabetic drugs, antimuscarinics, drugs used to lower blood pressure.

 movement disorders, muscle spasms, restlessness, shaking, dry mouth, heart rhythm disturbance, low blood pressure, weight gain, blurred vision, impotence, low body temperature, breast swelling, menstrual changes, blood, liver, eye, and skin changes, drowsiness, reduced reactions, dizziness, excitation, apathy, nightmares, sleep disturbances, depression, blocked nose, difficulty passing water, headache, ANTIMUSCARINIC effects. Rarely, fits, severe allergic reaction, noises in the ears, sensitivity to sunlight, confusion, depression, sweating, muscle pain, pins and needles, hair loss, NEUROLEPTIC MALIGNANT SYNDROME.

 in the elderly and in patients suffering from heart, lung, or circulation disorders, infections, difficulty passing urine, or some blood disorders. Should be withdrawn gradually.

---

trimethoprim *see* co-trimoxazole, Polytrim, trimethoprim

---

trimethoprim tablets/suspension

A tablet or suspension used as an ANTIBIOTIC to treat and prevent infections such as bronchitis or urine infections.

Strengths available: 100 mg and 200 mg tablets; 50 mg/5 ml suspension.
Dose: adults, 200 mg twice a day, children aged 6 weeks-5 months 25 mg (aged 6 months-5 years 50 mg, aged 6-12 years 100 mg) twice a day. For long-term prevention of infection adults 100 mg at night (children use reduced dose according to body weight).
Availability: NHS and private prescription.
Contains: trimethoprim.
Brand names: Monotrim, Trimopan.
Compound preparations: co-trimoxazole tablets/suspension.

 stomach upset, skin reactions, itching, blood changes. Rarely, meningitis.

 in young babies, women who are breastfeeding, and in patients suffering from kidney disease, folate deficiency (vitamin deficiency), PORPHYRIA. Your doctor may advise regular blood tests.

 infants under 6 weeks, pregnant women, or for patients suffering from severe kidney disorders or blood disorders.

 ANTICOAGULANTS, pyrimethamine, cyclosporin, azathioprine, methotrexate, digoxin.

Tri-Minulet *see* oral contraceptive (combined) (Wyeth Laboratories)

---

trimipramine tablets/capsules

A tablet or capsule used as a TRICYCLIC ANTIDEPRESSANT to treat depression and associated symptoms.

Strengths available: 10 mg and 25 mg tablets; 50 mg capsules.
Dose: adults 50-75 mg once a day (2 hours before bedtime) increasing to a maximum of 300 mg a day; elderly patients 10-25 mg three times a day at first.
Availability: NHS and private prescription.
Contains: trimipramine maleate.
Brand names: Surmontil.

dry mouth, noises in the ears, tiredness, constipation, difficulty passing urine, blurred vision, stomach upset, palpitations, drowsiness, sleeplessness, dizziness, shaking hands, low blood pressure, weight change, sweating, fever, behavioural changes in children, confusion in the elderly, skin reactions, jaundice or blood changes, interference with sexual function, changes in heart rhythm, rash, hormone disturbances, fits, movement disorders, blood changes, breast changes in women, menstrual disorders.

in the elderly, pregnant women, mothers who are breastfeeding, and in patients suffering from heart disease, liver and kidney disorders, thyroid disease, PHAEOCHROMOCYTOMA, epilepsy, diabetes, PORPHYRIA, glaucoma, urine retention, constipation, some other psychiatric conditions. Your doctor may advise regular blood tests.

children or for patients suffering from recent heart attacks, heart rhythm abnormalities, severe liver disease or elevated mood.

alcohol, sedatives, MAOIS, BARBITURATES, other antidepressants, ANTIHYPERTENSIVES, tranquillizers, anti-epileptic drugs, ritonavir, entacapone, selegiline, sotalol, halofantrine, drugs affecting heart rhythm, methylphenidate.

Trimopan *see* trimethoprim tablets/suspension (Berk Pharmaceuticals)

Trimovate *see* topical corticosteroid cream and nystatin ointment (GlaxoWellcome UK)

Trinordiol *see* oral contraceptive (combined) (Wyeth Laboratories)

TriNovum *see* oral contraceptive (combined) (Janssen-Cilag)

---

tripotassium dicitratobismuthate tablets

A tablet used as a cell surface protector to treat stomach ulcers.

Strengths available: 120 mg tablets.

cont.

T

Dose: adults, 2 tablets twice a day or 1 tablet four times a day before meals. Treatment continued for 1-2 months then leave at least 1 month before repeating.
Availability: NHS and private prescription, over the counter.
Contains: tripotassium dicitratobismuthate.
Brand names: De-Noltab.

black colour to tongue and stools, stomach upset.

children, pregnant women, or for patients with kidney disorders.

some ANTIBIOTICS.

---

triprolidine *see* Sudafed Plus

Triptafen/Triptafen M *see* amitriptyline tablets and perphenazine tablets
(Forley)
A mixed formulation used to treat depression with anxiety.

Strengths available: 25 mg + 2 mg and 10 mg + 2 mg tablets.
Dose: adults 1 tablets 3-4 times a day.

Trisequens/Trisequens Forte *see* hormone replacement therapy (combined)
(Novo Nordisk Pharmaceuticals)

Tritace *see* ramipril capsules
(Hoechst Marion Roussel)

Tropergen *see* co-phenotrope tablets
(Goldshield Healthcare)

Tropiovent Steripoules *see* ipratropium nebulizer solution
(Ashbourne Pharmaceuticals)

---

tropisetron capsules
A capsule used to prevent nausea and vomiting caused by chemotherapy treatment.

Strengths available: 5 mg capsules.
Dose: adults and children over 5 years, 5 mg each morning before food for 5 days.
Availability: NHS and private prescription.

upset stomach, headache, dizziness, tiredness, abdominal pain, flushed face, tight chest, difficulty breathing, low blood pressure, collapse, fainting, slow heart rate.

in patients suffering from heart conduction disorders, uncontrolled high blood pressure, or abnormal heart rhythm.

Contains: tropisetron hydrochloride.
Brand names: Navoban.

Not to be used for: children under 5 years, pregnant women, mothers who are breastfeeding.

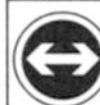

Caution needed with: drugs that affect the heart rhythm or the liver, BETA-BLOCKERS.

Tropium *see* chlordiazepoxide tablets/capsules
(DDSA Pharmaceuticals)

---

trospium tablets

A tablet used as an ANTIMUSCARINIC to treat bladder disorders that cause urgency or frequency of passing urine, or incontinence.

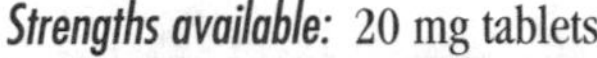

Strengths available: 20 mg tablets.
Dose: adults, 20 mg twice a day on an empty stomach.
Availability: NHS and private prescription.
Contains: trospium chloride.
Brand names: Regurin.

Side effects: antimuscarinic effects, dry mouth, upset stomach. Rarely, disorders of passing urine, disturbed vision, weakness, rash, chest pain, rapid heart rate, severe allergic reaction.

Caution: in pregnant women, mothers who are breast-feeding, and in patients suffering from blocked intestines, kidney disorders, hiatus hernia and reflux oesophagitis, overactive thyroid, heart failure, narrowed blood vessels in the heart, obstructed outflow from the bladder, some nerve disorders, or coeliac disease.

Not to be used for: children under 12 years or for patients suffering from liver disorders, difficulty passing urine, glaucoma, some heart rhythm abnormalities, kidney failure needing dialysis, MYASTHENIA GRAVIS, swollen or ulcerated intestines.

Caution needed with: other antimuscarinic drugs, TRICYCLIC ANTI-DEPRESSANTS, amantadine, quinidine, ANTIHISTAMINES, disopyramide, BRONCHODILATORS, colestipol, cholestyramine.

Trosyl *see* tioconazole nail solution
(Pfizer)

Trusopt *see* dorzolamide eye drops
(Merck Sharp and Dohme)

---

tryptophan tablets

A tablet used (in addition to other drugs) as an antidepressant to treat severe and disabling depression when other treatments have failed.

Strengths available: 500 mg tablets.
Dose: adults, 1000 mg three times a day (maximum of 6000 mg a day); elderly patients may require lower doses.
Availability: NHS and private prescription (specialist use only).

Side effects: drowsiness, nausea, light-headedness, headache, blood changes, muscle disorders.

cont.

Contains: tryptophan.
Brand names: Optimax.

 in pregnant women and mothers who are breastfeeding. Your doctor will advise regular check-ups.

 children or for patients who have previously developed muscle or blood disorders after treatment with this drug.

 alcohol, sedating drugs, other antidepressants.

---

tuberculosis vaccine (BCG)

An injection used to provide active immunity to tuberculosis. (Vaccination is carried out usually only after using a diagnostic test to determine suitability.)

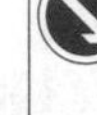 swollen glands, rash, fever, irritation and reddening at the injection site. Within 2-6 weeks a small swelling appears at the injection site and may progress to an ulcer that usually heals within 6-12 weeks.

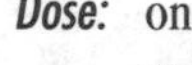

Dose: one dose only (babies under 3 months given half dose).
Availability: NHS and private prescription.
Contains: live *Mycobacterium bovis*.

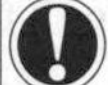 in pregnant women and in patients suffering from eczema.

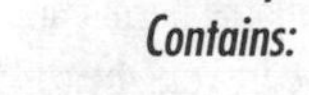

 patients suffering from feverish illness, HIV infection, infected skin conditions, or who have a poorly functioning immune system.

live vaccines, CORTICOSTEROIDS, drugs that suppress immunity, treatments for tuberculosis.

Tuinal *see* quinalbarbitone capsules and amylobarbitone capsules
(Flynn Pharma)

Strengths available: 50 mg + 50 mg capsules.
Dose: 1-2 at bedtime.

Twinrix *see* hepatitis A vaccine and hepatitis B vaccine
(SmithKline Beecham Pharmaceuticals)
A combined vaccine.

Dose: three doses (the second given 1 month after the first, and the third given 5 months after that). Children given half adult dose.

Tylex *see* co-codamol capsules/effervescent tablets
(Schwartz Pharma)

Typherix *see* typhoid vaccine
(SmithKline Beecham Pharmaceuticals)

Typhim Vi *see* typhoid vaccine
(Aventis Pasteur MSD)

typhoid vaccine (injectable)

A killed vaccine used to provide active immunization against typhoid.

Dose: 2 injections at 4-6 week intervals; children 1-10 years given half adult dose. Booster needed after 3 years.
Availability: NHS and private prescription.
Contains: killed *Salmonella typhi* vaccine.
Brand names: Typherix, Typhim Vi.
Compound preparations: Hepatyrix.
Other preparations: typhoid vaccine (oral).

 influenza-like symptoms of headache, fever, and general feeling of being unwell, irritation and swelling at injection site.

 in pregnant women and mothers who are breastfeeding.

 children under 1 year or for patients suffering from feverish illness or who have a poorly functioning immune system.

 drugs that affect immunity.

typhoid vaccine (oral)

A live vaccine enclosed in an E-C CAPSULE used to provide active immunization against typhoid.

Dose: adults and children over 6 years, 1 capsule on days 1, 3, and 5. Swallow the capsule with a cold drink 1 hour before a meal. Repeat the course after 1 year if continued protection required.
Availability: NHS and private prescription.
Contains: live *Salmonella typhi* vaccine.
Brand names: Vivotif.
Compound preparations: Hepatyrix.
Other preparations: typhoid vaccine (injectable).

 influenza-like symptoms of headache, stomach upset, fever, and general feeling of being unwell, irritation and swelling at injection site, severe allergic reaction.

 in pregnant women and mothers who are breastfeeding.

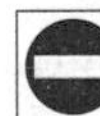 children under 6 years or for patients suffering from feverish illness, HIV infection, stomach disorder, or who have a poorly functioning immune system.

 drugs that affect immunity, ANTIBIOTICS, mefloquine, oral poliomyelitis vaccine, drugs used to treat cancer, ANTACIDS.

Ubretid *see* distigmine tablets
(Rhône-Poulenc Rorer)

Ucerax *see* hydroxyzine tablets/syrup
(UCB Pharma)

Ultec *see* cimetidine tablets
(Berk Pharmaceuticals)

Ultrabase *see* emollient cream
(Schering Health Care)

Ultralanum *see* topical corticosteroid cream/ointment
(Schering Health Care)

Ultraproct *see* rectal corticosteroid ointment/suppositories
(Schering Health Care)

Ultratard *see* insulin

---

undecenoic acid *see* Ceanel

Unguentum M *see* emollient cream
(Crookes Healthcare)

Unifine *see* insulin injection devices
(Owen Mumford)

Unilet GP SuperLite Lancets

(Owen Mumford)
Diabetics who need to test their blood regularly can use lancets to pierce the skin, either with or without the use of a finger-pricking device.

Lancet width and length: 21G/0.81 mm (Type A).
Availability: NHS and private prescription, over the counter.
Compatible finger-pricking devices: Autolet Lite Clinisafe, Autolet Mini, Hypolance, Penlet II Plus, Soft Touch.

Unilet G SuperLite Lancets

(Owen Mumford)
Diabetics who need to test their blood regularly can use lancets to pierce the skin, either with or without the use of a finger-pricking device.

Lancet width and length: 23G/0.66 mm (Type A).

Availability: NHS and private prescription, over the counter.
Compatible finger-pricking devices: Autoclix, Autolet Mini Hypolance, Penlet II Plus, Soft Touch.

Unilet SuperLite Lancets

(Owen Mumford)
Diabetics who need to test their blood regularly can use lancets to pierce the skin, either with or without the use of a finger-pricking device.

Lancet width and length: 23G/0.66 mm (Type B).
Availability: NHS and private prescription, over the counter.
Compatible finger-pricking devices: Autolet II, Autolet Lite, Autolet Lite Clinisafe, Glucolet.

Unilet Universal ComforTouch Lancets

(Owen Mumford)
Diabetics who need to test their blood regularly can use lancets to pierce the skin, either with or without the use of a finger-pricking device.

Lancet width and length: 26G/0.45 mm (Type A/B).
Availability: NHS and private prescription, over the counter.
Compatible finger-pricking devices: Autolet II, Autolet Lite, Autolet Lite Clinisafe, Autolet Mini, Glucolet, Hypolance, Microlet, Penlet II Plus, Soft Touch.

Uniphyllin Continus *see* theophylline modified-release tablets
(Napp Pharmaceuticals)

Uniroid HC *see* rectal corticosteroid ointment/suppositories
(Unigreg)

Unisept *see* chlorhexidine solution
(SSL International)

Unitulle *see* paraffin gauze dressing
(Hoechst Marion Roussel)

Univer *see* verapamil modified-release capsules
(Elan Pharma)

Urantoin *see* nitrofurantoin tablets
(DDSA Pharmaceuticals)

Urdox *see* ursodeoxycholic acid tablets
(C.P. Pharmaceuticals)

---

urea cream/lotion

A cream used as an EMOLLIENT to treat chronic dry skin condition, scaly and itchy skin.

Strengths available: 10% cream.
Dose: apply thinly and rub into affected area twice a day.
Availability: NHS and private prescription, over the counter.
Contains: urea.
Brand names: Aquadrate, Eucerin, Nutraplus.
Compound preparations: Alphaderm and Calmurid-HC (*see* topical corticosteroid cream), Calmurid (with lactic acid), emollient preparations.

---

urea hydrogen peroxide *see* Exterol

Uriben *see* nalidixic acid suspension
(Rosemont Pharmaceuticals)

Urispas *see* flavoxate tablets
(Shire Pharmaceuticals)

---

urofollitrophin injection

An injection used to treat infertility through failure of ovulation in women, and to stimulate the ovaries for *in vitro* fertilization treatment.

Strengths available: 75 unit and 150 unit injections.
Dose: as advised by doctor.
Availability: NHS and private prescription.
Contains: follicle stimulating hormone.
Brand names: Metrodin High Purity.
Compound preparations: human menopausal gonadotrophin injection.

skin reaction around injection site, overstimulation of ovaries, multiple pregnancies.

in patients with ADRENAL or thyroid disorders, or high levels of prolactin (a hormone) in the blood. Hormone or brain disorders must be treated before using this drug.

children, pregnant women, mothers who are breastfeeding, or for patients with some brain, ovary, uterus, or breast cancers, ovarian cysts, or undiagnosed vaginal bleeding.

---

urofollitropin *see* urofollitrophin (alternative name)

ursodeoxycholic acid tablets/capsules/suspension

A tablet, capsule, or suspension used as a bile acid to dissolve gallstones and to treat degeneration of the bile ducts.

Strengths available: 150 mg and 300 mg tablets; 250 mg capsules; 250 mg/5 ml suspension.
Dose: as advised by doctor (depends on body weight).
Availability: NHS and private prescription.
Contains: ursodeoxycholic acid.
Brand names: Destolit, Urdox, Ursofalk, Ursogal.

 some lipid-lowering drugs, oral contraceptives.

 upset stomach, itching, hardening of the stones (so that they cannot be dissolved).

 women must use non-hormonal methods of contraception.

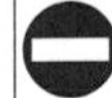 pregnant women, mothers who are breast-feeding, women not using adequate contraception, or for patients with liver disease, non-functioning gall bladder, stomach ulcers, inflammatory bowel conditions.

Ursofalk *see* ursodeoxycholic acid capsules/suspension
(Provalis Healthcare)

Ursogal *see* ursodeoxycholic acid tablets/capsules
(Galen)

Utinor *see* norfloxacin tablets
(Merck Sharp and Dohme)

Utovlan *see* norethisterone tablets
(Searle)

Vagifem *see* hormone replacement therapy (oestrogen-only)
(Novo Nordisk Pharmaceuticals)

---

valaciclovir tablets

A tablet used as an antiviral to treat shingles, and to treat and suppress herpes infections of the skin and mucous membranes such as genital herpes.

Strengths available: 500 mg tablets.
Dose: for shingles, 1000 mg three times a day for 7 days; for other herpes infections, 500 mg twice a day for

 upset stomach, headache, rash, dizziness, drowsiness, confusion, hallucinations.

 in pregnant women, mothers who are breast-feeding, and in patients suffering from kidney disorders.

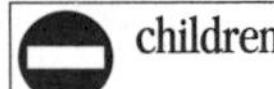 children.

cont.

5-10 days on first infection, then 5-day course only for subsequent attacks; to suppress herpes infection, 500 mg once a day (or 250 mg twice a day) with double dose in patients with poorly functioning immune system.

 alcohol, sedating drugs.

Availability: NHS and private prescription.
Contains: valaciclovir hydrochloride.
Brand names: Valtrex.

Valclair *see* diazepam suppositories
(Sinclair Pharmaceuticals)

Valium *see* diazepam tablets
(Roche Products)

Vallergan *see* trimeprazine tablets/syrup
(Distriphar)

Valoid *see* cyclizine tablets
(CeNeS)

---

valproic acid capsules *see* sodium valproate preparations

---

valsartan capsules

A capsule used as an ACE-II ANTAGONIST to treat high blood pressure.

Strengths available: 40 mg, 80 mg, and 160 mg capsules.
Dose: adults 80 mg once a day at first increasing gradually to a maximum of 160 mg a day if needed. Elderly patients start with 40 mg once a day.
Availability: NHS and private prescription.
Contains: valsartan.
Brand names: Diovan.

 low blood pressure, high potassium levels, severe allergic reaction, headache, dizziness, muscle or joint pain, tiredness, nose bleeds, blood disorders.

 in patients with liver or kidney disorders. Your doctor may advise regular blood tests.

 children, pregnant women, mothers who are breastfeeding, or for patients suffering from liver disorders, blocked bile duct.

 anaesthetics, NON-STEROIDAL ANTI-INFLAMMATORY DRUGS, cyclosporin, DIURETICS, potassium.

Valtrex *see* valaciclovir tablets
(GlaxoWellcome UK)

Vancocin Matrigel *see* vancomycin capsules
(Eli Lilly and Co.)

---

vancomycin capsules

A capsule used as an ANTIBIOTIC to treat intestinal infection and inflammation due to antibiotics.

Strengths available: 125 mg and 250 mg capsules.
Dose: adults, usually 125 mg four times a day (rarely up to 2000 mg a day) for 8-10 days; children use reduced doses according to body weight.
Availability: NHS and private prescription.
Contains: vancomycin hydrochloride.
Brand names: Vancocin Matrigel.

rarely, kidney or blood disorders, ear damage, severe allergic reaction, nausea, chills, fever, skin disorders, low blood pressure, breathing disorders, itching, flushing, pain, muscle spasm.

in the elderly, pregnant women, mothers who are breastfeeding, and in patients suffering from kidney disorders.

Vaqta *see* hepatitis A vaccine
(Aventis Pasteur MSD)

Vascace *see* cilazapril tablets
(Roche Products)

Vasogen

(Pharmax)
A cream used as a barrier preparation to treat nappy rash, pressure sores, and ileostomy/colostomy care.

Dose: apply as needed.
Availability: NHS and private prescription, nurse prescription, over the counter.
Contains: dimethicone, calamine, zinc oxide.

Vectavir *see* penciclovir cream
(SmithKline Beecham Pharmaceuticals)

Velosef *see* cephradine capsules/syrup
(Bristol-Myers Squibb Pharmaceuticals)

Velosulin *see* insulin

---

venlafaxine tablets/modified-release capsules

A tablet or M-R CAPSULE used as an antidepressant to treat depression.

Strengths available: 37.5 mg and 75 mg tablets; 75 mg and 150 mg m-r capsules.
Dose: 75 mg a day at first, increased if necessary to 150 mg a day (or up to 375 mg for severely depressed patients). Tablets taken as two doses through the day; m-r capsules taken as a single daily dose (maximum 225 mg).
Availability: NHS and private prescription.
Contains: venlafaxine hydrochloride.
Brand names: Efexor.

upset stomach, headache, dizziness, sleeplessness, drowsiness, sweating, low blood pressure on standing (occasionally high blood pressure), shaking, unsteadiness, nervousness, disturbance of sexual function, liver changes, weakness, fits, loss of appetite, abdominal pain, visual disturbance, pins and needles, abnormal dreams, widened blood vessels, chills, agitation, weight changes, palpitations, tense muscles, skin reactions, low blood sodium levels, liver changes, altered blood cholesterol levels.

in patients suffering from liver or kidney disorders or with a history of epilepsy, heart attack, heart disease, or drug abuse. Your doctor will advise regular blood pressure checks. Treatment should be withdrawn slowly.

MAOIS, entacapone, sedatives, alcohol.

children under 18 years, pregnant women, mothers who are breastfeeding, or for patients with severe liver or kidney disorders.

Ventide *see* salbutamol inhaler/rotacaps and beclomethasone inhaler/rotacaps
(Allen and Hanburys)

Strengths available: 100 mcg + 50 mcg inhaler; 200 mcg + 100 mcg and 200 mcg + 200 mcg rotacaps.
Dose: adults 2 puffs of inhaler (or 1 x 200 mcg + 200 mcg rotacap used in the rotahaler) 3-4 times a day; children 1-2 puffs of inhaler (or 1 x 200 mcg + 100 mcg rotacap used in the rotahaler) 2-4 times a day.

Ventmax *see* salbutamol modified-release capsules
(Trinity Pharmaceuticals)

Ventodisks *see* salbutamol disks
(Allen and Hanburys)

Ventolin *see* salbutamol accuhaler/inhaler/CFC-free inhaler/nebulizer solution/rotacaps/syrup
(Allen and Hanburys)

Veracur *see* formaldehyde gel
(Typharm)

verapamil tablets/modified-release tablets/modified-release capsules

A tablet, M-R TABLET, or M-R CAPSULE used as a CALCIUM-CHANNEL BLOCKER to treat angina, high blood pressure, and heart rhythm disturbances.

Strengths available: 40 mg, 80 mg, 120 mg, and 160 mg tablets; 120 mg and 240 mg m-r tablets; 120 mg, 180 mg, and 240 mg m-r capsules.

Dose: adults for heart rhythm disturbance, 120-360 mg a day; for angina 240-360 mg a day; for high blood pressure 240-480 mg a day. Doses for standard tablets divided into three doses through the day; doses for m-r tablets/capsules taken either as a single daily dose or divided into two depending on brand and condition. Children treated only with standard tablets according to doctor's advice.

Availability: NHS and private prescription.

Contains: verapamil hydrochloride.

Brand names: Cordilox, Ethimil, Half Securon SR, Securon, Univer, Verapress, Vertab.

Compound preparations: Tarka.

stomach upset, flushes, headache, dizziness, tiredness, swollen ankles, liver disorders, swollen breasts or gums, tiredness, skin disorders, severe allergic reaction, muscle or joint pain, pins and needles, hot and painful hands and feet, high prolactin levels in the blood. With high doses, low blood pressure, heart failure, slow heart rate, heart rhythm disturbance.

in pregnant women, mothers who are breast-feeding, and in patients suffering from some types of heart conduction disorders, liver or kidney disease, slow heart rate, heart attack, or low blood pressure.

patients suffering from severe heart conduction block, heart failure, very slow heart rates, some other heart disorders, very low blood pressure, PORPHYRIA. M-r products not suitable for use in children.

grapefruit juice, BETA-BLOCKERS, alcohol, anaesthetics, drugs used to treat heart rhythm disturbances, anti-epileptic treatments, ALPHA-BLOCKERS, ritonavir, BARBITURATES, digoxin, cyclosporin, lithium, theophylline, aminophylline, sedatives, rifampicin.

Verapress MR *see* verapamil modified-release tablets
(Cox Pharmaceuticals)

Vermox *see* mebendazole tablets/suspension
(Janssen-Cilag)

Verrugon *see* salicylic acid collodion
(J. Pickles and Sons)

V

Vertab SR *see* verapamil modified-release tablets
(Trinity Pharmaceuticals)

Vexol *see* rimexolone eye drops
(Alcon)

Viagra *see* sildenafil tablets
(Pfizer)

Viazem XL *see* diltiazem modified-release capsules
(Genus Pharmaceuticals)

Vibramycin *see* doxycycline capsules
(Invicta Pharmaceuticals)

Vibramycin-D *see* doxycycline dispersible tablets
(Invicta Pharmaceuticals)

Videx/Videx EC *see* didanosine tablets/enteric-coated capsules
(Bristol-Myers Squibb Pharmaceuticals)

Videne *see* povidone iodine alcoholic solution
(Adams Healthcare)

---

vigabatrin tablets/sachets

A tablet or sachet of powder used, in conjunction with other similar drugs, as an anti-epileptic treatment to control epilepsy. (Used without other drugs to control infant spasms.)

Strengths available: 500 mg tablets; 500 mg sachets.
Dose: adults, 1000 mg a day at first, then up to 3000 mg a day (in one single dose or divided into two); children use reduced doses according to body weight.
Availability: NHS and private prescription.
Contains: vigabatrin.
Brand names: Sabril.

 aggression, mental disorders, confusion, drowsiness, tiredness, dizziness, nervousness, irritability, memory disturbances, eye disorders, excitation, agitation, headache, unsteadiness, shaking, pins and needles, lack of concentration, weight gain, fluid retention, skin disorders, liver disorders, blood changes, depression, increased frequency of fits.

 in the elderly, pregnant women, and in patients with a history of mental or behavioural problems, or suffering from kidney damage. Your doctor will recommend regular eye examinations. (Report any eye symptoms to your doctor.) Treatment should be withdrawn gradually.

 mothers who are breastfeeding.

 other anti-epileptic treatments, alcohol, sedating drugs.

Vioform-HC *see* topical corticosteroid cream/ointment
(Novartis Consumer Health)

Vioxx *see* rofecoxib tablets/suspension
(Merck Sharp and Dohme)

Viracept *see* nelfinavir tablets/powder
(Roche Products)

Viramune *see* nevirapine tablets/suspension
(Boehringer Ingelheim)

Viridal Duo *see* alprostadil injection
(Schwartz Pharma)

Virormone *see* testosterone injection
(Ferring Pharmaceuticals)

Virovir *see* aciclovir tablets
(Opus Pharmaceuticals)

Visclair *see* methyl cysteine tablets
(Sinclair Pharmaceuticals)

Viscopaste *see* zinc paste bandage
(Smith and Nephew Healthcare)

Viscotears *see* carbomer eye drops
(CIBA Vision Ophthalmics)

V

Viskaldix
(Sovereign Medical)
A tablet used as a BETA-BLOCKER and DIURETIC to treat high blood pressure.

Strengths available: 10 mg + 5 mg tablets.
Dose: adults, 1 tablet each morning, increased gradually if necessary to a maximum of 3 tablets.
Availability: NHS and private prescription.
Contains: pindolol and clopamide.

cold hands and feet, sleep disturbance, slow heart rate, weakness, blood changes, low blood pressure, sensitivity to light, tiredness, wheezing, heart failure, low blood pressure, stomach upset. Rarely, dry eyes, rash, worsening of psoriasis.

in pregnant women, mothers who are breast-feeding, the elderly, and in patients suffering from diabetes, high lipid levels, gout, kidney or liver disorders, MYASTHENIA GRAVIS, or with a history of allergies. May need to be withdrawn before surgery. Withdraw gradually.

children or for patients suffering from heart block or failure, asthma, severe kidney or liver disorders, PHAEOCHROMOCYTOMA, or a history of breathing disorders.

general anaesthetics, CALCIUM-CHANNEL BLOCKERS, ALPHA-BLOCKERS, clonidine, ANTIHYPERTENSIVES, amiodarone, antidiabetics, thymoxamine, theophylline, aminophylline, NON-STEROIDAL ANTI-INFLAMMATORY DRUGS, drugs used to treat abnormal heart rhythm, halofantrine, pimozide, digoxin, lithium.

Visken *see* pindolol tablets
(Sovereign Medical)

Vista-methasone *see* betamethasone drops, corticosteroid nasal drops
(Martindale Pharmaceuticals)

Vista-methasone N *see* betamethasone drops and neomycin drops, corticosteroid nasal drops
(Martindale Pharmaceuticals)

Strengths available: 0.1% + 0.5% drops.
Dose: apply 2-3 drops twice a day to nose, every 3-4 hours to ear, or every 1-2 hours to eye. (Reduce frequency of application in ear and eye once symptoms subside.)

Vitalograph *see* peak flow meter (low range)
(Vitalograph)

---

vitamin A *see* Ketovite, Maxepa, Mothers' and Children's Vitamin Drops, multivitamin drops, vitamins A and D capsules, vitamins capsules BPC, Vitamin Tablets for Nursing Mothers

---

vitamin B_1 *see* Ketovite, multivitamin drops, vitamin B compound tablets, vitamins capsules BPC

---

vitamin B_2 *see* Ketovite, multivitamin drops, vitamin B compound tablets, vitamins capsules BPC

---

vitamin B_3 *see* Ketovite, multivitamin drops, nicotinamide tablets, vitamin B compound tablets, vitamins capsules BPC

---

vitamin B_5 *see* Ketovite

---

vitamin B_6 *see* Ketovite, multivitamin drops, pyridoxine tablets

---

vitamin B_{12} *see* cyanocobalamin, hydroxocobalamin, Ketovite

---

vitamin B compound tablets/vitamin B compound strong tablets

A tablet used as a source of B vitamins to prevent vitamin B deficiency.

Strengths available: 1 mg + 1 mg + 15 mg and 5 mg + 2 mg + 20 mg + 2 mg (strong) tablets.
Dose: adults 1-2 tablets a day.
Availability: NHS and private prescription, over the counter.
Contains: vitamins B_1, B_2, B_3; (strong tablets also contain vitamin B_6).

Not to be used for: children.

Caution needed with: levodopa (strong tablets only).

---

vitamin C *see* Ketovite, Mothers' and Children's Vitamin Drops, multivitamin drops, vitamins capsules BPC, Vitamin Tablets for Nursing Mothers

---

vitamin D *see* alfacaldidol capsules/drops, calciferol tablets, calcitriol tablets, calcium and vitamin D tablets, dihydrotachysterol solution, Ketovite, Maxepa, Mothers' and Children's Vitamin Drops, multivitamin drops, vitamins A and D capsules, vitamins capsules BPC, Vitamin Tablets for Nursing Mothers

---

vitamin E suspension/tablets

A tablet or suspension used as a vitamin E supplement to treat deficiency (e.g. in cystic fibrosis).

Strengths available: 50 mg and 200 mg tablets; 500 mg/5 ml suspension.
Dose: as advised by doctor (depends on age and condition).

diarrhoea and abdominal pain with high doses.

cont.

Availability: NHS and private prescription, over the counter.
Contains: vitamin E (alpha tocopheryl acetate).
Brand names: Ephynal.
Compound preparations: Ketovite.

 in patients with a tendency to blood clots and in infants with inflamed intestines.

V

vitamin H *see* Ketovite

vitamin K *see* menadiol tablets, phytomenadione tablets

vitamins A and D capsules

A capsule used as a vitamin supplement to correct deficiency.

Strengths available: 4000 units + 400 units per capsule.
Dose: as advised by doctor.
Availability: NHS and private prescription, over the counter.
Contains: vitamin A and vitamin D.
Other preparations: halibut-liver oil capsules.

 mothers who are breastfeeding.

 pregnant women.

vitamins capsules BPC

A capsule used as a multivitamin supplement.

 in pregnant women.

Strengths available: 2500 unit + 1 mg + 0.5 mg + 7.5 mg + 15 mg +300 unit capsules.
Dose: as advised by doctor or manufacturer.
Availability: NHS and private prescription, over the counter.
Contains: vitamins A, B_1, B_2, B_3, C, D.

Vitamin Tablets (with Calcium and Iodine) for Nursing Mothers

(Sussex Pharmaceuticals)
A tablet used as a multivitamin supplement for mothers who are breastfeeding.

Strengths available: 8 mg + 60 mg + 400 unit + 190 mg + 130 mcg tablets.
Dose: as advised by doctor.
Availability: NHS and private prescription, over the counter. Also available from maternity and child health clinics.
Contains: vitamins A, C, D, calcium hydrogen phosphate, potassium iodide.

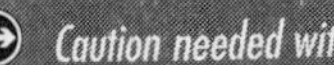

Vitrex Soft Lancets

(Vitrex Medical)
Diabetics who need to test their blood regularly can use lancets to pierce the skin, either with or without the use of a finger-pricking device.

Lancet width and length: 23G/0.65 mm and 28G/0.36 mm (Type A).
Availability: NHS and private prescription, over the counter.
Compatible finger-pricking devices: Autoclix, Autolet II, Autolet Lite and Autolet Lite Clinisafe, Autolet Mini, B-D Lancer 5, Glucolet, Hypolance, Microlet, Penlet II Plus, Soft Touch.

Vivazide *see* gliclazide tablets
(Viva Pharmaceuticals)

Vividrin *see* sodium cromoglycate eye drops and sodium cromoglycate nasal spray
(Nucare)

Vivotif *see* typhoid vaccine (oral)
(Masta)

Viz-On *see* sodium cromoglycate eye drops
(Opus Pharmaceuticals)

Volmax *see* salbutamol modified-release tablets
(Allen and Hanburys)

Volraman *see* diclofenac enteric-coated tablets
(Eastern Pharmaceuticals)

Volsaid Retard *see* diclofenac modified-release tablets
(Trinity Pharmaceuticals)

Voltarol/Voltarol Dispersible/Voltarol SR/Voltarol Rapid/Voltarol Retard *see* diclofenac enteric-coated tablets/modified-release capsules/modified-release tablets/suppositories/dispersible tablets
(Novartis Pharmaceuticals UK)

Voltarol Emulgel *see* non-steroidal anti-inflammatory drug (topical)
(Novartis Pharmaceuticals UK)

Voltarol Ophtha *see* diclofenac eye drops
(CIBA Vision Ophthalmics)

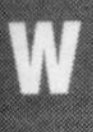

Volumatic

(Allen and Hanburys)
A two-piece spacer device used with Allen and Hanburys inhalers. Mask available for children and infants.

Availability: NHS and private prescription, over the counter.

warfarin tablets

A tablet used as an ANTICOAGULANT to treat and prevent blood clots.

Strengths available: 0.5 mg, 1 mg, 3 mg, and 5 mg tablets.
Dose: as advised by doctor.
Availability: NHS and private prescription.
Contains: warfarin sodium.
Brand names: Marevan.

alcohol, allopurinol, stanozolol, aspirin, NON-STEROIDAL ANTI-INFLAMMATORY DRUGS, cholestyramine, amiodarone, propafenone, quinidine, ANTIBIOTICS, some antidepressants, some antidiabetics, anti-epileptic treatments, antifungals, proguanil, clopidogrel, ticlopidine, ritonavir, chloral, primidone, CORTICOSTEROIDS, disulfiram, danazol, tamoxifen, thyroxine, lipid-lowering drugs, oral contraceptives, raloxifene, acitretin, testosterone, sucralfate, cimetidine, omeprazole, sulphinpyrazone, influenza vaccine, vitamin K, azathioprine, zafirlukast.

bleeding, liver damage, reversible hair loss, stomach upset, headache, skin disorders, inflamed pancreas, purple toes.

in mothers who are breastfeeding, the elderly, and in patients suffering from high blood pressure, reduced ability of protein in blood to bind drugs, severe heart failure, liver or kidney disease, stomach disorders, vitamin K deficiency. Your doctor will advise regular blood tests to determine correct dose.

children, pregnant women, or for patients suffering from stomach ulcers, severe high blood pressure, some heart disorders, poor liver or kidney function, some blood disorders.

Warticon/Warticon Fem *see* podophyllotoxin cream/solution
(Stiefel Laboratories (UK))

Waxsol *see* docusate ear drops
(Norgine)

Welldorm *see* chloral elixir/tablets
(Smith and Nephew Healthcare)

Wellvone *see* atovaquone suspension
(GlaxoWellcome UK)

white soft paraffin *see* emollient preparations, Lacri-Lube, liquid and white soft paraffin ointment NPF, Lubri-Tears, Metanium, paraffin gauze dressing, zinc ointment BP

whooping cough vaccine *see* pertussis vaccine

wool alcohols *see* emollient preparations, Lacri-Lube

wool fat *see* emollient preparations, Lubri-Tears, simple eye ointment, Sudocrem, zinc cream/ointment BP

Wright Pocket Peak Flow Meter 208/209 *see* peak flow meter
(Ferraris Medical)

Xalatan *see* latanoprost eye drops
(Pharmacia and Upjohn)

Xanax *see* alprazolam tablets
(Pharmacia and Upjohn)

Xanthomax *see* allopurinol tablets
(Ashbourne Pharmaceuticals)

Xatral/Xatral SR/XL *see* alfuzosin tablets
(Sanofi Synthelabo)

Xenazine 25 *see* tetrabenazine tablets
(Cambridge Laboratories)

Xenical *see* orlistat capsules
(Roche Products)

Xepin *see* doxepin cream
(Bioglan Laboratories)

---

xipamide tablets

A tablet used as a DIURETIC to treat high blood pressure and fluid retention.

Strengths available: 20 mg tablets.
Dose: for high blood pressure, 20 mg each morning; for fluid retention, 20-80 mg each morning.
Availability: NHS and private prescription.
Contains: xipamide.
Brand names: Diurexan.

 stomach upset, dizziness, low blood potassium levels. Rarely, other chemical disturbances in the blood, inflamed pancreas.

 in pregnant women, the elderly, and in patients suffering from liver or kidney disorders, enlarged prostate, narrowed blood vessels in the heart or brain, diabetes, gout, LUPUS.

 mothers who are breastfeeding or for patients suffering from severe kidney or liver disorders, Addison's disease, raised blood calcium/uric acid levels, low blood potassium/sodium levels, or PORPHYRIA.

 NON-STEROIDAL ANTI-INFLAMMATORY DRUGS, drugs that alter heart rhythm, antidiabetics, carbamazepine, halofantrine, pimozide, digoxin, lithium, ANTIHYPERTENSIVES.

---

xylitol *see* saliva (artificial)

Xylocaine *see* lignocaine gel
(AstraZeneca UK)

---

xylometazoline *see* Otrivine-Antistin, xylometazoline nasal drops/spray

---

xylometazoline nasal drops/spray

A nasal spray or nasal drops used as a SYMPATHOMIMETIC treatment for blocked nose.

Strengths available: 0.1% spray; 0.05% and 0.1% drops.
Dose: adults 2-3 drops (0.1%) or 1 spray in each nostril 2-3 times a day; children over 3 months 1-2 drops (0.05%) in each nostril

 itching or irritated nose, sleeplessness, headache, rapid heart rate. Congestion and less effect with continued use.

 use only in children under 2 years as advised by a doctor. Avoid excessive use.

 infants under 3 months.

once or twice a day. Treatment continued for a maximum of 7 days.

Availability: NHS (if prescribed generically) and private prescription, over the counter.
Contains: xylometazoline hydrochloride.
Brand names: Otrivine (not available on NHS).
Compound preparations: Rynacrom Compound.

Xyloproct *see* rectal corticosteroid ointment
(AstraZeneca UK)

---

yellow fever vaccine

A live vaccine used to prevent yellow fever.

Dose: one single dose given by injection.
Availability: available at designated centres only.
Contains: yellow fever virus.
Brand names: Arilvax.

 fever, headache, muscle pain, discomfort at site of injection. Rarely, severe allergic reaction, brain disorders.

 in pregnant women and infants under 9 months (vaccinate only if unavoidable).

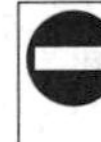 patients with feverish illness, poorly functioning immune system, HIV infection, some cancers, or who are allergic to eggs.

---

yellow soft paraffin *see* emollient preparations, simple eye ointment

---

Zacin *see* capsaicin cream
(Elan Pharma)

Zaditen *see* ketotifen tablets/capsules/elixir
(Novartis Pharmaceuticals UK)

Zaedoc *see* ranitidine tablets
(Ashbourne Pharmaceuticals)

---

zafirlukast tablets

A tablet used to prevent asthma.

Strengths available: 20 mg tablets.
Dose: adults, 20 mg twice a day.
Availability: NHS and private prescription.
Contains: zafirlukast.
Brand names: Accolate.

 stomach upset, headache, severe allergic reaction, liver and blood disorders, respiratory infection in the elderly, swollen ankles/legs, muscle or joint pain.

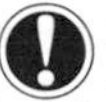 in the elderly, pregnant women, and in patients suffering from kidney disorders.

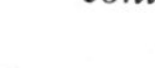
cont.

 children under 12 years, mothers who are breastfeeding, or for patients suffering from liver disorders, severe kidney disorders or Churg-Strauss syndrome (a condition involving breathing or nasal symptoms and blood vessel disorders.)

 warfarin, theophylline, aminophylline.

zalcitabine tablets

A tablet used in combination with other antiviral drugs, as an antiviral to treat HIV infection.

Strengths available: 375 mcg and 750 mcg tablets.
Dose: adults, 750 mcg every 8 hours.
Availability: NHS and private prescription.
Contains: zalcitabine.

 in pregnant women and in patients at risk of developing numb hands or feet or suffering from inflamed pancreas, heart disorders, kidney or liver disorders, alcoholism. Women should use effective contraception.

 children under 13 years, mothers who are breastfeeding, or for patients with numb hands and feet caused by nerve disorders.

Brand names: Hivid.

 numbness or pain in hands and feet (report to your doctor immediately), upset stomach, loss of appetite, abdominal pain, sore throat, headache, dizziness, muscle or joint pain, inflamed pancreas, skin disorders, itching, sweating, weight loss, tiredness, fever, chest pain, blood or liver disorders, disturbance of hearing or vision, fast heart rate, heart failure, heart muscle disorders, fits, shaking, sleep disturbance, mood change, movement disorders, hair loss, kidney disorders, high uric acid levels in the blood, ulcers in the mouth, rectum, or throat.

 drugs likely to cause numb hands and feet.

zaleplon capsules

A capsule used as a sedative for the short-term treatment of sleeplessness.

Strengths available: 5 mg and 10 mg capsules.
Dose: adults, 10 mg once each night at bedtime (or during the night as long as at least 4 hours of sleeping time remains); elderly patients use only 5 mg each night. Maximum treatment period 2 weeks.
Availability: NHS and private prescription.
Contains: zaleplon.
Brand names: Sonata.

 lessening effect and addiction with prolonged use, headache, weakness, drowsiness, dizziness, loss of memory, sleeplessness, and anxiety.

 in patients with breathing disorders, liver disorders, or a history of drug or alcohol abuse.

 children under 18 years, pregnant women, mothers who are breastfeeding, or for patients with severe liver disorders, MYASTHENIA GRAVIS, severe mental disorders, or who have stopped breathing while asleep.

 alcohol, other sedating drugs, rifampicin, ritonavir.

Zamadol/Zamadol SR *see* tramadol capsules/modified-release capsules
(ASTA Medica)

Zanaflex *see* tizanidine tablets
(Athena Neurosciences)

---

zanamavir disks

A powder contained in a disk for inhalation using a diskhaler device and used as an antiviral treatment to reduce the duration, severity, and complications of influenza.

Strengths available: 5 mg per dose.
Dose: adults, 2 doses inhaled twice a day for 5 days beginning within 2 days of the onset of influenza symptoms.
Availability: NHS and private prescription.
Contains: zanamavir.
Brand names: Relenza.

 stomach upset. Rarely, breathing difficulty, rash.

 in pregnant women, the elderly, and in patients suffering from asthma and other breathing disorders, impaired immunity, untreated long-term illnesses. BRONCHODILATORS should be used before this treatment if both are used.

 bronchodilators (*see* above).

 mothers who are breastfeeding.

Zanidip *see* lercanidipine tablets
(Napp Pharmaceuticals)

Zantac *see* ranitidine tablets/effervescent tablets/syrup
(GlaxoWellcome UK)

Zapain *see* co-codamol 30/500 tablets/capsules
(Goldshield Healthcare)

Zarontin *see* ethosuximide capsules/syrup
(Parke Davis and Co.)

Zeasorb
(Stiefel Laboratories (UK))
A dusting powder used to treat skin inflammation in areas such as between the thighs or beneath the breasts, excessive sweating, sweating brought on by using certain drugs.

cont.

Strengths available: 0.5% + 0.2% powder.
Dose: apply as required.
Availability: NHS and private prescription.
Contains: chloroxylenol and aluminium dihydroxyallantoinate.

Zeffix *see* lamivudine tablets/solution
(GlaxoWellcome UK)

Zelapar *see* selegiline tablets
(Athena Neurosciences)

Z

Zemtard XL *see* ditiazem modified-release capsules
(Galen)

Zerit *see* stavudine capsules/solution
(Bristol-Myers Squibb Pharmaceuticals)

Zestoretic *see* lisinopril tablets and hydrochlorothiazide tablets
(Zeneca Pharma)

Strengths available: 10 m g + 12.5 mg and 20 mg + 12.5 mg tablets.
Dose: adults 1-2 tablets a day.

Zestril *see* lisinopril tablets
(Zeneca Pharma)

Ziagen *see* abacavir tablets/solution
(GlaxoWellcome UK)

Zida-Co *see* co-amilozide tablets
(Opus Pharmaceuticals)

Zidoval *see* metronidazole vaginal gel
(3M Health Care)

---

zidovudine capsules/tablets/syrup
A capsule, tablet, or syrup used as an antiviral treatment for HIV infection. Used alone to treat pregnant

women, but in combination with other antiviral drugs for other patients.

Strengths available: 100 mg and 250 mg capsules; 300 mg tablets; 50 mg/5 ml syrup.
Dose: adults (in combination with other drugs) 500-600 mg a day in two or three divided doses; pregnant women 100 mg five times a day; children use reduced doses according to size.
Availability: NHS and private prescription.
Contains: zidovudine.
Brand names: Retrovir.
Compound preparations: Combivir.

blood disorders, headache, stomach upset or pain, rash, fever, nerve disorders, loss of appetite, muscle pain, sleeplessness, sleepiness, tiredness, weakness, anxiety, depression, fits, liver disorders, cough, difficulty breathing, frequent need to pass urine, chest pain, swollen breasts, influenza-like symptoms, taste disturbance, inflamed pancreas, loss of mental alertness, discoloration of nails, skin, and mouth.

in the elderly, pregnant women, and in patients suffering from kidney or liver disorders, blood disorders (such as anaemia) or vitamin B_{12} deficiency.

children under 3 months (unless infected by mother during pregnancy), mothers who are breastfeeding, or for patients with low numbers of white or red blood cells in the blood, some other blood disorders, or babies with jaundice who require treatment other than ultraviolet light.

anti-epileptic treatments, ganciclovir.

Zildil SR *see* diltiazem modified-release capsules (Chanelle Medical UK).

Zileze *see* zopiclone tablets (Opus Pharmaceuticals)

Zimbacol XL *see* bezafibrate modified-release tablets (Link Pharmaceuticals)

Zimovane/Zimovane LS *see* zopiclone tablets (Rhône-Poulenc Rorer)

Zinamide *see* pyrazinamide tablets (Merck Sharp and Dohme)

zinc acetate *see* Zineryt

---

zinc and castor oil ointment BP *see* zinc cream

---

zinc and coal tar paste *see* coal tar paste and zinc ointment

---

zinc cream/ointment BP

A cream or ointment used as a soothing and protecting preparation to treat nappy and urine rashes, and eczema.

Dose: apply as needed.
Availability: NHS and private prescription, over the counter.
Contains: zinc oxide, wool fat. Cream also contains arachis (peanut) oil, calcium hydroxide, and oleic acid. Ointment also contains hard paraffin, white soft paraffin, and cetostearyl alcohol.
Compound preparations: Vasogen, zinc and castor oil ointment BP (with castor oil for added protection – also contains peanut oil, and additionally available on nurse prescription), zinc and coal tar paste BP.

Not to be used for: cream not suitable for patients allergic to peanuts.

---

zinc oxide *see* Anusol, Sprilon, Sudocrem, rectal corticosteroid, Vasogen, zinc cream/ointment BP, zinc paste bandage, Zipzoc

---

zinc paste bandage BP 1993

A bandage used to treat eczema or dermatitis. Also used (in addition to compression bandages) to treat leg ulcers.

Strengths available: 10% or 15% bandages.
Availability: NHS and private prescription, nurse prescription, over the counter.
Contains: zinc oxide.
Brand names: Steripaste, Viscopaste PB7, Zincaband.
Compound preparations: zinc paste and calamine bandage; zinc paste, clioquinol, and calamine bandage; zinc paste and coal tar bandage; zinc paste and ichthammol bandage.
Other preparations: Zipzoc.

Side effects: irritation.

---

zinc paste, clioquinol, and calamine bandage BP 1993

A bandage used (in addition to compression bandages) to treat (and reduce the smell from) leg ulcers.

Availability: NHS and private prescription, over the counter.
Availability: NHS and private prescription, nurse prescription, over the counter.
Brand names: Quinaband.

zinc paste and calamine bandage

A bandage used to treat eczema or dermatitis. Also used (in addition to compression bandages) to treat leg ulcers.

Availability: NHS and private prescription, nurse prescription, over the counter.
Contains: zinc oxide, calamine.
Brand names: Calaband.

zinc paste and coal tar bandage BP 1993

A bandage used to treat eczema or dermatitis. Also used (in addition to compression bandages) to treat leg ulcers.

Availability: NHS and private prescription, nurse prescription, over the counter.
Contains: zinc oxide, coal tar.
Brand names: Tarband.

zinc paste and ichthammol bandage BP 1993

A bandage used to treat eczema or dermatitis. Also used (in addition to compression bandages) to treat leg ulcers.

Strengths available: 15% + 2% or 6% + 2% bandages.
Availability: NHS and private prescription, over the counter.
Contains: zinc oxide, ichthammol.
Brand names: Icthaband, Ichthopaste.

zinc pyrithione *see* coal tar shampoo

zinc sulphate *see* Efalith, zinc sulphate effervescent tablets, zinc sulphate eye drops

zinc sulphate effervescent tablets

An effervescent tablet used as a zinc supplement to treat zinc deficiency.

Strengths available: 125 mg effervescent tablets.
Dose: adults, 125 mg 1-3 times a day after meals; children over 10 kg half adult dose; children under

 stomach upset, abdominal pain.

 in patients suffering from kidney failure.

 TETRACYCLINE ANTIBIOTICS.

cont.

10 kg 62.5 mg once a day only.
Availability: NHS and private prescription, over the counter.
Contains: zinc sulphate.
Brand names: Solvazinc.

---

zinc sulphate eye drops

Eye drops used as an astringent to treat excessive tear production.

Strengths available: 0.25% drops.
Dose: as advised by doctor.
Availability: NHS and private prescription, over the counter.
Contains: zinc sulphate.

Zincaband *see* zinc paste bandage
(SSL International)

Zineryt *see* erythromycin lotion
(Yamanouchi Pharma)

Zinga *see* nizatidine capsules
(Ashbourne Pharmaceuticals)

Zinnat *see* cefuroxime tablets/suspension/sachets
(GlaxoWellcome UK)

Zip-zoc

A medicated stocking used to treat leg ulcers. May be used in conjunction with compression bandages or elastic stockings.

Strengths available: 20% stockings.
Availability: NHS and private prescription, nurse prescription, over the counter.
Contains: zinc oxide.
Compound preparations: zinc paste and calamine bandage; zinc paste, clioquinol, and calamine bandage; zinc paste and coal tar bandage; zinc paste and ichthammol bandage.

Zirtek *see* cetirizine tablets/solution
(UCB Pharma)

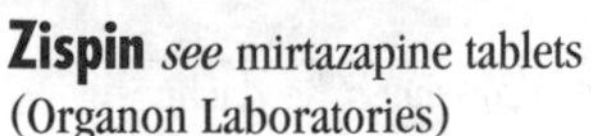

Zispin *see* mirtazapine tablets
(Organon Laboratories)

Zita *see* cimetidine tablets
(Eastern Pharmaceuticals)

Zithromax *see* azithromycin capsules/tablets/suspension
(Richborough Pharmaceuticals)

Zocor *see* simvastatin tablets
(Merck Sharp and Dohme)

Zofran/Zofran Melt *see* ondansetron tablets/syrup/suppositories
(GlaxoWellcome UK)

Zoladex/Zoladex LA *see* goserelin injection
(Zeneca Pharma)

Zoleptil *see* zotepine tablets
(Orion Pharma (UK))

---

zolmitriptan tablets

A tablet used to treat migraine attacks.

Strengths available: 2.5 mg tablets.
Dose: adults, 2.5 mg at start of attack. If migraine then clears but later recurs, another dose may be taken after 2 hours. (Do not take a second dose if the first fails to work.) Dose may be doubled to 5 mg if 2.5 mg inadequate. Maximum 15 mg in 24 hours.
Availability: NHS and private prescription.
Contains: zolmitriptan.
Brand names: Zomig.

sensations of warmth, tingling, pressure, tightness, or heaviness, dizziness, flushing, tiredness, weakness, stomach upset, heart rhythm disturbance.

in pregnant women, mothers who are breast-feeding, and in patients at risk of heart disease or who suffer from liver disorders.

children or for patients with some heart disorders, uncontrolled high blood pressure, or blood vessel disease.

other migraine treatments.

---

zolpidem tablets

A tablet used as a sedative for the short-term treatment of sleeplessness.

cont.

Z

Strengths available: 5 mg and 10 mg tablets.
Dose: adults, 10 mg (elderly or weak patients 5 mg) at bedtime.
Availability: NHS and private prescription.
Contains: zolpidem tartrate.
Brand names: Stilnoct.

 stomach upset, drowsiness, headache, dizziness, weakness, addiction, memory disturbances, shaking, confusion, disturbed perception, depression, nightmares, double vision, unsteadiness.

 in patients suffering from liver or kidney disorders, depression, or with a history of alcohol or drug abuse.

 alcohol, other sedating drugs, ritonavir.

children, pregnant women, mothers who are breastfeeding, or for patients with MYASTHENIA GRAVIS, severe liver disorders, mental disorders, breathing disorders, or who have stopped breathing while asleep.

Zomacton *see* somatropin injection
(Ferring Pharmaceuticals)

Zomig *see* zolmitriptan tablets
(Zeneca Pharma)

Zomorph *see* morphine modified-release capsules
(Link Pharmaceuticals)

Zonivent Aquanasal *see* corticosteroid nasal spray
(Ashbourne Pharmaceuticals)

zopiclone tablets

A tablet used as a sedative for the short-term treatment of sleeplessness.

Strengths available: 3.75 mg and 7.5 mg tablets.
Dose: adults, 7.5 mg (elderly patients initially 3.75 mg) at bedtime. Maximum treatment period 4 weeks.
Availability: NHS and private prescription.
Contains: zopiclone.
Brand names: Zileze, Zimovane.

 metallic aftertaste, stomach upset, confusion, depression, dizziness, light-headedness, lack of co-ordination, headache, addiction, hallucinations, nightmares, loss of memory, behavioural disorders, aggression, drowsiness, impaired judgement and ability.

children, pregnant women, mothers who are breastfeeding, or for patients suffering from MYASTHENIA GRAVIS, severe breathing difficulties, or who have stopped breathing while asleep.

 in the elderly and in patients suffering from liver or kidney disorders or with a history of mental disorders.

 alcohol, other sedating drugs, ritonavir, erythromycin.

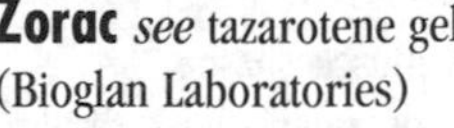

Zorac *see* tazarotene gel
(Bioglan Laboratories)

---

zotepine tablets

A tablet used as a sedative to treat schizophrenia.

Strengths available: 25 mg, 50 mg, and 100 mg tablets.
Dose: adults, 25 mg three times a day at first increasing at 4-day intervals to a maximum of 100 mg three times a day; elderly patients 25 mg twice a day at first, and maximum of 75 mg twice a day.
Availability: NHS and private prescription.
Contains: zotepine.
Brand names: Zoleptil.

 weight gain, dizziness, low blood pressure on standing, drowsiness, rapid heart rate, shaking hands, movement disorders, NEUROLEPTIC MALIGNANT SYNDROME, dry mouth, stomach upset, weakness, inflamed nasal passages, fever, anxiety, depression, headache, sleeplessness, high or low body temperature, increased salivation, blurred vision, sweating, muscle or joint pain, rash, heart rhythm abnormality, blood changes, liver disorders. More rarely, loss of appetite, high blood pressure, influenza-like symptoms, fits, confusion, difficulty breathing, decreased sexual desire, vertigo, speech disorders, fluid retention, thirst, impotence, incontinence or urine retention, inflamed eyes, acne, loss of consciousness, nose bleed, loss of memory, enlarged abdomen, diminished sensitivity, irregular periods, hair loss, sensitivity to light.

 in the elderly, pregnant women, and in patients with a history of epilepsy or suffering from heart or circulation disorders (including brain circulation), enlarged prostate, liver or kidney disorders, urine retention, some forms of glaucoma, non-functioning bowel, or Parkinson's disease.

 children under 18 years, mothers who are breastfeeding, or for patients suffering from intoxication, gout attack, or with a history of kidney stones.

 drugs which affect heart rhythm, other sedating drugs, alcohol, antidepressants, anti-epileptic treatments, halofantrine, ritonavir.

Zoton *see* lansoprazole capsules/suspension
(Wyeth Laboratories)

Zovirax *see* aciclovir cream, aciclovir eye ointment, aciclovir suspension/tablets/dispersible tablets
(GlaxoWellcome UK)

Z

cont.

zuclopenthixol tablets

A tablet used as a sedative to treat mental disorders, particularly schizophrenia.

Strengths available: 2 mg, 10 mg, and 25 mg tablets.
Dose: adults, 20-30 mg a day (in divided doses) at first, increasing to a maximum of 150 mg a day if needed.
Availability: NHS and private prescription.
Contains: zuclopenthixol dihydrochloride.
Brand names: Clopixol.

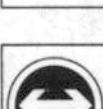
children, unconscious or withdrawn patients, or for those with severe kidney or liver impairment, or who are suffering from bone marrow depression, PORPHYRIA, or PHAEOCHROMOCYTOMA.

movement disorders, muscle spasms, restlessness, shaking, dry mouth, heart rhythm disturbance, low blood pressure, weight gain, blurred vision, impotence, low body temperature, breast swelling, menstrual changes, blood, liver, eye, and skin changes, drowsiness, apathy, nightmares, sleeplessness, depression, blocked nose, difficulty passing water. Rarely, fits.

in pregnant women, mothers who are breast-feeding, the elderly, and in patients suffering from heart, lung, or circulation disorders, epilepsy, Parkinson's disease, thyroid disorders, infections, MYASTHENIA GRAVIS, kidney or liver disease, glaucoma, enlarged prostate, or some blood disorders. Should be withdrawn gradually.

alcohol, sedatives, antidepressants, some antidiabetic drugs, anaesthetics, anti-epileptic medications, drugs affecting heart rhythm, ritonavir, halofantrine, sotalol, propranolol, lithium.

Zumenon *see* hormone replacement therapy (oestrogen-only)
(Solvay Healthcare)

Zyban *see* bupropion tablets
(GlaxoWellcome UK)

Zydol/Zydol SR/Zydol XL *see* tramadol capsules/modified-release tablets/soluble tablets
(Searle)

Zyloric *see* allopurinol tablets
(GlaxoWellcome UK)

Zyomet *see* metronidazole gel
(Goldshield Healthcare)

Zyprexa *see* olanzapine tablets
(Eli Lilly and Co.)

Addendum

Actiq
(Elan Pharma)
A lozenge containing 200-1600mcg fentanyl, which is absorbed via the lining of the mouth. The lozenge is moved around the mouth using the applicator provided and consumed over a 15-minute period.

ACWY Vax
(SmithKline Beecham Pharmaceuticals)
A vaccination used to provide active immunization against meningitis A, C, W135 and Y.

Adcal - *see* calcium carbonate chewable tablets
(Strakan Ltd)
Strengths available: 600mg chewable tablets.

---

alendronate tablets - additional 70mg tablet available (for use as once-weekly dose)

Almogran tablets
(Lundbeck)
A tablet containing almotriptan (similar to sumatriptan), used to treat migraine headache.

Strengths available: 12.5mg tablets.
Dose: adults (over 18 years only) 1 tablet, repeated after 2 hours if symptoms reappear. (Maximum of 2 tablets in 24 hours).

---

amisulpride tablets - 400mg strength also now available.

AS Saliva Orthana - *see* saliva (artificial) spray/lozenges
(AS Pharma)

Centyl K - *see* bendrofluazide tablets and potassium chloride tablets
(Leo Pharmaceuticals)
A combination product used to treat fluid retention, high blood pressure, or to prevent kidney stones.

Strengths available: 2.5mg+573mg tablets.
Dose: 2-4 tablets each morning at first, reducing to 1-4 tablets a day or on alternate days.

Climanor - *see* medroxyprogesterone tablets
(Chanelle Medical)

Co-aprovel - *see* hydrochlorothiazide tablets and irbesartan tablets
(Sanofi Synthelabo)
A combination product used to treat high blood pressure in patients not adequately controlled on either ingredient alone.

Strengths available: 12.5+150mg and 12.5+300mg tablets.
Dose: adults 1 tablet a day.

Depakote - *see* valproic acid tablets
(Sanofi Synthelabo)
A plain (uncoated) tablet of valproic acid used to treat manic episodes associated with bipolar disorder (where the mood swings from mania to depression).

Strengths available: 250mg and 500mg plain tablets.

Dermestril Septem - *see* hormone replacement therapy (oestrogen-only)
(Strakan)

Strengths available: 25mcg, 50mcg and 75mcg patches.
Dose: 1 patch applied to the skin and replaced every 7 days.

---

epoetin alfa injection - now also available as 6,000unit, 7,000unit, 8,000unit or 9,000unit prefilled syringes.

Feprapax - *see* lofepramine tablets
(Ashbourne Pharmaceuticals)

Indivina - *see* hormone replacement therapy (combined)
(Orion Pharma (UK))

Contains: medroxyprogesterone acetate and oestradiol valerate.

---

montelukast - now also available as 4mg chewable tablet

Dose: children aged 2-5 years, 4mg at night.

Neoclarityn tablets
(Schering-Plough)
A tablet containing desloratadine (similar to loratadine), used as an ANTIHISTAMINE to treat hayfever symptoms.

Strengths available: 5mg tablets.
Dose: 5mg once a day.

Oilatum cream – no longer contains arachis oil – main ingredients are now light liquid paraffin and white soft paraffin.

---

paroxetine tablets/liquid – now also used to treat post-traumatic stress syndrome.

Ranzac - *see* ranitidine tablets
(Eastern Pharmaceuticals)

Retalzem 60 - *see* diltiazem m/r tablets
(OPD Pharmaceuticals)

Saliva Stimulating Tablets (SST) - *see* saliva (artificial) tablets
(Sinclair Pharmaceuticals)
Tablets dissolved in the mouth to relieve dry mouth symptoms – maximum of 16 per day (adults) if required.

Syprol
(Rosemont Pharmaceuticals)
An oral solution containing PROPRANOLOL.

Strengths available: 5mg/5ml, 10mg/5ml or 50mg/5ml oral solution.

Tagadine - *see* cimetidine tablets
(OPD Pharmaceuticals)

---

telmisartan tablets - additional 20mg tablet available.

Tenkorex - *see* cephalexin tablets/capsules/suspension
(OPD Pharmaceuticals)

Thaden - *see* dothiepin capsules/tablets
(Opus Pharmaceuticals)

Trizivir - *see* abacavir tablets, lamivudine tablets and zidovudine tablets
(GlaxoWellcome UK)

Strengths available: 300mcg+150mg+300mg per tablet.
Dose: adults over 18 years, 1 tablet twice a day.

Vibrox - *see* doxycycline capsules
(OPD Pharmaceuticals)

Zyvox tablets/oral suspension

(Pharmacia and Upjohn)
A tablet containing linezolid, used as an ANTIBIOTIC to treat some forms of pneumonia, skin and soft tissue infections.

Strengths available: 600mg tablets; 20mg/ml oral suspension.
Dose: adults 400-600mg twice a day for 10-14 days.

Additional Information

anabolic steroid
Anabolic steroids are used to treat vascular disorders, thinning of the bones, and some bone marrow disorders. They may be abused by some athletes because of their body-building properties. Example, stanozolol tablets.

corticosteroid
corticosteroids are used to suppress inflammatory or allergic disorders, such as asthma, rheumatic conditions, or eczema. High doses may cause patients to develop a 'moon-face' appearance. After long treatment periods, the drug should be withdrawn gradually. Example, prednisolone tablets.

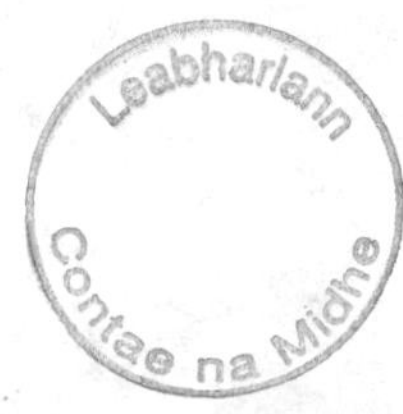